Strategies to Enhance Drug Permeability across Biological Barriers

Strategies to Enhance Drug Permeability across Biological Barriers

Editors

Jingyuan Wen
Yuan Huang

MDPI • Basel • Beijing • Wuhan • Barcelona • Belgrade • Manchester • Tokyo • Cluj • Tianjin

Editors

Jingyuan Wen
The School of Pharmacy
University of Auckland
Auckland
New Zealand

Yuan Huang
West China School of Pharmacy
Sichuan University
Chengdu
China

Editorial Office
MDPI
St. Alban-Anlage 66
4052 Basel, Switzerland

This is a reprint of articles from the Special Issue published online in the open access journal *Pharmaceutics* (ISSN 1999-4923) (available at: www.mdpi.com/journal/pharmaceutics/special_issues/drug_permeability_across_barrier).

For citation purposes, cite each article independently as indicated on the article page online and as indicated below:

LastName, A.A.; LastName, B.B.; LastName, C.C. Article Title. *Journal Name* **Year**, *Volume Number*, Page Range.

ISBN 978-3-0365-7463-9 (Hbk)
ISBN 978-3-0365-7462-2 (PDF)

Contents

About the Editors

Jingyuan Wen

Dr. Jingyuan Wen received a master's degree in 1991 at the School of Pharmacy, Shanghai Medical University (now Fudan University), China, and was awarded a PhD in Pharmaceutical Science in 2003 from the School of Pharmacy, Otago University of New Zealand. In 2005, she was appointed as a lecturer at the School of Pharmacy, University of Auckland, New Zealand. She was appointed as a research theme leader in drug delivery in 2014 and was promoted to an Associate Professor in 2015 (equal to a full professor in the USA). Her research expertise is the oral/transdermal and brain delivery of macromolecule compounds; she has facilitated over 250 peer-reviewed articles, patents and abstracts in drug delivery, nutraceutical, and biological science. She has served as a consultant for national and international pharmaceutical companies since 2005 and is an editor for several journals.

Yuan Huang

Dr. Yuan Huang is a professor and dean at West China School of Pharmacy, Sichuan University. Her research interests are the construction and mechanisms of efficient drug delivery systems, including oral protein–peptide drug delivery systems and tumor-targeting drug delivery systems. Her major research has been published in authoritative journals including *ACS Nano*, *Adv. Drug Deliver. Rev.*, *Adv. Funct. Mater.* and *Angew. Chem. Int. Ed.*, and she has been granted eight patents in China. She was named a High-Cited Scholar of China in *Elsevier* in 2020 and 2021.

Preface to "Strategies to Enhance Drug Permeability across Biological Barriers"

The delivery of therapeutic drugs to desired sites under required conditions is often challenged by numerous biological barriers in the body, such as the intestinal epithelium membrane, blood–brain barrier (BBB), and skin barrier. Each biological system presents a unique and formidable challenge; for example, the densely packed microvascular epithelial cells of the BBB block almost 100% of macromolecular drugs and 98% of small lipophilic drugs.

Biological systems have a fundamental way of limiting the effectiveness of therapeutic drugs. The collection of articles written by global experts featured in this Special Issue showcases a number of recent advancements which circumvent the barriers of the intestinal epithelium, skin barrier, the BBB, and other barriers such as the lung epithelium membrane.

This Special Issue will explore the wide range of advanced and innovative approaches, technologies, and drug delivery systems that have been implemented to overcome these biological barriers and improve drug permeability and absorption to achieve a wide range of therapeutical goals.

The development of this Special Issue, entitled "Strategies to Enhance Drug Permeability across Biological Barriers", has been a collaborative effort between Professor Wen and Professor Huang. Both editors have extensive experience with the study of the fabrication and mechanisms of efficient drug delivery systems, including oral/transdermal protein–peptide and tumour-targeting drug delivery systems, and they have facilitated many major publications in the field.

Acknowledgements

We are very grateful to all authors' contributions to this Special Issue and also are grateful to the reviewers for their enormous help and constructive comments. Additionally, we thank the *Pharmaceutics* management team for offering us the opportunity to edit this Special Issue. Finally, thank you to the readers; we hope you find this read discussing advanced technology to enhance drug permeability across biological barriers informative and enjoyable.

Jingyuan Wen and Yuan Huang
Editors

pharmaceutics

MDPI

Editorial

Strategies to Enhance Drug Permeability across Biological Barriers—A Summary of This Important Special Issue

Jingyuan Wen [1,*] and **Yuan Huang** [2,*]

[1] The School of Pharmacy, Faculty of Medical Health Science, University of Auckland, Auckland 1023, New Zealand
[2] West China School of Pharmacy, Sichuan University, Chengdu 610093, China
* Correspondence: j.wen@auckland.ac.nz (J.W.); huangyuan0@163.com (Y.H.); Tel.: +64-9-9232762 (J.W.); +86-28-85501617 (Y.H.)

This Special Issue, "Strategies to Enhance Drug Permeability across Biological Barriers", is hosted by Pharmaceutics and highlights the recent technological advancements for overcoming biological barriers and improving drug permeability and absorption.

The delivery of therapeutic drugs to desired sites at required rates/extents is limited by the numerous biological barriers in the body, including the intestinal epithelium membrane, blood–brain barrier (BBB), and skin barrier. The drug permeability of almost all macromolecular drugs and most small lipophilic drugs, across the intestinal membrane, for instance, will be severely limited by the physical barriers that are presented by the mucous layer, the epithelial membrane, and the tight junctions, in addition to the enzymatic barrier for unstable compounds. Experts in the drug delivery field need to find advanced, non-invasive methods to persistently overcome these biological barriers. This Special Issue highlights the recent advancements in overcoming these barriers and improving drug permeability. The 11 papers in this Special Issue, contributed by global experts to explore various advanced strategies, provide new insights on all aspects of the enhancement of drug penetration across biological barriers.

The first article of this Special Issue looks at the recent advances in cancer-targeting drug research, which have been made by overcoming the multiple biological barriers that are associated with mitochondrial targeting. Yi et al. established a 2-(dimethylamino) ethyl methacrylate (DEA)-modified N-(2-hydroxypropyl) methacrylamide (HPMA) copolymer–CPT conjugate (P-DEA-CPT) to mediate the mitochondrial accumulation of CPT [1]. This mitochondria-targeting P-DEA-CPT can quickly internalize into 4T1 cells, escaping from lysosomes and accumulating inside mitochondria. P-DEA-CPT has shown the successful in vivo inhibition of metastasis with decreased side effects, suggesting mitochondrial targeting as a promising treatment of metastatic tumors.

Similarly, Zhang et al. managed to overcome the barriers of cancer cells by using cholera toxic subunit b (CTB) [2]. A more significant in vivo targeting of lung metastasis, via a chemical conjugation of a CTB protein onto the surface of PEGylated liposomes (CTB-sLip), was observed when compared to unmodified PEGylated liposomes (sLip).

Li et al. tackled the skin barrier by developing a niosomal nano carrier system to deliver green tea catechins and their analogue, epigallocatechin gallate (EGCG), to the dermis layer, in order to achieve a greater antioxidant effect [3]. In this study, a drug-loaded niosomal delivery system delivered EGCG to the dermal layer and effectively prolonged its release, demonstrating a much deeper skin penetration and deposition than free EGCG. The resulting antioxidant effects, in comparison to those of free EGCG, were seen through an increased cell survival after UVA irradiation, a reduced lipid peroxidation, and increased antioxidant enzyme activities in the human dermal fibroblasts (Fbs).

Eedara et al. reviewed the application of dry powder inhalation to treat lung diseases such as asthma, cystic fibrosis, and lung infections, by crossing the lung barrier [4]. Due to

Citation: Wen, J.; Huang, Y. Strategies to Enhance Drug Permeability across Biological Barriers—A Summary of This Important Special Issue. *Pharmaceutics* **2023**, *15*, 1189. https://doi.org/10.3390/pharmaceutics15041189

Received: 24 March 2023
Revised: 28 March 2023
Accepted: 31 March 2023
Published: 8 April 2023

a lack of a standard dissolution methods and absorption models, this review looked into various dissolution systems and evaluated their performances in crossing the lung barrier.

Ryall et al. reviewed the approaches and techniques from the last two decades for the topical delivery of wound-healing bioactives [5]. Many natural products have desirable biological properties that are applicable to wound healing, but are limited by their inability to cross the stratum corneum to access the wound. Such natural products and their reapplication, through the use of modern delivery methods such as niosomes and microneedles, were summarized in this review. The molecular mechanism of wound healing was also examined in detail.

He et al. reviewed our understanding of membrane proteins and drug permeability by editing the expression of these membrane proteins using the CRISPR-Cas9 system, which is the most developed and used CRISPR-associated Cas system [6]. Both methods of genome editing that use CRISPR-Cas9 and their applications for improving our understanding of biological barriers were compiled in this paper.

There are many ways to overcome biological barriers and deliver a drug to its intended location. Crowe and Hsu compiled the recent research on completely bypassing the BBB through the intranasal route, which will be an essential step towards the treatment of patients with neurological diseases [7]. Methods for improving the safety and efficacy of intranasal formulations were reviewed in this paper, including the use of nasal permeability enhancers, gelling agents, and nanocarrier formulations.

Alternatively, another way to overcome biological barriers is to increase their permeability through a conjugation with lipid moieties. Tran et al. summarized the cellular internalization effects of hydrophobic moieties that were bound to oligonucleotides [8]. The common hydrophobic moieties in this paper included fatty acids, cholesterol, tocopherol, and squalene. Tran et al. also looked into the clinically successful oligonucleotide conjugates that are currently in use.

The final three reviews looked into the advances in conquering the BBB. Han reviewed the multitude of methods that are currently used to modulate the BBB's permeability, such as opening tight junctions, inhibiting active efflux, and/or enhancing transcytosis [9]. This review outlined the strategies, mechanisms, and safety of such BBB permeability modulators for a better pre-clinical and clinical study design.

Rechberger et al. bibliometrically summarized the efforts and trends of intra-arterial therapy for brain tumors that have emerged over the past several decades [10]. This bibliographical review of the recent clinical trials and publications in this field of research aimed to provide an idea of the future trends in this field.

Finally, Gandhi et al. took an in-depth dive into the modulation of the BBB's permeability by using an ultrasound to deliver normally impenetrable drugs into the brain [11]. This review featured information from diverse ultrasound parameters that had already used to achieve an increase in the BBB's permeability. Microbubbles, transducer frequency, peak-negative pressure, pulse characteristics, and the dosing of ultrasound applications were also included in this review. In total, 107 articles and their protocols, parameters, safety, and efficacy were identified and summarized to help in achieving the standardization of these protocols and parameters in future preclinical and clinical studies.

This special issue features a comprehensive array of approaches and technologies developed to deliver drugs through a variety of biological barriers. These articles showcased in this issue illuminate the challenges posed by these barriers and provide insight into the latest advanced technologies used to overcome them. We are confident that the content of this issue will prove informative and engaging to readers, and we extend our sincere appreciation to all contributors who have made this special issue possible. Thank you for your interest in Pharmaceutics, and we hope you find this special issue enlightening.

Author Contributions: Writing—original draft preparation, J.W.; writing—review and editing J.W. and Y.H. All authors have read and agreed to the published version of the manuscript.

Funding: Many thanks to New Zealand Pharmacy Education and Research Foundation (NZPERF grant number: 332) and NZ-China Biomedical Research Alliance Grant (grant number: 21/815).

Conflicts of Interest: The authors declare no conflict of interest.

References

1. Yi, X.; Yan, Y.; Shen, X.; Li, L.; Huang, Y. Mitochondria-Targeted delivery of camptothecin based on HPMA copolymer for metastasis suppression. *Pharmaceutics* **2022**, *14*, 1534. [CrossRef] [PubMed]
2. Zhang, X.; Tang, W.; Wen, H.; Wu, E.; Ding, T.; Gu, J.; Lv, Z.; Zhan, C. Evaluation of CTB-sLip for targeting lung metastasis of colorectal cancer. *Pharmaceutics* **2022**, *14*, 868. [CrossRef] [PubMed]
3. Li, D.; Martini, N.; Wu, Z.; Chen, S.; Falconer, J.R.; Locke, M.; Zhang, Z.; Wen, J. Niosomal nanocarriers for enhanced dermal delivery of epigallocatechin gallate for protection against oxidative stress of the skin. *Pharmaceutics* **2022**, *14*, 726. [CrossRef] [PubMed]
4. Eedara, B.B.; Bastola, R.; Das, S.C. Dissolution and absorption of inhaled drug particles in the lungs. *Pharmaceutics* **2022**, *14*, 2667. [CrossRef] [PubMed]
5. Ryall, C.; Duarah, S.; Chen, S.; Yu, H.; Wen, J. Advancements in skin delivery of natural bioactive products for wound management: A brief review of two decades. *Pharmaceutics* **2022**, *14*, 1072. [CrossRef] [PubMed]
6. He, J.; Biswas, R.; Bugde, P.; Li, J.; Liu, D.-X.; Li, Y. Application of CRISPR-Cas9 System to study biological barriers to drug delivery. *Pharmaceutics* **2022**, *14*, 894. [CrossRef] [PubMed]
7. Crowe, T.P.; Hsu, W.H. Evaluation of recent intranasal drug delivery systems to the central nervous system. *Pharmaceutics* **2022**, *14*, 629. [CrossRef] [PubMed]
8. Tran, P.; Weldemichael, T.; Liu, Z.; Li, H.-Y. Delivery of oligonucleotides: Efficiency with lipid conjugation and clinical outcome. *Pharmaceutics* **2022**, *14*, 342. [CrossRef] [PubMed]
9. Han, L. Modulation of the Blood–Brain barrier for drug delivery to brain. *Pharmaceutics* **2021**, *13*, 2024. [CrossRef] [PubMed]
10. Rechberger, J.S.; Thiele, F.; Daniels, D.J. Status quo and trends of Intra-Arterial therapy for brain tumors: A bibliometric and clinical trials analysis. *Pharmaceutics* **2021**, *13*, 1885. [CrossRef] [PubMed]
11. Gandhi, K.; Barzegar-Fallah, A.; Banstola, A.; Rizwan, S.B.; Reynolds, J.N.J. Ultrasound-Mediated Blood–Brain barrier disruption for drug delivery: A systematic review of protocols, efficacy, and safety outcomes from preclinical and clinical studies. *Pharmaceutics* **2022**, *14*, 833. [CrossRef] [PubMed]

pharmaceutics

Article

Mitochondria-Targeted Delivery of Camptothecin Based on HPMA Copolymer for Metastasis Suppression

Xiaoli Yi †, Yue Yan †, Xinran Shen, Lian Li and Yuan Huang *

Key Laboratory of Drug-Targeting and Drug Delivery System of the Education Ministry, Sichuan Engineering Laboratory for Plant-Sourced Drug and Sichuan Research Center for Drug Precision Industrial Technology, West China School of Pharmacy, Sichuan University, No. 17, Block 3, South Renmin Road, Chengdu 610041, China; yixiaoli728@126.com (X.Y.); xinwen93696@126.com (Y.Y.); yy18224019649@163.com (X.S.); liliantripple@163.com (L.L.)

* Correspondence: huangyuan0@163.com

† These authors contributed equally to this work.

Abstract: Poor anti-metastasis effects and side-effects remain a challenge for the clinical application of camptothecin (CPT). Mitochondria can be a promising target for the treatment of metastatic tumors due to their vital roles in providing energy supply, upregulating pro-metastatic factors, and controlling cell-death signaling. Thus, selectively delivering CPT to mitochondria appears to be a feasible way of improving the anti-metastasis effect and reducing adverse effects. Here, we established a 2-(dimethylamino) ethyl methacrylate (DEA)-modified *N*-(2-hydroxypropyl) methacrylamide (HPMA) copolymer–CPT conjugate (P-DEA-CPT) to mediate the mitochondrial accumulation of CPT. The mitochondria-targeted P-DEA-CPT could overcome multiple barriers by quickly internalizing into 4T1 cells, then escaping from lysosome, and sufficiently accumulating in mitochondria. Subsequently, P-DEA-CPT greatly damaged mitochondrial function, leading to the reactive oxide species (ROS) elevation, energy depletion, apoptosis amplification, and tumor metastasis suppression. Consequently, P-DEA-CPT successfully inhibited both primary tumor growth and distant metastasis in vivo. Furthermore, our studies revealed that the mechanism underlying the anti-metastasis capacity of P-DEA-CPT was partially via downregulation of various pro-metastatic proteins, such as hypoxia induction factor-1α (HIF-1α), matrix metalloproteinases-2 (MMP-2), and vascular endothelial growth factor (VEGF). This study provided the proof of concept that escorting CPT to mitochondria via a mitochondrial targeting strategy could be a promising approach for anti-metastasis treatment.

Keywords: camptothecin; metastasis; mitochondria; 2-(dimethylamino) ethyl methacrylate

Citation: Yi, X.; Yan, Y.; Shen, X.; Li, L.; Huang, Y. Mitochondria-Targeted Delivery of Camptothecin Based on HPMA Copolymer for Metastasis Suppression. *Pharmaceutics* **2022**, *14*, 1534. https://doi.org/10.3390/pharmaceutics14081534

Academic Editors: Emanuela Fabiola Craparo and Marta Gonzá-lez-Álvarez

Received: 16 May 2022
Accepted: 20 July 2022
Published: 23 July 2022

1. Introduction

CPT is a promising chemotherapeutic agent due to its potent inhibitory effect against DNA topoisomerase [1]. Although targeted delivery of CPT has been reported to improve its cytotoxicity, the anti-metastasis effect is poor [2–4]. Furthermore, recent studies disclosed that nuclear DNA damage by CPT could induce a massive release of double-stranded DNA (dsDNA), which could subsequently stimulate a strong immune response to initiate the intestinal diarrhea, a life-threatening side-effect of camptothecin [5,6]. Thus, exploring new strategies to improve its anti-metastasis efficacy while reducing its side-effects is needed.

Due to the imperative roles in regulating cellular metabolism and cell-death signaling [7,8], mitochondria not only provide various metabolites and antiapoptotic proteins for rapid tumor growth but also facilitate the migration and invasion of tumor cells by offering abundant energy and upregulating pro-metastatic factors [9–11]. Increasing evidence has shown that targeted induction of mitochondria dysfunction by therapeutics (i.e., doxorubicin, lonidamine, and metformin) hold tremendous potential for suppressing both primary tumors and metastases [12–14]. Notably, CPT can be a cellular respiration inhibitor to impair mitochondrial without causing side-effects such as diarrhea [15,16].

Thus, selectively delivering CPT to mitochondria appears to be a feasible way of improving the anti-metastasis effect and reducing adverse effects.

Free drugs rely on simple diffusion to randomly interact with the organelles of tumor cells [17]. Thus, the amount of CPT that accumulates in mitochondria is very limited due to the multiple intracellular barriers to reaching mitochondria and the extremely poor permeability of the mitochondrial inner membrane, which represent formidable hurdles [18,19]. Recently, various ligands have been reported to improve mitochondrial accumulation, such as triphenylphosphonium bromide, mitochondrial penetration peptide, and mitochondrial targeting sequence [20–22]. However, those lipophilic moieties might deteriorate the solubility of the highly hydrophobic CPT. 2-(Dimethylamino) ethyl methacrylate, a hydrophilic small molecular containing a tertiary amino group, might be a promising ligand to facilitate the transport of CPT to mitochondria [23]. Nevertheless, the modification content of DEA for effective mitochondria targeting remains unknown.

Herein, we designed a DEA-modified HPMA copolymer–CPT conjugate (P-DEA-CPT) consisting of (1) HPMA copolymer acting as a carrier and (2) DEA acting as the mitochondria-targeting moiety (Scheme 1). DEA was decorated on the side-chain, and its modification degree was screened to ensure sufficient mitochondria accumulation. P-DEA-CPT greatly enhanced mitochondrial location of CPT in cancer cells. Subsequently, P-DEA-CPT induced mitochondrial dysfunction, thereby efficiently curbing the growth and metastasis of breast cancer. Thus, our study unleashed the potential for anti-metastasis treatment of CPT via a mitochondria-targeted delivery system.

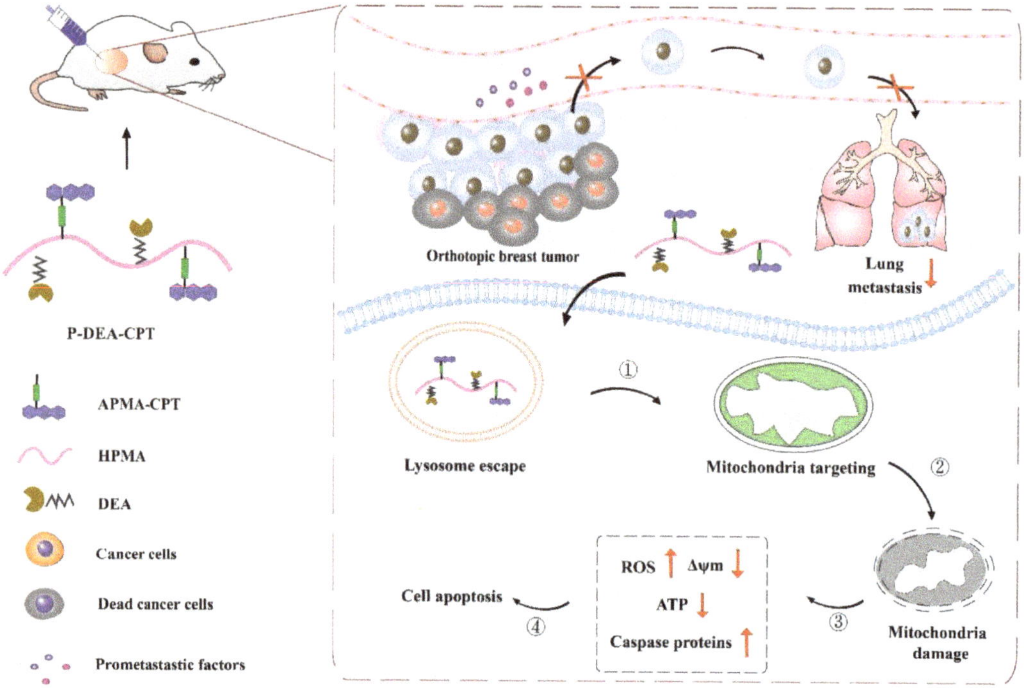

Scheme 1. Schematic illustration of P-DEA-CPT for damaging mitochondria and suppressing metastasis. After internalized into cancer cells, P-DEA-CPT ① escaped from lysosome, ② targeted mitochondria, ③ damaged mitochondria and ④ finally induced cell apoptosis.

2. Materials and Methods

2.1. Materials

Camptothecin (CPT) (>98%) and 2-(dimethylamino) ethyl methacrylate (DEA) were acquired from Giant Medical Technology Co., Ltd. (Chengdu, China), whereas *N*-(3-aminopropyl) methacrylamide hydrochloride was purchased from Bide Pharmaceutical Technology Co., Ltd. (Shanghai, China). Lyso-tracker Red was provided by Thermo Fisher Scientific (Shanghai, China). MitoTracker Red, Mitochondrial Membrane Potential Assay Kit, Reactive Oxygen Species Assay Kit, ATP Assay Kit, Caspase 3 and Caspase 9 Activity Assay Kit, and Tissue Mitochondria Isolation Kit were all obtained from Beyotime Biotechnology Co., Ltd. (Shanghai, China). All other reagents were of analytical grade or above.

2.2. Cells and Animals

Murine breast cancer cells (4T1) and human umbilical vein endothelial cells (HUVECs) were obtained from Icell Biotech Co., Ltd. (Shanghai, China) and the Chinese Academy of Science Cell Bank for Type Culture Collection (Shanghai, China), respectively. Cells were incubated in a homothermal cell incubator (37 °C) with 5% CO_2. RPMI 1640 medium (Gibco, Invitrogen Co., Grand Island, NY, USA) supplemented with 10% (*v*/*v*) fetal bovine serum (FBS) and 1% (*v*/*v*) antibiotics (penicillin–streptomycin) was used for 4T1 cells, and Dulbecco's modified Eagle's medium (Gibco, Invitrogen) supplemented with 10% (*v*/*v*) fetal bovine serum (FBS) and 1% (*v*/*v*) antibiotics (penicillin–streptomycin) was used for HUVECs.

Female BALB/c mice (6 to 10 weeks) were provided by Chengdu Dashuo Experimental Animal Co., Ltd. (Chengdu, China). All animal experiments strictly abided by the Guidelines of Medical Ethics Committee of Sichuan University.

2.3. Synthesis, Characterization, and Mitochondria-Targeting Capacity of HPMA Copolymers with Different Modification Ratios of DEA

FITC-labeled HPMA copolymers conjugated with different 2-(dimethylamino) ethyl methacrylate (DEA) ratios were synthesized, and their mitochondrial accumulation was evaluated. Firstly, *N*-(2-hydroxypropyl) methacrylamide (HPMA) and *N*-(3-aminopropyl) methacrylamide–fluorescein isothiocyanate monomer (APMA–FITC) were synthesized in the same way as our previous study [24]. Then, FITC-labeled HPMA polymers with various DEA modification amounts were obtained by direct radical polymerization of monomers. Briefly, the monomers (APMA–FITC:DEA:HPMA = 5:0~13:95~82 mol.%) and azobisisobutyronitrile (2 wt.%) as the initiator were dissolved in dimethyl sulfoxide and stirred for 24 h at 50 °C under argon atmosphere. Products were precipitated into diethyl ether and freeze-dried after being purified by dialysis. The obtained HPMA conjugates modified with 0%, 5%, 10% and 13% molar ratios of DEA were defined as PFITC, P-DEA (5%)-FITC, P-DEA (10%)-FITC, and P-DEA (13%)-FITC, respectively. Next, a Fast Protein Liquid Chromatograph (FPLC, GE Healthcare Life Science, Piscataway, NJ, USA) was used to detect the molecular weight and polydispersity of these copolymers. The zeta potential of the copolymers was estimated by Zetasizer Nano ZS90 at 25 °C (Malvern Instruments, Malvern, UK). The amount of FITC contained in these copolymers was determined via ultraviolet spectroscopy GENESYS 180 (Thermo fisher technologies, South San Francisco, CA, USA).

Then, mitochondria-targeting capacity of various HPMA copolymers was evaluated in 4T1 cells. Briefly, after being incubated with the above-obtained copolymers (FITC dose, 10 $\mu g \cdot mL^{-1}$) for 4 h, the mitochondria of 4T1 cells were extracted by grinding the cells in mitochondria extraction reagent under ice bath 20 times, and cell debris was removed by centrifuging at 600× *g* for 10 min at 4 °C. Next, the obtained supernatant containing mitochondria was centrifuged at 11,000× *g* for 15 min at 4 °C, and the mitochondria pellets were collected. Finally, the fluorescence intensity of FITC in mitochondria was quantitatively determined via flow cytometry (FACS Calibur, BD, Franklin Lakes, NJ, USA).

Furthermore, the safety of these copolymers was investigated in both 4T1 tumor cells and HUVECs. After seeding in 96-well plates, 4T1 cells and HUVEC were treated with P-FITC, P-DEA (5%)-FITC, P-DEA (10%)-FITC, and P-DEA (13%)-FITC at various predetermined concentrations for 48 h. Then, fresh MTT agent was added and cultured for another 4 h. Finally, the amount of formazan in each well was determined by Varioskan Flash 902-ULTS (Thermo Scientific, Sunnyvale, CA, USA) after being dissolved in 200 μL of dimethyl sulfoxide (DMSO). The relative cell viability was calculated as the absorption value of experimental wells reverse that in the drug-free medium treated group.

2.4. *Synthesis and Characterization of HPMA Copolymer-CPT Conjugates*

The azelaic acid–camptothecin conjugate (LA–CPT) and *N*-(3-aminopropyl) methacrylamide hydrochloride–azelaic acid–camptothecin (APMA–LA–CPT) monomer were synthesized as described in our previous study [23]. Subsequently, CPT-loaded HPMA copolymers with (13% molar ratio, P-DEA-CPT) or without DEA modification (P-CPT) were synthesized according to the same procedure mentioned above. The molecular weight, polydispersity, zeta potential, and CPT loading capacity of P-CPT and P-DEA-CPT were evaluated using the same method in Section 2.3.

2.5. *Cellular Uptake, Lysosome Escape, and Mitochondrial Targeting of HPMA Copolymer–CPT Conjugates*

The 4T1 cells were treated with free CPT, P-CPT and P-DEA-CPT (equivalent CPT dose, 20 $\mu g \cdot mL^{-1}$) for 4 h. Then, 4T1 cells were harvested, and the fluorescence intensity of CPT was qualitatively observed via a laser scanning confocal microscope (CLSM, Zeiss LSM 800, Oberkochen, Germany) and quantitatively detected via flow cytometry.

Then, whether HPMA copolymer–camptothecin conjugates could escape from lysosome and accumulate in mitochondria was investigated. The 4T1 cells were incubated with P-CPT or P-DEA-CPT (equivalent CPT dose, 20 $\mu g \cdot mL^{-1}$) for 4 h. After being labeled with Mito-Tracker Red or Lyso-Tracker Red, cells were visualized under CLSM.

2.6. *In Vitro Mitochondrial Damage by HPMA Copolymer–Camptothecin Conjugates*

2.6.1. Reactive Oxygen Species Detection

The level of reactive oxygen species in cancer cells after CPT polymeric conjugate treatment was detected using a DCFH-DA probe. The 4T1 cells were seeded in 12-well plates and then treated with free CPT, P-CPT, and P-DEA-CPT (equivalent CPT dose, 20 $\mu g \cdot mL^{-1}$) for 8 h. Afterward, cells were harvested and incubated with DCFH-DA solution for 30 min at 37 °C followed by flow cytometry analysis.

2.6.2. Mitochondrial Membrane Potential Detection

Mitochondrial membrane depolarization in 4T1 cells was measured by JC-1 probe, which is a cationic lipophilic dye that can form red fluorescent complexes known as J-aggregates in the mitochondrial matrix under normal mitochondrial membrane potential ($\Delta\psi m$). In contrast, $\Delta\psi m$ loss can induce decreased J-aggregates in the mitochondria and increased monomeric form (J-monomer) emitting green fluorescence in the cytosol. Therefore, the red (J-aggregate)/green (J-monomer) fluorescence intensity ratio is a direct evaluation of the $\Delta\psi m$ depolarization. The 4T1 cells received the same drug treatments as in ROS detection assay and were stained with JC-1 probe for 30 min at 37 °C in the dark before being measured by flow cytometry.

2.6.3. Measurement of ATP Level

Adenosine 5′-triphosphate (ATP) could offer energy and catalyze luciferase to generate fluorescence. On this basis, intracellular ATP can be quantitatively detected by measuring the bioluminescence of luciferase. The 4T1 cells were seeded in 24-well plates and then treated with free CPT, P-CPT, and P-DEA-CPT (equivalent CPT dose, 20 $\mu g \cdot mL^{-1}$) for 24 h.

Afterward, cells were harvested and treated according to the standard protocol of the ATP assay kit.

2.6.4. Detection of Caspase 9 and Caspase 3

To investigate the initiation of mitochondrial-related apoptosis pathway, the levels of caspase 9 and caspase 3 were detected. The 4T1 cells were treated with free CPT, P-CPT, and P-DEA-CPT (equivalent CPT dose, 20 μg mL^{-1}) for 24 h. Afterward, cells were harvested and treated according to the manufacturer's illustration of Caspase 9 Activity Assay Kit and Caspase 3 Activity Assay Kit.

2.7. *Cell Proliferation Suppression Efficacy of HPMA Copolymer–Camptothecin Conjugates*

The cell proliferation suppression efficacy of CPT polymeric conjugates was investigated by MTT assay and cell apoptosis assay. For the MTT assay, the 4T1 cells were seeded into a 96-well plate (3×10^3 cells per well) and incubated with free CPT, P-CPT, or P-DEA-CPT at various predetermined concentrations for 48 h. Then, cell viability was determined by MTT reagent. For the apoptosis assay, the 4T1 cells were incubated with CPT, P-CPT, or P-DEA-CPT (equivalent CPT dose, 20 μg mL^{-1}) for 24 h. Afterward, the cells were collected and used for apoptosis analysis according to the standard protocols of the Annexin V-FITC/7-AAD Apoptosis Detection kit (BioLegend, San Diego, CA, USA).

2.8. *In Vitro Anti-Metastasis Assay*

The in vitro anti-metastasis effect of CPT polymeric conjugates was evaluated via a migration assay, wound healing assay, and invasion assay. For the migration assay, the 4T1 cells (1×10^5) were suspended in 200 μL of serum-free RPMI 1640 medium and seeded into the upper chamber of transwell inserts. After 4 h incubation, the upper medium was replaced with free CPT, P-CPT, or P-DEA-CPT (equivalent CPT dose, 4 μg·mL^{-1}) and incubated for another 24 h. Subsequently, transwell inserts were fixed with 4% paraformaldehyde followed by staining with crystal violet solution (0.1%). The cells that remained in the upper chamber were wiped out, and the cells that migrated to the lower membranes were imaged under the microscope (Leica Microsystems, Wetzlar, Germany) and dissolved with 33% acetic acid aqueous solution for quantitative determination by Varioskan Flash at 590 nm (Thermo Scientific Varioskan Flash, Waltham, MA, USA).

For the wound healing assay, 4T1 cells were seeded in 24-well plates to grow into a monolayer and scratched with a sterile pipette. Then, cells were incubated with different drug solutions for 24 h. The widths of the wounds at 0 h and 24 h were recorded under microscopy at the same scratched location, and the distance migrated was calculated using Image J software. Furthermore, Matrigel (BD Biosciences, San Diego, CA, USA) was added into the inner bottom of the chamber for 4 h ahead of 4T1 cell seeding, and the invasion assay was performed corresponding to the migration assay.

2.9. *Intratumoral Mitochondria Targeting Assay*

To establish the orthotopic breast cancer mice model, the 4T1 cells (4×10^5 cells) were carefully inoculated into one mammary fat pad of female BALB/c mice. When the tumor size reached about 200–300 mm^3, mice were intratumorally administrated with free CPT, P-CPT, or P-DEA-CPT (equivalent CPT dose, 5 mg·kg^{-1}). Then, 12 h post injection, tumor tissues were dissected and cut into small pieces followed by trypsin digestion for 15 min. Subsequently, mitochondria in tumor cells were collected according to the standard protocol of Tissue Mitochondria Isolation Kit. A fraction of the collected mitochondria were stained with Mito-Tracker Red (100 nM) for 45 min at 37 °C and visualized under CLSM. Finally, the total fluorescence intensity of CPT in the rest of mitochondria (TFL) was determined via Varioskan Flash and the amount of mitochondrial protein was detected using the Bradford Protein Assay Kit (Keygen Biotechnology, Nanjing, China). The mitochondria accumulation in each group was calculated as the TFL divided by the concentration of mitochondrial protein.

2.10. *In Vivo Antitumor and Anti-Metastasis Evaluation*

When the tumor volume reached about 100 mm^3 (defined as day 0), orthotopic breast tumor-bearing mice were randomly divided into four groups ($n = 5$) and intratumorally administered saline, free CPT, P-CPT, or P-DEA-CPT (equivalent CPT dose of 5 $mg \cdot kg^{-1}$, 25 μL) every 3 days for a total of five times. Tumor volumes of mice were detected using a vernier caliper, and the changes in body weight were recorded every 2 days. Tumor volumes were calculated as the following formula: tumor volume (mm^3) = $width^2 \times length/2$. For the evaluation of the anti-metastasis effect, mice were sacrificed on day 18, and the excised lungs were immersed in Bouin's Fluid overnight to count the number of pulmonary metastatic nodules. Subsequently, tumors and the excised organs were fixed in 4% paraformaldehyde for at least 48 h and embedded in paraffin for hematoxylin and eosin (H&E) staining and immunohistochemistry analysis of matrix metalloproteinase-2 (MMP-2), hypoxia inducible factor-1α (HIF-1α), and vascular endothelial growth factor (VEFG).

2.11. *Statistical Analysis*

Student's *t*-test and one-way analysis of variance (ANOVA) were used to test the significant difference between two groups or multiple groups via SPSS 19.0 software (SPSS, Chicago, IL, USA). Data were expressed as the mean ± standard deviation. Statistical significance was implied using asterisks (* $p < 0.05$, ** $p < 0.01$, *** $p < 0.001$).

3. Results and discussion

3.1. *DEA Content-Dependent Mitochondrial Targeting Capacity of HPMA Conjugates*

To guarantee efficient mitochondria-targeting capacity, we prepared FITC-labeled HPMA polymers with various proportions of DEA decorated on the side-chains to select an optimal amount of DEA. FITC-labeled HPMA polymers containing 0–13% molar ratio of DEA (P-FITC, P-DEA (5%)-FITC, P-DEA (10%)-FITC, and P-DEA (13%)-FITC) were prepared via one-step radical homo-polymerization according to our previous reports [25] (Figure 1A). As depicted in Figure 1B,C, the molecular weights of these copolymers were in the range of 15.2 to 29.5 kDa, and the PDIs were in the range of 1.16 to 1.46. The FITC loading (5.44–6.23 wt.%) of each group was at a similar level. Furthermore, the gradually increased zeta potentials of these polymers revealed the different modification degrees of the positively charged DEA (Figure 1C). Notably, the DEA content-dependent mitochondria-targeting capacity was observed, and P-DEA (13%)-FITC mediated approximately 24-fold higher mitochondrial accumulation than P-FITC (Figure 1D). In addition, the cell viabilities of HUVECs and 4T1 cells were both over 90% at concentrations of P-DEA (13%)-FITC up to 1000 $\mu g \cdot mL^{-1}$ (Figure 1E,F). These results strongly verified that the 13% molar proportion of DEA was optimal to induce efficient mitochondria location of HPMA polymers with good cytocompatibility.

3.2. *Synthesis and Characterization of HPMA Copolymer–CPT Conjugates*

HPMA copolymer–CPT conjugates were synthesized as shown in Figure 2A. Briefly, CPT polymeric conjugate decorated with 13 mol.% of DEA (P-DEA-CPT) was synthesized via direct radical polymerization of HPMA, DEA, and APMA–CPT and initiation of azobisisobutyronitrile. Furthermore, a CPT polymeric conjugate without DEA modification (P-CPT) was prepared as a control. As displayed in Figure 2B,C, the molecular weight of P-DEA-CPT was 23.3 kDa with a PDI of around 1.1. P-DEA-CPT displayed a successful CPT loading of ~10 wt.%. Similar properties were also observed in P-CPT. Moreover, zeta potentials revealed that P-DEA-CPT with DEA modification had a significantly stronger positive charge as compared with P-CPT.

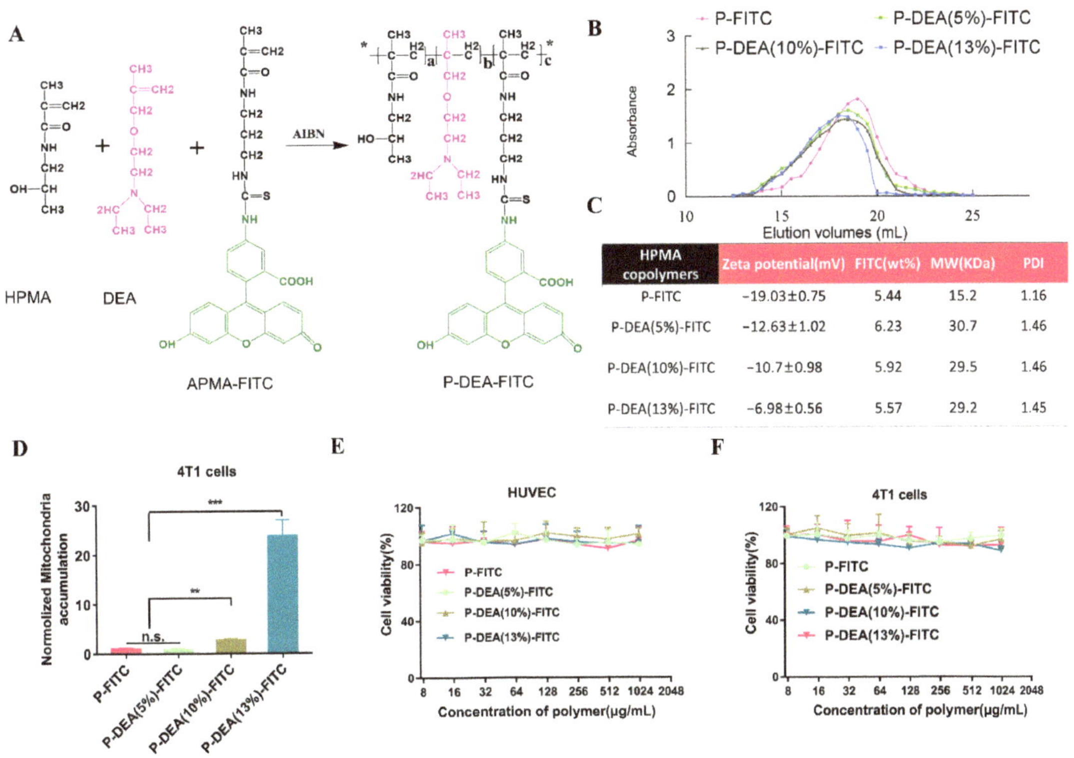

HPMA copolymers	Zeta potential(mV)	FITC(wt%)	MW(KDa)	PDI
P-FITC	−19.03±0.75	5.44	15.2	1.16
P-DEA(5%)-FITC	−12.63±1.02	6.23	30.7	1.46
P-DEA(10%)-FITC	−10.7±0.98	5.92	29.5	1.46
P-DEA(13%)-FITC	−6.98±0.56	5.57	29.2	1.45

Figure 1. Characterization, mitochondrial targeting capacity, and cytotoxicity of HPMA polymers modified with variable DEA content. (**A**) Graphic illustration of the synthesis route of FITC-labeled HPMA polymers decorated with different proportions of DEA. (**B**) The fast protein liquid chromatography (FPLC) curves and (**C**) the detailed characterizations of FITC-labeled HPMA polymers. (**D**) Mitochondrial accumulation of HPMA polymers with different content of DEA; mean ± SD (n = 3). Cell viability of HPMA polymers with different modification degrees of DEA in (**E**) HUVECs and (**F**) 4T1 cells; * $p < 0.05$, ** $p < 0.01$, *** $p < 0.001$, n.s. (no significance); mean ± SD (n = 5).

3.3. Cellular Uptake, Lysosome Escape, and Mitochondrial Targeting of P-DEA-CPT

To investigate whether DEA could facilitate internalization of HPMA copolymer-CPT conjugates in cancer cells, cellular uptake of P-DEA-CPT was investigated in 4T1 cells. CLSM observation displayed that the fluorescence intensity of FITC was significantly stronger in the P-DEA-CPT group than that in the P-CPT group (Figure 3A). Consistently, quantitative analysis by flow cytometry indicated a 5.7-fold higher internalization of P-DEA-CPT over P-CPT (Figure 3B). After entering cancer cells, P-DEA-CPT was expected to escape from lysosome and accumulate in mitochondria. To verify this, the subcellular trafficking of the internalized polymers was examined. The results displayed that most of the P-CPT was trapped in the lysosome (Rr = 0.85, between CPT and lysosome, Figure 3C), whereas a small proportion of P-CPT was localized in the mitochondria (Rr = 0.55, between CPT and mitochondria, Figure 3D). Encouragingly, P-DEA-CPT could largely escape from lysosome (Rr = 0.44, between CPT and lysosome, Figure 3C) and subsequently accumulate in the mitochondria (Rr = 0.70, between CPT and mitochondria, Figure 3D). Thus, the modification of DEA not only improved the internalization of copolymer conjugates but also facilitated lysosome escape and mitochondrial colocalization.

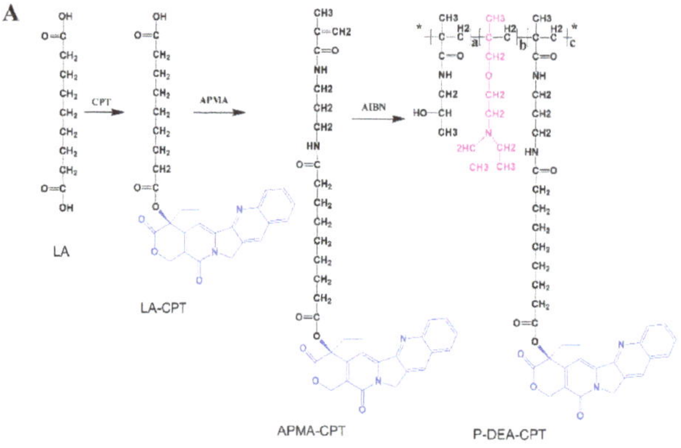

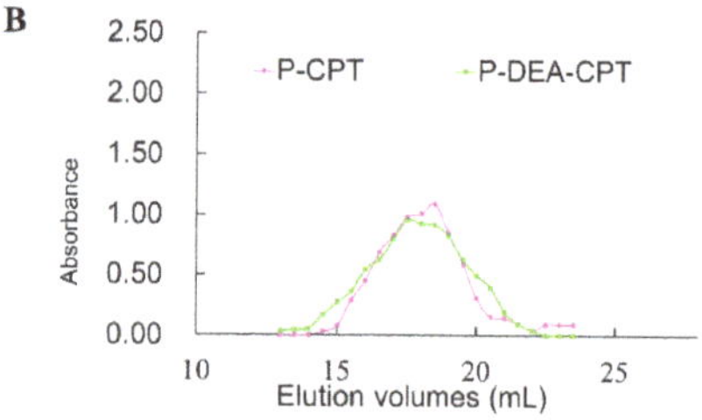

C

Copolymers	Zeta potential (mV)	Mw (KDa)	PDI	CPT (wt %)
P-CPT	−2.36 ± 0.52	24.6	1.18	10.26%
P-DEA-CPT	19.75± 0.21	24.3	1.15	10.78%

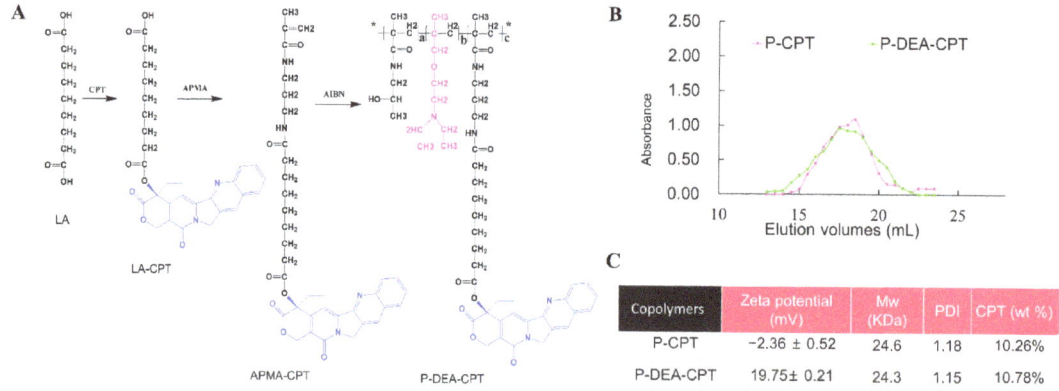

Figure 2. Synthesis and characterization of HPMA copolymer–CPT conjugates. (**A**) Schematic representation of the synthesis route of P-DEA-CPT. (**B**) The fast protein liquid chromatography (FPLC) curves and (**C**) detailed characterizations of P-CPT and P-DEA-CPT; * $p < 0.05$; mean ± SD ($n = 3$).

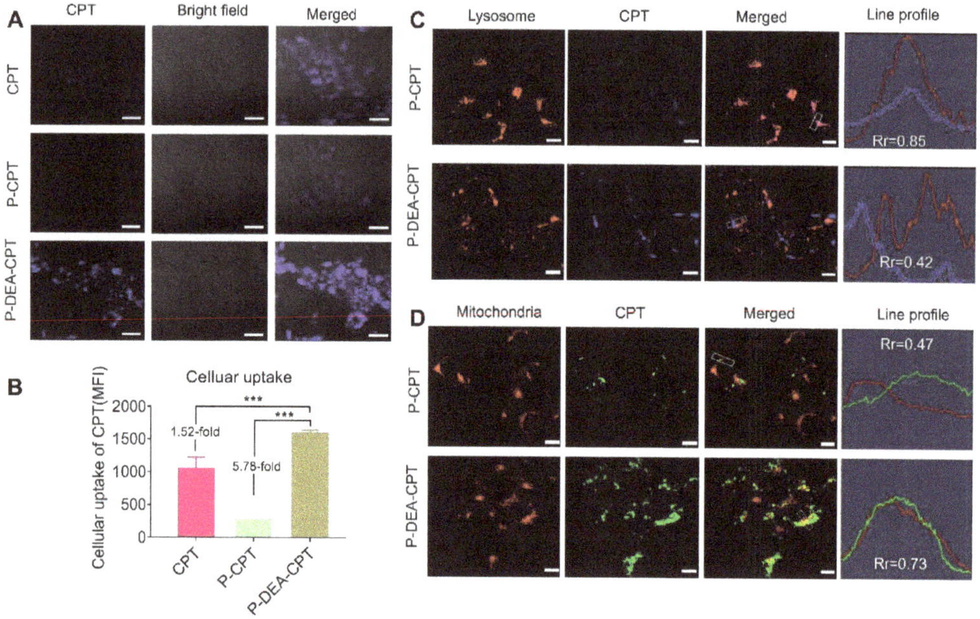

Figure 3. Subcellular trafficking of HPMA copolymer–CPT conjugates in cancer cells. (**A**) Qualitative CLSM and (**B**) quantitative flow cytometry analysis of the cellular uptake in 4T1 cells. Scale bar: 20 μm; mean ± SD ($n = 3$). (**C**) Lysosome escape and (**D**) mitochondria localization of HPMA copolymer–CPT conjugates in 4T1 cells observed under CLSM. Scale bar: 10 μm. *** $p < 0.001$; mean ± SD ($n = 3$).

3.4. In Vitro Mitochondrial Damage-Induced Apoptosis and Cytotoxicity of P-DEA-CPT

Mitochondria perform pivotal roles in determining cancer cell fate. The damage can directly cut down the energy supply and activate a variety of key events to initiate intrinsic pathways of apoptosis [26,27]. We investigated whether the enhanced delivery of CPT to mitochondria could result in mitochondria dysfunction. Notably, a significant increase in ROS was observed in the P-DEA-CPT group compared with P-CPT (Figure 4A). Once CPT inhibited the mitochondrial respiratory chain complexes, the electron transfer in the electron transfer chain would be blocked and unstable oxygen would leak out from mitochondria, subsequently forming ROS [28,29]. Thus, the overload of intracellular ROS induced by P-DEA-CPT revealed the impaired mitochondrial function by CPT. Moreover, mitochondrial membrane potential depolarization is another sign of mitochondrial dysfunction. JC-1 is a cationic lipophilic probe with $\Delta\psi$m-dependent aggregation in the mitochondria, and the transition from the red J-aggregate to the green J-monomer is a direct measurement of the decreased mitochondrial membrane potential. As displayed in Figure 4B, P-DEA-CPT caused a sharper drop in the red (aggregate)/green (monomer) fluorescence intensity ratio than both free CPT and P-CPT, indicating the significant $\Delta\psi$m loss (52.6% decrease compared to control). Furthermore, the majority of ATP in tumor cells is produced by the mitochondria aerobic respiration. Therefore, the dysfunction of mitochondria would inevitably reduce ATP production. As shown in Figure 4C, P-DEA-CPT exhibited maximum ATP decline in the 4T1 cells among all the groups, suggesting the most severe mitochondrial dysfunction.

It has been reported that mitochondria play crucial roles in regulating the intrinsic apoptotic pathways of cancer cells [30]. Upon inducing mitochondrial apoptosis, caspase 9 and caspase 3 would be activated, subsequently amplifying the apoptotic cascade [31]. Thus, caspase 9 and caspase 3 were determined to investigate whether mitochondrial dysfunction could activate the mitochondrial apoptotic pathway. After being incubated with P-DEA-CPT for 24 h, the expressions of caspase 9 and caspase 3 in 4T1 cells were both significantly upregulated as compared with P-CPT (Figure 4D,E). Consequently, P-DEA-CPT induced significantly stronger cytotoxicity (Figure 4F) with much higher cell apoptosis than P-CPT (Figure 4G). DNA-damaging drugs that cause apoptosis also rely on the initiation of caspase proteins [32,33]. Thus, free CPT-induced dose-dependent cytotoxicity was ascribed to the direct destruction of nuclear DNA, resulting in the elevated release of caspase 9 and caspase 3. Taken together, by impairing mitochondrial function, P-DEA-CPT efficiently blocked the energy generation and curbed proliferation of cancer cells, ultimately potentiating the therapeutic outcomes in cancer therapy.

3.5. *In Vitro Anti-Metastasis Effect of P-DEA-CPT*

Cancer metastasis involves complex cell biological cascades. Tumor cells migrate into the surrounding tumor stroma and invade through basement membranes, followed by entering blood circulation [34–36]. Thus, whether this mitochondria-targeting strategy could impede the processes of tumor-metastasis was investigated. As shown in Figure 5A, P-CPT only displayed a slight migration inhibitory effect (~75% of migration rate). In stark contrast, a much lower migration rate (~50%) was observed in P-DEA-CPT group. The wound healing assay also displayed that P-DEA-CPT exhibited a significantly stronger inhibitory effect on the mobility of 4T1 cells than P-CPT (52.9% vs. 25.5%, Figure 5B). Furthermore, P-DEA-CPT induced potent invasion restraint of 4T1 cells, and the invasion rate decreased to 36.45% (Figure 5C). Although free CPT inhibited the migration and invasion of 4T1 cells due to its certain cytotoxicity and anti-proliferation capacity, it might also cause unexpected side-effects. These results validated that P-DEA-CPT could potently suppress the migration, mobility, and invasion of 4T1 cells, providing great promise for inhibiting cancer cells from disseminating into circulation.

3.6. *Intratumoral Mitochondrial Targeting of P-DEA-CPT*

Due to the cationic feature afforded by DEA modification on the side-chain, the polymer P-DEA-CPT could achieve enhanced internalization into tumor cells due to the affinity to the negatively charged tumor cell membrane upon intratumoral injection [37]. Then, P-DEA-CPT could achieve lysosome escape due to the "proton sponge effect" [38]. Lastly, according to the negative nature of mitochondrial inner membrane ($\Delta\Psi = -150$ to

−180 mV), P-DEA-CPT could effectively target mitochondria in tumor cells [39]. To verify this, whether P-DEA-CPT could locate in mitochondria within tumor tissues was then further evaluated. Intratumoral mitochondrial targeting experiments displayed that P-CPT exhibited negligible mitochondria colocation under CLSM observation, whereas the strong dotted blue signals of P-DEA-CPT overlapped well with the red signals of mitochondria (Figure 6A). Consistently, quantitative analysis revealed a 4.7-fold higher mitochondrial accumulation of P-DEA-CPT as compared with P-CPT (Figure 6B). These results confirmed that P-DEA-CPT could successfully accumulate in the mitochondria within tumor tissues, laying the foundations for in vivo treatment.

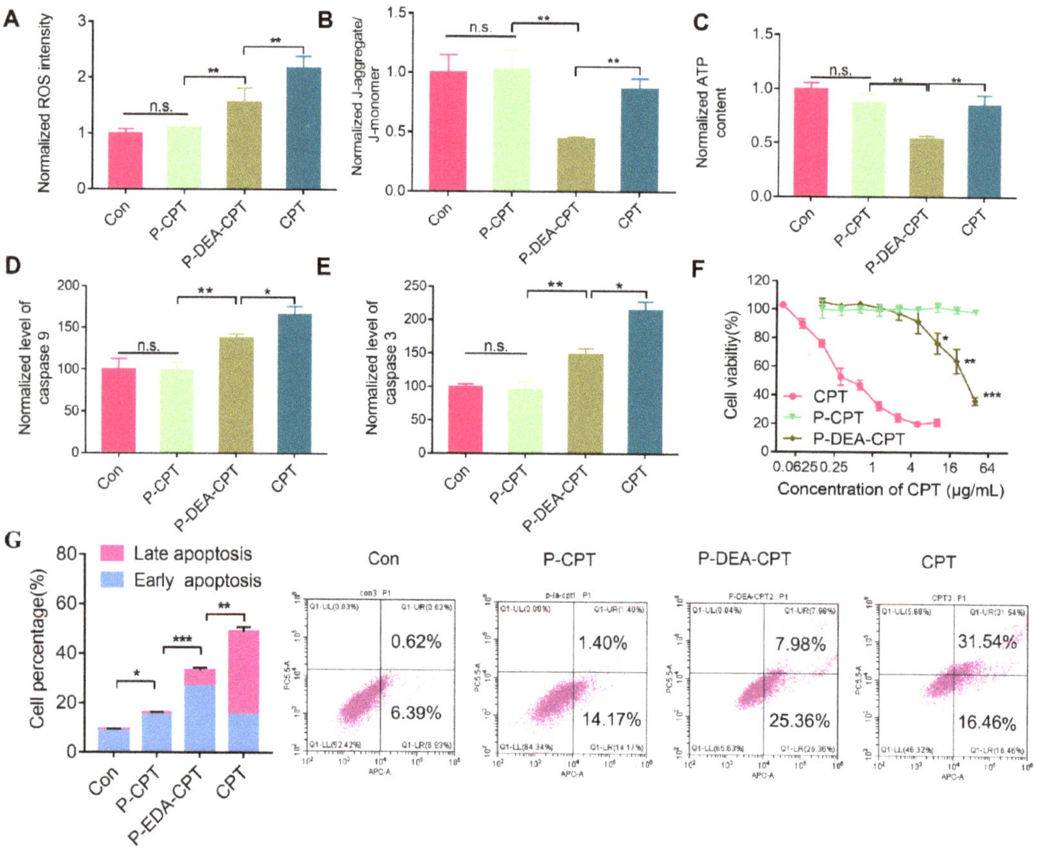

Figure 4. P-DEA-CPT damaged the mitochondria, initiated the mitochondrial apoptosis pathway, and caused cancer cell death. (**A**) Intracellular ROS level, (**B**) mitochondrial membrane potential depolarization, (**C**) ATP generation, (**D**) caspase-9 expression, and (**E**) caspase-3 expression in 4T1 cells were determined after different treatments. (**F**) Cell viability of 4T1 cells after being treated with different CPT polymers for 48 h. (**G**) The mean value and representative images of apoptotic and necrotic 4T1 cells induced by CPT polymers, as tested by flow cytometry. * $p < 0.05$, ** $p < 0.01$, *** $p < 0.001$, n.s. (no significance); mean ± SD ($n = 3$).

3.7. *In Vivo Antitumor and Anti-Metastasis Effect of P-DEA-CPT*

Triple-negative breast cancer (TNBC) orthotopic murine models can simulate multiple phases of metastasis formation [40,41]. Motivated by the potent anti-metastasis capacity in vitro, the orthotopic 4T1 breast tumor model was established as the method mentioned above to evaluate the in vivo antitumor and anti-metastasis effect of P-DEA-CPT. When tumor volume reached around 100 cm^3, free CPT, P-CPT, and P-DEA-CPT (equivalent CPT dose of 5 $mg \cdot kg^{-1}$, 25 μL) were intratumorally injected every 3 days for a total of five times. At the end of the treatment, P-CPT displayed a negligible tumor growth-inhibitory effect. In sharp contrast, P-DEA-CPT potently curbed tumor growth (inhibition rate of 61.2%) with the slowest tumor growth rate and lowest tumor weight among all the groups (Figure 7A–C). It is also worth noting that free CPT only exhibited a moderate antitumor effect despite its much stronger cytotoxicity than P-DEA-CPT in vitro. This might be attributed to its rapid clearance in tumor tissues via vascular leakage, whereas the high-molecular-weight polymer remained in tumor tissue for a longer time [42,43]. Hematoxylin and eosin (H&E) staining results further validated the best tumor growth suppression capacity of P-DEA-CPT with a larger area of apoptosis (Figure 7D). At the end of the assay, the excised lungs were immersed in Bouin's fluid, and the metastatic nodules were counted to evaluate the lung metastasis formation in each treatment group. Obviously, mice in the saline group developed serious lung metastasis, and an imperceptible metastasis suppression effect was observed in both P-CPT and free CPT groups (Figure 7E,F). Comparably, P-DEA-CPT greatly decreased lung metastasis with the fewest lung nodules among all the groups (Figure 7E,F). In addition, all the groups exhibited favorable safety with no weight loss and histopathological changes in major organs during the treatment period (Figure 8A,B). These results manifested that P-DEA-CPT attained the efficient anti-tumor and anti-metastasis capacity with considerable safety.

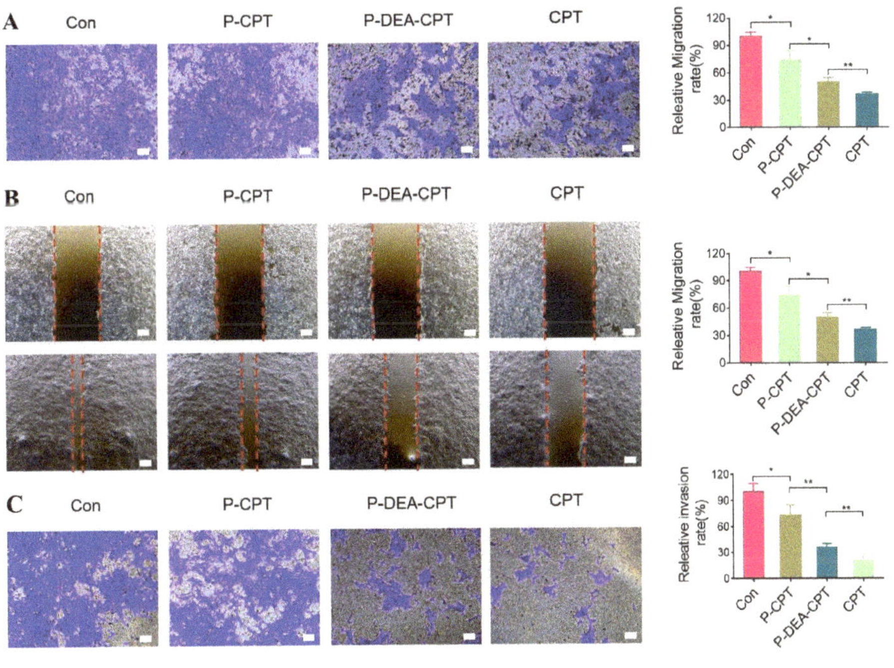

Figure 5. Anti-metastasis effect of P-DEA-CPT in vitro. (**A**) Migration, (**B**) wound healing, and (**C**) invasion of 4T1 cell lines after being treated with free CPT, P-CPT, and P-DEA-CPT for 24 h, as displayed via representative images and quantitative results. Migrant or invasive cells (at the outer bottom of the transwell chamber) were stained with crystal violet and measured by the microplate reader. Scale bar: 200 μm. * $p < 0.05$, ** $p < 0.01$; mean ± SD ($n = 3$).

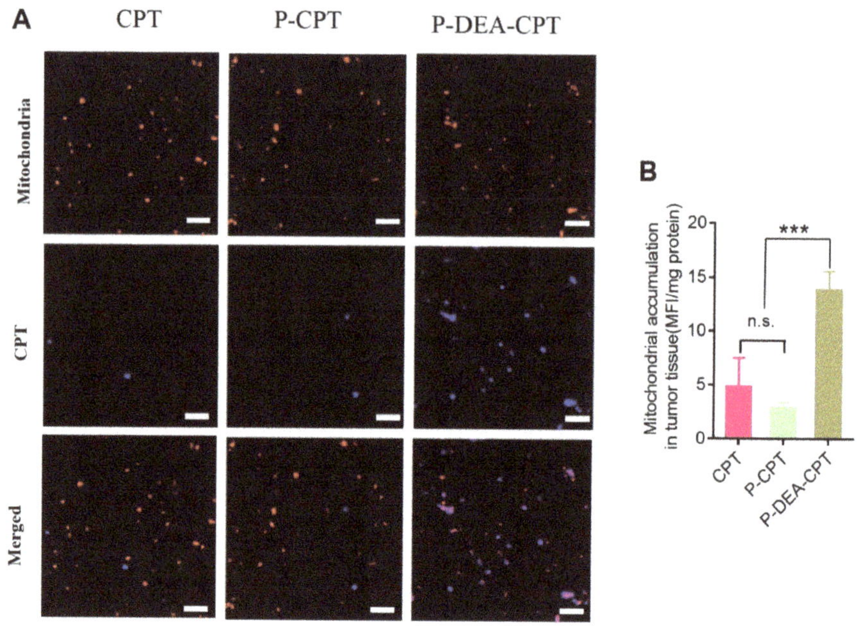

Figure 6. Intratumoral mitochondrial targeting of P-DEA-CPT in 4T1 orthotopic breast tumor. Mitochondria-specific colocalization of HPMA copolymer conjugates and free CPT in 4T1 cells as (**A**) observed under CLSM and (**B**) quantitatively detected via microplate reader. Red, mitochondria; blue, CPT. Scale bar: 10 µm. *** $p < 0.001$, n.s. (no significance); mean ± SD ($n = 3$).

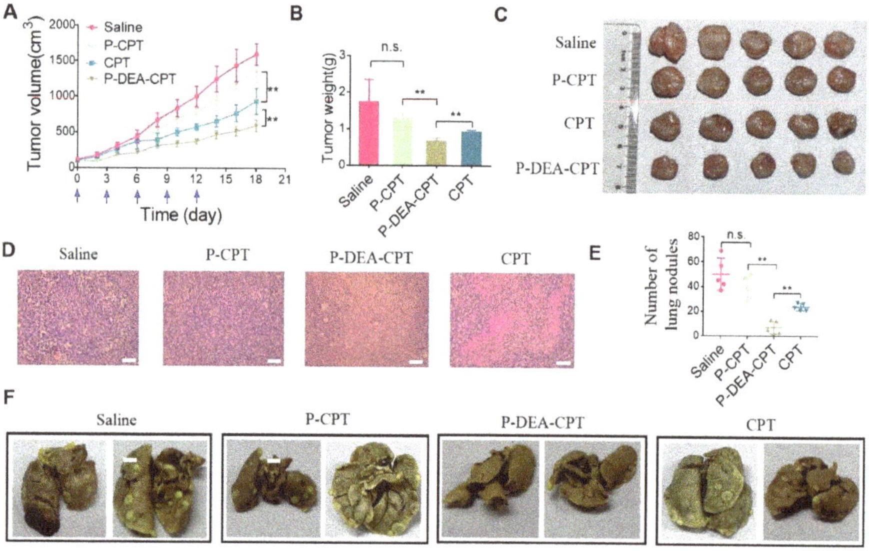

Figure 7. In vivo antitumor and anti-metastasis effect of P-DEA-CPT in 4T1 orthotopic breast tumor. (**A**) Average tumor growth curves, (**B**) tumor weight at the end of the assay, (**C**) representative images of the excised tumor tissues, and (**D**) H&E results of tumor sections in each treatment group. Scale bar: 200 µm. (**E**) The number of metastatic nodules and (**F**) representative images of excised lung stained by Bouin's fluid in each treatment group. ** $p < 0.01$, n.s. (no significance); mean ± SD ($n = 5$).

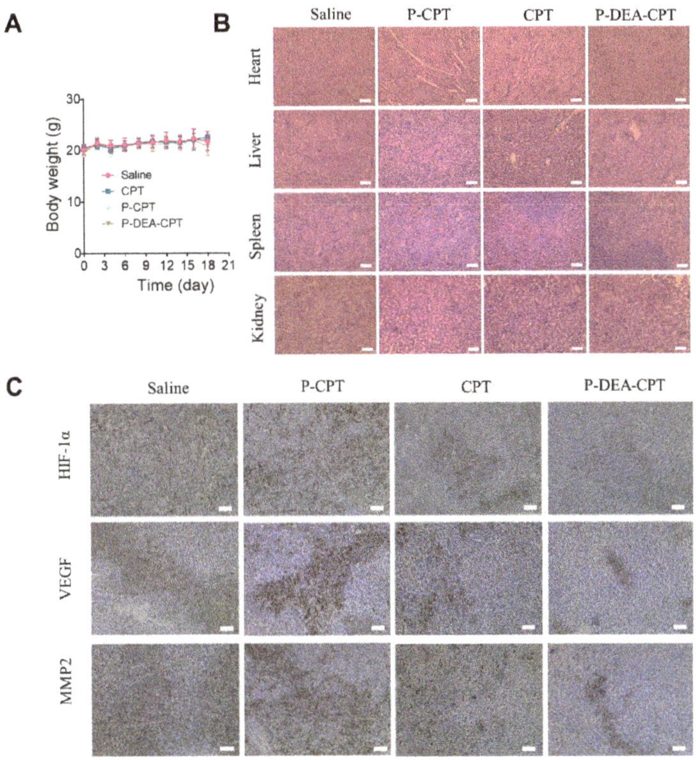

Figure 8. (**A**) Body weight changes and (**B**) H&E staining of major organs of all the groups during the treatment period in 4T1 orthotopic breast tumor. (**C**) Immunohistochemistry staining of tumor sections for analysis of the expression of HIF-1α, MMP-2, and VEGF at the endpoint. The brown area indicates the positive expression of these proteins. Scale bar: 200 μm.

The potent anti-metastasis effect of P-DEA-CPT could be partially ascribed to its energy depletion and enhanced apoptosis caused by impairing mitochondria. Moreover, mitochondria dysfunction was reported to alleviate hypoxia and downregulate hypoxia-inducible factor (HIF-1α) [44,45], the key regulator for various pro-metastasis downstream signaling pathways, resulting in the expressions of vascular endothelial growth factor (VEGF) and matrix metalloproteinases (MMPs) [46,47]. To verify this, the expression of crucial factors for tumor metastasis (HIF-1α, MMP2, and VEGF) was investigated via immunohistochemistry assay. As shown in Figure 8C, remarkably downregulated expressions (lighter brown) of HIF-1α, MMP-2, and VEGF were observed in P-DEA-CPT group. Collectively, the great efficacy of our mitochondrial targeting strategy to inhibit tumorigenesis and metastasis largely originates from multiple mechanisms, including cutting down energy supply, activating the intrinsic apoptotic pathway, and downregulating HIF-1α and its downstream pro-metastasis factors (MMP2 and VEGF).

4. Conclusions

In summary, we fabricated a mitochondria-targeting CPT delivery platform based on water-soluble HPMA copolymers with an optimal content of DEA modified on the side-chain. Firstly, the water-soluble DEA sufficiently escorted the CPT conjugates located in the mitochondria both in 4T1 cells and in tumor tissues. Secondly, P-DEA-CPT elicited serious mitochondrial dysfunction with the decline in ATP and activation of proapoptotic caspase proteins, thereby resulting in the restraint of cancer cell proliferation, migration, and invasion. Furthermore, the expressions of HIF-1α and its downstream metastasis-associated proteins including MMP-2 and VEGF in tumor sites were notably inhibited. Consequently, both primary breast cancers and distant pulmonary metastases were largely impeded. Overall, our study revealed that DEA is a promising candidate to escort CPT to accumulate in the mitochondria. Furthermore, selectively delivering CPT to the mitochondria provides a feasible way of improving the anti-metastasis effect.

Author Contributions: Conceptualization, X.Y., Y.Y., L.L. and Y.H.; formal analysis, X.Y.; investigation, Y.Y. and X.S.; methodology, X.Y; resources, X.Y., X.S. and Y.H.; supervision, L.L. and Y.H.; validation, X.S. and Y.H.; writing—original draft, X.Y. and Y.Y.; writing—review and editing, Y.Y., X.S. and L.L. All authors have read and agreed to the published version of the manuscript.

Funding: This work was supported by the National Natural Science Foundation of China (Grant No. 81625023).

Institutional Review Board Statement: This study was approved by institutional ethical review board of our institution (Medical Ethics Committee of Sichuan University, Chengdu, China). (Protocol code: SYXK(Chuan)2018-113, date of approval: 18 May 2018). All of the animal experiments were approved by the Medical Ethics Committee of Sichuan University, and the animal experiments were performed in the Animal Laboratory of West China School of Pharmacy in Sichuan University.

Informed Consent Statement: Not applicable.

Data Availability Statement: Not applicable.

Acknowledgments: We gratefully acknowledge financial support from the National Natural Science Foundation for Distinguished Young Scholars (81625023).

Conflicts of Interest: The authors declare no conflict of interest.

References

1. Barua, S.; Mitragotri, S. Synergistic targeting of cell membrane, cytoplasm, and nucleus of cancer cells using rod-shaped nanoparticles. *ACS Nano* **2013**, *7*, 9558–9570. [CrossRef] [PubMed]
2. Cheng, Z.; Huang, Y.; Shen, Q.; Zhao, Y.; Wang, W.; Yu, J.; Lu, W. A camptothecin-based, albumin-binding prodrug enhances efficacy and safety in vivo. *Eur. J. Med. Chem.* **2021**, *226*, 113851. [CrossRef]
3. Ghanbari-Movahed, M.; Kaceli, T.; Mondal, A.; Farzaei, M.H.; Bishayee, A. Recent advances in improved anticancer efficacies of camptothecin nano-formulations: A systematic review. *Biomedicines* **2021**, *9*, 480. [CrossRef] [PubMed]
4. Sadalage, P.S.; Patil, R.V.; Havaldar, D.V.; Gavade, S.S.; Santos, A.C.; Pawar, K.D. Optimally biosynthesized, PEGylated gold nanoparticles functionalized with quercetin and camptothecin enhance potential anti-inflammatory, anti-cancer and anti-angiogenic activities. *J. Nanobiotechnol.* **2021**, *19*, 84. [CrossRef] [PubMed]
5. Lian, Q.; Xu, J.; Yan, S.; Huang, M.; Ding, H.; Sun, X.; Geng, M. Chemotherapy-induced intestinal inflammatory responses are mediated by exosome secretion of double-strand DNA via AIM2 inflammasome activation. *Cell Res.* **2017**, *27*, 784–800. [CrossRef] [PubMed]
6. Swami, U.; Goel, S.; Mani, S. Therapeutic targeting of CPT-11 induced diarrhea: A case for prophylaxis. *Curr. Drug Targets* **2013**, *14*, 777–797. [CrossRef]
7. Roth, K.G.; Mambetsariev, I.; Kulkarni, P.; Salgia, R. The mitochondrion as an emerging therapeutic target in cancer. *Trends Mol. Med.* **2020**, *26*, 119–134. [CrossRef]
8. Vyas, S.; Zaganjor, E.; Haigis, M.C. Mitochondria and Cancer. *Cell* **2016**, *166*, 555–566. [CrossRef]
9. Reichard, A.; Asosingh, K. The role of mitochondria in angiogenesis. *Mol. Biol. Rep.* **2019**, *46*, 1393–1400. [CrossRef]
10. LeBleu, V.S.; O'Connell, J.T.; Gonzalez Herrera, K.N.; Wikman, H.; Pantel, K.; Haigis, M.C.; Kalluri, R. PGC-1α mediates mitochondrial biogenesis and oxidative phosphorylation in cancer cells to promote metastasis. *Nat. Cell Biol.* **2014**, *16*, 992–1003. [CrossRef]
11. Weinberg, S.E.; Chandel, N.S. Targeting mitochondria metabolism for cancer therapy. *Nat. Chem. Biol.* **2015**, *11*, 9–15. [CrossRef] [PubMed]
12. Chen, C.; Li, Q.; Xing, L.; Zhou, M.; Luo, C.; Li, S.; Huang, Y. Co-delivery of mitochondrial targeted lonidamine and PIN1 inhibitor ATRA by nanoparticulate systems for synergistic metastasis suppression. *Nano Res.* **2022**, *15*, 3376–3386. [CrossRef]
13. Fulda, S.; Galluzzi, L.; Kroemer, G. Targeting mitochondria for cancer therapy. *Nat. Rev. Drug Discov.* **2010**, *9*, 447–464. [CrossRef] [PubMed]
14. Yi, X.; Yan, Y.; Li, L.; Li, Q.; Xiang, Y.; Huang, Y. Sequentially targeting cancer-associated fibroblast and mitochondria alleviates tumor hypoxia and inhibits cancer metastasis by preventing "soil" formation and "seed" dissemination. *Adv. Funct. Mater.* **2021**, *31*, 2010283. [CrossRef]

15. Zhang, W.; Hu, X.; Shen, Q.; Xing, D. Mitochondria-specific drug release and reactive oxygen species burst induced by polyprodrug nanoreactors can enhance chemotherapy. *Nat. Commun.* **2019**, *10*, 1704. [CrossRef] [PubMed]
16. Wang, Y.; Zhang, T.; Hou, C.; Zu, M.; Lu, Y.; Ma, X.; Xu, Z. Mitochondria-specific anticancer drug delivery based on reduction-activated polyprodrug for enhancing the therapeutic effect of breast cancer chemotherapy. *ACS Appl. Mater. Interfaces* **2019**, *11*, 29330–29340. [CrossRef]
17. Ma, X.; Gong, N.; Zhong, L.; Sun, J.; Liang, X.J. Future of nanotherapeutics: Targeting the cellular sub-organelles. *Biomaterials* **2016**, *97*, 10–21. [CrossRef]
18. Li, Q.; Yang, J.; Chen, C.; Lin, X.; Zhou, M.; Zhou, Z.; Huang, Y. A novel mitochondrial targeted hybrid peptide modified HPMA copolymers for breast cancer metastasis suppression. *J. Control. Release* **2020**, *325*, 38–51. [CrossRef]
19. Zhou, M.; Li, L.; Li, L.; Lin, X.; Wang, F.; Li, Q.; Huang, Y. Overcoming chemotherapy resistance via simultaneous drug-efflux circumvention and mitochondrial targeting. *Acta Pharm. Sin. B* **2019**, *9*, 615–625. [CrossRef]
20. Zielonka, J.; Joseph, J.; Sikora, A.; Hardy, M.; Ouari, O.; Vasquez-Vivar, J.; Kalyanaraman, B. Mitochondria-targeted triphenylphosphonium-based compounds: Syntheses, mechanisms of action, and therapeutic and diagnostic applications. *Chem. Rev.* **2017**, *117*, 10043–10120. [CrossRef]
21. Qin, J.; Gong, N.; Liao, Z.; Zhang, S.; Timashev, P.; Huo, S.; Liang, X.J. Recent progress in mitochondria-targeting-based nanotechnology for cancer treatment. *Nanoscale* **2021**, *13*, 7108–7118. [CrossRef] [PubMed]
22. Wang, Y.; Zheng, J.; Lin, J.; Ye, K.; Wei, P. Mitochondria-targeting and ROS-responsive nanocarriers via amphiphilic TPP-PEG-TK-Ce6 for nanoenabled photodynamic therapy. *Adv. Polym. Technol.* **2022**, *2022*, 1178039. [CrossRef]
23. Yi, X.; Yan, Y.; Li, L.; Zhou, R.; Shen, X.; Huang, Y. Combination of mitochondria impairment and inflammation blockade to combat metastasis. *J. Control. Release* **2022**, *341*, 753–768. [CrossRef] [PubMed]
24. Wang, F.; Sun, W.; Li, L.; Li, L.; Liu, Y.; Zhang, Z.R.; Huang, Y. Charge-reversible multifunctional HPMA copolymers for mitochondrial targeting. *ACS Appl. Mater. Interfaces* **2017**, *9*, 27563–27574. [CrossRef] [PubMed]
25. Sun, W.; Li, L.; Li, L.J.; Yang, Q.Q.; Zhang, Z.R.; Huang, Y. Two birds, one stone: Dual targeting of the cancer cell surface and subcellular mitochondria by the galectin-3-binding peptide G3-C12. *Acta Pharmacologica. Sin.* **2017**, *38*, 806–822. [CrossRef] [PubMed]
26. Murphy, M.P.; Hartley, R.C. Mitochondria as a therapeutic target for common pathologies. *Nat. Rev. Drug Discov.* **2018**, *17*, 865–886. [CrossRef]
27. Lakhani, S.A.; Masud, A.; Kuida, K.; Porter Jr, G.A.; Booth, C.J.; Mehal, W.Z.; Flavell, R.A. Caspases 3 and 7: Key mediators of mitochondrial events of apoptosis. *Science* **2006**, *311*, 847. [CrossRef]
28. Zorov, D.B.; Juhaszova, M.; Sollott, S.J. Mitochondrial reactive oxygen species (ROS) and ROS-induced ROS release. *Physiol. Rev.* **2014**, *94*, 909–950. [CrossRef]
29. Kudryavtseva, A.V.; Krasnov, G.S.; Dmitriev, A.A.; Alekseev, B.Y.; Kardymon, O.L.; Sadritdinova, A.F.; Snezhkina, A.V. Mitochondrial dysfunction and oxidative stress in aging and cancer. *Oncotarget* **2016**, *7*, 44879–44905. [CrossRef]
30. Bock, F.J.; Tait, S.W.G. Mitochondria as multifaceted regulators of cell death. *Nat. Rev. Mol. Cell Biol.* **2020**, *21*, 85–100. [CrossRef]
31. Kumar, S.; Eroglu, E.; Stokes III, J.A.; Scissum-Gunn, K.; Saldanha, S.N.; Singh, U.P.; Mishra, M.K. Resveratrol induces mitochondria-mediated, caspase-independent apoptosis in murine prostate cancer cells. *Oncotarget* **2017**, *8*, 20895–20908. [CrossRef] [PubMed]
32. Dilshara, M.G.; Jayasooriya, R.G.P.T.; Karunarathne, W.A.H.M.; Choi, Y.H.; Kim, G.Y. Camptothecin induces mitotic arrest through Mad2-Cdc20 complex by activating the JNK-mediated Sp1 pathway. *Food Chem. Toxicol.* **2019**, *127*, 143–155. [CrossRef] [PubMed]
33. Pang, W.J.; Xiong, Y.; Wang, Y.; Tong, Q.; Yang, G.S. Sirt1 attenuates camptothecin-induced apoptosis through caspase-3 pathway in porcine preadipocytes. *Exp. Cell Res.* **2013**, *319*, 670–683. [CrossRef] [PubMed]
34. Wan, L.; Pantel, K.; Kang, Y. Tumor metastasis: Moving new biological insights into the clinic. *Nat. Med.* **2013**, *19*, 1450–1464. [CrossRef] [PubMed]
35. Friedl, P.; Alexander, S. Cancer invasion and the microenvironment: Plasticity and reciprocity. *Cell* **2011**, *147*, 992–1009. [CrossRef]
36. Valastyan, S.; RWeinberg, A. Tumor metastasis: Molecular insights and evolving paradigms. *Cell* **2011**, *147*, 275–292. [CrossRef]
37. Jin, Q.; Deng, Y.; Chen, X.; Ji, J. Rational design of cancer nanomedicine for simultaneous stealth surface and enhanced cellular uptake. *Acs Nano* **2019**, *13*, 954–977. [CrossRef]
38. Wang, R.; Yin, C.; Liu, C.; Sun, Y.; Xiao, P.; Li, J.; Jiang, X. Phenylboronic acid modification augments the lysosome escape and antitumor efficacy of a cylindrical polymer brush-based prodrug. *J. Am. Chem. Soc.* **2021**, *143*, 20927–20938. [CrossRef]
39. Liberman, E.A.; Topaly, V.P.; Tsofina, L.M.; Jasaitis, A.A.; Skulachev, V.P. Mechanism of coupling of oxidative phosphorylation and the membrane potential of mitochondria. *Nature* **1969**, *222*, 1076–1078. [CrossRef]
40. Jiang, T.; Chen, L.; Huang, Y.; Wang, J.; Xu, M.; Zhou, S.; Chen, J. Metformin and docosahexaenoic acid hybrid micelles for premetastatic niche modulation and tumor metastasis suppression. *Nano Lett.* **2019**, *19*, 3548–3562. [CrossRef]
41. Arroyo-Crespo, J.J.; Armiñán, A.; Charbonnier, D.; Deladriere, C.; Palomino-Schätzlein, M.; Lamas-Domingo, R.; Vicent, M.J. Characterization of triple-negative breast cancer preclinical models provides functional evidence of metastatic progression. *Int. J. Cancer* **2019**, *145*, 2267–2281. [CrossRef] [PubMed]
42. Xiang, Y.; Chen, L.; Li, L.; Huang, Y. Restoration and enhancement of immunogenic cell death of cisplatin by coadministration with digoxin and conjugation to HPMA copolymer. *ACS Appl. Mater. Interfaces* **2020**, *12*, 1606–1616. [CrossRef] [PubMed]

43. Huang, A.; Pressnall, M.M.; Lu, R.; Huayamares, S.G.; Griffin, J.D.; Groer, C.; Berkland, C.J. Human intratumoral therapy: Linking drug properties and tumor transport of drugs in clinical trials. *J. Control. Release* **2020**, *326*, 203–221. [CrossRef] [PubMed]
44. Mai, X.; Zhang, Y.; Fan, H.; Song, W.; Chang, Y.; Chen, B.; Teng, G. Integration of immunogenic activation and immunosuppressive reversion using mitochondrial-respiration-inhibited platelet-mimicking nanoparticles. *Biomaterials* **2020**, *232*, 119699. [CrossRef]
45. Yang, Z.; Wang, J.; Liu, S.; Li, X.; Miao, L.; Yang, B.; Guan, W. Defeating relapsed and refractory malignancies through a nano-enabled mitochondria-mediated respiratory inhibition and damage pathway. *Biomaterials* **2020**, *229*, 119580. [CrossRef]
46. Steeg, P.S. Targeting metastasis. *Nat. Rev. Cancer* **2016**, *16*, 201–218. [CrossRef]
47. Rankin, E.B.; Giaccia, A.J. Hypoxic control of metastasis. *Science* **2016**, *352*, 175–180. [CrossRef]

pharmaceutics

Article

Evaluation of CTB-sLip for Targeting Lung Metastasis of Colorectal Cancer

Xiaoying Zhang [1,†], Wenjing Tang [2,†], Haoyu Wen [3], Ercan Wu [4], Tianhao Ding [2], Jie Gu [3], Zhongwei Lv [1,*] and Changyou Zhan [2,4,*]

1 Department of Nuclear Medicine, The Affiliated Shanghai Tenth People's Hospital of Nanjing Medical University, Shanghai 200072, China; yingzx2002@126.com
2 Center of Medical Research and Innovation, Shanghai Pudong Hospital & Department of Pharmacology, School of Basic Medical Sciences, Fudan University, Shanghai 201399, China; 16111030025@fudan.edu.cn (W.T.); 18111010017@fudan.edu.cn (T.D.)
3 Department of Thoracic Surgery, Zhongshan Hospital, Fudan University, Shanghai 200032, China; 20211210051@fudan.edu.cn (H.W.); gu.jie3@zs-hospital.sh.cn (J.G.)
4 School of Pharmacy, Fudan University & Key Laboratory of Smart Drug Delivery (Fudan University), Ministry of Education, Shanghai 201203, China; 20211030020@fudan.edu.cn
* Correspondence: lvzwjs2020@163.com (Z.L.); cyzhan@fudan.edu.cn (C.Z.); Tel.: +86-21-66302714 (Z.L.)
† These authors contributed equally to this work.

Abstract: Lung metastasis of colorectal cancer is common in the clinic; however, precise targeting for the diagnosis and therapy purposes of those lung metastases remains challenging. Herein, cholera toxin subunit b (CTB) protein was chemically conjugated on the surface of PEGylated liposomes (CTB-sLip). Both human-derived colorectal cancer cell lines, HCT116 and HT-29, demonstrated high binding affinity and cellular uptake with CTB-sLip. In vivo, CTB-sLip exhibited elevated targeting capability to the lung metastasis of colorectal cancer in the model nude mice in comparison to PEGylated liposomes (sLip) without CTB modification. CTB conjugation induced ignorable effects on the interaction between liposomes and plasma proteins but significantly enhanced the uptake of liposomes by numerous blood cells and splenic cells, leading to relatively rapid blood clearance in BALB/c mice. Even though repeated injections of CTB-sLip induced the production of anti-CTB antibodies, our results suggested CTB-sLip as promising nanocarriers for the diagnosis of lung metastasis of colorectal cancer.

Keywords: lung metastasis; targeting; colorectal cancer; liposome; immunogenicity

Citation: Zhang, X.; Tang, W.; Wen, H.; Wu, E.; Ding, T.; Gu, J.; Lv, Z.; Zhan, C. Evaluation of CTB-sLip for Targeting Lung Metastasis of Colorectal Cancer. *Pharmaceutics* **2022**, *14*, 868. https://doi.org/10.3390/pharmaceutics14040868

Academic Editors: Gert Fricker and Francesco Grossi

Received: 28 February 2022
Accepted: 13 April 2022
Published: 15 April 2022

1. Introduction

Colorectal cancer has become an increasing burden in public health, firmly ranking in the top three of both the morbidity and the cause of death from malignant tumors [1]. Even worse, remote spreading of colorectal cancer is of high occurrence, which accelerates the pathological progression and exacerbates the difficulty of clinical treatments. Lung metastasis is among the most common in colorectal cancer patients even after surgical resection [2], readily leading to rapid recurrence and disease progression. However, the early stage of lung metastasis of colorectal cancer remains challenging to track even using positron emission tomography [3]. Targeting the lung metastasis of colorectal cancer is of crucial importance for the diagnosis and therapy purposes [4].

There are numerous ligands being developed to target colorectal cancer cells by recognizing the corresponding receptors or antigens, including small molecules [5], peptides [6], antibodies [7], and aptamers [8]. Such targeting ligands are conjugated with nanocarriers for the delivery of imaging probes [9], therapeutic agents [10], or even both. Unfortunately, none of them have been successfully approved for the clinical use. There are multiple biological barriers hampering the efficient delivery of those targeted delivery systems [11]. We [12,13] and other groups [14,15] previously reported that ligand modification could severely alter the bio-nano surface properties, thus affecting the formation of protein corona and enhancing the mononuclear phagocyte system recognition. Conversely, the biological media that the targeted delivery systems encounter during in vivo circulation can also destroy the ligands to compromise the bioactivity [16,17], leading to the loss of targeting capability.

GM1 ganglioside is expressed on the membrane of various types of cells [18], acting as the receptor for cholera toxin by strongly binding with the subunit b (CTB) [19]. In our previous study [20,21], the CTB protein was conjugated on the surface of poly (lactic-co-glycolic acid) (PLGA) nanoparticles to penetrate the blood–brain barrier and to target glioma cells and neovasculature by recognizing GM1. The CTB protein not only preserved bioactivity in the presence of mouse serum but also exhibited nonsignificant impacts on the absorption of plasma proteins after conjugation on the surface of PLGA nanoparticles. These results suggested that the CTB protein may be an appropriate ligand to efficiently circumvent the biological barriers in blood circulation by mitigating the reciprocal influences between delivery systems and biological media.

The CTB protein was found to demonstrate high binding with intestinal cells in the human histological sections [22,23], suggestive of the potential of the CTB protein for targeting colorectal cancer. Liposomes are a class of commonly used nanocarriers in both basic research [24,25] and the clinic [26], representing a class of versatile tools for the delivery of imaging probes and therapeutic agents [27]. In the present study, the CTB protein was chemically conjugated on the surface of PEGylated liposomes (CTB-sLip). We investigated the targeting capability of CTB-sLip to colorectal cancer cells in vitro and lung metastasis of colorectal cancer in vivo. In particular, the effects of serum were emphasized on the bioactivity of the CTB protein, as well as the immunogenicity and in vivo fate of CTB-sLip.

2. Materials and Methods

2.1. Animals and Cells

Adult male BALB/c mice and nude mice were purchased from Shanghai Laboratory Animal Research Center (Shanghai, China) and raised under Specific Pathogen Free (SPF) conditions. HCT116 and HT-29 cell lines were purchased from Shanghai Institute of Cell Biology. Cells were cultured with McCoy'5A medium containing 10% fetal bovine serum (FBS) at 37 °C with 5% CO_2.

2.2. Materials

Cholesterol, mPEG$_{2000}$-DSPE, Mal-PEG$_{3500}$-DSPE, and HSPC were acquired from Shanghai A.V.T. Pharmaceutical company (Shanghai, China). DiI (1,1′-Dioctadecyl-3,3,3′,3′-tetramethylindocarbo-cyanine perchlorate), 2-iminothiolane hydrochloride (Traut's Reagent), and Sephadex® G50 were obtained from Sigma (St. Louis, MO, USA). Doxorubicin HCl/Adriamycin (MB1087-S), DiO dye (MB4239), and DiR dye (MB12482) were bought from Meilunbio Co. Ltd. (Dalian, China). HisSep Ni-NTA Agarose Resin 6FF (20503ES50) and Ampicillin Sodium (60203ES10) were acquired from YEASEN Biotech Co., Ltd. (Shanghai, China). One-Step™ ABTS Substrate Solution (37615), Zeba™ Spin Desalting Columns (7 kDa MWCO) and a Pierce TM BCA Protein Assay Kit (23225) were obtained from Thermo Fisher Scientific (Rockford, IL, USA). TMB Substrate Solution for ELISA was obtained from Beyotime Biotech Co. Ltd. (Shanghai, China). Anti-His tag antibody [M2] (HRP) (ab9108), anti-mouse serum albumin (ab19194), and donkey polyclonal secondary antibody to Rabbit IgG-H&L (Alexa Fluor® 647) (ab150075) were obtained from Abcam (Cambridge, MA, USA). Mini-PROTEAN® TGXTM Precast Protein Gel 4–20% (4561093) was purchased from Bio-Rad Laboratories Co., Ltd. (Shanghai, China). Polymyxin B sulfate (A610318), IPTG (Isopropyl-beta-D-thiogalactopyranoside), and MOPS (4-Morpholinepropanesulfonic acid) were purchased from Sangon Biotech Co., Ltd. (Shanghai, China). Tryptone (LP0042) and yeast extract (LP0021) were obtained from Oxid Co., Ltd. (Hants, UK). Ganglioside GM1 was purchased from Avanti Co., Ltd. (Birmingham, UK). McCoy'5A medium

(L630KJ) was obtained from Basal Media Co., Ltd. (Shanghai, China), and FBS was obtained from Cytiva Co., Ltd. (Marlborough, MA, USA). APC anti-mouse CD3 antibody (100235), Brilliant Violet 421™ anti-mouse CD19 antibody (115537), APC anti-mouse/human CD11b antibody (101211), Brilliant Violet 421™ anti-mouse Ly-6G antibody (127627), APC anti-mouse CD146 antibody (134711), Brilliant Violet 421™ anti-mouse F4/80 antibody (123131), anti-mouse CD11c recombinant antibody (161102), and Brilliant Violet 421™ anti-human CD326 (EpCAM) Antibody (369821) were purchased from BioLegend. Co., Ltd. (San Diego, CA, USA).

2.3. Expression and Characterization of the CTB Protein

The plasmid was successfully constructed and cloned into PET-28a (kanamycin resistance) containing a C-terminal His (6×) tag. The *E. Coli* cells were amplified at 37 °C and induced at 15 °C by IPTG (1 mM) for 12 h. The crude protein was obtained by centrifugation at 6000× *g* for 10 min and dissolved in buffer containing 50 mM Tris, 500 mM NaCl, 2 M urine, and 10 mM 2-hydroxy-1-ethanethiol. The crucial protein was folded by dialysis for 48 h and subsequently loaded in a Ni-NTA column according to manufacturer's instructions (Yisen Co. Ltd., Shanghai, China). The CTB protein was collected with elution buffer (250 mM imidazole in PBS) and ultrafiltrated at 8000× *g* with PBS three times until complete replacement of the storing buffer by PBS. The gradient (4–20%) polyacrylamide SDS-PAGE gel and Fast sliver staining kit were used to characterize the purity and molecular weight of the CTB protein.

ELISA was used to determine the binding activity of CTB to GM1. GM1 was coated on 96-well microplates with 1 µg per well at 4 °C overnight. After blockade with 5% BSA (in PBS), serial dilutions of CTB in 0.1% BSA were added and incubated at 37 °C for 1 h. HRP conjugated anti-His antibody was used to detect CTB at 405 nm (ABTS).

2.4. Preparation and Characterization of Liposomes

Plain PEGylated liposomes (sLip) were prepared by the lipid-film hydration method. HSPC, cholesterol, and mPEG$_{2000}$-DSPE (52:43:5 in molar ratio) were dissolved in chloroform and formed a thin film through vacuum evaporation. Any residual chloroform was removed overnight under vacuum. The film was hydrated with saline and extruded through polycarbonate membranes (400 nm, 200 nm, and 100 nm) at 60 °C. The DiI-, DiR-, and DiO-labelled sLip (sLip/DiI, sLip/DiR, and sLip/DiO) were prepared according to the same procedure as above except by adding 100 µg mL^{-1} DiI, DiR, and DiO, respectively. The 5-FAM-loaded sLip (sLip/FAM) were prepared using the same procedure as that used for plain sLip, except using 5-FAM solution (2 mg mL^{-1} in deionized water) to hydrate the film. A Sephadex-G50 column was used to remove the unloaded fluorescence dye. Maleimide functionalized sLip were prepared by adding 1% mol Mal-PEG$_{3500}$-DSPE before vacuum evaporation.

CTB (775 µg, 14 nmol) was dissolved in 1.5 mL PBS (containing 5 mM EDTA, pH adjusted to 8.0), and 9.7 µL Traut's Reagent (14.5 mM in PBS) was added. The mixture was reacted for 45 min at room temperature. A desalting column was used to remove un-reacted Traut's Reagent, and the thiolated CTB was collected by centrifugation. Mal-sLip (1 mL, with 10 µmol HSPC) were mixed with thiolated CTB (1–4 nmol, resulted in a molar ratio of 0.1–0.4‰ CTB to HSPC). The mixture was reacted at room temperature for 3 h. The reaction solution was collected, and CTB-sLip were purified using a Sephadex-G50 column. The size and zeta potential of liposomes (50 times dilution with deionized water) were measured by a Zetasizer Nano ZS (Malvern Instruments, Malvern, UK).

2.5. Characterization of Liposome Stability in Mouse Serum

sLip/DiI and CTB-sLip/DiI were incubated with the same volume of BALB/c serum for 24 h at room temperature, and PBS was set as a control. Liposomes were diluted 1000 times and detected by Nanoparticle Tracking Analysis (NTA 3.4 Build 3.4.003).

2.6. Binding Activity of CTB-sLip with GM1 In Vitro

GM1 or BSA was coated in 96-well microplates with 1 μg per well. After blockade with 5% BSA in PBS, serial dilutions of CTB-sLip/DiI were added and reacted at 37 °C for 1 h; sLip/DiI were set as the controls. DiI was quantified by a microplate reader at Ex/Em = 540/580 nm. To evaluate the effect of serum on GM1 binding, CTB-sLip were pre-incubated with BALB/c serum or PBS for 24 h. Serial dilutions were added and incubated with GM1-immoblized wells at 37 °C for 1 h. HRP conjugated anti-His antibody was used to detect CTB at 450 nm (TMB).

2.7. Protein Corona Separation and Characterization

CTB-sLip with different CTB modification degrees or sLip were incubated with the same volume of BALB/c plasma at 37 °C for 1 h. After centrifugation at 14,000× *g* for 30 min, the pellet was rinsed with cold PBS twice. The pellet was boiled in a mixture containing SDS-PAGE 5 × sample buffer (5 μL), PBS (20 μL) and β-mercaptethanol (2 μL) at 95 °C for 5 min. Electrophoresis was performed using gradient polyacrylamide gel, which was stained with a Fast Silver Stain Kit.

2.8. Pharmacokinetic Profile of CTB-sLip/DiI

Male BALB/c aged 4–5 weeks were intravenously injected with CTB-sLip or sLip (50 mg kg^{-1} lipid), and blood was sampled at 10 min, 30 min, 1 h, 2 h, 4 h, 8 h, 12 h, and 24 h. The fluorescence of DiI in plasma was detected by a microplate reader at 540/580 nm.

2.9. Cellular Uptake and Binding of CTB-sLip/FAM In Vitro

HCT116 and HT-29 cells were cultured with McCoy'5A medium (10% FBS) at 5% CO_2. Cells were seeded into 12-well plates and incubated with CTB-sLip/FAM or sLip/FAM (5 μM of FAM) in 0.1% BSA or 10% BALB/c serum for 2 h at 37 °C. Cells were harvested and analyzed by flow cytometry. To assess the binding ability of CTB-sLip/FAM or sLip/FAM with cells, liposomes (5 μM of FAM) in 0.1% BSA or 10% BALB/c serum were incubated with HCT116 and HT-29 cells for 2 h at 4 °C.

2.10. Uptake of CTB-FITC to Colorectal Cancer Cell Lines

HCT116 and HT-29 cells were cultured and seeded as aforementioned. The FITC-labeled CTB protein (CTB-FITC, 1 μM) was added and incubated with cells in the presence of BSA or BALB/c serum for 2 h at 37 °C. FITC labeled BSA (BSA-FITC) was set as the control. Flow cytometry was used to evaluate the uptake ability of the CTB protein in colorectal cancer cells.

2.11. Uptake of Liposomes by Blood Cells of BALB/c Mice In Vivo

To investigate the cellular uptake of CTB-sLip in peripheral blood cells, male BALB/c mice aged 4–5 weeks were intravenously injected with CTB-sLip/DiO (50 mg kg^{-1} lipid, $n = 3$), and sLip/DiO were set as the control. Peripheral whole blood was sampled at 2 h or 24 h after injection and collected into PBS with 10 mM EDTA. Red blood cells were then lysed twice with ACK Lysis Buffer. Fluorescent antibodies, including anti-mouse CD3/APC for T cells, anti-mouse CD19/BV421 for B cells, anti-mouse CD11b/APC, and anti-mouse Ly6G/BV421 for monocytes and neutrophils, were incubated with white blood cells at 4 °C for 30 min. The fluorescence of internalized DiO-labeled liposomes was evaluated by flow cytometry.

2.12. Cellular Uptake of Liposomes in Liver and Splenic Cells In Vivo

BALB/c mice were intravenously injected with CTB-sLip/DiO (50 mg kg^{-1} lipid, $n = 3$); sLip/DiO were the control group. Mice were sacrificed at 2 h or 24 h, and the corresponding livers and spleens were dissected after perfusion with HBSS via postcava. The livers were gently mashed and sieved through a 70 μm cell strainer. Hepatocytes were collected by centrifugation (4 °C, 50× *g*, 3 min), and the supernatant containing nonparenchymal cells was collected and centrifuged at 650× g for 7 min. Kupffer cells and liver sinusoidal endothelial cells (LSECs) were enriched in the middle layer by Percoll gradient centrifugation (25%/50%). Hepatocytes were fixed in 4% PFA and permeabilized with 0.5% Triton-X 100. Collected cells were strained with anti-mouse albumin and Alexa Fluor 647 donkey anti-Rabbit IgG antibody. The enriched nonparenchymal cells were strained with anti-mouse F4_80/BV421 and anti-mouse CD146/APC to mark Kupffer cells and liver sinusoidal endothelial cells (LSEC).

The dissected spleens were sieved through a 70 μm cell strainer, and spleen cell suspensions were incubated with anti-mouse CD3/APC, anti-mouse CD19/BV421, anti-mouse F4_80/BV421, and anti-mouse CD11c antibody at 4 °C for 30 min to mark T cells, B cells, Macrophages (Mϕ), and DC cells. The fluorescence of internalized liposomes was evaluated by flow cytometry (Agilent Technologies, Novocyte3000, Santa Clara, CA, USA).

2.13. Distribution of Liposomes in BALB/c Nude Mice with Lung Metastasis of Colorectal Cancer

Male BALB/c nude mice aged 6–8 weeks were injected with 2 × 10^6 HCT116 or HT-29 cells per mice in the left lung, and distribution of liposomes was determined after 9–14 days. CTB-sLip/DiR or sLip/DiR (50 mg kg^{-1} lipid) were intravenously injected, and organs were dissected at 24 h after administration. Opti-Scan Viewn Vivo superior optics (vie-works, for HT-29 cells animal model) and Visque InVivio Elite (for HCT116 cells animal model) were applied to quantify the fluorescence intensity of organs. DiO-labeled liposomes (50 mg kg^{-1} lipid per kg body weight of mice) were applied to evaluate cellular distribution in vivo. Lungs were dissected at 24 h after injection and digested with IV collagenase. The tumor cells were labeled with BV421 conjugated anti-CD236, and DiO in tumor cells was analyzed by flow cytometry (Agilent Technologies, Novocyte3000, Santa Clara, CA, USA).

2.14. Immunogenicity of Liposomes

Male BALB/c nude mice weighing ~20 g were intravenously injected through the tail vein with CTB-sLip or sLip (50 mg kg^{-1}) per week for 21 days, and the corresponding serum of each group was sampled. sLip or CTB-sLip (20 μg lipid per well) were coated in 96-well microplates, and serial dilutions of corresponding serum were added and incubated at 37 °C for 1 h. HRP-conjugated anti-mouse IgM and IgG antibody were utilized to detect anti-PEG IgG/IgM and anti-CTB IgG/IgM in serum, respectively.

2.15. Statistical Analysis

Data are presented as the means ± standard deviations (SD) and were analyzed by GraphPad Prism software 8.0.1 (GraphPad Software, San Diego, CA, USA). $p < 0.05$ was considered statistically significant (ns: $p > 0.05$, * $p < 0.05$, ** $p < 0.01$, *** $p < 0.001$).

3. Results and Discussion

3.1. Preparation and Characterization of CTB-Conjugated Liposomes (CTB-sLip)

The CTB protein is a homopentamer that binds GM1 in each monomer (Figure 1a). A His (6×) tag was constructed in the CTB protein molecule for purification. After expression via the *E. coli* system and protein refolding (see Methods), the CTB protein was purified by the Ni-NTA column with good purity and correct molecular weight according to the SDS-PAGE silver staining results (Figure 1b). The purified CTB protein was quantified by the BCA method, demonstrating an expression yield of 10–15 mg L^{-1} in the present study. The expressed CTB protein was further ascertained by measuring its binding affinity with GM1 using the ELISA method (see Methods). As shown in Figure 1c, the expressed CTB protein demonstrated high binding affinity with GM1, registering an equilibrium dissociation constant (K_d) of 39.2 pM. In contrast, the negative control protein, BSA, exhibited no obvious binding with GM1.

To chemically conjugate the CTB protein on the surface of PEGylated liposomes, the CTB protein was thiolated using Traut's Reagent (see Methods) and reacted with the maleimide group of PEGylated liposomes (Figure 2a). As shown in Figure 2b, all populations of liposomes demonstrated a mean diameter ~130 nm with narrow size distributions. The conjugation of CTB slightly increased particle sizes and zeta potentials. The binding of CTB-sLip with GM1 was measured in the 96-well ELISA plates by reading the fluorescence of DiI encapsulated in liposomes (Figure 2c). CTB-sLip demonstrated increasing fluorescence intensity of the encapsulated DiI in a concentration-dependent manner, indicating preservation of CTB bioactivity after chemical conjugation with PEGylated liposomes. In contrast, sLip and Mal-sLip (without CTB modification) displayed no binding with GM1. Meanwhile, the nonspecific binding of all populations of liposomes was excluded by measuring the interactions of liposomes with BSA-coated plates (Figure 2d).

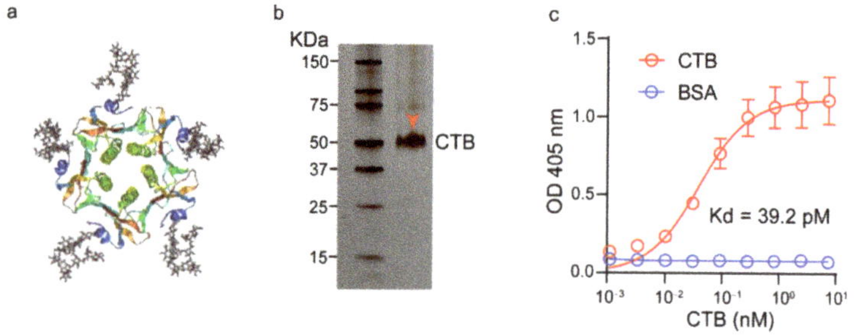

Figure 1. Expression and characterization of the CTB protein. (**a**) Schematically illustration of the structure of CTB. (**b**) Characterization of the expressed and refolded CTB by SDS-PAGE. (**c**) Binding activity of the expressed CTB to GM1; BSA was set as the control. The K_d value was calculated using GraphPad Prism 8.0.1. Data are means ± SDs, $n = 3$.

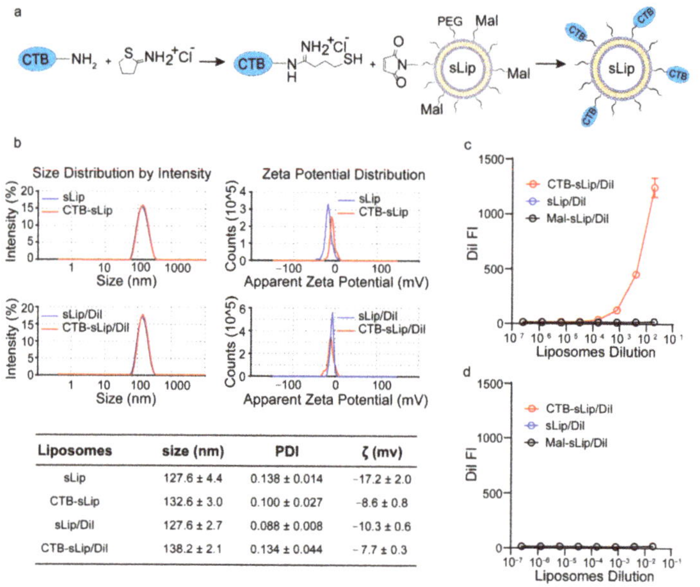

Liposomes	size (nm)	PDI	ζ (mv)
sLip	127.6 ± 4.4	0.138 ± 0.014	−17.2 ± 2.0
CTB-sLip	132.6 ± 3.0	0.100 ± 0.027	−8.6 ± 0.8
sLip/DiI	127.6 ± 2.7	0.088 ± 0.008	−10.3 ± 0.6
CTB-sLip/DiI	138.2 ± 2.1	0.134 ± 0.044	−7.7 ± 0.3

Figure 2. Preparation and characterization of CTB-conjugated PEGylated liposomes (CTB-sLip). (**a**) Schematic illustration of the conjugation method of CTB to the maleimide group grafted on the surface of PEGylated liposomes. (**b**) Size and zeta potential characterization of the prepared CTB-sLip and fluorescence dye DiI-loaded CTB-sLip. The binding activities of CTB-sLip/DiI to GM1 coated (**c**) and BSA coated (**d**) were performed by ELISA; sLip/DiI and Mal-sLip/DiI were set as the controls. Data are means ± SDs, $n = 3$.

3.2. *Effects of Serum on the Targeting Capability of CTB-sLip*

The effects of mouse serum on CTB-sLip were investigated in vitro. After incubation with BALB/c serum for 24 h, liposomal size and distribution were measured using Nanoparticle Tracking Analysis (NTA). As shown in Figure S1, all particles in various media displayed a major size distribution ranging from 50 nm to 300 nm. Pre-incubation of CTB-sLip or sLip with BALB/c serum did not significantly alter the size distribution. The effect of serum on CTB bioactivity was also determined. In comparison to PBS (Figure 3a), pre-incubation with BALB/c serum only slightly affected the CTB binding to GM1. The formed protein coronas on the surface of CTB-sLip and sLip were separated, and their compositions were analyzed using SDS-PAGE. As shown in Figure 3b, the CTB protein at different modification degrees did not induce obvious differences in the composition of the formed protein corona in comparison to sLip. These results are consistent with our previous report [20], where the CTB protein on the surface of the polymeric nanoparticles preserved bioactivity with GM1 after interaction with serum.

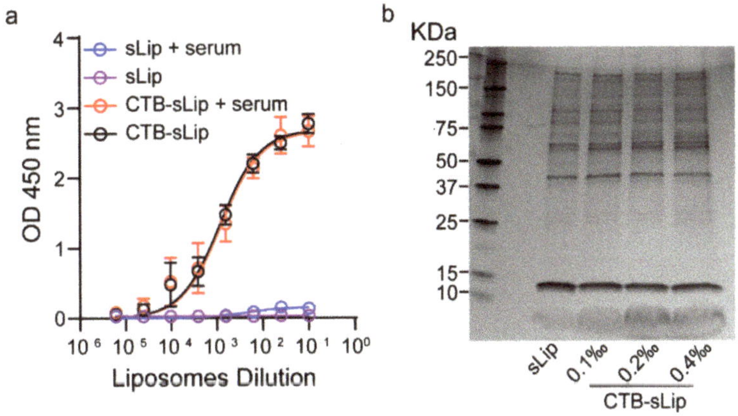

Figure 3. Effects of BALB/c plasma proteins on the bioactivity of CTB-sLip. (**a**) Affinity characterization of CTB-sLip (pre-incubation with BALB/c serum and PBS for 24 h) to GM1 based on ELISA; sLip were set as a control. Data are means ± SDs, $n = 3$. (**b**) Evaluation of protein corona of CTB-sLip (with 0.1‰, 0.2‰ or 0.4‰ molar ratio CTB modification) by SDS-PAGE.

To study the targeting capability of CTB-sLip, two human-derived colorectal cancer cell lines, HCT116 and HT-29, were cultured. As shown in Figure S2, both cell lines demonstrated high uptake of CTB, suggesting GM1 expression on the cell membrane. The binding of CTB-sLip with cells was studied at 4 °C. After 2 h incubation with FAM-encapsulated CTB-sLip or sLip, the FAM fluorescence-positive cells were counted using a flow cytometer. As shown in Figures S3 and S4, both HCT116 and HT-29 cells demonstrated significantly higher binding with CTB-sLip than with sLip, suggesting the targeting capability of CTB-sLip to human-derived colorectal cancer cells. The presence of BALB/c serum dramatically decreased the binding of all populations of liposomes with cancer cells. However, CTB-sLip still exhibited significant enhancement of cell binding compared with sLip, which is consistent with the results shown in Figure 3. Cellular uptake of liposomes by cancer cells was conducted at 37 °C (Figure 4). As expected, CTB demonstrated high targeting capability to both HCT116 and HT-29 cells.

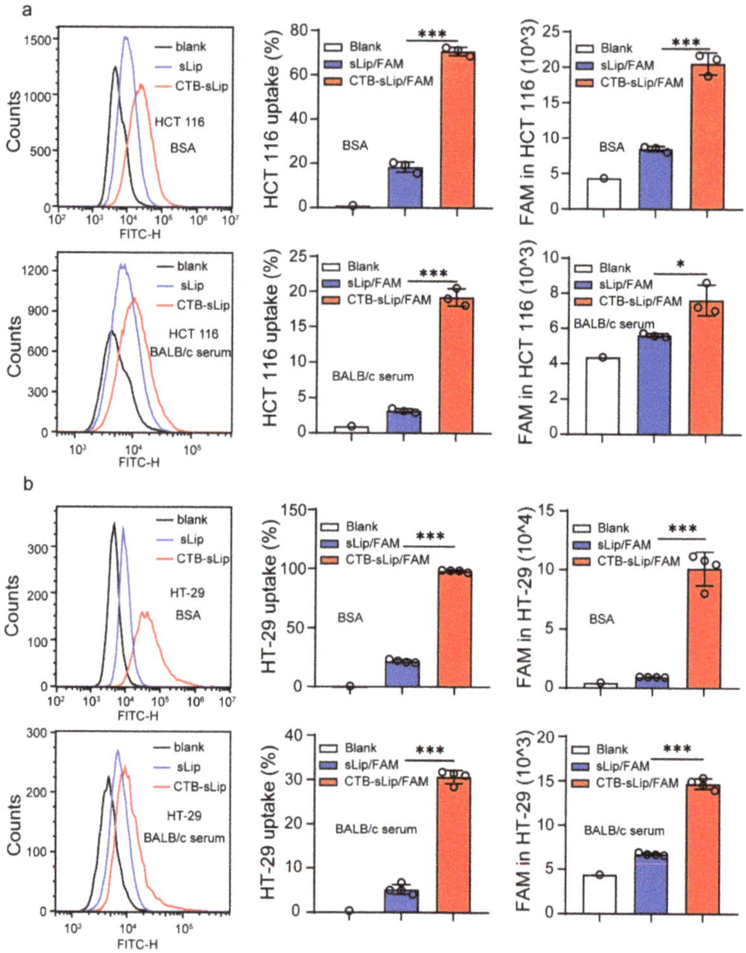

Figure 4. Effect of BALB/c serum on the targeting capability of CTB-sLip to human-derived colorectal cancer cells. CTB-sLip/FAM (5 μM 5-FAM) were prepared to study the in vitro uptake by HCT116 cell ((**a**), $n = 3$) and HT-29 cell ((**b**), $n = 4$) at 37 °C after 2 h incubation, in 0.1% BSA and 10% BALB/c serum, respectively. Data are means ± SDs. * $p < 0.05$ and *** $p < 0.001$ based on one-way ANOVA with Prism.8.0.1.

3.3. Pharmacokinetic Profiles of CTB-sLip

To study the in vivo fate of liposomes, the pharmacokinetic profiles and biodistribution of both CTB-sLip and sLip were investigated in BALB/c mice. Liposomes at a dose of 50 mg kg^{-1} (lipid to mouse body weight) were injected into the tail vein, and blood was sampled at the predetermined time points. As shown in Figure 5a, CTB-sLip demonstrated a significant decrease of the area under the curve (AUC) in the plasma concentration–time curve, suggesting relatively rapid clearance of CTB-sLip in mice. At the last time point (24 h after injection), the biodistribution of liposomes in the main organs was measured (Figure 5b). Most liposomes were, as expected, found in the liver and spleen, and CTB-sLip still demonstrated higher distribution in both organs in comparison to sLip.

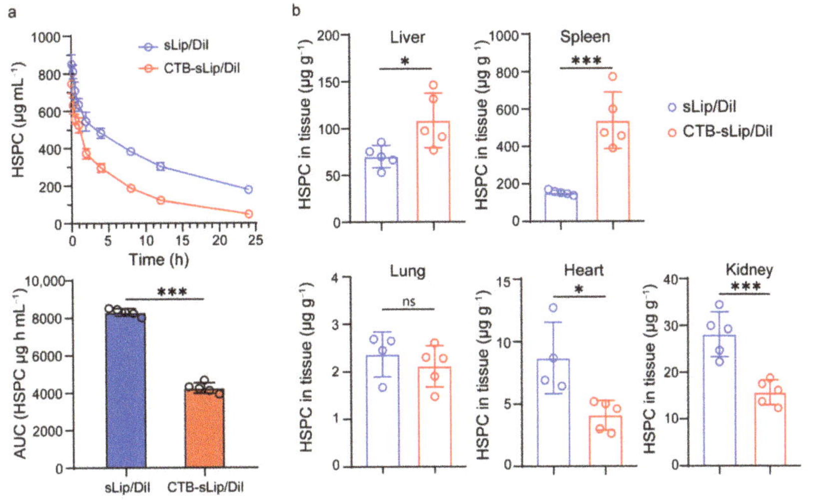

Figure 5. Pharmacokinetic profiles (**a**) and biodistribution (**b**) of sLip/DiI and CTB-sLip/DiI in major organs of BALB/c mice over 24 h after intravenous injection with 50 mg kg^{-1} lipids. Data are means ± SDs, $n = 5$. * $p < 0.05$, *** $p < 0.001$; ns indicates non-significant based on Student's *t*-tests.

To further understand the interaction of CTB-sLip with the body, the uptake of liposomes by blood cells was measured. At 2 h and 24 h after injection of DiO-labeled liposomes, blood cells were collected and labeled with respective specific antibodies. The uptake of liposomes was determined using a flow cytometer. As shown in Figure 6, CTB-sLip demonstrated higher uptake of neutrophils, monocytes, B cells, and T cells to some extent, suggesting extensive binding of CTB-sLip with cells in vivo.

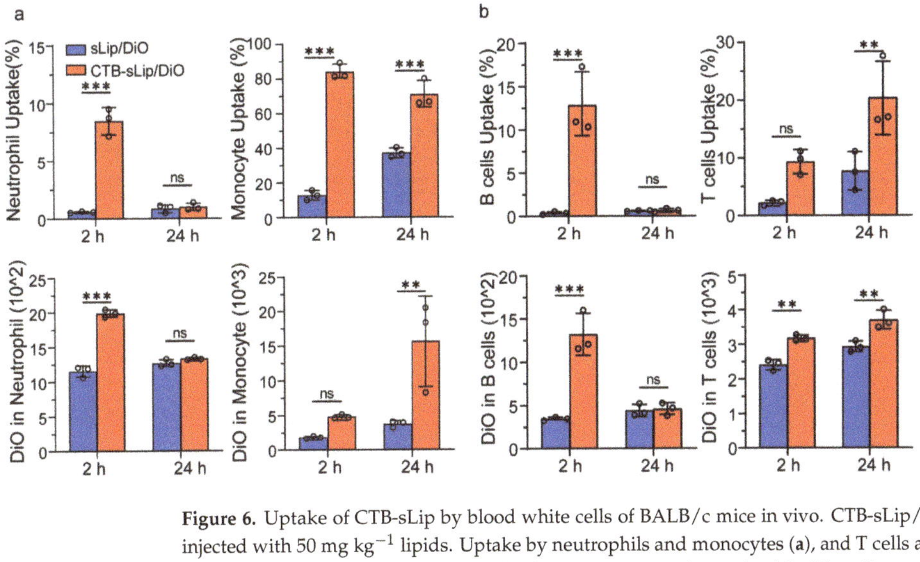

Figure 6. Uptake of CTB-sLip by blood white cells of BALB/c mice in vivo. CTB-sLip/DiO were injected with 50 mg kg^{-1} lipids. Uptake by neutrophils and monocytes (**a**), and T cells and B cells (**b**) in peripheral blood at 2 h and 24 h after injection was determined by Flow Cytometry. Data are means ± SDs ($n = 3$). ** $p < 0.01$, *** $p < 0.001$; ns indicates nonsignificant based on grouped two-way ANOVAs.

The biodistribution of liposomes in the liver and spleen of BALB/c mice was also carefully studied. The hepatocytes, Kupffer's cells, and liver sinusoidal endothelial cells (LSECs) were separated according to the previously reported protocol with minor modification [28] (see Methods) and labeled with respective markers or antibodies. It was interesting that only CTB-sLip demonstrated significant enhancement (88% vs. 70%) of uptake by Kupffer's cells in comparison to sLip (Figure 7a), while the other cells did not exhibit significant uptake of CTB-sLip at both time points. In contrast, CTB-sLip displayed significant enhancement of uptake by splenic cells, including splenic microphages, dendritic cells, and B cells (Figure 7b), which is consistent with the data shown in Figure 5b. At 24 h after injection, CTB-sLip exhibited higher accumulation in the spleen than sLip. These data also indicated that interaction of CTB-sLip with blood cells and splenic cells may majorly contribute to the relatively rapid clearance of CTB-sLip (Figure 5a).

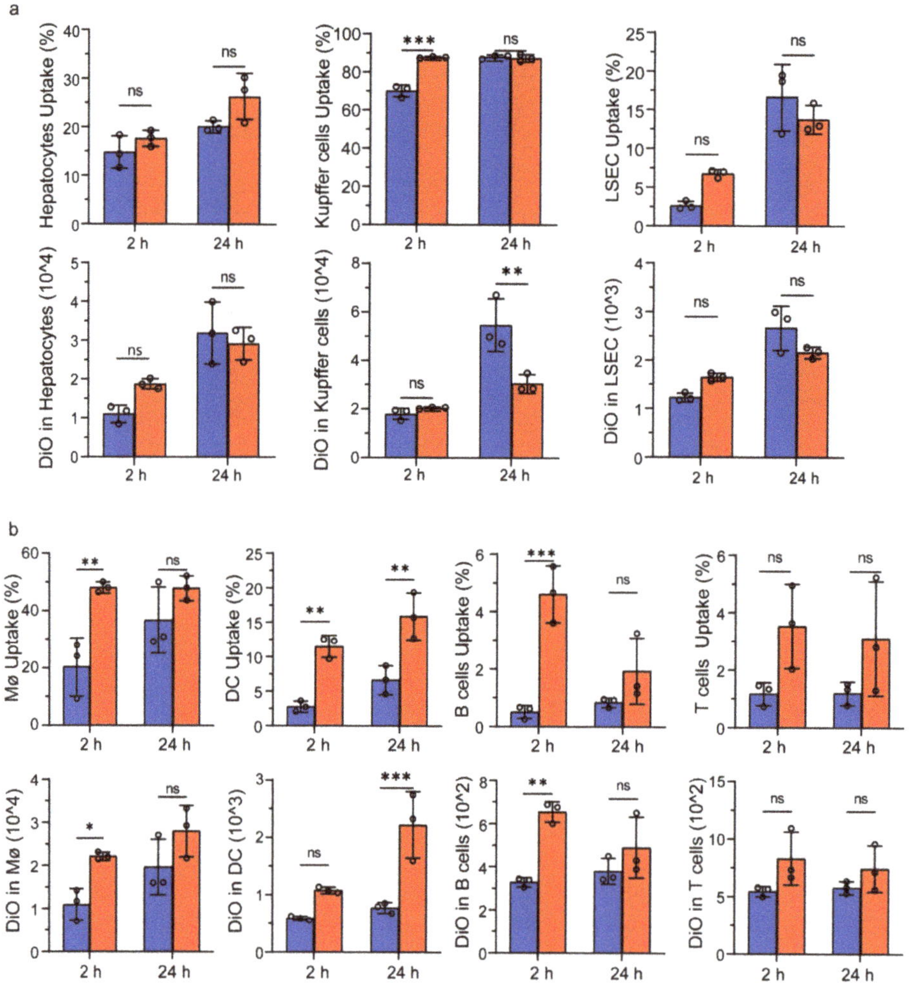

Figure 7. Uptake of CTB-sLip/DiO by hepatic cells and splenic cells. (**a**) Kupffer's cells and liver sinusoidal endothelial cells (LSECs) were marked with F4/80 and CD146, respectively. (**b**) Splenic macrophages (MΦ), DC cells, splenic B cells, and T cells were marked with F4/80, CD11c, CD19, and CD3, respectively. Data are means ± SDs ($n = 3$). * $p < 0.05$, ** $p < 0.01$, *** $p < 0.001$; ns represents nonsignificant based on grouped two-way ANOVAs.

3.4. Lung Metastasis Targeting of Colorectal Cancer by CTB-sLip

To evaluate the targeting capability of CTB-sLip to lung metastasis of colorectal cancer, male BALB/c nude mice were injected with 2×10^6 HT-29 cells per mice in the left lung. At nine days after injection, fluorescent dye (DiO for cellular study and DiR for in situ imaging)-labeled liposomes (50 mg kg^{-1} lipid of mice body weight) were intravenously injected, and the left lung with implanted colorectal cancer cells was dissected for in situ imaging. As shown in Figure 8a,b, CTB-sLip demonstrated significant enhancement in the cancer tissues compared with sLip. The cells were further separated, and cellular uptake of liposomes was determined by a flow cytometer (Figure 8c,d). As shown in Figure S6, BALB/c nude mice with lung metastasis of HCT116 also demonstrated significantly higher distribution with CTB-sLip than with sLip at 24 h after injection, suggesting the targeting capability of CTB-sLip to human-derived colorectal cancer cells. Both CTB-sLip and sLip demonstrated higher uptake by cancer cells than the paracancerous lung tissues, which may be attributed to the enhanced permeability and retention effect. As for the cancer cells, CTB-sLip displayed significantly higher targeting capability than sLip, suggestive of the targeting capability of the former for lung metastasis of colorectal cancer.

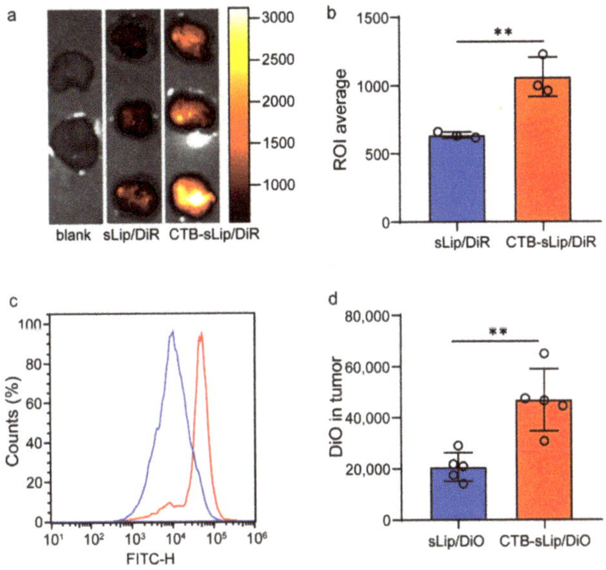

Figure 8. Targeting capability of CTB-sLip to lung metastasis of colorectal cancer in vivo. Male BALB/c nude mice planted with HT-29 cells in left lungs were injected with CTB-sLip/DiR ((**a**,**b**), $n = 3$) for in situ imaging and CTB-sLip/DiO ((**c**,**d**), $n = 5$) for cellular uptake study; sLip/DiR and sLip/DiO were set as the controls. Data are means ± SDs. ** $p < 0.01$ based on Student's *t*-tests.

3.5. Immunogenicity of CTB-sLip

Considering the high uptake of CTB-sLip by the splenic cells, immunogenicity was investigated by detecting the antibodies. Both CTB-sLip and sLip were intravenously injected via the tail vein weekly, and blood was sampled one week after the third injection. The anti-PEG and anti-CTB antibodies were measured using the ELISA methods (see Methods). As shown in Figure 9, sequential injections of CTB-sLip induced significant anti-CTB IgG and slight anti-CTB IgM antibodies. Meanwhile, CTB-sLip demonstrated slight enhancement of anti-PEG IgG antibody in comparison to sLip, with no significant generation of anti-PEG IgM antibody. These data suggested the immunogenicity of CTB-sLip, warning the repeated injection when CTB-sLip were exploited as the targeted delivery system.

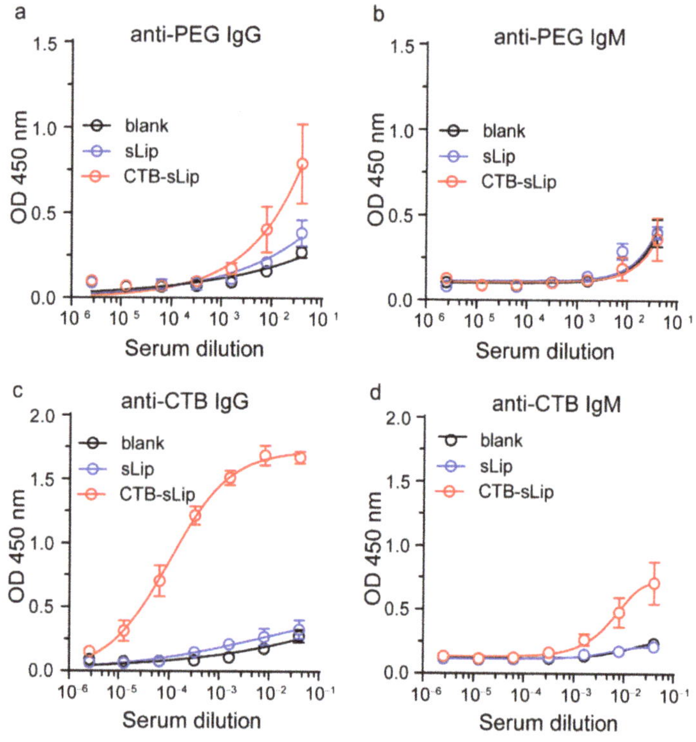

Figure 9. Immunogenicity of CTB-sLip in vivo. BALB/c mice were sequentially injected with sLip or CTB-sLip (50 mg kg^{-1} lipids) per week for 21 days. Anti-PEG IgG/M (**a**,**b**) and anti-CTB IgG/M (**c**,**d**) in serum on day 21 were detected by ELISA. Data are means ± SDs (n = 3).

4. Conclusions

Herein, the CTB protein was chemically conjugated on the surface of PEGylated liposomes, and their potential for targeting lung metastasis of colorectal cancer was evaluated. Chemical conjugation of CTB did not significantly alter the interaction between liposomes and plasma proteins. CTB-sLip demonstrated good stability in the presence of mouse serum, which may be attributed to the high stability of the homopentamer structure and low plasma protein binding on the surface of CTB-sLip. The presence of serum induced the decrease of binding with colorectal cancer cells to some extent, while CTB-sLip still retained targeting capability in comparison to sLip. As expected, CTB demonstrated high targeting capability to lung metastasis of colorectal cancer. The extensive interaction of CTB-sLip with blood cells and splenic cells may contribute to their relatively rapid blood clearance from BALB/c mice. Even though immunogenicity of CTB-sLip warned their applications when repeated treatments were indispensable, the present study provided a potential tool to achieve lung metastasis targeting of colorectal cancer for diagnostic purposes.

Supplementary Materials: The following supporting information can be downloaded at: https://www.mdpi.com/article/10.3390/pharmaceutics14040868/s1, Figure S1: Characterization of liposomes stability in BALB/c serum in vitro. Figure S2: The uptake capability of CTB protein to HCT 116 and HT-29 cells in vitro. Figure S3: The binding capability of CTB-sLip to HCT 116 cells in vitro. Figure S4: The binding capability of CTB-sLip to HT-29 cells in vitro. Figure S5: Characterization of antibody strained cells by flow-cytometry. Figure S6: Targeting capability of CTB-sLip to lung metastasis of colorectal cancer in vivo.

Author Contributions: Conceptualization, X.Z., W.T., Z.L. and C.Z.; methodology, X.Z., W.T., H.W., E.W. and T.D.; investigation, X.Z., W.T., H.W., E.W. and T.D.; writing—original draft preparation, X.Z., W.T. and C.Z.; writing—review and editing, X.Z., W.T., J.G., Z.L. and C.Z.; supervision, Z.L. and C.Z.; funding acquisition, Z.L. All authors have read and agreed to the published version of the manuscript.

Funding: This work was financially supported by the Shanghai Leading Talent Program of Shanghai Human Resources and Social Security Bureau (grant number: 2019) and the key discipline construction project of the three-year action plan of the Shanghai public health system of Shanghai Municipal Health Commission (grant number: GWV-10.1-XK09).

Institutional Review Board Statement: The animal study protocol was approved by the Ethics Committee of Shanghai Pudong Hospital (protocol code: 2019-M-15; date of approval: March 2019).

Conflicts of Interest: The authors declare no conflict of interest.

References

1. Siegel, R.L.; Miller, K.D.; Sauer, A.G.; Fedewa, S.A.; Butterly, L.F.; Anderson, J.C.; Cercek, A.; Smith, R.A.; Jemal, A. Colorectal cancer statistics. *CA Cancer J. Clin.* **2020**, *70*, 145–164. [CrossRef] [PubMed]
2. Hiratsuka, S.; Watanabe, A.; Aburatani, H.; Maru, Y. Tumour-mediated upregulation of chemoattractants and recruitment of myeloid cells predetermines lung metastasis. *Nat. Cell Biol.* **2006**, *8*, 1369–1375. [CrossRef] [PubMed]
3. Li, J.; Yuan, Y.; Yang, F.; Wang, Y.; Zhu, X.; Wang, Z.; Zheng, S.; Wan, D.; He, J.; Wang, J.; et al. Expert consensus on multidisciplinary therapy of colorectal cancer with lung metastases. *J. Hematol. Oncol.* **2019**, *12*, 16. [CrossRef] [PubMed]
4. Zhang, N.; Ng, A.S.; Cai, S.; Li, Q.; Yang, L.; Kerr, D. Novel therapeutic strategies: Targeting epithelial–mesenchymal transition in colorectal cancer. *Lancet Oncol.* **2021**, *22*, e358–e368. [CrossRef]
5. Song, L.; Li, Y.; He, B.; Gong, Y. Development of Small Molecules Targeting the Wnt Signaling Pathway in Cancer Stem Cells for the Treatment of Colorectal Cancer. *Clin. Colorectal Cancer* **2015**, *14*, 133–145. [CrossRef]
6. Carvalho, M.R.; Carvalho, C.R.; Maia, F.R.; Caballero, D.; Kundu, S.C.; Reis, R.L.; Oliveira, J.M. Peptide-Modified Dendrimer Nanoparticles for Targeted Therapy of Colorectal Cancer. *J. Adv. Ther.* **2019**, *2*, 1900132. [CrossRef]
7. Sartore-Bianchi, A.; Martini, M.; Molinari, F.; Veronese, S.; Nichelatti, M.; Artale, S.; di Nicolantonio, F.; Saletti, P.; de Dosso, S.; Mazzucchelli, L.; et al. PIK3CA mutations in colorectal cancer are associated with clinical resistance to EGFR-targeted monoclonal antibodies. *Cancer Res.* **2009**, *69*, 1851–1857. [CrossRef]
8. Go, G.; Lee, C.-S.; Yoon, Y.M.; Lim, J.H.; Kim, T.H.; Lee, S.H. PrPC aptamer conjugated–gold nanoparticles for targeted delivery of doxorubicin to colorectal cancer cells. *Int. J. Mol. Sci.* **2021**, *22*, 1976. [CrossRef]
9. Yang, H.; Fu, Y.; Jang, M.-S.; Li, Y.; Lee, J.H.; Chae, H.; Lee, D.S. Interfaces, Multifunctional Polymer Ligand Interface CdZnSeS/ZnS Quantum Dot/Cy3-Labeled Protein Pairs as Sensitive FRET Sensors. *J. ACS Appl. Mater.* **2016**, *8*, 35021–35032. [CrossRef]
10. Morales-Cruz, M.; Delgado, Y.; Castillo, B.; Figueroa, C.M.; Molina, A.M.; Torres, A.; Milian, M.; Griebenow, K. Smart Targeting To Improve Cancer Therapeutics. *Drug Des. Dev. Ther.* **2019**, *13*, 3753–3772. [CrossRef]
11. Zhang, J.; Wei, K.; Shi, J.; Zhu, Y.; Guan, M.; Fu, X.; Zhang, Z. Biomimetic Nanoscale Erythrocyte Delivery System for Enhancing Chemotherapy via Overcoming Biological Barriers. *ACS Biomater. Sci. Eng.* **2021**, *7*, 1496–1505. [CrossRef] [PubMed]
12. Zhang, Z.; Guan, J.; Jiang, Z.; Yang, Y.; Liu, J.; Hua, W.; Mao, Y.; Li, C.; Lu, W.; Qian, J.; et al. Brain-targeted drug delivery by manipulating protein corona functions. *Nat. Commun.* **2019**, *10*, 3561. [CrossRef] [PubMed]
13. Guan, J.; Shen, Q.; Zhang, Z.; Jiang, Z.; Yang, Y.; Lou, M.; Qian, J.; Lu, W.; Zhan, C. Enhanced immunocompatibility of ligand-targeted liposomes by attenuating natural IgM absorption. *Nat. Commun.* **2018**, *9*, 2982. [CrossRef] [PubMed]
14. Zhang, H.; Wu, T.; Yu, W.; Ruan, S.; He, Q.; Gao, H. Ligand Size and Conformation Affect the Behavior of Nanoparticles Coated with in Vitro and in Vivo Protein Corona. *ACS Appl. Mater. Interfaces* **2018**, *10*, 9094–9103. [CrossRef]
15. Cai, R.; Ren, J.; Ji, Y.; Wang, Y.; Liu, Y.; Chen, Z.; Sabet, Z.F.; Wu, X.; Lynch, I.; Chen, C. Corona of Thorns: The Surface Chemistry-Mediated Protein Corona Perturbs the Recognition and Immune Response of Macrophages. *ACS Appl. Mater. Interfaces* **2020**, *12*, 1997–2008. [CrossRef]
16. Yoo, J.; Park, C.; Yi, G.; Lee, D.; Koo, H. Active Targeting Strategies Using Biological Ligands for Nanoparticle Drug Delivery Systems. *Cancers* **2019**, *11*, 640. [CrossRef]
17. Wei, X.; Zhan, C.; Shen, Q.; Fu, W.; Xie, C.; Gao, J.; Peng, C.; Zheng, P.; Lu, W. A D-peptide ligand of nicotine acetylcholine receptors for brain-targeted drug delivery. *Angew. Chem.* **2015**, *54*, 3023–3027. [CrossRef]
18. Ledeen, R.W.; Wu, G. The multi-tasked life of GM1 ganglioside, a true factotum of nature. *Trends Biochem. Sci.* **2015**, *40*, 407–418. [CrossRef]
19. Ruhlman, T.; Ahangari, R.; Devine, A.; Samsam, M.; Daniell, H. Expression of cholera toxin B-proinsulin fusion protein in lettuce and tobacco chloroplasts—Oral administration protects against development of insulitis in non-obese diabetic mice. *Plant Biotechnol. J.* **2007**, *5*, 495–510. [CrossRef]
20. Guan, J.; Zhang, Z.; Hu, X.; Yang, Y.; Chai, Z.; Liu, X.; Liu, J.; Gao, B.; Lu, W.; Qian, J.J.A.h.m. Cholera Toxin Subunit B Enabled Multifunctional Glioma-Targeted Drug Delivery. *Adv. Healthc. Mater.* **2017**, *6*, 1700709. [CrossRef]

21. Guan, J.; Qian, J.; Zhan, C. Preparation of Cholera Toxin Subunit B Functionalized Nanoparticles for Targeted Therapy of Glioblastoma. *Methods Mol. Biol.* **2020**, *2059*, 207–212. [PubMed]
22. Holmgren, J.; Lonnroth, I.; Mansson, J.; Svennerholm, L. Interaction of cholera toxin and membrane GM1 ganglioside of small intestine. *Proc. Natl. Acad. Sci. USA* **1975**, *72*, 2520–2524. [CrossRef] [PubMed]
23. Sánchez, J.; Holmgren, J. Cholera toxin—A foe & a friend. *Indian J. Med. Res.* **2011**, *133*, 153. [PubMed]
24. Tang, W.; Zhang, Z.; Li, C.; Chu, Y.; Qian, J.; Ying, T.; Lu, W.; Zhan, C. Facile Separation of PEGylated Liposomes Enabled by Anti-PEG scFv. *Nano Lett.* **2021**, *21*, 10107–10113. [CrossRef] [PubMed]
25. Zhang, Z.; Chu, Y.; Li, C.; Tang, W.; Qian, J.; Wei, X.; Lu, W.; Ying, T.; Zhan, C. Anti-PEG scFv corona ameliorates accelerated blood clearance phenomenon of PEGylated nanomedicines. *J. Control. Release* **2021**, *330*, 493–501. [CrossRef]
26. Lamichhane, N.; Udayakumar, T.S.; D'Souza, W.D.; Simone, C.B., 2nd; Raghavan, S.R.; Polf, J.; Mahmood, J. Liposomes: Clinical Applications and Potential for Image-Guided Drug Delivery. *Molecules* **2018**, *23*, 288. [CrossRef]
27. Bozzuto, G.; Molinari, A. Liposomes as nanomedical devices. *Int. J. Nanomed.* **2015**, *10*, 975–999. [CrossRef]
28. Aparicio-Vergara, M.; Tencerova, M.; Morgantini, C.; Barreby, E.; Aouadi, M. Isolation of Kupffer Cells and Hepatocytes from a Single Mouse Liver. *Methods Mol. Biol.* **2017**, *1639*, 161–171.

pharmaceutics

Article

Niosomal Nanocarriers for Enhanced Dermal Delivery of Epigallocatechin Gallate for Protection against Oxidative Stress of the Skin

Danhui Li [1], Nataly Martini [1], Zimei Wu [1], Shuo Chen [1], James Robert Falconer [2], Michelle Locke [3], Zhiwen Zhang [4] and Jingyuan Wen [1,*]

1 School of Pharmacy, Faculty of Medical and Health Sciences, The University of Auckland, Auckland 1023, New Zealand; danhui.li@auckland.ac.nz (D.L.); n.martini@auckland.ac.nz (N.M.); z.wu@auckland.ac.nz (Z.W.); shuo.chen@auckland.ac.nz (S.C.)
2 Department of Plastic, School of Pharmacy, The University of Queensland, Pharmacy Australia Centre of Excellence, Brisbane, QLD 4102, Australia; j.falconer@uq.edu.au
3 Reconstructive Surgery, Middlemore Hospital, Counties Manukau District Health Board, Auckland 2104, New Zealand; m.locke@auckland.ac.nz
4 Shanghai Institute of Materia Medica, Chinese Academy of Sciences, Shanghai 201203, China; zwzhang0125@simm.ac.cn
* Correspondence: j.wen@auckland.ac.nz

Citation: Li, D.; Martini, N.; Wu, Z.; Chen, S.; Falconer, J.R.; Locke, M.; Zhang, Z.; Wen, J. Niosomal Nanocarriers for Enhanced Dermal Delivery of Epigallocatechin Gallate for Protection against Oxidative Stress of the Skin. *Pharmaceutics* **2022**, *14*, 726. https://doi.org/10.3390/pharmaceutics14040726

Academic Editors: Alyssa Panitch and Montse Mitjans Arnal

Received: 30 January 2022
Accepted: 23 March 2022
Published: 28 March 2022

Abstract: Among green tea catechins, epigallocatechin gallate (EGCG) is the most abundant and has the highest biological activities. This study aims to develop and statistically optimise an EGCG-loaded niosomal system to overcome the cutaneous barriers and provide an antioxidant effect. EGCG-niosomes were prepared by thin film hydration method and statistically optimised. The niosomes were characterised for size, zeta potential, morphology and entrapment efficiency. Ex vivo permeation and deposition studies were conducted using full-thickness human skin. Cell viability, lipid peroxidation, antioxidant enzyme activities after UVA-irradiation and cellular uptake were determined. The optimised niosomes were spherical and had a relatively uniform size of 235.4 ± 15.64 nm, with a zeta potential of −45.2 ± 0.03 mV and an EE of 53.05 ± 4.46%. The niosomes effectively prolonged drug release and demonstrated much greater skin penetration and deposition than free EGCG. They also increased cell survival after UVA-irradiation, reduced lipid peroxidation, and increased the antioxidant enzymes' activities in human dermal fibroblasts (Fbs) compared to free EGCG. Finally, the uptake of niosomes was via energy-dependent endocytosis. The optimised niosomes have the potential to be used as a dermal carrier for antioxidants and other therapeutic compounds in the pharmaceutical and cosmetic industries.

Keywords: niosomes; catechin; dermal delivery; antioxidant activity; oxidative stress; skin barrier; penetration; cellular uptake

1. Introduction

The skin is the largest organ of the human body, which makes it the direct target of oxidative stress due to the exposure to reactive oxygen species (ROS) from the surrounding environment. The most important function of human skin is protection by providing a barrier from pathogens, and physical and chemical damages. It also plays a crucial role in thermoregulation and endocrine function such as vitamin D synthesis [1,2]. The skin comprises three layers: the epidermis, which consists of keratinocytes; the dermis consisting of connective tissue, and the subcutaneous layer [3]. The epidermis can be divided into four layers, including the stratum corneum (SC), stratum granulosum, stratum spinosum and stratum basale. The dermis is composed of connective tissues, which are also rich in glands, white blood cells and blood vessels [4,5]. SC is the highly hydrophobic surface layer that contains 18 to 21 cell layers and is composed of corneocytes that are terminally differentiated keratinocytes anchored in a lipophilic matrix [3,4]. The 'bricks and mortar' model is often employed to describe the structure of SC, in which intercellular lipid accounts for 10% of the dry weight of this layer, and the rest is an intracellular protein (mainly keratin). Keratins are a family of alpha-helical polypeptides with a molecular weight ranging from 40,000 to 70,000 Daltons, making the corneocyte layers dense and relatively impervious to external compounds [6].

The skin is continuously exposed to environmental threats such as UV radiation, pollution, micro-organisms, and viruses, which lead to ROS production. ROS are also formed during the normal cellular metabolism and immune reactions. More than 80% of environmental ROS that damage the skin is produced by UV [7]. Antioxidants such as glutathione, ubiquinol and thiols inhibit oxidation reactions by donating electrons to free radicals [7]. Our bodies also produce enzymatic antioxidants, such as superoxide dismutase and glutathione peroxidases. Other non-enzymatic antioxidants such as vitamin E (alpha-tocopherol) and vitamin C (ascorbic acid) are obtained from the diet [8]. However, the antioxidants produced by our bodies are inadequate to protect against oxidative stress, and antioxidants are often used as dietary supplements to replenish the level of endogenous antioxidants and hence help to delay the onset of aging or diseases [8].

Catechins are a group of powerful antioxidants with health-promoting effects, and epigallocatechin gallate (EGCG) is one of the catechins found in green tea. EGCG has several beneficial effects on the skin, including anti-aging, anti-inflammatory, and anti-cancer properties. According to a study, treating normal human epidermal keratinocytes with EGCG prevented UVB-induced intracellular release of hydrogen peroxide while also inhibiting UVB-induced oxidative stress-mediated skin damage [9]. EGCG has been shown to inhibit UV-induced collagen production and collagenase transcription in human dermal fibroblasts [10]. In addition, on the human model, catechins were shown to have anti-aging functions [9]. A double-blind, placebo-controlled experiment of adult women found that catechins can reduce total sun damage when given as oral catechins supplements [11]. The oral administration route is generally the most accepted for drug administration, particularly for long-term prevention purposes. However, when administered orally, catechins readily undergo several metabolic transformations by intestinal microflora and enzymes; therefore, they are poorly bioavailable [12]. The application of EGCG is also limited by its unstable physiochemical properties, which can be degraded quickly. Many studies have reported that green tea catechins were vulnerable to degradation caused by the elevation of temperature, pH, and metal ions of incubation media [13]. The instability is part of the reason for the poor bioavailability and also presents as an issue in the manufacturing process. Therefore, the oral bioavailability of catechin represents a big challenge. Topical application of these bioactive compounds may be able to overcome the problem, as this route bypasses metabolism by the liver and gastrointestinal track with relatively low enzymatic degradation. However, the skin barrier, which is due to the SC layer, impedes the transport of exogenous compounds into the skin and restricts diffusion of external substances into the deeper dermis layer. Therefore, we hypothesise that loading EGCG into a drug carrier would help overcome the skin barrier, improve penetration into the deeper skin layers and improve their stability. The compound can therefore exert its beneficial effect at the site of interest.

Niosomes are versatile drug carrier systems that have been administered via various routes; they are surfactant-based nanocarriers that are mainly composed of non-ionic surfactant and cholesterol [14–17]. Niosomes have been extensively studied in topical drug delivery due to their ability to significantly improve penetration across the skin barrier and deposition in the dermis layer [18–24]. Drugs with a variety of physicochemical properties have been investigated for topical and transdermal delivery using niosomes, for example, diacerein [25], itraconazole [26], tretinoin [27], salidroside [28] and finasteride [29], demonstrating their advantages in topical delivery. In addition, a range of bioactive compounds has also been loaded into niosomes, such as curcumin, rutin, and Ginkgo biloba extract [30–32]. Silymarin-loaded niosomes demonstrated superior antioxidant activity over silymarin suspension in vitro [33].

In formulation development, various factors might impact the final product's performance. Design of Experiment (DOE) is a planned set-up of experiments to acquire information efficiently and precisely. It applies to any process that has quantifiable inputs and outputs. DOE was first designed for agricultural applications, but it has since become a frequently used technique in process sectors, including the chemical, food and pharmaceutical industries [34]. It may be used to explore the effect of multiple variables on responses by altering them all at once in a small number of tests. By this strategy, the costs and time involved with the research and production of medicine may be significantly decreased [34,35]. Furthermore, it aids in the creation of the "best possible" formulation composition and gives a comprehensive knowledge of the process and product behaviors [36]. This study aimed to develop an optimal niosome formulation using the DOE methodology and evaluate the formulation for topical administration of EGCG for protecting the skin from external oxidative stress. An ex vivo investigation on human skin was carried out to evaluate drug deposition and the antioxidant activity of the EGCG-niosomes. The uptake of niosomes by human skin fibroblasts was also investigated.

2. Materials and Methods

2.1. Materials

Span® 60, EGCG $\geq$ 98% (HPLC), cholesterol (CH), Triton™ X-100, dihexadecyl phosphate (DCP), Fluorescein 5(6)-isothiocyanate (FITC), Sulforhodamine B (SRB), trichloroacetic acid (TCA), dimethyl sulphoxide (DMSO), methanol and acetonitrile (ACN) were purchased from Merck (Merck, Kenilworth, NJ, USA). Dulbecco's Modified Eagle Medium (DMEM) with high glucose and L-glutamine, Phosphate-Buffered Saline (PBS), Hank's Balanced Salt Solution (HBSS), penicillin-streptomycin, fetal bovine serum of New Zealand origin (FBS), trypsin-EDTA, DAPI and CellTracker were purchased from Thermo Fisher Scientific (Auckland, New Zealand). Malondialdehyde (MDA), glutathione peroxidase (GSH-px) and superoxide dismutase (SOD) kits were purchased from Biovision (Biovision Inc., Milpitas, CA, USA). Trifluoroacetic acid (TFA) was purchased from Fluka (Fluka, Darmstadt, Germany). Distilled, deionised water was used throughout and was obtained from a Millipore water purifier.

2.2. High-Pressure Liquid Chromatography Method for Quantification of EGCG

An Angilent Technologies 1100 series high pressure liquid chromatography (HPLC) system equipped with a vacuum degasser, autosampler, thermostatted column compartment and photodiode-array detector (PDA) was used. A C18 column (Jupiter, 250 × 4.6 mm, 5 mm, Phenomenex, Torrance, CA, USA) was used for HPLC method development for EGCG. The mobile phase consisted of Milli Q water (0.1% TFA) and methanol at 75:25 ratio. EGCG was analysed at flow rate of 0.8 mL/min, with an injection volume of 20 μL and wavelength of 280 nm at 25 °C.

2.3. Preparation of EGCG Loaded Niosomes

A total of 150 mmol of surfactant, cholesterol and DCP (2 μmol) was dissolved in organic solvents (methanol/chloroform, 4:1, *v*/*v*) and then the mixture rotatory evaporated to form a thin lipid film on the wall at 45 °C. The the lipid film was purged with nitrogen to remove any organic solvents. The thin film was then hydrated with PBS (pH 7.4, 10% ethanol) containing 2 mg of EGCG at 58 °C to form EGCG-niosomes. The niosome suspension was then extruded through a 400 nm polyester membrane with an ER-1 extruder (Eastern Scientific, Rockville, MD, USA) for 10 cycles and then stored at 20–25 °C for the niosome membrane to anneal.

2.4. Optimisation of Formulation with Design of Experiment

2.4.1. Formulation Optimisation by 2^{6-2} Fractional Factorial Design

Based on the preliminary experiments and literature study, six independent variables (factors), namely surfactant type (X_1), drug amount (X_2), molar ratio of CH to surfactant (X_3), DCP amount (X_4), hydration medium volume (X_5) and hydration time (X_6) were selected to be evaluated for their effect on drug entrapment efficiency (EE), which was the dependable variable (response). The six factors were examined on two levels: low and high, which were represented by transform codes of -1 and +1, respectively. A one-quarter two-level six-factor (2^{6-2}) fractional factorial design comprising 16 runs as highlighted in the design display table was constructed by Design-Expert® 7.0 (Stat-Ease, Minneapolis, MN, USA). The factors and levels employed in the design are listed in Table 1. In order to estimate the experimental error and check the response curvature, duplicates were added at two centre points (one for each surfactant type), totally giving 20 runs. The batches were produced in random order. Data analysis was performed by using Design-Expert® 7.0 statistical software. The main effect of variables and interactions were determined according to the Equation (1) listed below:

$$E_X = \overline{y_{(+1)}} - \overline{y_{(-1)}} \quad (1)$$

Table 1. $2^{(6-2)}$ screening design, providing values and coded units with centre points.

Factors	Factor Setting		
	Low (−1)	**Centre (0)**	**High (+1)**
Surfactant type (X_1)	Tween 40	nil	Span 60
Drug amount (mg) (X_2)	1	5.5	10
Molar ratio of CH to surfactant (X_3)	1:4	7:8	3:2
DCP content (μmol) (X_4)	2	6	10
Hydration medium amount (mL) (X_6)	10	17.5	25
Hydration time (min) (X_6)	30	75	120

Contribution was used to determine which factors were larger contributors than others and it is calculated as:

$$Contribution_{x_i}(\%) = \frac{SS_{xi}}{SS_{total}} \times 100$$

where SS_{xi} is the sum of square of factor X_i; SS_{total} is the total sum of square. The data was tested for significance by analysis of variance (ANOVA) with a level of significance of 5% ($p = 0.05$).

2.4.2. Optimisation of Entrapment Efficiency by Central Composite Design (CCD)

The key variables that were identified to have significant effects on the EE were subjected to the optimisation step. A CCD was used to determine the optimum conditions and to investigate how sensitive the response was to the changes in the settings of the independent variables. The CCD, as described previously, consists of a full factorial design with centre and star points, which generates enough information to fit a second-order polynomial model. The two influential factors, namely drug amount (X_1) and ratio of CH to surfactant (X_2) were chosen as independent variables and EE was assessed as dependent variable, the other factors were fixed based on the findings obtained from the screening design. A total of 13 experiments were performed, including five replicates on the centre point which improved the assessment of the response surface curvature and simplified the estimation of the model error. The levels of the factors in EGCG-niosome optimisation are shown in Table 2.

Table 2. Optimisation of epigallocatechin gallate (EGCG)-niosome by central composite design.

Factors	Factor Setting				
	−1.4	**−1**	**Centre (0)**	**+1**	**+1.4**
Drug amount (mg) (X_1)	0.58	1	2	3	3.4
Molar ratio of CH to surfactant (X_2)	3:1	1:2	1:1	3:2	17:10

Data analysis was performed by using Design-Expert® 7.0 statistical software. The data were tested for significance by analysis of variance (ANOVA) with a level of significance of 5% ($p = 0.05$). The second-order Equation (2) generated is described as:

$$y = \beta_o + \beta_1 X_1 + \beta_2 X_2 + \beta_{11} X_1^2 + \beta_{22} X_2^2 + \beta_{12} X_1 X_2 \quad (2)$$

where y stands for the predicted response (dependent variable), β_o is the intercept; $\beta_1 - \beta_{22}$ are the regression coefficients; X_1 and X_2 stand for the main effect of the two factors; X_1X_2 is the interactions between the main effects; and X_1^2 X_2^2 are quadratic terms of the independent variables that are used to simulate the curvature of the designed space.

Checkpoint analyses were carried out to establish the reliability of the CCD regression model in describing composition parameters' effect on entrapment efficiency. The optimum point was chosen according to the prediction based on the second-order equation. Predicted and experimental values were compared to determine the correlation extent between the actual and predicted responses.

2.5. Characterisation Studies

2.5.1. Particle Size, Size Distribution and Zeta Potential Analysis

The mean particle size and polydispersity index (PDI) of the optimised EGCG niosome was determined by dynamic light scattering using the photon correlation spectroscopy (PCS) technique using a Zetasizer (Malvern instruments, Malvern, UK). A dilute suspension of the niosomes was prepared with Milli Q water. The size measurement was performed in triplicate at 25 °C.

The zeta potential (ζ), is an indicator of particle surface charge, which may arise from the adsorption of a charged species and/or from ionization of groups that at the surface of the formed particles. It determines particles' stability in dispersion. To measure zeta potential of the optimised EGCG niosome, they were dispersed into Milli Q water (pH 7) and measured in triplicate using the Malvern Zetasizer.

2.5.2. Entrapment Efficiency (EE%)

To separate the free and entrapped drugs, ultracentrifugation was used. In summary, the niosomal dispersion was centrifuged for 1 h at 4 °C at 41,000 rpm using a WX80 centrifuge (Beckman Sorvall, Waltham, MA, USA). The amount of EGCG in the supernatant was measured with HPLC (Agilent LC1100, Santa Clara, CA, USA) after particle separation by centrifugation. Then the niosome pellets were gently rinsed with PBS and then dissolved in a methanol solution containing 10% Triton™X-100 solution and then sonicated in a water bath sonicator for 10 min. The resulting liquid was filtered and then subjected to concentration determination by HPLC. The following Equation (3) was used to calculate the entrapment efficiency:

$$Entrapment\ efficiency = \frac{(Total\ drug - Free\ drug)}{Total\ drug\ added} \times 100\% \quad (3)$$

2.5.3. Morphology by Scanning Electron Microscopy (SEM)

SEM (XL30S FEG, Philips, Eindhoven, Netherlands) was used to study the optimised niosomes' morphology. The niosome dispersion was diluted 20 times with Milli Q water before being dried on the grid. Gold and palladium sputter coating was applied before morphological evaluation at 25 kV.

2.5.4. Differential Scanning Calorimetry (DSC) and Fourier Transform Infra-Red Spectroscopy (FTIR)

IR spectroscopy and DSC were used to investigate the drug's interaction and entrapment in the vesicular structure. DSC (TA Instruments, New Castle, DE, USA, Q2000+ RCS40) was used to analyse the thermal properties of the optimised niosomes. Span60®, cholesterol, pure drug, and a physical mixture of these components and the lyophilised niosomes were placed into T-zero aluminum pans and hermetically sealed. The temperature rises to 200 °C at a rate of 10 °C/min from a starting temperature of 20 °C for all experimental runs.

FTIR spectra of the individual and mixture of formulation components and lyophilized niosomes were determined using a Bruker FTIP tensor 37 (Bruker Optics, Billerica, MA, USA) at a 4 cm^{-1} resolution between 500 and 4000 cm^{-1}.

2.6. In Vitro Drug Release

In vitro release of drug-loaded EGCG-niosomes was studied using a Franz diffusion apparatus (FDC-6, Logan Instrument Corp, Somerset, NJ, USA). EGCG solution containing the equivalent quantity of EGCG as the drug loaded niosomes was used as a control. EGCG-niosomes and drug solution were added to the donor compartment of the Franz diffusion cell, with a cellulose membrane (MW 12,000–14,000, Membra-Cel ®, Viskase, Lombard, IL, USA) sandwiched between the donor and receptor chambers. The receptor chamber was filled with PBS (pH 5.5) and the temperature was maintained at 37 ± 1 °C. Aliquots (400 µL) were withdrawn at pre-determined time points (15 min, 30 min, 1 h, 2 h, 3 h, 4 h, 6 h, 8 h, 12 h and 24 h) and replaced with fresh PBS (400 µL). The samples were centrifuged at 13,000 rpm for 30 min, and the supernatant was filtered (0.22 µm) and analysed with the HPLC method.

To determine the release mechanism, the release data were fitted into the Korsmeyer–Peppas model:

$$Q_t = K_k t^n$$

where Q_t is the cumulative drug released at time t, k_k is a kinetic constant characteristic of the drug/polymer system, and n is an exponent describing the release mechanism.

2.7. Ex Vivo Skin Permeation and Deposition Studies

2.7.1. Skin Permeation Studies

The full-thickness skin samples were kindly donated by patients who underwent elective skin reduction surgeries at Middlemore hospital, Auckland. This project has been approved by the University of Auckland's Human Participants Ethics Committee (approval number: 010990). The skin samples were stored at −20 °C immediately after the surgeries and used within one month.

The ex vivo skin permeation and deposition studies were carried out using Franz diffusion apparatus (FDC-6, Logan Instrument Corp, Somerset, NJ, USA). EGCG-niosomes and drug solution were added to the donor compartment of the Franz diffusion cell, with a piece of full-thickness human skin sandwiched between the donor and receptor chambers (effective diffusional area: 1.77 cm^2). The receptor chambers were filled with PBS (pH 5.5) and the temperature was maintained at 37 ± 1 °C. Prior to the experiments, the integrity of the skin samples was verified by a Millicell-ERS equipment (Millipore, Burlington, MA, USA) to determine the electrical resistance (ER) across the skin. The skin samples that had an ER value above the cut-off value of 27.4 kΩ·cm^2 were used in the study and equilibrated in PBS for 4 h before the study. For the permeation test, EGCG-niosome suspension and EGCG solution (containing an equivalent amount of EGCG as the drug loaded niosomes) were added to the donor compartments. Aliquots (400 μL) were withdrawn at 12 h and 24 h and replaced with fresh PBS (400 μL). The samples were centrifuged at 13,000 rpm for 30 min, and the supernatant was filtered (0.22 μm) and the drug concentration was determined by HPLC.

2.7.2. Drug Deposition in the Skin

The skin tissues were removed from the Franz diffusion cells after 12 h and 24 h of the deposition study, and the surface of the skin tissue was thoroughly cleaned with methanol and then placed on a tissue cutting board. The SC layer of the skin was removed by a tape-stripping method with Scotch® Magic tapes (3M, Maplewood, MN, USA) [37]. A tape and a 2 kg weight were placed on each skin sample for 10 s, then peeled with forceps, and 15 strippings were applied consecutively to remove the SC. Subsequently, the skin was cut into smaller pieces and 60 mg of skin tissue was placed in a MACS™ tube (Mitenyi Biotec Inc, Cambridge, MA, USA) with methanol, then dissociated using a dissociator (Mitenyi Biotec Inc, Cambridge, MA, USA). Protein was precipitated by adding TCA, then centrifuged at 13,000 rpm for 30 min, and the supernatants were filtered and analysed by HPLC.

2.7.3. Visualisation of Skin Penetration and Deposition

FITC was added to the hydration medium to prepare FITC-labelled niosomes. Full-thickness human skin was placed between the donor and the receptor chamber of the Franz cells, and FITC labelled niosomes were added to the donor compartment. The skin samples were removed after 12 h and thoroughly cleaned. They were frozen and directly embedded in wax and then cut into sections with a microtome. The tissue sections were fixed on glass slides and then observed using a fluorescence microscope (DMIL LED, Leica, Wetzlar, Germany), and the images were captured.

2.8. Antioxidant Effect of EGCG Loaded Niosomes on Human Fibroblasts

2.8.1. Cell Culture

The primary human fibroblasts (Fbs) were obtained from the American Type Culture Collection (ATCC, Manassas, VA, USA). Cells were routinely maintained in complete DMEM medium in T-75 tissue culture flasks (Corning, Phoenix, AZ, USA) at 37 °C in an atmosphere of 5% CO^2 and 95% relative humidity. Complete DMEM medium was prepared by adding 10% fetal bovine serum, 1% penicillin-streptomycin-glutamine, and 1% nonessential amino acids. Culture medium was changed every 2 days until cells grew to 90% confluence.

2.8.2. Cellular Viability after UVA-Irradiation Using Sulforhodamine B (SRB) Assay

Optimised EGCG-loaded niosomes were prepared and centrifuged as per the above-mentioned method and were resuspended in cell culture medium. Fbs were seeded in 96-well plates (5000 cells/well) 24 h before UVA-irradiation to allow cells to attach. To administer UVA-irradiation, a UVA lamp (EN-160 L/FE, Spectroline, Melville, NY, USA) with a dose of 0.72 J/cm^2 and wavelength of 320–400nm and wave peak at 365 nm was used. After irradiation, EGCG niosome suspension and free EGCG in culture medium solution were added to the 96-well and incubated for 24 h. The SRB assay was used to assess the cell viability. Briefly, the cells were gently washed with ice-cold PBS and fixed with 10% TCA, then 0.1 mL of 0.4% (*w*/*v*) SRB in acetic acid was added to stain the cellular proteins. The cell-bound dye was extracted using 0.1 mL 10 mM unbuffered Tris base solution (pH 10.5), and absorbance was measured at 596 nm with a plate reader (SpectraMax® Plus, Molecular Devices, San Jose, CA, USA). Cell viability was expressed as a percentage of the control.

2.8.3. Intracellular MDA Level and the Antioxidant Enzyme Activities

EGCG and EGCG niosomes were diluted with a serum-free medium and then added to the cells after being irradiated by UV light and then cultured for 24 h. After incubation, cells were removed from the 6-well plate and the amount of MDA was determined by the MDA assay kits. The antioxidant enzyme activities of SOD and GSH-px were determined using the same method described above, and the cellular enzymatic activities were determined using the respective assay kits.

2.9. Cellular Uptake of Niosomes by Human Fibroblasts

FITC was added to the hydration medium to prepare FITC-labelled niosomes, then subjected to centrifugation to remove free FITC. The niosome pellets were then resuspended in the medium and diluted to the predetermined concentrations. The control solution was prepared by dissolving FITC in DMSO and then diluted with the medium. For the uptake studies, Fbs suspension (5×10^5 cell in 5 mL) was seeded onto Petri dishes (100 mm, Corning, Phoenix, AZ, USA), fed with completed DMEM every 2 days and incubated at 37 °C in an atmosphere of 5% CO2 and 95% relative humidity to allow cells to attach and proliferate. On reaching 90% confluence, the culture medium was replaced with 2 mL of HBSS. After incubation at 37 °C for 15 min, the HBSS was replaced with FTIC-labelled niosomes at concentrations from 50 to 2000 μg/mL to determine the effect of concentration on cellular uptake; to study the effected of incubation temperature and duration, FITC-labelled niosomes were incubated with Fbs at 4 and 37 °C for 0.5–24 h and at 37 °C for 0.5–24 h, respectively. Then the cells were washed with ice-cold HBSS for three times and then the cells were collected into a tube containing lysis medium (Methanol with 10% Triton™ X-100 solution), followed by ultrasonication for 15 min. Finally, 25 μL of the cell lysates was subjected to BCA protein assay using a Pierce® BCA protein assay kit (Thermo Fisher Scientific, Waltham, MA, USA) to determine the amount of protein in the cells. The remainder of the cell lysates were subjected for quantitative measurement using a fluorescein spectrophotometer (PerkinElmer Precisely, Waltham, MA, USA), at excitation wavelength of 495 nm, emission wavelength of 525 nm.

A Confocal Laser Scanning Microscope (CLSM) was used to examine whether niosomes were taken up and localised intracellularly or were simply adsorbed onto the cell surface. Fbs were transferred into 2-well chamber slides (BD Falcon, Phoenix, AZ, USA) at a density of 2×10^5 cells/well (5×10^4 cells/cm^2) and grown in complete DMEM culture medium. The cells were treated with FITC-labeled niosome (2 mL) at the given doses for 2 h at 37 °C. After incubation, the cells were washed with ice-cold HBSS and then incubated with serum free medium for 15 min. Then the medium was withdrawn and a cytoplasm dye (CellTracker, Invitrogen, Auckland, New Zealand) (5 μM) in serum-free medium for 30 min in a cell incubator at 37 °C. After incubation, the cells were washed with PBS followed by a fixation solution of 3% paraformaldehyde for 30 min at room temperature. Then nuclei staining dye, DAPI (100 nM) (Invitrogen, Auckland, New Zealand) was added to the cells for 3 min. The culture chambers were removed, and the slides were rinsed and mounted with CITI-Fluor (Electron Microscopy Sciences, Hatfield, PA, USA). Coverslips were cemented in place with application of nail polish around their edges. Then the slides were observed by a confocal microscope FV1000 (Olympus, Hamburg, Germany).

2.10. Statistical Analysis

Statistical analysis was performed using the GraphPad Prism® (GraphPad, San Diego, CA, USA) version 8.0 software via one-way ANOVA. A p-value of < 0.05 was considered the minimum level of significance. All data were expressed as mean ± SD.

3. Results

3.1. Formulation Development and Optimisation

Six formulation variables: surfactant type (X_1), drug amount (X_2), molar ratio of CH to surfactant (X_3) and DCP (X_4), hydration medium amount (X_5) and hydration time (X_6) were selected, and their effect on drug entrapment efficiency (Y) was evaluated. The experimental matrix for EGCG-niosome and responses of different batches obtained are presented in Table 3. The EE of EGCG in the niosomes had a range from 2.3 to 49%, suggesting that the factors investigated were influential on the drug encapsulation. Calculations were carried out based on the responses to determine the main effects of the factors and the interaction effects

Table 3. Screening design of EGCG-niosome showing variables in coded values and response EE (%).

Run Number	Variables						Response (Y); EE (%)
	X_1	X_2	X_3	X_4	X_5	X_6	
1	1	1	−1	−1	1	1	2.3
2	1	1	1	1	1	1	47.9
3	1	1	1	−1	1	−1	24.5
4	−1	1	1	1	−1	1	5.7
5	−1	1	1	−1	−1	−1	12.6
6	−1	1	−1	1	1	−1	27.8
7	1	−1	1	−1	−1	1	49.0
8	1	−1	−1	1	1	1	15.8
9	1	−1	1	1	−1	−1	45.8
10	−1	0	0	0	0	0	18.3
11	−1	−1	1	1	1	1	22.7
12	−1	−1	−1	1	−1	1	17.0
13	1	1	−1	−1	−1	1	30.0
14	1	0	0	0	0	0	42.7
15	−1	0	0	0	0	0	24.6
16	−1	−1	−1	−1	1	1	46
17	1	−1	−1	−1	1	−1	48.7
18	−1	−1	−1	−1	−1	−1	21
19	1	1	−1	1	−1	−1	38.7
20	1	0	0	0	0	0	24.8

The results calculated to determine the main effects of the factors and the interaction effect are shown in Table 4.

After the estimation of the main effects, ANOVA was performed to determine the significant factors. The ANOVA results of the EGCG-niosome are shown in Table 5. A p value less than 0.05 ($p < 0.05$) indicated the effect was statistically significant. In this screening, surfactant type (X_1), drug amount (X_2), and the ratio of CH to surfactant (X_3) were significantly influential on the response. The ANOVA showed that none of the two-factor interactions had a significant effect in the EGCG-niosome screening experiment. Surfactant type (X_1), drug amount (X_2) and the ratio of CH to surfactant (X_3) were significantly influential factors on EE. Surfactant type (X_1) played an important role in determining EE, and therefore, in the optimisation step, Span 60 was used, whereas drug amount (X_2) and the ratio of CH to surfactant (X_3) were optimised.

Table 4. Main effects of single factors and two-factor interactions in EGCG-niosome variable screening.

Factor	Response (EE%)	
	Standardized Effect	Contribution (%)
X_1-Surfactant	15.58	28.64
X_2-Drug amount	−6.98	5.74
X_3-Molar ratio of CH to surfactant	−9.20	9.99
X_4-DCP content	−1.00	0.12
X_5-Hydration amount	−0.06	0.04
X_6-Hydration time	−0.93	0.01
$[X_1 X_2] = X_1 X_2 + X_3 X_5$	2.60	0.80
$[X_1 \times 3] = X_1 X_3 + X_2 X_5$	−0.52	0.03
$[X_1X_4] = X_1 X_4 + X_5X_6$	1.82	0.39
$[X_1X_5] = X_1 X_5 + X_2 X_3 + X_4 X_6$	−6.22	4.57
$[X_1X_6] = X_1X_6 + X_4 X_5$	−2.65	0.83
$[X_2X_4] = X_2 X_4 + X_3 X_6$	6.48	4.83
$[X_2X_6] = X_2 X_6 + X_3 X_4$	1.50	0.27

Table 5. Summary of analysis of variance (ANOVA) for the $2^{(6-2)}$ factorial design for EGCG-niosome variable screening.

Source	Sum of Squares	Df **	Mean Square	F Value	*p*-Value
Model	4566.98	13	352.25	9.12	0.023
X_1-Surfactant	32.49	1	32.49	0.84	0.411
X_2-Drug amount	2213.7	1	2213.7	57.32	0.002 *
X_3-Molar ratio of CH to surfactant	566.40	1	566.44	14.67	0.019 *
X_4-DCP content	257.60	1	257.60	6.67	0.061
X_5-Hydration amount	277.22	1	277.22	7.18	0.055
X_6-Hydration time	707.56	1	707.56	18.32	0.013 *
$[X_1 X_2] = X_1 X_2 + X_3 X_5$	31.56	1	31.36	0.81	0.419
$[X_1X_3] = X_1 X_3 + X_2 X_5$	58.52	1	58.52	1.52	0.286
$[X_1X_4] = X_1 X_4 + X_5X_6$	102.01	1	102.01	2.64	0.179
$[X_1X_5] = X_1 X_5 + X_2 X_3 + X_4 X_6$	72.25	1	72.25	1.87	0.243
$[X_1X_6] = X_1X_6 + X_4 X_5$	238.70	1	238.70	6.18	0.068
$[X_2X_4] = X_2 X_4 + X_3 X_6$	12.60	1	12.60	0.33	0.598
$[X_2X_6] = X_2 X_6 + X_3 X_4$	13.69	1	13.69	0.35	0.584
Lack of fit	21.84	2	10.92	0.16	0.859
Pure Error	123.73	2	61.86		
Cor Total ***	5784.34	19			

* statistically significant $p < 0.05$, R-Squared = 0.96, Adj R-Squared = 0.861, Pred R-Squared = 0.598. ** df: degree of freedom. *** Cor Total: corrected total sum of square.

3.2. Optimisation of EE by CCD

In this step, significant factors detected by the screening design were optimised using a CCD. This design provides a solid foundation for generating a response surface plot, from which it is possible to get a target response. In the current study, it was the maximum EE% that the optimisation aimed to achieve. Transformed values of all the batches along with results of EGCG-niosome are shown in Table 6.

Table 6. Optimisation design of EGCG-niosome showing variables in coded values and responses.

Run Number	Type	X_2	X_3	Response Entrapment Efficiency (%)
1	Center	0	0	49.1
2	Axial	0	−1.4	47.5
3	Fractional	−1	+1	11.6
4	Center	0	0	54
5	Center	0	0	39.1
6	Axial	0	+1.4	7.3
7	Fractional	−1	−1	43.6
8	Axial	+1.4	0	12.1
9	Center	0	0	46
10	Fractional	+1	−1	34.6
11	Fractional	+1	+1	12.8
12	Axial	−1.4	0	30.5
13	Center	0	0	47.1

Equation (4) below represents the polynomial model for EGCG-niosome as obtained from the above experiment.

$$Y(EE\%) = 47.06 - 3.98X_2 + 2.61X_3 - 4.30X_2^2 - 2.14X_3^2 - 0.61X_2X_3 \quad (4)$$

The correlation coefficient (r^2) of 0.92 indicated that the model fitted the data very well and the ANOVA of the model reported a high significance ($p < 0.001$) (Table 7). The three-dimensional response surface and contour plots showing the variation in the entrapment efficiency with changes in drug amount (X_2) and CH to surfactant ratio (X_3) are presented in Figure 1. The highest EE was predicted to be achieved when drug amount (X_2) is 1.4 mg and the molar ratio of CH to surfactant (X_3) is 0.9.

Table 7. Analysis of Variance (ANOVA) of the drug entrapment efficiency.

Source	Sum of Squares	Df **	Mean Square	F Value	*p*-Value
Model	3232.04	5	646.81	27.8	0.0002
X_2-drug amount	1530.47	1	1530.47	65.78	0.0001 *
X_3-Molar ratio of CH to surfactant	142.99	1	142.99	6.15	0.0423 *
X_2X_3	26.01	1	26.01	1.12	0.3255
X_2^2	1096.54	1	1096.54	47.13	0.0002
X_3^2	628.49	1	628.49	27.01	0.0013

Table 7. *Cont.*

Source	Sum of Squares	Df **	Mean Square	F Value	p-Value
Residual	162.86	7	23.27		
Lack of fit	46.05	3	15.35	0.53	0.6879
Pure Error	116.81	4	29.20		
Cor Total ***	3396.90	12			

* statistically significant $p < 0.05$; ** df: degree of freedom; *** Cor Total: corrected total sum of square.

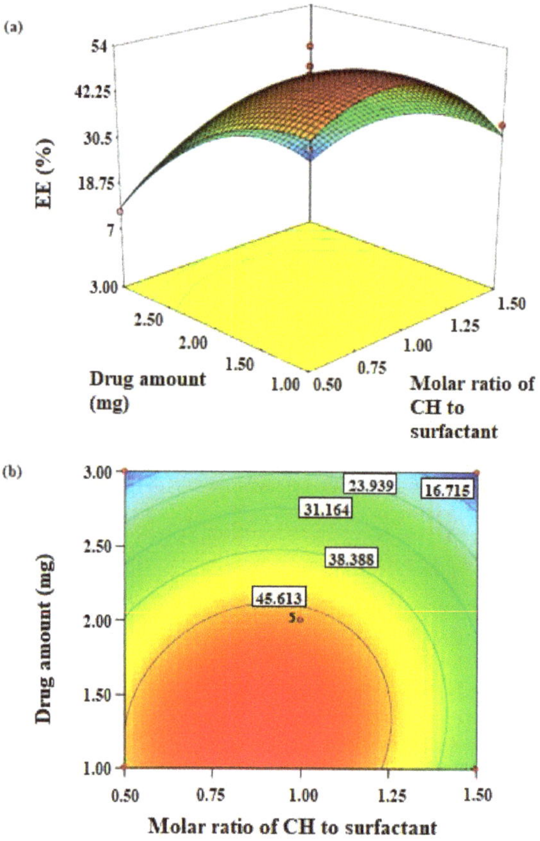

Figure 1. (**a**) Three-dimensional surface plot for EE of EGCG-niosome as a function of the formulation variables. (**b**) Contour plot for EE of EGCG-niosome as a function of the formulation variables.

3.3. Check Point Analysis

Having studied the effect of independent variables on the response, EE%, the levels of the factors were further determined by the optimisation process. Check points were evaluated to confirm the mathematic models' predictivity by comparing the experimental EE (mean value out of four experiments) with the predicted value. In EGCG-niosome, the average experimental EE was 53.05 ± 4.46%, which was close to the predicted value EE of 53% with low percentage of bias (0.4%), suggesting that the optimised formulation parameters were reliable. The optimised formulation composition for EGCG-niosome is shown in Table 8, and the following characterisation studies were carried out on the optimised EGCG-niosome.

Table 8. Optimised formulation composition for EGCG-niosome.

Formulation Variables	EGCG-Niosome
Surfactant (X_1)	Span 60
Drug amount (mg) (X_2)	1.4
Molar ratio of CH to surfactant (X_3)	0.9
DCP amount (μmol) (X_4)	2
Hydration medium volume (mL) (X_5)	10
Hydration time (h) (X_6)	2
EE (%)	53.05 ± 4.46

3.4. *Characterisation of EGCG-Loaded Niosomes*

The developed HPLC method was validated for linearity, repeatability, accuracy and sensitivity as per International Conference on Harmonisation (ICH) Q2(R1) guidelines. The standard curve was linear in the range between 1.93 to 145 μg/mL with a correlation coefficient (r^2) of 0.999. Percentage of coefficient of variation (% CV) was determined to assess instrumental precision; both instrumental precision and intra-assay precision had % CV of less than 1.5%, indicating the method for EGCG is precise. Intermediate precision of the method was determined by assessing intra-day and inter-day repeatability; the % CV values were below 2.5%, which is acceptable according to the ICH guidelines. The sensitivity of the method was determined by limit of detection (LOD) and limit of quantification (LOQ), which were 0.33 μg/mL and 0.98 μg/mL, respectively.

3.5. *Particle Size, Size Distribution, Zeta Potential Analysis and EE%*

The average particle size of optimised EGCG-niosomes was 235.4 ± 15.64 nm, and the PDI value was 0.267 ± 0.053. A PDI of less than 0.5 indicates a narrow distribution of the particles [17]. EGCG-niosomes had a zeta potential of −45.2 ± 0.03 mV and EE% of 53.05 ± 4.46%.

3.6. *Morphological Study*

As shown in Figure 2, the niosomes were 200 to 300 nm, spherical in shape with a closed vesicular structure and narrow size distribution. These findings were consistent with the size determined by the Zetasizer.

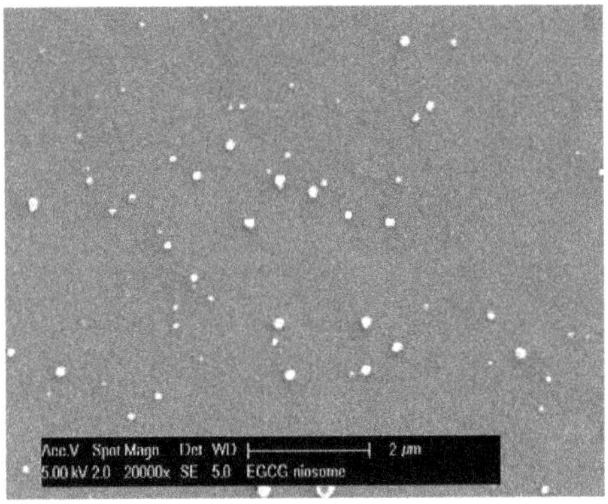

Figure 2. Scanning Electron Microscopy (SEM) image of the optimised EGCG niosomes.

3.7. *DSC and FTIR*

The DSC curves of the optimised EGCG niosomes, physical mixture of the formulation components, cholesterol, surfactant and EGCG are shown in Figure 3a. The endothermic peaks for Span 60 and cholesterol were 53 °C and 149 °C, respectively, which correspond to their melting points. The endothermic transition of EGCG (120 and 225 °C) are also reported in other studies. The physical mixture of formulation components showed similar transitions as EGCG and surfactant, where the characteristic peaks were not observed with EGCG niosomes. Additional peaks were found in EGCG niosomes between 100 to 150 °C, indicating there were interactions between the excipients. A large peak that appeared between 200 and 300 °C in EGCG-niosomes may suggest drug and excipient breakdown. FTIR spectroscopy verified the above results (Figure 3b. The FTIR graph showed the characteristic peaks for EGCG such –C–O stretching at 1200–1000 cm^{-1} and –C=C stretching at 1600–1500 cm^{-1}. The spectrum of EGCG niosomes was similar to the surfactant; the other characteristic peaks were not observed, which confirmed the encapsulation of EGCG.

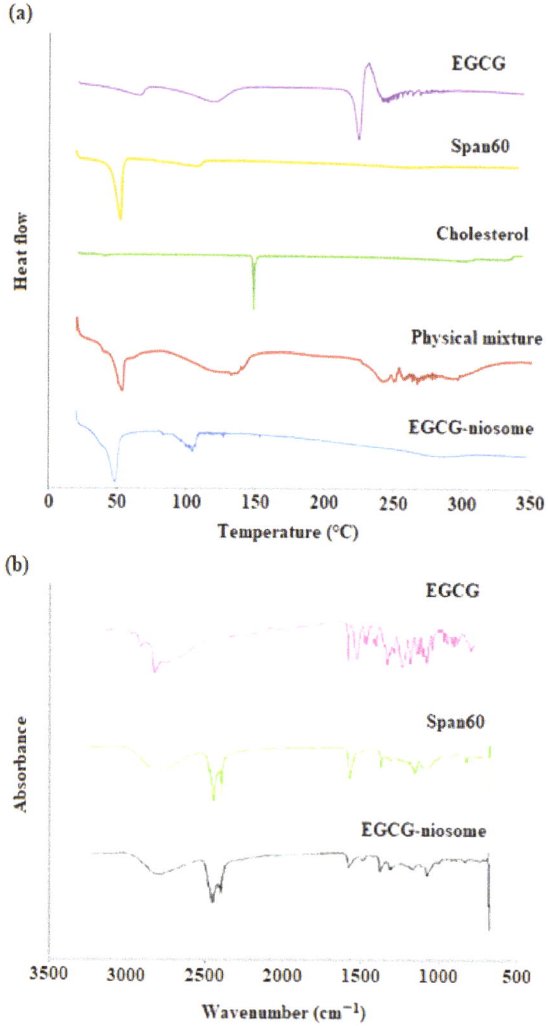

Figure 3. (**a**) Differential Scanning Calorimetry (DSC) thermograms and (**b**) Fourier Transform Infra-red Spectroscopy (FTIR) spectra of EGCG, Span 60 and EGCG-niosomes.

3.8. *In Vitro Drug Release Profile*

The in vitro drug release of EGCG from niosomes was examined using Franz diffusion cells. Figure 4 shows the release profile for control (EGCG solution) and EGCG-niosomes. Within 2 h, the EGCG solution was released immediately. The EGCG-niosomes, on the other hand, displayed a biphasic phase; around 35% of EGCG were released from the niosomes within the first 3 h, and then a sustained release was observed over 21 h, with 73% of EGCG was release at the end of the study. As shown in Table 9, the release data was fitted in several mathematical models of release kinetics. Based on the results, EGCG release from niosomes followed the Korsmeyer–Peppas model (r^2 = 0.996). The release exponents were found to be 0.461, which indicates the drug release was governed by an anomalous diffusion mechanism with multiple steps.

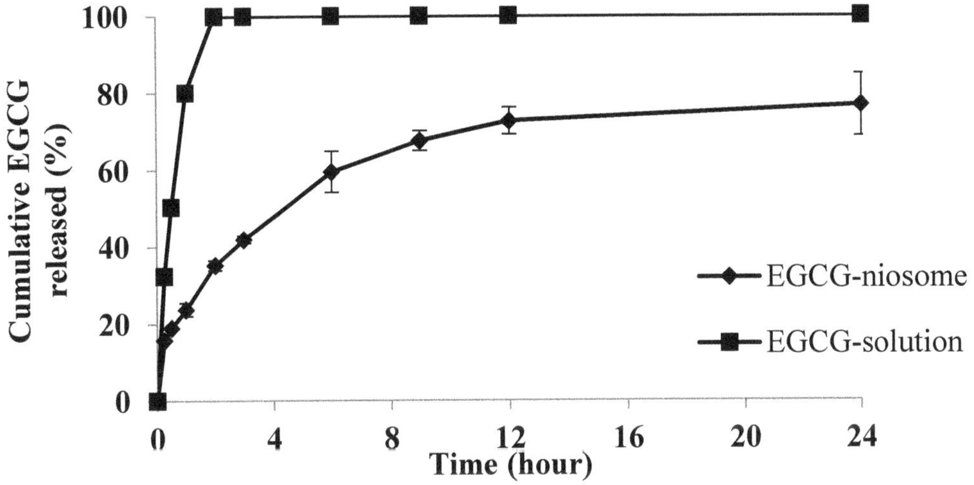

Figure 4. In vitro drug release of EGCG-niosomes and EGCG solution (mean ± SD, n = 3).

Table 9. Drug release kinetic parameters of EGCG niosomes.

Formulation	Korsmeyer-Peppas Model			Higuchi Model		First-Order		Zero-Order	
	r^2	n	k_k	r^2	k_h	r^2	k_1	r^2	k_0
EGCG-niosomes	0.996	0.461	3.885	0.876	2.555	0.832	0.002	0.521	0.077

3.9. *Ex Vivo Skin Permeation and Deposition Studies*

No drug was found in the receptor chamber at the end of the permeation study, and this could be caused by hydrolysis of EGCG in the aqueous medium and the limited sensitivity of the HPLC method. Figure 5 shows the amount of EGCG deposited in the human skin from niosomes and EGCG solution at 12 and 24 h. The deposition of EGCG-solution were 30.02 ± 2.45 µg/cm^2, 29.00 ± 1.36 µg/cm^2 at 12 h and 24 h, respectively. The drug deposition levels of EGCG-niosome were 69.0 ± 13.87 µmg/cm^2 and 54.38 ± 8.86 µmg/cm^2 at 12 h and 24 h, respectively. When the deposition of the EGCG-niosome and the drug solution was compared at 12 and 24 h, it was discovered that the deposition from the EGCG-niosome was about 2-fold higher than that of the drug solution.

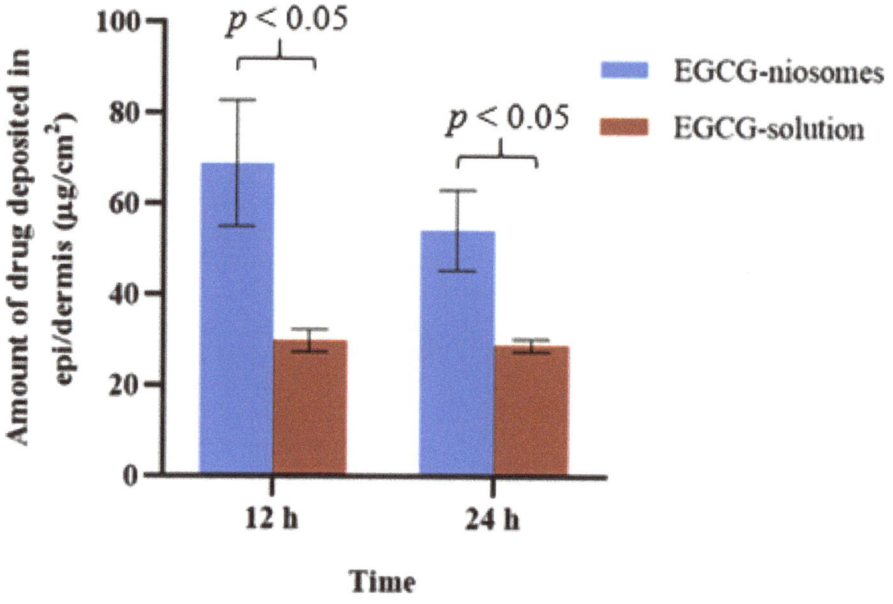

Figure 5. The amount of drug deposited in the human skin layers from EGCG-niosomes and EGCG-solution (mean ± SD, $n = 3$).

3.10. Visualisation of Skin Penetration and Deposition

A small amount of fluorescence was seen in the epidermis after 12 h of ethanol solution application (Figure 6). On the other hand, the niosome carrier improved fluorescence penetration through the SC and greater fluorescence intensity can be observed in the epidermis and dermis. This result matched with the results obtained from the deposition studies and confirmed that niosome could increase drug deposition into the human skin layers.

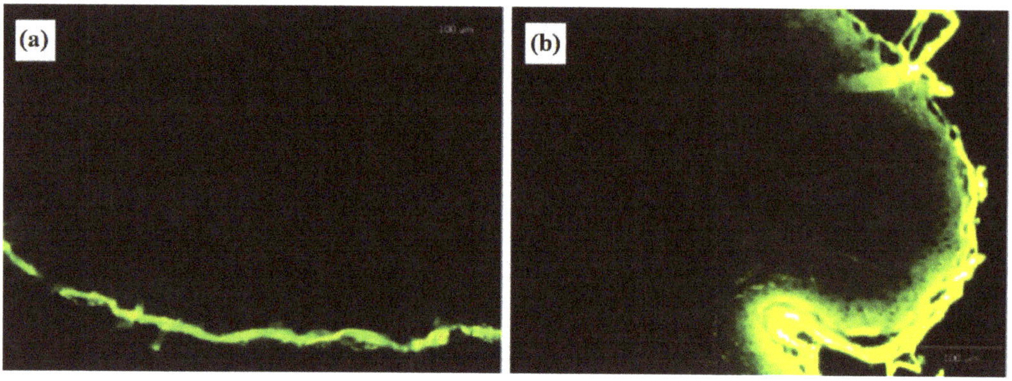

Figure 6. Sections of the full-thickness human skin after been treated with Fluorescein 5(6)-isothiocyanate (FITC) solution (**a**) and FITC-loaded niosomes (**b**) after 12 h.

3.11. The Pharmacological Effects of EGCG-Niosomes on Fbs

3.11.1. Cell Viability after UVA-Irradiation

UVA-irradiation caused substantial reduction in cell viability of 40% when compared to control ($p < 0.05$) (Figure 7a). Fbs treated with EGCG-niosomes demonstrated higher viability, ($p < 0.05$) as compared to the UVA-irradiation group, considerably greater than the group treated with EGCG ($p < 0.05$).

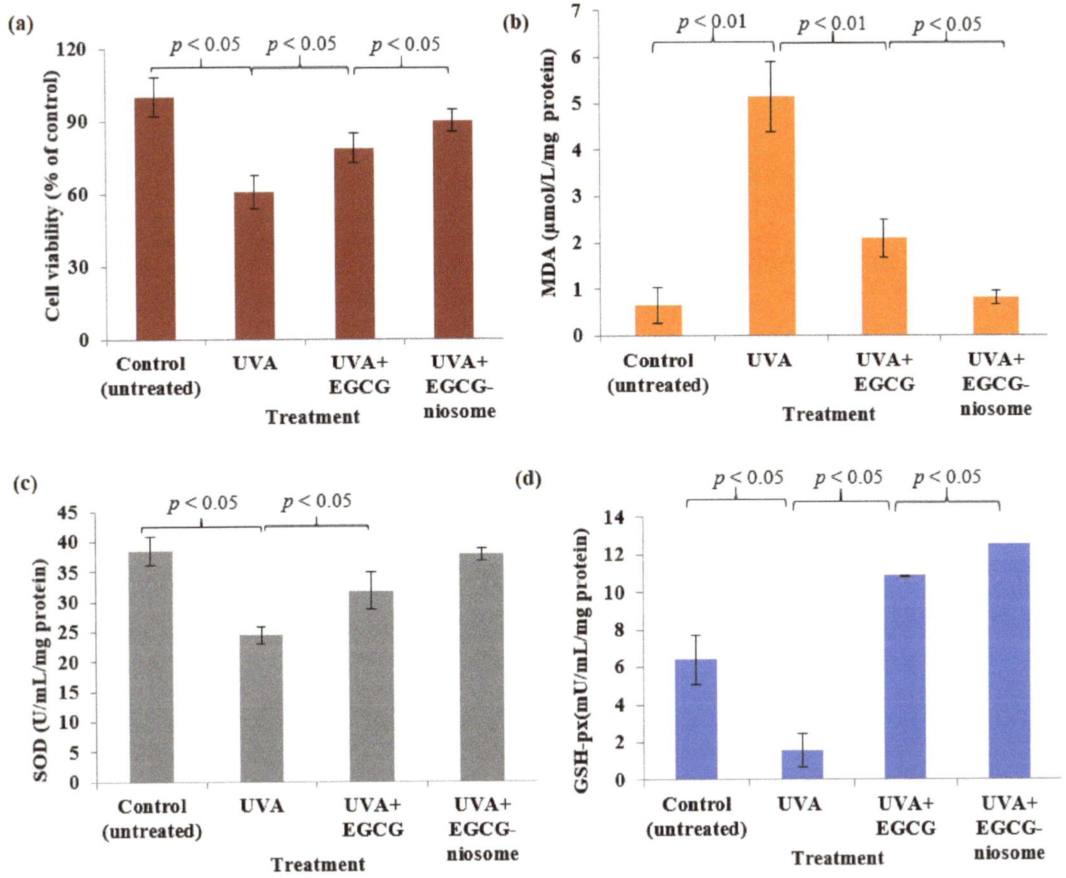

Figure 7. (**a**) Cellular viability after UVA-irradiation and treatment with EGCG and EGCG-niosomes. The effect of EGCG and EGCG niosomes on (**b**) intracellular malondialdehyde (MDA) level (**b**), (**c**) superoxide dismutase (SOD) and (**d**) glutathione peroxidase (GSH)-px after UVA-irradiation (mean ± SD, $n = 3$).

3.11.2. Intracellular MDA Level and the Antioxidant Enzyme Activities

The extent of cellular lipid peroxidation can be determined by measuring intracellular MDA levels. As shown in Figure 7b, intracellular MDA levels after UVA-irradiation was 5.12 ± 0.76 µmol/L/mg protein, which was significantly higher compared to untreated cells ($p < 0.01$), showing that UVA has a strong oxidative effect on skin cells. The intracellular MDA levels of Fbs treated with EGCG-niosomes were much lower (0.80 ± 0.33 µmol/L/mg protein) compared to Fbs treated with free EGCG (2.08 ± 0.33 mol/L/mg protein). Figure 7c,d shows that the activity of the intracellular antioxidant enzymes following UVA-irradiation were reduced significantly for both SOD and GSH-px. EGCG-niosome had a greater enhancing effect on the SOD activity compared to the pure drug, but the difference was insignificant ($p > 0.05$) (Figure 7c), the level of SOD was 36.48 ± 1.98 μ/L/mg protein, the group treated with free EGCG was 31.92 ± 1.67 μ/L/mg protein. The GSH-px level in Fbs after UVA irradiated was increased by EGCG-niosomes to 12.53 ± 0.01 mU/L/mg protein, significantly higher when compared to the group treated with free EGCG (10.88 ± 0.55 mU/L/mg protein) ($p < 0.05$) (Figure 7d).

3.12. Cellular Uptake of Niosome by Fbs Cells

Three factors influenced cellular uptake including niosome concentration, exposure duration, and incubation temperature were studied. Figure 8a shows that increasing the concentration from 50 to 500 μg/mL enhanced cellular uptake, but a further increase from 500 μg/mL did not lead to further increase. Figure 8b shows that cellular uptake was time dependent. Maximum uptake was reached after 3 h before it was declining. At 37 °C, cellular absorption was 6.89 μg FITC/mg protein, 6-fold higher than at 4 °C (0.90 μg FITC/mg protein), which indicated that this process requires energy. No cellular uptake was observed in cells incubated free FITC and no intercellular fluorescence was detected. Confocal microscopy was used to examine whether niosomes were taken up into the cells; it provides the observation of a three-dimensional cross-sectional images of the cells and the location of niosomes within the cells. Labelling the cells with CellTracker and DAPI allowed the cells to be visible under the microscope.

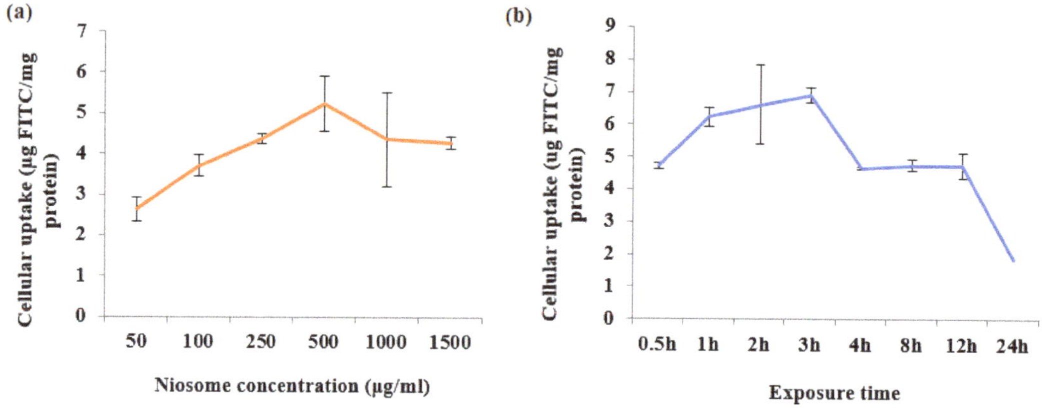

Figure 8. (**a**) Effects of niosome concentrations and (**b**) duration of exposure on the uptake of vesicles by Fbs.

Figure 9a,b illustrates the distribution of green FITC-labelled niosomes inside Fbs after 2 h of uptake. The images indicated that the niosomes were distributed throughout the cytoplasm and perinuclear region. The planar section observation confirmed that FITC was internalised rather than just adsorbing on the cell membranes.

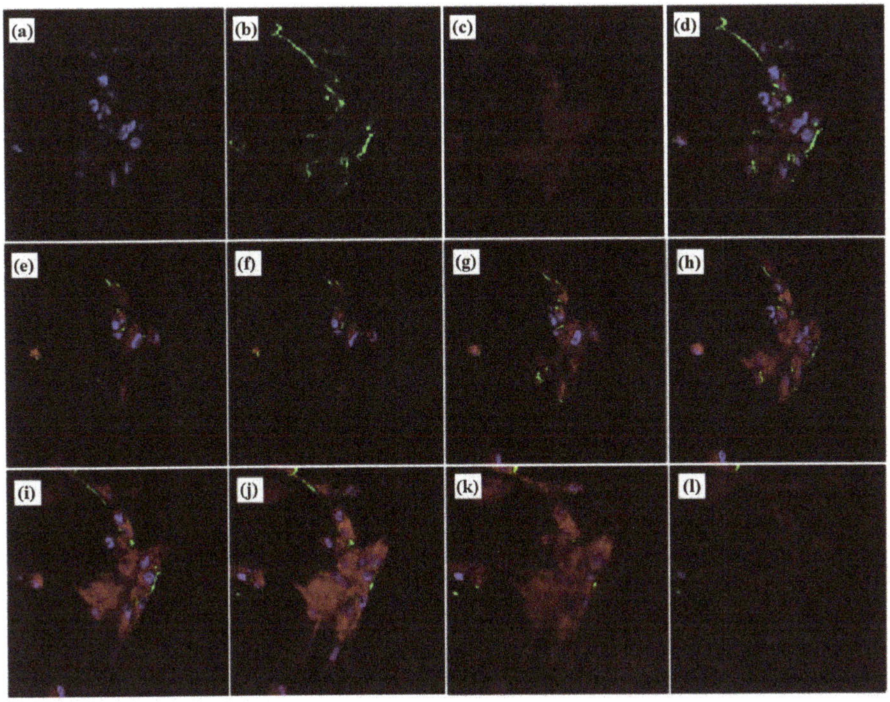

Figure 9. Confocal laser scanning microscopy images of Fbs after incubation with FITC-labelled niosomes for 2 h at 37 °C showing perinuclear accumulation of particles. Nuclei: blue (**a**), FITC-labelled niosomes: green (**b**), cytoplasm: red (**c**), merged images (**d**) confirming uptake of intake niosomes. Eight images of optical sections taken in the vertical axis at interval of 1 µm from the apical surface (**e**–**l**) from left to right; top to bottom, depths 0, 1, 2, 3, 4, 5, 6 and 7 µm, demonstrating particle internalisation. Magnification (600×).

4. Discussion

In this study, EGCG-loaded niosomes were fabricated and optimised by using first a 2^{6-2} fractional factorial design followed by a central composite design. The development of niosomes involves many factors, which may affect their properties such as size and encapsulation of the drug in niosomes. The traditional experimental approach implies altering one factor at a time while keeping the other constant. In this case, to evaluate a certain number of factors, a great effort and long period of time are required. In contrast to the traditional method, utilisation of fractional factorial design is able to provide the maximum amount of information with the least experiments [38]. From a pharmaceutical viewpoint, EE is one of the most important attributes of niosome formulation; a high EE would result in less time and effort spent removing unentrapped material and a greater therapeutic effect of the product [39].

The effect of drug content used in preparation on EE% was statistically significant. Generally, increasing drug amount led to improved EE, but in the EGCG-niosomes, further increase in the drug amount above 1.4 mg showed a decrease of EE. This might be due to saturation of drug entrapment, i.e., further addition of the drug was not able to induce more drug entrapped. The ratio of CH to surfactant was found to significantly influence the entrapment of the EGCG-niosome. CH acts as a membrane stabiliser. It increases rigidity of the bilayer and reduces leakage of drugs from the vesicles; it has been reported that as the amount of CH increases in the formulation, the entrapment efficiency of the drug also increases [40]. Nevertheless, the addition of CH above a certain level may cause disruption of the regular vesicle structure, thus decreasing the entrapment [41]. This finding is consistent with those reported by other researchers. Incorporation of CH into Span 60 niosome loaded with flurbiprofen resulted in an increase of EE from 55% to 67%, but EE was reduced by 30% when CH was increased to 60% [42]. The EE of caffeine decreased from 80% to 50% when the molar ratio of CH to surfactant increased from 3:7 to 3:5 [43]. In the current CCD study, it was obvious that the response surface had curvature in the optimisation phase of both niosome formulations. It indicated that in both niosome preparation, as the CH amount in preparation increased, the EE increased at first, whereas after a certain level, further increase of CH caused a decrease of EE.

The optimised nano-size EGCG-niosomes had an average particle size of 235.4 ± 15.64 nm and a zeta potential of −45.2 ± 0.03 mV. SEM confirmed the findings obtained from Zetasizer, that niosomes were in the 200 to 300 nm size range with a narrow distribution. In topical drug delivery, the particle size of the carriers plays an important role in penetration across the skin barrier. Studies have shown that when the particle size of carriers is greater than 600 nm, no skin deposition was observed. Carriers with a smaller particle size, such as 300 nm promote dermal delivery, while a size lower than 300 nm may result in excessive transdermal drug transport [17]. The zeta potential is an extremely useful measure of a formulation's stability. A zeta potential of less than −30 mV indicates high stability [44]. Adding DCP in the EGC-niosomes resulted in a much lower zeta potential than −30 mV.

The EGCG-niosomes achieved a high EE of 53.05 ± 4.46%, and DSC and FTIR showed that EGCG was successfully encapsulated in the niosomes. In EGCG-niosomes, an additional peak was observed between 100 to 150 °C, indicating a surfactant-cholesterol interaction. This interaction is crucial, as CH acts as a membrane stabiliser in niosomes. Drug release from EGCG-niosomes showed a biphasic pattern, where an initial burst release and a subsequent slow release were observed. The release kinetics followed the Korsmeyer release model, (r^2 = 0.996), demonstrating an anomalous diffusion mechanism regulated by many processes [45,46]. When it comes to topical drug delivery, this type of release pattern is appealing because the initial fast release improves drug penetration, while the subsequent sustained release provides the drug delivery over a longer period to maintain a therapeutic level in the skin and reduces the frequency of reapplication [47–49].

According to research, the use of the niosome carrier has a considerable impact on enhancing topical drug penetration, as well as increasing drug deposition in the human skin, which are both advantageous for dermal formulations. As such, niosomes have been extensively used in topical treatments [17,21,28,50,51]. A number of theories have been put forward to explain their ability to enhance penetration, firstly the adsorption and fusion of carriers onto the skin's surface results in a significant thermodynamic activity gradient of the drug at the surface of the carriers and the skin's surface, which serves as a driving force for drug penetration into the skin [52–54]. Secondly, disruption of the tightly packed lipids that occupy the extracellular spaces of the SC increases drug permeability through structural alteration of the SC. Thirdly, the carrier may disturb the densely packed lipids of the SC to promote drug penetration by modifying the SC structure. Lastly nonionic surfactants may act as penetration enhancers, increasing membrane fluidity [26,32,52,55]. Finally, niosomes alter the SC characteristics by reducing trans-epidermal water loss, increasing SC hydration and leading to the relaxation of its tightly packed cellular structure and, hence, better penetration [52,53]. Ethanol is also known as a penetration enhancer [56]. It reduces the phase transition temperature of SC lipids, improving fluidity of SC. In addition, ethanol imparts soft properties to the carrier's membrane, facilitating vesicle skin penetration [17]. On the other hand, no drug was detected in the receptor chamber of the Franz diffusion cells, indicating that EGCG did not permeate across the skin. The entrapped EGCG and released EGCG molecules may partition into and diffuse through the SC. A drug depot may be formed in the SC, and then the remaining free drug and vesicles penetrate farther into the epidermis until they reach the interface between the SC and the epidermis. The free drug, as well as any remaining intact vesicles, are subsequently released into the skin layers. It is possible that the drug was metabolised by the enzymes in the skin. Catechin is unstable in aqueous environments, and it has been shown that it is rapidly hydrolyzed or degraded. Based on these findings, it may be feasible to explain why no drug was detected in the receptor chamber.

The assay is based on the ability of the dye sulforhodamine B to bind electrostatically and pH-dependently on protein basic amino acid residues of TCA fixed cells. A significant reduction in cellular viability was observed after UVA-irradiation; however, the Fbs viability was significantly improved by both EGCG solution and EGCG-niosomes, with the EGCG-niosomes showing greater protective effects against UVA-irradiation. ROS may cause cell and tissue dysfunction, which is partly manifested as lipid peroxidation. Malondialdehyde (MDA) is the main product of lipid peroxidation, and it reveals the level of cell damage under oxidation [57]. In addition, antioxidant molecules in the skin interact with ROS or their by-products such as MDA to minimise the deleterious oxidation effect. After being exposed to oxidative stress, the antioxidants in the skin SOD and GSH-px are activated [58]. UV irradiation causes an accumulation of ROS in the skin, overwhelming the tissue antioxidants, and thus it causes oxidative stress-related skin problems [6]. ROS may be alleviated by SOD and GSH-px. The decrease in SOD and GSH-px levels observed after UV irradiation might be attributed to the formation of a large number of free radicals that exceeded the antioxidant enzymes' scavenging capacity [59]. Furthermore, the reduction in enzymatic activity might be related to enzyme inactivation caused by ROS damage to DNA. MDA content, which indicates the lipid peroxidation state, increases following UV irradiation, showing damage induced by oxidative stress. EGCG is a polyphenol compound with a wide range of pharmacological actions. This compound has strong antioxidant properties. It is capable of scavenging ROS or their precursors, blocking ROS synthesis and upregulating antioxidant enzymes [60]. Following UV irradiation, skin Fbs treated with EGCG-niosomes had higher SOD and GSH-px activity compared to UV-treated cells. Furthermore, the MDA levels in the EGCG solution-treated group were lower than in the UV group. EGCG-niosomes showed significantly higher antioxidant activity, which might be due to the following explanations: when in cell culture, the medication is subject to autooxidation, but within a vesicle, it is somewhat shielded from destruction [61]. Furthermore, the drug-loaded niosomes produced prolonged release, keeping the level of the drug constant, resulting in an increased antioxidant effect. Furthermore, the carrier may influence drug internalisation by cells [62]. The improved antioxidant activity of EGCG encapsulated in the niosome carrier prompted researchers to investigate niosome-cell interactions.

Since free FITC had difficulties penetrating cells, the increased FITC intake should be attributed to the niosome carriers. Many studies have indicated greater drug absorption mediated by drug carriers; tamoxifen citrate loaded niosomes showed in an in vitro study on MCF-7 breast cancer cells that the amount of cellular uptake and cytotoxicity of tamoxifen were greatly enhanced when it was loaded in niosomes. Incorporating antimicrobial agents into carrier systems, such as nanoparticles or microemulsions, might be a successful technique for increasing cellular uptake [62]. Furthermore, niosomes loaded with salidroside improved the drug's intracellular absorption by both human epidermal immortal keratinocytes and human embryonic skin fibroblasts [53].

Endocytosis is a primary mechanism through which cells internalise chemicals and macromolecules. It is essential for cell-to-cell communication and cell-to-microenvironment communication [63]. To internalise foreign particles, human cells employ multiple endocytosis processes. Phagocytosis, macropinocytosis, clathrin-mediated endocytosis, and caveolae-mediated endocytosis are all examples of endocytic processes [64–66]. Endocytosis demands energy, as opposed to passive transport, which does not involve any expenditure of energy [64]. According to a study, depending on their size, liposomes are mostly endocytosed by clathrin- or caveolae-mediated endocytosis [65]. Recent findings have revealed that endocytosis of niosomes is an energy-dependent process, follows a concentration- and time-dependent pattern and has a saturation point [66]. As a result, it is likely that cell surface proteins are involved in the process of niosome endocytosis.

Niosome carriers have the potential to increase cellular absorption of encapsulated compounds, even if the medication has a low permeability into the cells. Further studies are required to fully understand the uptake process.

5. Conclusions

In this work, the niosome-carrier system was fabricated to encapsulate EGCG for cutaneous administration. Based on the findings, we can conclude that EGCG-niosomes can penetrate the skin barrier and improve drug deposition in the viable layers. Because of increased cellular absorption and based on the studies of the antioxidant enzymes, EGCG-niosomes demonstrated an improved antioxidant effect on skin cells. Because antioxidants have numerous roles in skin health, this topical formulation has the potential to be used in the treatment of skin diseases. Furthermore, in both the pharmaceutical and cosmetic industries, this carrier has the potential to be used as a dermal drug carrier for a variety of bioactive compounds.

Author Contributions: Conceptualization, J.W.; methodology, D.L., N.M., Z.W., M.L. and J.W.; software, D.L.; formal analysis, D.L., N.M. and Z.W.; investigation, D.L. and M.L.; resources, D.L., M.L., Z.Z. and J.W.; data curation, D.L., S.C. and J.R.F.; writing—original draft preparation, D.L. and S.C.; writing—review and editing, J.W., D.L., N.M., Z.W., S.C., J.R.F. and Z.Z.; visualization, D.L and S.C.; supervision, J.W. and Z.Z.; project administration, D.L., N.M. and Z.W. All authors have read and agreed to the published version of the manuscript.

Funding: This research was funded by New Zealand Pharmacy Education Foundation (NZPERF), grant number is 236.

Institutional Review Board Statement: The full-thickness skin samples were kindly donated by patients who underwent elective skin reduction surgeries at Middlemore hospital, Auckland. This project has been approved by the University of Auckland's Human Participants Ethics Committee (approval number: 010990).

Informed Consent Statement: Informed consent was obtained from all subjects involved in the study.

Data Availability Statement: The data presented in this study are available on request from the corresponding author.

Conflicts of Interest: The authors declare no conflict of interest.

References

1. Michalak, M. Plant-Derived Antioxidants: Significance in Skin Health and the Ageing Process. *Int. J. Mol. Sci.* **2022**, *23*, 585. [CrossRef] [PubMed]
2. Tiwari, N.; Osorio-blanco, E.R.; Sonzogni, A.; Esporrín-ubieto, D.; Wang, H.; Calderón, M. Nanocarriers for Skin Applications: Where Do We Stand? *Angew. Chem. Int. Ed. Engl.* **2021**, *61*, 1–26.
3. Hemrajani, C.; Negi, P.; Parashar, A.; Gupta, G.; Jha, N.K.; Singh, S.K.; Chellappan, D.K.; Dua, K. Overcoming drug delivery barriers and challenges in topical therapy of atopic dermatitis: A nanotechnological perspective. *Biomed. Pharmacother.* **2022**, *147*, 112633. [CrossRef]
4. Uchida, N.; Yanagi, M.; Hamada, H. Physical Enhancement? Nanocarrier? Current Progress in Transdermal Drug Delivery. *Nanomaterials* **2021**, *11*, 335. [CrossRef] [PubMed]
5. Ng, K.W.; Lau, W.M. Skin Deep: The Basics of Human Skin Structure and Drug Penetration. In *Percutaneous Penetration Enhancers Chemical Methods in Penetration Enhancement*; Springer: Berlin, Germany, 2015; pp. 1–7.
6. Gu, Y.; Han, J.; Jiang, C.; Zhang, Y. Biomarkers, oxidative stress and autophagy in skin aging. *Ageing Res. Rev.* **2020**, *59*, 101036. [CrossRef]
7. Yin, Z.; Zhu, M. Free radical oxidation of cardiolipin: Chemical mechanisms, detection and implication in apoptosis, mitochondrial dysfunction and human diseases. *Free Radic. Res.* **2012**, *46*, 959–974. [CrossRef] [PubMed]
8. Sangiovanni, E.; Di Lorenzo, C.; Piazza, S.; Manzoni, Y.; Brunelli, C.; Fumagalli, M. Vitis Vinifera, L. Leaf Extract Inhibits In Vitro Mediators of Inflammation and Oxidative Stress Involved in Inflammatory-Based Skin Diseases. *Antioxidants* **2019**, *16*, 134. [CrossRef]
9. Chotphruethipong, L.; Sukketsiri, W.; Battino, M.; Benjakul, S. Conjugate between hydrolyzed collagen from defatted seabass skin and epigallocatechin gallate (EGCG): Characteristics, antioxidant activity and cellular bioactivity. *RSC Adv.* **2021**, *11*, 2175–2184. [CrossRef]

10. Kim, J.; Hwang, J.; Cho, Y.; Han, Y.; Jeon, Y.; Yang, K. Protective Effects of (−)-Epigallocatechin-3-Gallate on UVA- and UVB-Induced Skin Damage. *Skin Pharmacol. Physiol.* **2001**, *14*, 11–19. [CrossRef] [PubMed]
11. Janhua, R.; Munoz, C.; Gorelle, E.; Rehums, W.; Egbert, B.; Kern, D.; Chang, A.L.S. A Two-Year, Double-Blind, Randomized Placebo-Controlled Trial of Oral Green Tea Polyphenols on the Long-Term Clinical and Histologic Appearance of Photoaging Skin. *Dermatol. Surg.* **2009**, *35*, 1057–1065. [CrossRef] [PubMed]
12. Qiao, J.; Kong, X.; Kong, A.; Han, M. Pharmacokinetics and Biotransformation of Tea Polyphenols. *Curr. Drug Metab.* **2014**, *15*, 30–36. [CrossRef] [PubMed]
13. Xu, Y.; Yu, P.; Zhou, W. Combined effect of pH and temperature on the stability and antioxidant capacity of epigallocatechin gallate (EGCG) in aqueous system. *J. Food Eng.* **2019**, *250*, 46–54. [CrossRef]
14. Pham, T.T.; Jaafar-Maalej, C.; Charisset, C.; Fessi, H. Liposome and niosome preparation using a membrane contactor for scale-up. *Colloids Surf. B* **2012**, *94*, 15–21. [CrossRef] [PubMed]
15. Mehta, S.K.; Jindal, N. Formulation of Tyloxapol niosomes for encapsulation, stabilization and dissolution of anti-tubercular drugs. *Colloids Surf. B* **2013**, *101*, 434–441. [CrossRef] [PubMed]
16. Alomrani, A.H.; Al-Agamy, M.H.; Badran, M.M. In vitro skin penetration and antimycotic activity of itraconazole loaded niosomes: Various non-ionic surfactants. *J. Drug Deliv. Sci. Technol.* **2015**, *28*, 37–45. [CrossRef]
17. Chen, S.; Hanning, S.; Falconer, J.; Locke, M.; Wen, J.Y. Recent advances in non-ionic surfactant vesicles (niosomes): Fabrication, characterization, pharmaceutical and cosmetic applications. *Eur. J. Pharm. Biopharm.* **2019**, *144*, 18–39. [CrossRef]
18. Zeng, W.; Li, Q.; Wan, T.; Liu, C.; Pan, W.; Wu, Z.; Zhang, G.; Pan, J.; Qin, M.; Lin, Y.; et al. Hyaluronic acid-coated niosomes facilitate tacrolimus ocular delivery: Mucoadhesion, precorneal retention, aqueous humor pharmacokinetics, and transcorneal permeability. *Colloids Surf. B* **2016**, *141*, 28–35. [CrossRef]
19. Ojeda, E.; Puras, G.; Agirre, M.; Zarate, J.; Grijalvo, S.; Eritja, R.; Martinez-Navarrete, G.; Soto-Sánchez, C.; Diaz-Tahoces, A.; Aviles-Trigueros, M.; et al. The influence of the polar head-group of synthetic cationic lipids on the transfection efficiency mediated by niosomes in rat retina and brain. *Biomaterials* **2015**, *77*, 267–279. [CrossRef]
20. Manosroia, P.; Jantrawuta, P.; Manosroia, J. Anti-inflammatory activity of gel containing novel elastic niosomes entrapped with diclofenac diethylammonium. *Ned. Tijdschr. Diabetol.* **2008**, *360*, 156–163. [CrossRef]
21. El-Menshawe, S.F. A novel approach to topical acetazolamide/PEG 400 ocular niosomes. *J. Drug Deliv. Sci. Technol.* **2012**, *22*, 295–299. [CrossRef]
22. Pando, D.; Matos, M.; Gutiérrez, G.; Pazos, C. Formulation of resveratrol entrapped niosomes for topical use. *Colloids Surf. B* **2015**, *128*, 398–404. [CrossRef]
23. Elhissi, A.; Hidayat, K.; Phoenix, D.A.; Mwesigwa, E.; Crean, S.; Ahmed, W.; Faheem, A.; Taylor, K.M.G. Air-jet and vibrating-mesh nebulization of niosomes generated using a particulate-based proniosome technology. *Int. J. Pharm.* **2013**, *444*, 193–199. [CrossRef] [PubMed]
24. Jigar, S.; Nair, A.B.; Hiral, S.; Jacob, S.; Shehata, T.M.; Morsy, M.A. Enhancement in antinociceptive and anti-inflammatory effects of tramadol by transdermal proniosome gel. *Asian J. Pharm. Sci.* **2019**, *15*, 786–796.
25. Moghddam, R.M.; Ahad, A.; Aqil, M.; Imam, S.S.; Sultana, Y. Formulation and optimization of niosomes for topical diacerein delivery using 3-factor, 3-level Box-Behnken design for the management of psoriasis. *Mater. Sci. Eng. C* **2016**, *69*, 789–797. [CrossRef]
26. Maheshwari, C.; Pandey, R.S.; Chaurasiya, A.; Kumar, A.; Selvam, D.T.; Prasad, G.B.K.S.; Dixit, V.K. Non-ionic surfactant vesicles mediated transcutaneous immunization against hepatitis B. *Int. Immunopharmacol.* **2011**, *11*, 1516–1522. [CrossRef] [PubMed]
27. Ammar, H.O.; Ghorab, M.; El-Nahhas, S.A.; Higazy, I.M. Proniosomes as a carrier system for transdermal delivery of tenoxicam. *Int. J. Pharm.* **2011**, *405*, 142–152. [CrossRef]
28. Kong, M.; Park, H.; Feng, C.; Hou, L.; Cheng, X.; Chen, X. Construction of hyaluronic acid noisome as functional transdermal nanocarrier for tumor therapy. *Carbohydr. Polym.* **2013**, *94*, 634–641. [CrossRef]
29. Tabbakhian, M.; Tavakoli, N.; Jaafari, M.R.; Daneshamouz, S. Enhancement of follicular delivery of finasteride by liposomes and niosomes. *Int. J. Pharm.* **2006**, *323*, 16837150. [CrossRef]
30. Kamel, R.; Basha, M.; Abd, S.H. Development of a novel vesicular system using a binary mixture of sorbitan monostearate and polyethylene glycol fatty acid esters for rectal delivery of rutin. *J. Liposome Res.* **2013**, *23*, 28–36. [CrossRef]
31. Jin, Y.; Wen, J.; Garg, S.; Zhang, W.; Lr, T.; Liu, D.; Zhou, Y. Development of a novel niosomal system for oral delivery of Ginkgo biloba extract. *Int. J. Nanomed.* **2013**, *8*, 421–430. [CrossRef]
32. Tavano, L.; Muzzalupo, R.; Picci, N.; De, C.B. Co-encapsulation of lipophilic antioxidants into niosomal carriers: Percutaneous permeation studies for cosmeceutical applications. *Colloids Surf. B* **2014**, *114*, 144–149. [CrossRef] [PubMed]
33. Bragagni, M.; Mennini, N.; Ghelardini, C.; Mura, P. Development and characterization of niosomal formulations of doxorubicin aimed at brain targeting. *J. Pharm. Pharm. Sci.* **2012**, *15*, 184–196. [CrossRef] [PubMed]
34. Grangeia, H.B.; Silva, C.; Simões, S.P.; Reis, M.S. Quality by design in pharmaceutical manufacturing: A systematic review of current status, challenges and future perspectives. *Eur. J. Pharm. Biopharm.* **2020**, *147*, 19–37. [CrossRef]
35. Mishra, V.; Thakur, S.; Patil, A.; Shukla, A. Quality by design (QbD) approaches in current pharmaceutical set-up. Expert Opin. *Drug Deliv.* **2018**, *15*, 737–758.

36. Garg, N.K.; Sharma, G.; Singh, B.; Nirbhavane, P.; Tyagi, R.K.; Shukla, R.; Katare, O.P. Quality by Design (QbD)-enabled development of aceclofenac loaded-nano strctured lipid carriers (NLCs): An improved dermatokinetic profile for inflammatory disorder(s). *Int. J. Pharm.* **2017**, *517*, 413–431. [CrossRef]
37. Goh, C.F.; Craig, M.; Hadgraft, J.; Lane, M.E. The application of ATR-FTIR spectroscopy and multivariate data analysis to study drug crystallisation in the stratum corneum. *Eur. J. Pharm. Biopharm.* **2017**, *111*, 16–25. [CrossRef] [PubMed]
38. Araújo, J.; Vega, E.; Lopes, C.; Egea, M.A.; Garcia, M.L.; Souto, E.B. Effect of polymer viscosity on physicochemical properties and ocular tolerance of FB-loaded PLGA nanospheres. *Colloids Surf. B* **2009**, *72*, 48–56. [CrossRef]
39. Aboelwafa, A.A.; El-Setouhy, D.A.; Elmeshad, A.N. Comparative Study on the Effects of Some Polyoxyethylene Alkyl Ether and Sorbitan Fatty Acid Ester Surfactants on the Performance of Transdermal Carvedilol Proniosomal Gel Using Experimental Design. *AAPS Pharm. Sci. Tech.* **2010**, *11*, 1591–1602. [CrossRef]
40. Azeem, A.; Anwer, M.K.; Talegaonkar, S. Niosomes in sustained and targeted drug delivery: Some recent advances. *J. Drug Target* **2009**, *17*, 671–689. [CrossRef]
41. Hamishehkar, H.; Rahimpour, Y.; Kouhsoltani, M. Niosomes as a propitious carrier for topical drug delivery. *Expert Opin. Drug Deliv.* **2013**, *10*, 261–272. [CrossRef]
42. Mokhtar, M.; Sammour, O.A.; Hammad, M.A.; Megrab, N.A. Effect of some formulation parameters on flurbiprofen encapsulation and release rates of niosomes prepared from proniosomes. *Int. J. Pharm.* **2008**, *361*, 104–111. [CrossRef] [PubMed]
43. Khazaeli, P.; Pardakhty, A.; Shoorabi, H. Caffeine-Loaded Niosomes: Characterization and in Vitro Release Studies. *Drug Deliv.* **2007**, *14*, 447–452. [CrossRef] [PubMed]
44. Jacobs, C.; Müller, R.H. Production and Characterization of a Budesonide Nanosuspension for Pulmonary Administration. *Pharm. Res.* **2002**, *19*, 189–194. [CrossRef]
45. Rasul, A.; Khan, M.I.; Rehman, M.U.; Abbas, G.; Aslam, N.; Ahmad, S.; Abbas, S.; Shah, P.A.; Iqbal, M.; Al Subari, A.M.A. In vitro Characterization and Release Studies of Combined Nonionic Surfactant-Based Vesicles for the Prolonged Delivery of an Immunosuppressant Model Drug. *Int. J. Nanomed.* **2020**, *15*, 7937–7949. [CrossRef] [PubMed]
46. Katrolia, A.; Chauhan, S.B.; Shukla, V.K. Formulation and evaluation of Metformin Hydrochloride-loaded Curcumin–Lycopene Niosomes. *SN Appl. Sci.* **2019**, *12*, 1703. [CrossRef]
47. El-Feky, G.S.; El-Banna, S.T.; El-Bahy, G.; Abdelrazek, E.M.; Kamal, M. Alginate coated chitosan nanogel for the controlled topical delivery of Silver sulfadiazine. *Carbohydr. Polym.* **2017**, *177*, 194–202. [CrossRef]
48. Patel, D.; Dasgupta, S.; Dey, S.; Ramani, Y.R.; Ray, S.; Mazumder, B. Nanostructured lipid carriers (NLC)-based gel for the topical delivery of aceclofenac: Preparation, characterization, and in vivo evaluation. *Sci. Pharm.* **2012**, *80*, 749–764. [CrossRef]
49. Bom, S.; Santos, C.; Barros, R.; Martins, A.M.; Paradiso, P.; Cláudio, R.; Pinto, P.C.; Ribeiro, H.M.; Marto, J. Effects of Starch Incorporation on the Physicochemical Properties and Release Kinetics of Alginate-Based 3D Hydrogel Patches for Topical Delivery. *Pharmaceutics* **2020**, *12*, 719. [CrossRef]
50. Manosroi, A.; Chankhampan, C.; Manosroi, W.; Manosroi, J. Transdermal absorption enhancement of papain loaded in elastic niosomes incorporated in gel for scar treatment. *Eur. J. Pharm. Sci.* **2013**, *48*, 474–483. [CrossRef]
51. Manosroi, W.; Manosroi, J.; Manosroi, A.; Lohcharoenkal, W.; Götz, F.; Werner, R.G. Transdermal Absorption Enhancement of *N*-Terminal Tat–GFP Fusion Protein (TG) Loaded in Novel Low-Toxic Elastic Anionic Niosomes. *J. Pharm. Sci.* **2011**, *100*, 1525–1534. [CrossRef]
52. Kassem, A.; Abd, S.H.; Asfour, M.H. Enhancement of 8-methoxypsoralen topical delivery via nanosized niosomal vesicles: Formulation development, in vitro and in vivo evaluation of skin deposition. *Int. J. Pharm.* **2017**, *517*, 256–268. [CrossRef] [PubMed]
53. Zhang, Y.; Zhang, K.; Wu, Z.; Guo, T.; Ye, B.; Lu, M.; Zhao, J.; Zhu, C.; Feng, N. Evaluation of transdermal salidroside delivery using niosomes via in vitro cellular uptake. *Int. J. Pharm.* **2015**, *478*, 138–146. [CrossRef] [PubMed]
54. Priprem, A.; Janpim, K.; Nualkaew, S.; Mahakunakorn, P. Topical Niosome Gel of Zingiber cassumunar Roxb. Extract for Anti-inflammatory Activity Enhanced Skin Permeation and Stability of Compound D. *AAPS PharmSciTech* **2015**, *17*, 631–639. [CrossRef] [PubMed]
55. Jiang, T.; Wang, T.; Li, T.; Ma, Y.; Shen, S.; He, B.; Mo, R. Enhanced Transdermal Drug Delivery by Transfersome-Embedded Oligopeptide Hydrogel for Topical Chemotherapy of Melanoma. *ACS Nano* **2018**, *12*, 9693–9701. [CrossRef] [PubMed]
56. Muzzalupo, R.; Tavano, L.; Cassano, R.; Trombino, S.; Ferrarelli, T.; Picci, N. A new approach for the evaluation of niosomes as effective transdermal drug delivery systems. *Eur. J. Pharm. Biopharm.* **2011**, *79*, 28–35. [CrossRef] [PubMed]
57. Xu, G.; Gu, H.; Hu, B.; Tong, F.; Liu, D.; Yu, X.; Zheng, X.; Gu, J. PEG-b-(PELG-g-PLL) nanoparticles as TNF-α nanocarriers: Potential cerebral ischemia/reperfusion injury therapeutic applications. *Int. J. Nanomed.* **2017**, *12*, 2243–2254. [CrossRef]
58. Amjadi, S.; Mesgari, A.M.; Shokouhi, B.; Ghorbani, M.; Hamishehkar, H. Enhancement of therapeutic efficacy of betanin for diabetes treatment by liposomal nanocarriers. *J. Funct. Foods* **2019**, *59*, 119–128. [CrossRef]
59. Ahsanuddin, S.; Lam, M.; Baron, E.D. Skin aging and oxidative stress. *AIMS Mol. Sci.* **2016**, *3*, 187–195. [CrossRef]
60. Bernatoniene, J.; Kopustinskiene, D.M.K. The Role of Catechins in Cellular Responses to Oxidative Stress. *Molecules* **2018**, *23*, 965. [CrossRef] [PubMed]
61. Katiyar, S.K.; Afaq, F.; Azizuddin, K.; Mukhtar, H. Inhibition of UVB-Induced Oxidative Stress-Mediated Phosphorylation of Mitogen-Activated Protein Kinase Signaling Pathways in Cultured Human Epidermal Keratinocytes by Green Tea Polyphenol (−)-Epigallocatechin-3-gallate. *Toxicol. Appl. Pharmacol.* **2001**, *176*, 110–117. [CrossRef]

62. Shaker, D.S.; Shaker, M.A.; Hanafy, M.S. Cellular uptake, cytotoxicity and in-vivo evaluation of Tamoxifen citrate loaded niosomes. *Int. J. Pharm.* **2015**, *493*, 285–294. [CrossRef] [PubMed]
63. Canton, I.; Battaglia, G. Endocytosis at the nanoscale. *Chem. Soc. Rev.* **2012**, *41*, 2718–2739. [CrossRef] [PubMed]
64. Hillaireau, H.; Couvreur, P. Nanocarriers' entry into the cell: Relevance to drug delivery. *Cell Mol. Life Sci.* **2009**, *66*, 2873–2896. [CrossRef] [PubMed]
65. Abdel-Bar, H.M.; Basset, S.; Rania, A. Endocytic pathways of optimized resveratrol cubosomes capturing into human hepatoma cells. *Biomed. Pharm.* **2017**, *93*, 561–569. [CrossRef] [PubMed]
66. Santiwarangkool, S.; Akita, H.; Khaalil, I.A.; Abd, E.M.; Sato, Y.; Kusumoto, K.; Harashima, H. A study of the endocytosis mechanism and transendothelial activity of lung-targeted GALA-modified liposomes. *J. Control. Release* **2019**, *307*, 55–63. [CrossRef] [PubMed]

pharmaceutics

Review

Dissolution and Absorption of Inhaled Drug Particles in the Lungs

Basanth Babu Eedara [1,2], Rakesh Bastola [1] and Shyamal C. Das [1,*]

[1] School of Pharmacy, University of Otago, Dunedin 9054, New Zealand
[2] Center for Translational Science, Florida International University, Port St. Lucie, FL 34987, USA
* Correspondence: shyamal.das@otago.ac.nz

Abstract: Dry powder inhalation therapy has been effective in treating localized lung diseases such asthma, chronic obstructive pulmonary diseases (COPD), cystic fibrosis and lung infections. In vitro characterization of dry powder formulations includes the determination of physicochemical nature and aerosol performance of powder particles. The relationship between particle properties (size, shape, surface morphology, porosity, solid state nature, and surface hydrophobicity) and aerosol performance of an inhalable dry powder formulation has been well established. However, unlike oral formulations, there is no standard dissolution method for evaluating the dissolution behavior of the inhalable dry powder particles in the lungs. This review focuses on various dissolution systems and absorption models, which have been developed to evaluate dry powder formulations. It covers a summary of airway epithelium, hurdles to developing an in vitro dissolution method for the inhaled dry powder particles, fine particle dose collection methods, various in vitro dissolution testing methods developed for dry powder particles, and models commonly used to study absorption of inhaled drug.

Keywords: dissolution; absorption; inhalation; dry powders; fine particle dose

Citation: Eedara, B.B.; Bastola, R.; Das, S.C. Dissolution and Absorption of Inhaled Drug Particles in the Lungs. *Pharmaceutics* **2022**, *14*, 2667. https://doi.org/10.3390/pharmaceutics14122667

Academic Editors: Yuan Huang and Jingyuan Wen

Received: 30 September 2022
Accepted: 25 November 2022
Published: 30 November 2022

1. Introduction

Although pulmonary drug delivery by inhalation has been used for many years, research in dry powder inhalers (DPIs) has undergone rapid advancements during the last decade for both local and systemic delivery of drugs [1–4]. DPIs are monophasic solid particulate mixtures, introduced in the 1970s. DPIs are easy to process, portable, more stable, eco-friendly due to the absence of propellants, patient compliance and cost-effective [5–10]. Most of the DPIs available in the market are suffering from short residence time and low drug bioavailability locally in the lungs, resulting in suboptimal local therapeutic effect [11,12].

The rapid dissolution of micron-sized particles and subsequent absorption of the drug into the systemic circulation is one of the clearance mechanisms of inhaled drug particles from the lungs [13–15]. Therefore, many formulation strategies have been followed to prolong the residence time of inhaled drugs at the site of action with reduced dosing and to avoid unwanted toxicities [16,17]. Some of the approaches to prolong the residence time of the inhaled drug particles in the lung are drug encapsulation in a particulate carrier system (liposomes, polymeric and lipid microparticles), increase the molecular mass of the drug by conjugating with a ligand and decrease the solubility of the drug by conjugation with a low water-soluble, hydrophobic material [18].

In vitro dissolution testing is a traditional and standardized quality control tool in all the pharmacopoeias used to evaluate the batch-to-batch consistency, differentiate immediate and controlled release formulations and also to approximate in vivo release profiles [19]. There are many well-established pharmacopeial dissolution methods for oral solid dosage forms, however, there is no accepted standardized method for inhaled products, although many dissolution methods for testing aerosols have been developed [20–28].

This review describes the dissolution of inhaled respirable size particles and absorption of dissolved drug through lung epithelium. It covers a summary of airway epithelium, hurdles to develop an in vitro dissolution method for the inhaled dry powder particles, fine particle dose collection methods, various in vitro dissolution testing methods developed for dry powder particles, and various models commonly used to study the absorption of inhaled drugs.

2. Airway Epithelium

Dense core-granulated cells, basal cells, Clara cells, serous cells, ciliated cells, and mucus goblet cells are six distinct cell types present in the epithelium of the respiratory tract (Figure 1). At all levels of the airway, ciliated cells are the most abundant cells. Their primary function is to propel mucus towards the proximal direction, in simple term the process is known as mucociliary clearance. The ciliated cells in the bronchial pseudostratified epithelium are interspersed by secretory cells (mainly mucus-secreting goblet cells), whereas ciliated cells are interspersed mainly by Clara cells in the bronchiolar cuboidal epithelium. Two types of pneumocytes namely, type I and type II pneumocyte alveolar cells are found in the alveolar squamous epithelium (Figure 1). The luminal surface of the alveoli is mainly lined with alveolar type I cells. In addition, alveoli contain alveolar type II pneumocytes that possess microvilli and are cuboidal secretory cells [29]. Epithelial cells in the airway contribute to the secretion of respiratory tract lining fluid (RTLF) that lies on the surfaces of airways from nasal airways to alveolar regions [30]. RTLF is mainly composed of mucins in the conducting airways (trachea, bronchi, bronchioles and terminal bronchioles) whereas it mainly contains phospholipid-rich surfactants in respiratory zone (respiratory bronchioles, alveolar ducts and alveolar sacs) [31].

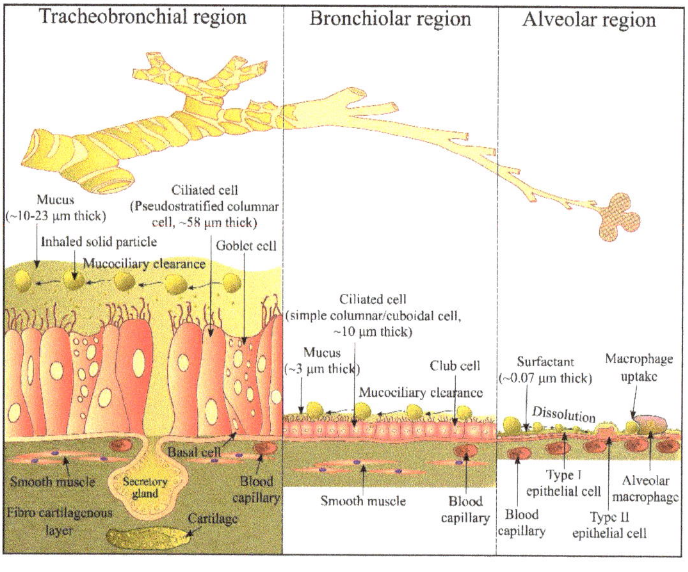

Figure 1. Comparison of the tracheobronchial, bronchiolar and alveolar regions of the lungs [32]. Reproduced with permission from Ref. [32]. 2015, McGraw Hill.

Particles inhaled in the respiratory tract have to overcome the non-epithelial pulmonary barriers (such as RTLF, mucociliary clearance, macrophage uptake) before they come in contact with the epithelial cells. Different types of transport systems occur in the epithelium of the airways such as paracellular transport, receptor-mediated transport and transporter-mediated transport [33]. Such transport systems translocate inhaled particles into epithelial cells and/or across the epithelia into the interstitium and to the blood and lymph [34].

3. In Vitro Dissolution Testing of Inhalable Dry Powder Particles

In vitro characterization of dry powder formulations includes the determination of physicochemical nature and aerosol performance of powder particles. The relationship between particle properties (size, shape, surface morphology, porosity, solid state nature, and surface hydrophobicity) and aerosol performance of an inhalable dry powder formulation has been well established [18,35–38]. However, unlike oral formulations, there is no standard dissolution method for evaluating the dissolution behaviour of the inhalable dry powder particles in the lungs.

3.1. Hurdles to Develop an In Vitro Dissolution Method for Inhalable Dry Powder Particles

One region of the lung differs from another in its anatomy and physiology (Figure 1). In addition, the RTLF where the inhaled particles dissolve varies regionally in composition, thickness and volume. A mucus gel (~3–23 μm) covers the airway region (trachea, bronchi, bronchioles) of the lungs over an area of 1–2 m^2. Composition of the mucus gel includes 95% of water, 2–3% of mucins, 0.3–0.5% lipids, 0.1–0.5% non-mucin proteins and other cellular debris [39,40]. However, an extremely thin (estimated thickness ~0.07 μm) film of the lung surfactant covers the alveolar region (>100 m^2) of the lungs. Lung surfactant contains 90.0% lipids (85.0% phospholipids: dipalmitoyl phosphatidylcholine (47.0%), unsaturated phosphatidylcholine (29.3%) and other lipids (23.7%); 5.0% neutral lipids: cholesterol) and 10.0% proteins (surfactant protein-SP) [41–43]. Hydrophilic SP comprises 3–5% SP-A, and <0.5% SP-D whereas hydrophobic SP contains 0.5–1.0% of SP-B and SP-C each. Gradual decrease in the thickness and volume of the RTLF along a respiratory tract is a major challenge for the development of an in vitro dissolution method that can accurately mimic the conditions of the lungs.

3.2. Fine Particle Dose (FPD) Collection

During inhalation, only a fine particle dose (FPD) with the particle size 1–5 μm deposits in the deeper lung regions [44,45]. Therefore, estimation of the FPD dissolution profile seems to be more applicable than the whole dose of the powder formulation. To this end, the Andersen Cascade Impactor (ACI), Next Generation Impactor (NGI), Twin Stage Impinger (TSI) and PreciseInhale system (Figure 2) have been used to collect the fine particle dose (FPD). Table 1 summarizes the FPD collection methods for dissolution testing of respirable particles.

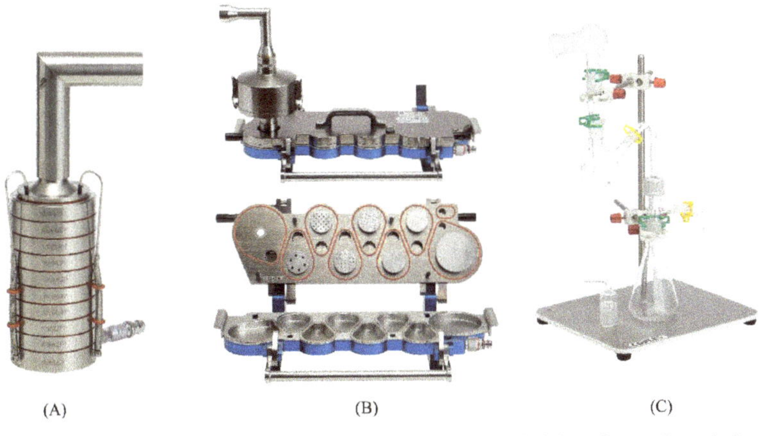

(A) (B) (C)

Figure 2. Various approaches to collect fine particle dose (FPD). (**A**) Andersen Cascade Impactor (ACI), (**B**) Next Generation Impactor (NGI; top- closed view and bottom- open view of NGI), and (**C**) Twin Stage Impinger (TSI). Figures (**A–C**) were reproduced with permission from Driving Results in Inhaler Testing [Brochure, 2020 edition] [46], Copley Scientific Limited.

Table 1. Summary of the fine particle dose (FPD) collection methods for dissolution testing of dry powder particles.

Apparatus	Drugs	Inhaler and Loading Dose	Collection Method	Ref.
Andersen Cascade Impactor (ACI)	Budesonide (BD), Fluticasone propionate (FP), Triamcinolone acetonide (TA)	Pulmicort Turbuhaler, BD, 200 μg Flixotide Accuhaler®, FP, 250 μg Azmacort®, TA, 200 μg	Collected onto a GF filter at the connection point of the induction port and inlet of ACI	[21]
	Flunisolide (FN), TA, BD, FP, Beclomethasone dipropionate (BDP)	Aerobid®, FN, 250–2500 μg Azmacort®, TA, 200–2000 μg Pulmicort Turbuhaler®, BD, 50–500 μg Flovent® HFA and Diskus, FP, 150–1250 μg Vanceril® and QVAR® (BDP, 350–700 μg)	Collected onto 6 PVDF membranes placed at the stage 4 of ACI operated at an air flow of 28.3 L/min	[20]
	BD, Fenoterol HBr (FNH), Substance A dibromide (SAD), Substance A crystalline base (SAC), Substance A amorphous base (SAA)	Micronized BD, FN, SAD and SAC; spray dried SA (SAA) HandiHaler® (1 mg (BD, SA) 10 mg (FN))	Collected onto the RC membrane (pore size 0.45 μm) at standard USP conditions (4 kPa, 4 L)	[25]
	BD, SAD, SAC, SAA	Micronized BD, SAD and SAC; spray dried SA (SAA) HandiHaler® (0.5 to 4 mg)	Collected onto the RC membrane at standard USP conditions (4 kPa, 4 L) using ACI with stage extension between stage 1 and filter stage, and modified/standard filter stage	[47]
	BD, SAD, SAC, SAA	Micronized BD, SAD and SAC; spray dried SA (SAA) HandiHaler® (0.5 to 4 mg)	Collected onto the PE, PC, IPC and RC membranes at standard USP conditions (4 kPa, 4 L) using ACI with stage extension between stage 1 and F, and modified/standard filter stage	[48]
	BD, Ciclesonide (CIC), FP	Symbicort® (BD) Alvesco® (CIC) Flixotide® (FP), (5 doses (BD-80 μg/dose, CIC-60 μg/dose and FP-110 μg/dose))	Collected onto the 24 mm GF filters or Fisherbrand Q8 filter papers at the stage 4 of ACI at an air flow of 28.3 L/min	[26]
	Salbutamol sulfate (SS), FP, Salmeterol xinafoate (SX)	Micronized SS blend, Rotahaler® (6–10 doses (2% w/w SS blend, 30 mg/dose) Seretide® 50/100 Diskus® (FP and SX, 50 μg SX and 100 μg FP/dose))	Collected onto an adhesive tape using the truncated ACI with a PTFE funnel and a collection plate at the filter stage (Stage F) operated at a pressure drop of 4 kPa at 60 L/min air flow rate	[49]
Next Generation Impactor (NGI)	Hydrocortisone (HC)	Bulk HC (50 mg) micronized HC blend Aerolizer® (150 mg micronized HC blend, ~10 mg of HC)	Collected onto the PC (0.05 μm) and CA (MWCO 3500, 12,000) at each dose plate of NGI	[28]
	Albuterol sulfate (AS), BD	Ventolin HFA® (AS,15–20 doses) Pulmicort Flexhaler® (BD, 1–10 doses)	Collected onto the impaction inserts at stage 2–5 of NGI at 30 L/min (AS) or 60 L/min (BD) air flow rate	[50]
	Rifampicin (RIF)	Microparticles; Aerolizer® (7 mg to 20 mg)	Collected onto the impaction insert at stage 3 of NGI operated at 60 L/min air flow rate for 4 s	[51]
	Itraconazole (ITZ)	Spray dried solid dispersions, Axahaler®	Collected onto the impaction inserts at each dose plate of NGI operated at 60 L/min air flow rate	[52]
	Tobramycin Clarithromycin	Nanoparticulate spray dried powders (TCn2), Physical blend (TCb), Axahaler®	Collected onto the impaction insert at stage 3 of NGI operated at 100 L/min air flow rate	[53]
	Pyrazinamide (PYR), RIF, Isoniazid (IZD)	Spray dried powders, Aerolizer® (Two 20 mg doses)	Collected onto a NC membrane at stage 3 of NGI operated at 100 L/min air flow rate	[54]
	FP	Flixotide® (FP, 5 doses of 110 μg/dose)	Collected onto the 24 mm Fisherbrand Q8 filter papers at stage 2 and 4 of NGI	[26]

Table 1. *Cont.*

Apparatus	Drugs	Inhaler and Loading Dose	Collection Method	Ref.
Twin Stage Impinger (TSI)	Dextrans labelled with fluorescein isothiocyanate (FITC-dex; 4, 10, 20, 40 and 70 kDa)	A custom-made glass dry powder insufflator (5 mg)	Collected onto the Calu-3 bronchial epithelial cells in a Transwell® insert using TSI at 60 L/min air flow rate for 5 s	[55]
	BDP	QVAR® and Sanasthmax® (100–250 µg/dose; 1.2 ± 0.12 mg deposited)	Collected on a NC membrane (0.45 µm) at stage 2 of a modified TSI	[56]
	Salbutamol base (SB), SS	Micronized SB and SS (5 mg)	Collected onto a Transwell® PE insert (0.4 µm) using modified TSI at 60 L/min air flow rate for 4 s	[57]
	Moxifloxacin Ethionamide	Aerolizer® device (20 mg)	Collected on a glass coverslip at 60 L/min air flow rate for 4 s	[58]
PreciseInhale system	BD, FP	Micronized powders (2.5 mg)	Collected onto the glass coverslips of 13 mm diameter at 1.2 L/min air flow rate	[23, 59]

CA—cellulose acetate; GF—glass fibre; IPC—isopore polycarbonate; NC—nitrocellulose; PC—polycarbonate; PE—polyester; PTFE—polytetra fluoroethylene; PVDF—polyvinylidene difluoride; RC—regenerated cellulose; USP—united states pharmacopoeia.

3.2.1. Andersen Cascade Impactor (ACI)

The Andersen cascade impactor (ACI, Figure 2A) is one of the high flow rate cascade impactors used to assess the aerodynamic size distribution of particles for both pharmaceutical and toxicological applications [60]. It consists of a standard tubular induction port (IP) with a 90° curvature, stages from 0–7 and a filter stage (stage-F). Each impactor stage comprises several nozzles with a decreasing size as the stage number increases, which directs air and particles onto the collection plates.

Davies and Feddah, 2003 [21] collected dry powder particles onto a glass fibre filter at the connection point of the induction port and inlet part of ACI using a custom designed stainless steel ring with a stainless steel screen support filter. The ACI assembly consists of an induction port and base of the impactor with only stage number zero. The main drawback of this collection method is that the whole emitted dose is collected over the filter, which does not mimic the size of the particles deposited in the deeper lung regions.

Later, Arora et al., 2010 [20] collected aerodynamically classified particles with diameters of 4.7–5.8 µm and 2.1–3.3 µm on the filter membranes from stage 2 and stage 4 of ACI. In this study, they used a 8-stage ACI with stage 2 and stage 4 collecting plates turned upside down to arrange six polyvinylidene difluoride (PVDF) filter membranes (25 mm in diameter; 0.22 µm pore size) for dose collection.

In another study, May et al., 2012 [25] collected particles onto the regenerated cellulose membrane filters at stage-F of an abbreviated ACI. In this study, the ACI assembly consisted of an induction port, pre-separator, stages 0, 1 and F. Later they modified this assembly by adding a cylindrical stage extension of 5.8 cm in between stage 1 and stage-F to attain a homogenous particle distribution on the membrane [47]. Further, a modified filter stage comprising of only three small bars was used to change the flow and deposition pattern of aerosolized particles. The modifications in ACI resulted in homogenous deposition of particles on the membrane compared to unmodified ACI.

Rohrschneider et al., 2015 [26], collected aerosolized particles onto the filter papers positioned at stage 4 of an 8-stage ACI connected to an external humidifier to maintain the humidity.

3.2.2. Next Generation Impactor (NGI)

Next generation impactor (NGI, Figure 2B) is a high flow rate cascade impactor specially designed for pharmaceutical inhaler testing. NGI was constructed with seven distinct stages plus a micro-orifice collector (MOC, a final filter) with a minimum stage overlap. The airflow passes with increasing velocity in a saw tooth pattern through a series of nozzles containing progressively reducing jet diameters. Out of seven, five stages give a particle size cut-off diameter of 0.54–6.13 μm at flow rates from 30 to 100 L min^{-1}.

Son et al., 2009 [28], collected aerodynamically separated particles on a polycarbonate membrane (PC) using a modified NGI. At each collection plate of NGI, a polycarbonate (PC) membrane was placed and covered with a plate-shaped wax paper which consists of a rectangular opening (2.0 × 2.5 cm) at the centre. The powder samples were dispersed into the NGI using an Aerolizer® device at an air flow rate of 60 L min^{-1} for 15 s per capsule. The limited size of the prototype holder frame only collects a fraction of powder particles over a rectangular area of the membrane. To overcome this, they designed a special membrane holder which fit in with the NGI cup and collected the whole dispersed particles [51,61]. However, the particles collected using the NGI either with a prototype holder frame or a special membrane holder were not homogenously distributed over the membrane.

3.2.3. Twin Stage Impinger (TSI)

The Twin stage impinger (TSI, Figure 2C) is a simplified device to multistage liquid impinger with only two stages. It was developed to assess drug delivery from meter dose inhalers. TSI is made up of a series of glassware components such as an inlet, a glass bulb which simulates oropharynx, upper (stage 1) and lower (stage 2) impinger stages. TSI separates the actuated aerosol into a coarse oropharyngeal fraction (non-respirable fraction) and a fine pulmonary fraction with an aerodynamic diameter of ≤6.4 μm [60].

Grainger et al., 2009 [55] modified the TSI (mTSI) to deposit the respirable particles of dextrans onto the Calu-3 bronchial epithelial cells in a Transwell® insert. A Transwell® insert containing the cells was attached in the place of an adapter piece to the TSI conducting tube in the lower stage without any medium. The powder (~5 mg) was loaded into the dry powder insufflator and aerosolised at 60 L min^{-1} air flow rate for 5 s. The particles collected using the TSI are homogenously distributed with a geometric diameter of <6.4 μm. Later they used the same mTSI to collect the beclomethasone dipropionate (BDP) respirable particles for in vitro dissolution testing [56]. The BDP particles emitted from each of the commercial pressurized metered dose inhalers [pMDI): QVAR and Sanasthmax, were collected (1.2 ± 0.12 mg) on a hydrated nitrocellulose membrane (0.45 μm pore size).

Haghi et al., 2012 [57] collected the micronized salbutamol base (SB) and salbutamol sulfate (SS) particles using the mTSI as described by Grainger et al., 2009 [55] for in vitro dissolution studies using the Franz cell. Five milligrams of powder sample was actuated using a Cyclohaler DPI device at 60 L min^{-1} for 4 s. The emitted particles were collected in a Transwell® polyester insert (0.4 μm pore size and 0.33 cm^2 area) at stage-2 of mTSI.

Eedara et al., 2019 [62] modified the stage 2 (lower impingement chamber) of TSI (mTSI, Figure 3) with a screw cap at its bottom to collect aerosolized powder particles onto the glass coverslips. Magnetic passe-partouts were used to hold glass coverslip (24 mm diameter) in position as it makes a boundary to collect the particles over an area of ~200 mm^2 (16 mm diameter) during aerosolization. Hard gelatin PEG capsule (size 3; Qualicaps, Osaka, Japan) was used to fill the drug powders (20 mg). Capsule was dispersed using an Aerolizer® device (Novartis, Surrey, UK) at a flow rate of 60 L min^{-1} for 4 s into stage 1 (upper impingement chamber) filled with 7 mL of water. The non-respirable fraction of dose gets separated in the stage 1 of TSI. Three capsules were actuated one after another and the mTSI was disassembled to collect coverslips with deposited powders.

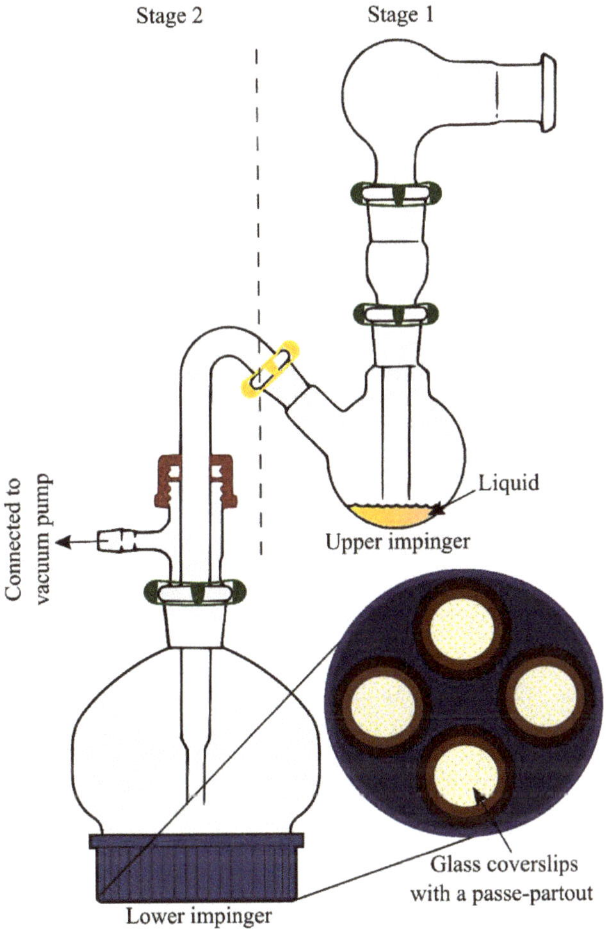

Figure 3. A modified Twin Stage Impinger (mTSI) to collect fine particle dose (FPD). Reproduced with permission from Eedara et al., 2019 [62], Springer Nature.

In a recent study, a modified version of Twin Stage Impinger and in vitro dissolution experiment were used to examine in vitro in vivo correlation of budesonide and salbutamol. Comparison using both the actual and predicted in vivo pharmacokinetic values of the mentioned drugs and the pattern of their Concentration-Time profiles illustrated a good similarity [63].

3.2.4. PreciseInhale System

The PreciseInhale system (Inhalation Sciences, Sweden) is a new aerosol delivery technique that is able to generate a dry powder aerosol in a free flowing state [64]. This system is a combination of a highly efficient aerosol generator and a precision dosing aerosol exposure unit. In brief, the powder to be aerosolized is placed in a powder chamber and suspended in a compressed gas passing from a pressure chamber to the powder chamber. The suspended powder agglomerates in the powder chamber ejects through the narrow conduit into a holding chamber with an ambient pressure and produces an aerosol cloud of deagglomerated particles. The aerosol of deagglomerated particles is transferred by airflow to the animal or collected for analysis.

Gerde et al., 2017 [23] collected the aerosolized dry powder particles of budesonide (BD) and fluticasone propionate (FP) on circular microscope glass coverslips using the PreciseInhale aerosol generator for in vitro dissolution testing by the Dissolv*It* system. Nine circular glass coverslips (13 mm diameter) were placed in a ring-shaped holder and covered with a thin steel passe-partout to limit the area of powder coating to the surface that will be in contact with the model barrier during the dissolution study. The coverslips were exposed to a single generation cycle of the powder (2.5 mg) aerosol produced using the PreciseInhale system at an air flow rate of 1.2 L min^{-1}. The amount of drug deposited on the coverslips was in the range from 0.99 to 1.20 mg with a mass median aerodynamic diameter (MMAD) of 1.7 mm for BD and of 3.4 mm for FP.

3.3. *In Vitro Dissolution Methods*

In vitro dissolution studies by conventional dissolution methods using USP apparatus 1 (basket) [65,66] and 2 (paddle) [27,67–69] have several limitations. Primarily these methods provide well-stirred environments contrasting with the in vivo condition in the alveolar region of the lungs. Homogenous dispersion of the particles into the vessel/basket is challenging, and dispersed particles adhere to the dissolution apparatus components and inadvertently enter the aliquots during the sampling procedure. To make up for some of the deficits of commercial USP 1 and 2 dissolution systems, various in vitro dissolution methods using compendial (USP 2) paddle apparatus, flow-through cell apparatus, dialysis bag, Franz diffusion cell, Transwell® and DissolvIt systems (Table 2) have been developed and applied to evaluate the drug release characteristics of the inhaled dry powder even though they are limited in mimicking the in vivo situation.

Table 2. Summary of various in vitro dissolution testing methods for dry powder particles.

Dissolution Apparatus	Membrane (Pore Size, µm or MWCO, kDa)	Dissolution Medium and Conditions	Ref.
USP 1 (basket) apparatus	Glass fiber filters, GF/F grade	PBS, pH 7.4, basket rotation- 150 rpm	[65]
	-	PBS, pH 7.4, 900 mL, basket rotation- 100 rpm	[66]
USP 2 [paddle) apparatus	-	Water, 300 mL, paddle rotation- 50 rpm	[68]
	-	Buffer, pH 1.2 or pH 6.8, 1000 mL, paddle rotation- 100 rpm	[67]
	-	PBS, pH 6.8, 1000 mL, paddle rotation- 50 rpm	[69]
Modified USP 2 (paddle over disc) apparatus	-	PBS, pH 7.4, 1000 mL, paddle rotation- 50 rpm	[27]
	Polycarbonate membranes (0.05 and 1 µm) Cellulose acetate membranes (3.5, 12 kDa)	SLF and modified SLF with DPPC (0.02% *w*/*v*), pH 7.4, 100 mL, paddle rotation- 50 rpm	[28]
	Polycarbonate membrane (0.05 µm)	SLF, 0.2 M PB, pH 7.4, PBS, modified PBS with DPPC, tween 80 (0.02 and 0.2% *w*/*v*), pH 7.4, 300 mL, paddle rotation- 50, 75, 100 rpm	[50]
	Polycarbonate membrane (0.05 µm)	PBS, pH 7.4 or 0.2 M citrate buffer with ascorbic acid (0.02% *w*/*v*), pH 5.2, 300 mL, paddle rotation- 75 rpm	[51]
	Polycarbonate membrane (0.4 µm)	Water with SLS (0.3%), buffer, pH 1.2, 300 mL, paddle rotation- 75 rpm	[52]
	Regenerated cellulose membrane (0.45 µm)	PBS, pH 7.4, 1000 mL, paddle rotation- 50, 100, and 140 rpm	[25,47]
	Polycarbonate membrane (0.4 µm)	PBS, pH 7.4, 300 mL, paddle rotation- 75 rpm	[53,70]
	Dialysis membrane (>900 kDa)	Gamble's solution, pH 7.4 and alveolar lung fluid, pH 4.5, 900 mL, paddle rotation- 150 rpm	[71]
	-	Modified SLF with tween 80 (0.2% *v*/*v*), 50 mL; paddle rotation- 50 rpm	[49]

Table 2. *Cont.*

Dissolution Apparatus	Membrane (Pore Size, μm or MWCO, kDa)	Dissolution Medium and Conditions	Ref.
Dialysis bag	Dialysis membrane (12 kDa)	10 mM PBS with tween 80 (0.1% *v/v*), pH 7.4, 20 mL, rotation- 900 rpm	[72]
	Dialysis membrane (12–14 kDa)	SLF, pH 7.4, 50 mL	[73]
	Dialysis membrane (12–14 kDa)	SLF, pH 7.4, 30 mL,	[74]
	Dialysis membrane (14 kDa)	PBS, pH 7.4, 250 mL, rotation- 100 rpm	[75]
Flow-through cell system	Cellulose acetate membrane (0.45 μm)	SLF, modified SLF with DPPC (0.02% *w/v*), flow rate- 0.7 mL/min,	[21]
	-	Deionized water, pH 5.5, medium flow rate- 5–16 mL/min,	[76]
	Nitrocellulose membrane (0.45 μm)	0.05 M PBS, pH 7.4, 1000 mL, medium flow rate- 0.5 mL/min	[27]
	Regenerated cellulose membrane (0.45 μm)	PBS, pH 7.4, medium flow rate- 0.5 mL/min	[25]
Franz diffusion cell	Nylon membrane (0.45 μm)	Degassed 0.05 M PB, pH 7.4, 17.5 mL, rotation- 240 rpm	[77]
	Nitrocellulose membrane (0.45 μm)	0.05 M PBS, pH 7.4, 1000 mL, medium flow rate- 5 mL/min	[27]
	MF™ membrane (0.45 μm)	PB, pH 7.4, 250 mL, medium flow rate- 5 mL/min	[78]
	Nitrocellulose membrane (0.45 μm)	PB, pH 7.4 containing 0.1% *w/v* SDS	[56]
	Polyester membrane (0.4 μm)	HBSS or SLF with DPPC (0.02% *w/v*), 50 mL, medium flow rate- 5 mL/min	[57]
	Regenerated cellulose membrane (0.45 μm)	PBS, pH 7.4, 1000 mL, magnet rotation- 100 rpm	[25]
	Regenerated cellulose membrane (0.45 μm)	Water, PB, pH 7.4, or modified SLF, pH 7.4, 10 mL, 75 rpm	[79]
	Cellulose acetate membrane (0.2 μm)	0.05 M degassed PB, pH 7.4, or SLF, 0.15 mL in donor compartment and 27 mL in receiver compartment	[80]
	Nitrocellulose membrane (0.45 μm)	SLF, pH 7.4, 22.7 mL	[54]
	Polycarbonate membrane (0.4 μm)	SLF with SDS (0.5% *w/v*), 4.2 mL	[81]
	Filter paper	PBS, pH 7.4, 21.5 mL	[82]
Transwell® system	Polyester membrane (0.4 μm)	PBS, pH 7.4 or distilled deionized water, pH 7.0, 0.04 mL in donor compartment and 1.4 mL in well plate	[20]
	Polycarbonate membrane (0.4 μm) or Polyester membrane (0.4 μm)	PBS, pH 7.4, 2.6 mL or 3.85 mL	[48]
	Polyester membrane (0.4 μm)	PBS with SDS (0.5% *w/v*), 0.1 mL in donor compartment and 1.5 mL in well plate	[26]
Dissolvit®	Polycarbonate membranes (0.03 μm)	1.5% *w/v* PEO in 0.1 M PB with DPPC (0.02 and 0.4% *w/w*)	[23]
Custom-made flow perfusion cell	dialysis membrane (MWCO = 12,400 Da)	1.0, 1.5, 2.0% *w/v* PEO in PBS, pH 7.4 1.5% *w/v* PEO in PBS, pH 7.4 with Curosurf®	[58]

DPPC—di-palmitoylphosphatidylcholine; HBSS—Hanks balanced salt solution; PB—phosphate buffer; PBS—phosphate-buffered saline; PEO—polyethylene oxide; SDS—sodium dodecyl sulfate; SLF—simulated lung fluid; SLS—sodium lauryl sulfate.

3.3.1. Modified USP 2 (Paddle over Disc) Apparatus

The paddle-over-disc dissolution setup consists of a round bottom glass vessel of 150 mL capacity with rotating mini-paddles and a membrane cassette. The membrane cassette is a powder holding device contains two membranes with sandwiched powder particles inside a modified histology cassette frame. Son and McConville 2009 [28], evaluated the dissolution properties of hydrocortisone inhalable powders using a mini-paddle dissolution apparatus containing a membrane cassette (Figure 4). Aerodynamically classified particles collected over a polycarbonate membrane (PC) using NGI were sandwiched using another pre-soaked PC membrane and inserted into the cassette frame. Then, this membrane cassette was placed into a dissolution vessel containing 100 mL of dissolution medium (SLF and mSLF; 37 °C), and drug release was evaluated at a paddle rotation speed of 50 rpm. In this method, the sandwiched dispersed particles in the membrane cassette undergo dissolution in the small volumes of the medium that enters through the pores in the membrane followed by diffusion of the dissolved drug into the bulk reservoir medium. This new method of dissolution studies showed a significant difference in the dissolution profiles between bulk hydrocortisone (HC) and an aerodynamically classified HC. However, the dissolution tests were performed for only a portion of dose collected on the rectangular portion of the membrane due to the holder frame limitations.

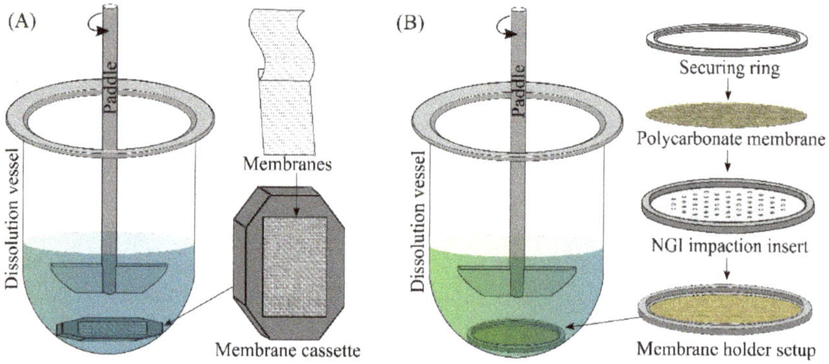

Figure 4. Schematic of paddle-over-disc apparatus with (**A**) membrane cassette, (**B**) NGI membrane holder. (**A**) reproduced with permission from Son and McConville 2009 [28], Elsevier. (**B**) reproduced with permission from Son et al., 2010 [50] Dissolution Technologies, Inc.

Later this research group designed a new, easy to use membrane holder (Figure 4B) to evaluate the dissolution behaviour of the whole dose collected in each NGI plate [50,51]. This new membrane holder consists of a NGI dissolution cup with a removable impaction insert, a securing ring, two sealing o-rings, and a PC membrane. A pre-soaked PC membrane was placed over the impaction insert with dispersed particles and secured in the designed membrane holder. The secured membrane holder with sandwiched particles was transferred into the dissolution vessel containing 300 mL of dissolution medium with membrane side up facing the rotating paddle.

3.3.2. Dialysis Bag

Dialysis is a separation technique which works by diffusion, a process that results from the thermal motion of molecules in solution from a region of higher to lower concentration until an equilibrium is reached. A dialysis bag made of a semipermeable membrane and had small pores. The bag filled with solid dry powder particles is suspended in a dialysate medium (Figure 5A). The large dry powder particles cannot pass through the pores of the membrane. Upon dissolution of the dry powder particles, the drug molecules are small enough to diffuse through the pores of the membrane into the dialysate medium.

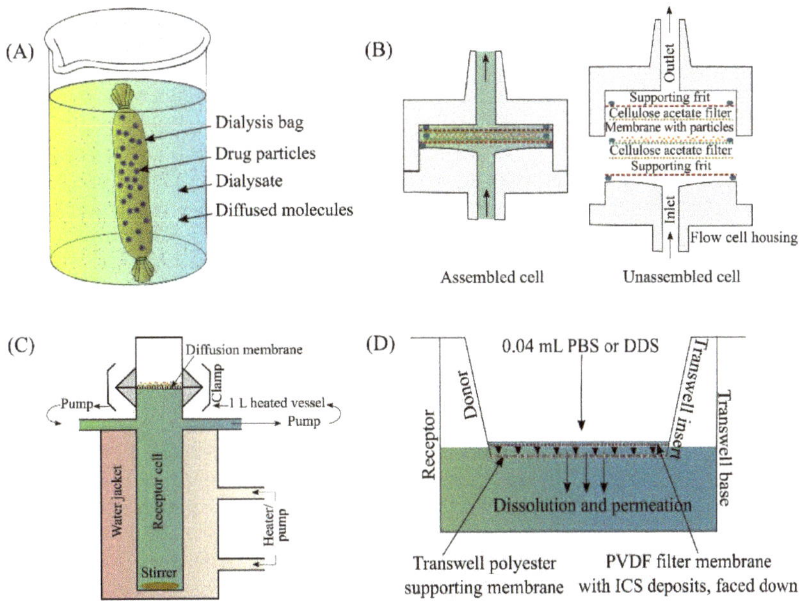

Figure 5. Schematic diagrams of (**A**) dialysis bag method, (**B**) flow-through cell [21], (**C**) Franz diffusion cell [27] and (**D**) Transwell® system [20].. (**B**) reproduced with permission from Davies and Feddah 2003 [21], Elsevier. (**C**) reproduced with permission from Salama et al., 2008 [27], Elsevier. (**D**) reproduced with permission from Arora et al., 2010 [20], Springer Nature.

Arora et al., 2015 [72] investigated the voriconazole release from the polylactide microparticles by the dialysis bag (MWCO: 12 kDa) method using 20 mL of phosphate-buffered saline (pH 7.4, 10 mM) containing 0.1% Tween 80 at 37 ± 0.5 °C and 900 rpm. Several other researchers also used dialysis bag method to evaluate the drug release from dry powder particles [73–75].

3.3.3. Flow-Through Cell Apparatus

The flow-through dissolution system (Figure 5B) was introduced in 1957 as a flowing medium dissolution apparatus [83] and in 1990, it was officially accepted by the United States, and European Pharmacopoeia for the evaluation of drug release behaviour from various dosage forms. The flow-through cell apparatus is a modified USP apparatus 4 which comprises a filter holder containing a membrane with the loaded powder particles and a pump that forces the dissolution medium from a reservoir into a vertically positioned flow cell. The flow-through system has several advantages: maintenance of sink conditions by the continuous flow of fresh medium; reduced influence of diffusion during dissolution testing [84].

Kanapilly et al., 1973 [85] evaluated the in vitro dissolution patterns of radioactive aerosol particles using two flowing systems (a flow-through system and parallel flow system) with adjustable solvent flow rates and a static system. In the flow-through systems, the aerosol particles were collected on a 0.8 μm membrane filter (sample filter) using a 7-stage round jet cascade impactor and sandwiched between a 0.1 μm membrane (backup filter) and 0.8 μm membrane filter (top cover filter) in a high-pressure steel filter holder. The solvent was pumped vertically to flow through the top cover filter, sample filter, and the backup filter.

Davies and Feddah 2003 [21] adapted the flow through system for in vitro dissolution testing of dry powder particles. In this study, aerodynamically classified aerosol particles were collected over membrane filters using ACI as described earlier and sandwiched using another membrane with a Teflon ring (1 mm thickness) in between the membranes. These sandwiched membranes were placed into the flow through cell held by two stainless steel support filters at both ends and dissolution medium was pumped at a flow rate of 0.7 mL/min in the upward direction to flow through the particles sandwiched in between the membranes.

Taylor et al., 2006 [76] prepared sustained release respirable spray coated particles of ipratropium bromide and evaluated for in vitro drug release behaviour using a flow-through cell method. In this study, the powder samples were placed directly onto a wire mesh screen and inserted into a flow cell of 22.6 mm in diameter. Deionized water (pH 5.5; 37 °C) was passed through the flow cell using a Sotax CY7 piston pump.

3.3.4. Franz Diffusion Cell

Another method which has been commonly used to investigate the in vitro dissolution of inhaled dry powder particles is the Franz diffusion cell. The Franz diffusion cell consists of two compartments, donor and receptor compartments, separated by a membrane as shown in Figure 5C. The donor compartment is exposed to the air while the receptor compartment filled with dissolution medium. The dissolution medium in the receptor compartment is continuously mixed with a magnetic stir bar. An advantage of the Franz diffusion cell is that it provides an air-liquid interface, as present in the lung [25]. However, in a Franz diffusion cell, it may be difficult to distinguish between dissolution rate and diffusion effects through the membrane [86].

A modified Franz diffusion cell was used by Salama et al. [27] to conduct the dissolution test for controlled released microparticles containing disodium cromoglycate (DSCG) and polyvinyl alcohol (PVA) for inhalation. This study compared several different methods of dissolution and found that a modified Franz diffusion cell was able to discriminate dissolution rates better than the flow through cell and the USP apparatus 2.

In another study, May et al. [25] conducted dissolution studies for unnamed drug substance A dibromide and amorphous base, fenoterol and budesonide in PBS (pH 7.4, 1 L) at 37 °C using a modified Franz diffusion cell. A regenerated cellulose membrane filter with a pore size of 0.45 µm was placed into the membrane holder, with the particles collected using the NGI facing upwards. In contrast to the results of Salama et al. [27], this study found that although the Franz diffusion cell was able to discriminate between substances of different solubilities in the dissolution media, it was not as sensitive and as reproducible as the USP dissolution apparatus 2. They speculated that the possible reasons for the variation in the results might be due to the difference in the method set up, membrane type and thickness, and loading dose.

3.3.5. Transwell® System

The Transwell® system (Figure 5D) consists of an upper (donor compartment) and lower (acceptor compartment) chambers separated by a membrane which is made out of either polyester (PET) or polycarbonate (PC) or collagen coated polytetrafluoroethylene (PTFE). Such systems are used in drug transport studies to characterize the permeability in apical-to-basolateral direction. Due to the lower volume of dissolution medium, the Transwell® system could provide more bio-relevant conditions in comparison to the Franz diffusion cell.

Arora et al., 2010 [20] developed a dissolution method for size classified respirable particles using a Transwell® system with limited volumes of stationary aqueous dissolution medium. Aerodynamically dispersed particles were collected on the filter membrane as reported by Davies and Feddah [21] from stage 4 (2.1–3.3 µm) and stage 2 (4.7–5.8 µm) of compendial Andersen cascade impactor. Then, the filter membranes with deposited aerosol powder were placed with particles facing in the downward direction on a semi-permeable polyester membrane of the Transwell® insert. Immediately after these inserts were transferred into a receptor compartment containing 1.4 mL of dissolution medium, 0.04 mL of the dissolution medium was placed in the donor compartment to initiate the particle dissolution. The system was then placed in an incubator maintained at 37 °C and an aliquot of 0.5 mL was collected (with replacement) from the receptor compartment at different time. At the end of the experiment, the donor compartment was thoroughly washed to recover the undissolved portion of the drug.

Rohrschneider et al., 2015 [26] evaluated the in vitro dissolution behaviour of orally inhalable products using a commercial Transwell® system with polycarbonate membrane and a modified Transwell® system in which polycarbonate membrane was replaced with a glass microfiber filter. In a modified system, incorporating a more permeable membrane, the drug transfer from donor to acceptor compartment was limited by the dissolution of the particles and not by the diffusion through the membrane.

3.3.6. DissolvIt System

Dissolv*It* system (Figure 6) is a recent in vitro dissolution testing method which simultaneously determines the dissolution and absorption of a drug from respirable size dry powder particles [23]. The system consists of a mucus layer (50 μm thick 1.5% *w/v* polyethylene oxide in 0.1 M PBS) on a polycarbonate membrane to mimic the air-blood barrier in the tracheobronchial region of the lung with a blood simulant (0.1 M PBS containing 4% *w/v* albumin) flowing on the other side of the membrane. The fine particle dose (0.99 to 1.20 μg) of respirable size particles was collected on glass coverslips using the PreciseInhale system as discussed in Section 3.2.4. The dissolution behavior of respirable size particles of budesonide and fluticasone propionate was studied by simultaneous observation of particle disappearance under microscope and quantification of drug in the perfusate on the vasular side of the membrane. This new system, in which the blood simulant buffer pumped in singlepass mode through the dissolution cell, enables the generation of in vitro dissolution/absorption curves of drugs from inhaled dry powders.

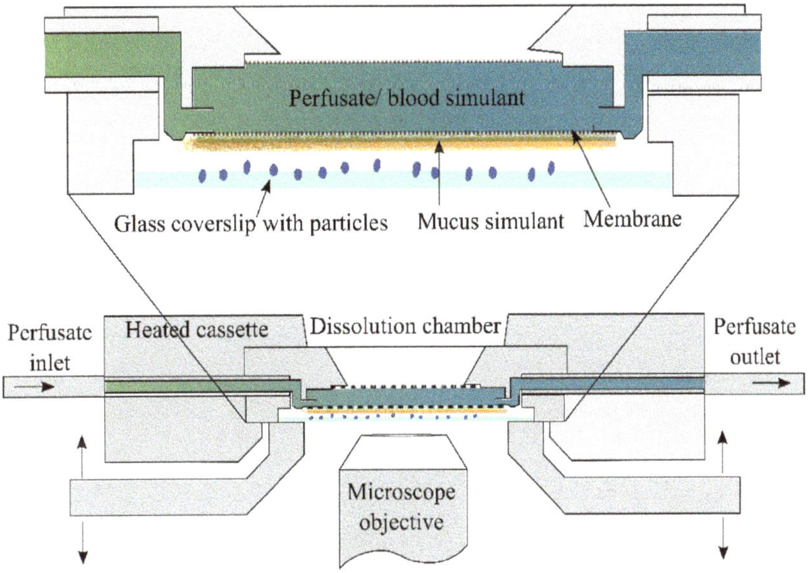

Figure 6. Schematic diagram of DissolvIt® system. Reproduced with permission from Börjel et al., 2014 [59], Respiratory Drug Delivery 2014, Virginia Commonwealth University.

In a recent study, Dissolv*It* system was used to assess the impact of dissolution medium on dissolution of fluticasone proprionate aerosol particles. A synthetic simulated lung lining fluid, 1.5% poly(ethylene oxide) + 0.4% L-alphaphosphatidyl choline and Survanta were three different media used in the Dissolv*It* chamber. It was illustrated that biorelevant dissolution studies can generate input parameters for physiologically based pharmacokinetic modeling of inhaled drug products [87].

3.3.7. Custom Made Flow Perfusion Cell

Eedara et al. [58] custom made a flow perfusion cell which resembles an air-blood perfusion model to evaluate the dissolution behaviour of respirable size particles. The flow perfusion cell was connected to a syringe pump (100 DM syringe pump, Teledyne ISCO, Lincoln, NE, USA) to collecte the perfusate and an optical microscope equipped with a digital camera (OPTIKA SRL, Ponteranica BG, Italy) to capture the images of respirable size particle dissolution [18,58,62,62]. Using this apparatus, the dissolution behaviours of fine particle doses (collected using mTSI) of moxifloxacin and ethionamide in 25 µL of mucus simulant were evaluated. The respirable size particles of moxifloxacin dissolved quickly (<30 min) compared to the ethionamide.

Similarly, Saha et al. conducted in vitro experiments using custom made flow perfusion cell and showed that ~68% of ivermectin got permeated in 30 h from dry powder formulation. The dissolution medium was polyethylene oxide (1.5% *w*/*w*) + Curosurf® (0.4% *w*/*w*) in phosphate-buffered saline (PBS) and Tween 80 (0.2% *w*/*v*) in PBS was perfusate. 50 µL of the dissolution medium was loaded on the apparatus and the flow rate of the perfusate was fixed at 0.05 mL/min [88].

A major drawback of the dialysis bag, Franz-type diffusion cell, Transwell®, Dissolv*It*® and custom made flow perfusion cell methods is that the mass of the drug released into the donor compartment is limited. The advantages and disadvantages/limitations of all the above methods are summarized in Table 3. Even though various dissolution apparatus has been developed for inhaled dry powder particles, maintaining very limited volumes of the dissolution media to simulate the lung conditions is still a challenge. Therefore, the development of a standardized in vitro dissolution method for dry powder particles is still an interesting topic to research.

Table 3. Advantages and disadvantages/limitations of the apparatus used to evaluate the dissolution behaviour of the inhaled products. Reproduced with permissions from Eedara et al., 2019 [58], Elsevier.

Apparatus	Advantages	Disadvantages/limitations
Paddle over disc apparatus	- Easy handling - Sink conditions maintained by large dissolution medium volumes	- Absence of an air-liquid interface - Large volumes of the dissolution medium and paddle agitation are not reflective of the actual in vivo dissolution process of inhaled particles
Dialysis bag	- Static and sink conditions maintained - Dissolution medium replacement possible	- Absence of an air-liquid interface - The powder particles might adhere to the sides of the bag or aggregate
Flow through cell	- Sink conditions maintained by the continuous flow of fresh medium - Reduced influence of diffusion during dissolution testing - Continuous sampling, a flow rate change and dissolution medium change possible during the run	- Absence of an air-liquid interface - The high fluid velocity applied does not represent the agility of the fluid in the lung, which is rather stationary - The flat geometry of the filter holders potentially generates a high fluid velocity at the centre but decreasing flow gradient towards the periphery causing diffusion effects and a local non-sink condition - Handling of this setup is sensitive to entrapped air in the membrane-drug substance sandwich and in the dead volume of the flow-through cell - The drug release is flow-rate controlled

Table 3. *Cont.*

Apparatus	Advantages	Disadvantages/limitations
Franz diffusion cell	- Represent the in vivo non-agitated situation - Consists of an air-liquid interface	- Presence of air bubbles at the membrane liquid interface and the difficulty or even failure of removing them - Difficult to distinguish between diffusion effects through the membrane and the dissolution rate
Transwell® system	- Represent the in vivo non-agitated situation - Consists of an air-liquid interface - Lower volumes of stationary dissolution media	- Difficult to distinguish between diffusion effects through the membrane and the dissolution rate - Saturation of the limited volume of dissolution medium causes decreased dissolution
Dissolv*It*® system	- Simulates the air-blood barrier of the upper airways of the lungs with low volumes of stationary mucus simulant - Particle dissolution is visualized under microscope as disappearance - Simulates the dissolution and absorption of drugs from inhaled dry powders	- The microscopic observation is limited by an optical resolution of around 0.2 µm - The thickness of the stationary mucus and membrane simulates the absorption kinetics in the tracheobronchial region rather than the deep lung regions

It has always been fascinating to explore the interactions of inhaled drugs and components of RTLF that ultimately affect their dissolution and absorption in the lungs. For instance, Langmuir monolayer technique enables the formation of a lipid film on the water subphase and facilitates characterization of lipid–water, lipid–lipid or lipid–drug interactions [89]. However, understanding the interactions of inhaled drug molecules and RTLF components is out of the scope of this current review.

4. Models for Pulmonary Drug Absorption

In vitro, ex vivo and in vivo models are commonly used to study absorption of inhaled drug particles. Table 4 summarizes the various models used to study pulmonary drug absorption.

Table 4. Summary of various models for pulmonary drug absorption.

Models		Drugs	Ref.
In vitro	Air-liquid interfaced layers Calu-3/Transwell system	Salbutamol Indomethacin	[90]
	DissolvIt system	Budesonide Fluticasone propionate	[23]
	Custom made flow perfusion cell	Moxifloxacin Ethionamide	[58]
Ex vivo	Isolated perfused rat lung	AZD5423 (developmental nonsteroidal glucocorticoid) Budesonide Fluticasone furoate Fluticasone propionate	[91]
In vivo	Rats	Rifampicin	[92]
	Guinea pigs	Rifampicin	[93]
	Cynomolgus monkeys (non-human primates)	Erythropoietin Fc fusion protein	[94]
	Patients with cystic fibrosis (Clinical study)	Colistin	[95]

In vitro air-to-blood barrier is reconstructed using cell models in the Transwell or Snapwell system under cell culture [96]. Table 5 summarizes different types of cells used for in vitro lung barrier models. Stem cell-derived lung epithelial cells and "lung-on-a-chip" models have grabbed the interest of many researchers. Most importantly, differentiation of human embryonic stem cells (ESC) or induced pluripotent stem cells (iPSC) to alveolar epithelial type II-like cells facilitates large-scale alveolar epithelial cell production. Air-liquid interface (ALI) culture can induce differentiation further to alveolar epithelial type I-like cells. Furthermore, a microfluidic device, "lung-on-a-chip" has been developed as lung model to study biological development and pathogenic responses of lungs. The utility of a unique six-well "lung-on-a-chip" prototype that can integrate an in vitro aerosol deposition system is currently being examined. This attempt looks interesting as it includes the presence of air, media flow and breathing-like stretching that resembles the movement of lungs [96].

Table 5. In vitro models for absorption of inhaled drug particles [33].

Alveolar Epithelial Models	Tracheobronchial Epithelial Models
Primary alveolar epithelial cell cultures	Primary cell cultures • Small airway epithelial cells • Normal human bronchial epithelial cells
Alveolar epithelial cell lines • A549 • NCI-H441 human bronchiolar epithelial cell	Bronchial epithelial cell lines • BEAS-2B • NuLi-1 • 16HBE14o • Calu-3 • Models of cystic fibrosis airway epithelium (NCF3, CFT1, CFBE41o, CuFi)
	Co-culture models or human bronchial/alveolar cells

When in vivo or in vitro models cannot clearly explain the mechanism of drug transport or lung disposition kinetics, ex vivo tissue models are used. Isolated perfused lung (IPL) is one of the most used method, where the lung is isolated from the body and kept in an artificial system maintaining certain experimental conditions. This separates distribution, metabolism and elimination from lung specific assessments. Architecture and functionality of the tissue is closely maintained in an isolated organ experiment enhancing its resemblance to in vivo state in comparison to in vitro monolayer models from a single cell type. An IPL prepared from small rodents has commonly been employed for lung disposition studies [97].

In vivo studies in intact animal models are used for investigating the absorption, distribution, and pharmacodynamics of inhaled drug particles. In such models, formulations are administered to conscious or anesthetized animals using different types of delivery devices with or without surgical intervention. Small animals such as mice and rats have been commonly used to study pulmonary pharmacokinetics. However, because of higher cost and logistics required for handling and housing, the use of larger animals such as guinea pigs, rabbits, dogs, sheep and monkeys are limited [98]. In larger animals, regional delivery/distribution of drugs can be achieved by the appropriate selection of aerosol size and inspiratory manoeuvres facilitating the study of region dependent lung absorption and disposition [96].

5. Future Perspectives

We have summarized various instruments and methods used for dissolution studies of inhaled drug particles, however there is no standard method that can be recommended for routine studies. Therefore, there is a need for sophisticated instrument for testing inhalable formulations. Moreover, currently available small volume dissolution apparatus only accounts for dissolution studies in stagnant medium (simulated RTLF) ignoring the fact that mucociliary clearance occurs in the upper airways and breathing results in the movement of alveoli and air sacs of the lungs. Therefore, small volume dissolution instruments should be developed or upgraded in such a way to incorporate fluid movement in them [30]. In addition, in vitro cell-based models that are being used for absorption studies are inconvenient to conduct routine testing of formulations. Therefore, automated cell free systems are always preferred over them.

On the other hand, various simulated RTLFs (dissolution media) [99] that are being used for in vitro dissolution studies do not closely resemble the human RTLF [30]. Composition and thickness of RTLF vary regionally from one region of respiratory tract to another and individually from healthy to diseased. RTLF is rich in mucus in upper respiratory tract whereas, it is rich in surfactant in lower respiratory tract [30]. For instance, in pulmonary disease like cystic fibrosis (CF), patients have highly tenacious (adhesive and cohesive) sputum. Along with mucin (regular component of normal mucus), CF sputum contains large amounts of DNA and filamentous actin [100] in comparison to RTLF of healthy person. Therefore, there is a need for region-specific and disease-specific simulated RTLFs. Determination of absolute concentration of components of RTLF is a must to mimic them but it is a challenging task. Therefore, there is a need for sophisticated method (technology) to accurately determine them. Moreover, components of simulated RTLF should always be chosen keeping in mind about their cost and availability that in turn will help commercialization in future [30].

6. Conclusions

In vitro dissolution testing is a well-established quality control test in characterizing the performance of a solid oral dosage form. However, no approved methods are available for evaluating the dissolution behaviour of inhaled dry powder particles even though many studies proved the relationship between dissolution and pharmacokinetics of inhaled drugs. The complex nature of the lungs with anatomical and physiological differences in the tracheobronchial region and alveolar region make a great challenge in the development of an in vitro dissolution method which mimics the lung conditions.

In this review, we summarized various dissolution methods and absorption models developed for the evaluation of dissolution and absorption behaviour of inhaled drug particles. Even though the recent methods used a small volume of dissolution medium, it represents only a particular region of the lung. A further improvement in the dissolution methods which mimic the different regions of the lungs is necessary.

Author Contributions: Invitation received, S.C.D.; conceptualization, B.B.E. and S.C.D.; writing and original draft preparation, B.B.E. and R.B.; writing, reviewing, and editing, B.B.E., R.B. and S.C.D. All authors have read and agreed to the published version of the manuscript.

Funding: This research was funded by School of Pharmacy's Marsden Fund near miss grant.

Acknowledgments: Basanth Babu Eedara would like to acknowledge the University of Otago, Dunedin, New Zealand for a doctoral scholarship.

Conflicts of Interest: The authors declare no conflict of interest.

References

1. Mehta, P. Dry Powder Inhalers: A Focus on Advancements in Novel Drug Delivery Systems. *J. Drug Deliv.* **2016**, *2016*, 8290963. [CrossRef] [PubMed]
2. Eedara, B.B.; Alabsi, W.; Encinas-Basurto, D.; Polt, R.; Ledford, J.G.; Mansour, H.M. Inhalation Delivery for the Treatment and Prevention of COVID-19 Infection. *Pharmaceutics* **2021**, *13*, 1077. [CrossRef] [PubMed]
3. Eedara, B.B.; Alabsi, W.; Encinas-Basurto, D.; Polt, R.; Mansour, H.M. Spray-Dried Inhalable Powder Formulations of Therapeutic Proteins and Peptides. *AAPS PharmSciTech* **2021**, *22*, 185. [CrossRef] [PubMed]
4. Alabsi, W.; Eedara, B.B.; Encinas-Basurto, D.; Polt, R.; Mansour, H.M. Nose-to-Brain Delivery of Therapeutic Peptides as Nasal Aerosols. *Pharmaceutics* **2022**, *14*, 1870. [CrossRef] [PubMed]
5. Frijlink, H.W.; De Boer, A.H. Dry powder inhalers for pulmonary drug delivery. *Expert Opin. Drug Deliv.* **2004**, *1*, 67–86. [CrossRef]

6. Muralidharan, P.; Hayes, D.; Mansour, H.M. Dry powder inhalers in COPD, lung inflammation and pulmonary infections. *Expert Opin. Drug Deliv.* **2015**, *12*, 947–962. [CrossRef]
7. Newman, S.P. Inhaler treatment options in COPD. *Eur. Respir. Rev.* **2005**, *14*, 102–108. [CrossRef]
8. Smith, I.J.; Parry-Billings, M. The inhalers of the future? A review of dry powder devices on the market today. *Pulm Pharmacol. Ther.* **2003**, *16*, 79–95. [CrossRef]
9. Svedsater, H.; Dale, P.; Garrill, K.; Walker, R.; Woepse, M.W. Qualitative assessment of attributes and ease of use of the ELLIPTA™ dry powder inhaler for delivery of maintenance therapy for asthma and COPD. *BMC Pulm Med.* **2013**, *13*, 72. [CrossRef]
10. Eedara, B.B.; Alabsi, W.; Encinas-Basurto, D.; Polt, R.; Hayes, D.; Black, S.M.; Mansour, H.M. Pulmonary Drug Delivery. In *Organelle and Molecular Targeting*; CRC Press: Boca Raton, FL, USA, 2021; pp. 227–278.
11. El-Sherbiny, I.M.; El-Baz, N.M.; Yacoub, M.H. Inhaled nano- and microparticles for drug delivery. *Glob. Cardiol. Sci. Pract.* **2015**, *2015*, 2. [CrossRef]
12. Newman, S.P. Dry powder inhalers for optimal drug delivery. *Expert Opin. Biol. Ther.* **2004**, *4*, 23–33. [CrossRef]
13. Olsson, B.; Bondesson, E.; Borgström, L.; Edsbäcker, S.; Eirefelt, S.; Ekelund, K.; Gustavsson, L.; Hegelund-Myrbäck, T. Pulmonary drug metabolism, clearance, and absorption. In *Controlled Pulmonary Drug Delivery*; Springer: Berlin/Heidelberg, Germany, 2011; pp. 21–50.
14. Patton, J.S.; Brain, J.D.; Davies, L.A.; Fiegel, J.; Gumbleton, M.; Kim, K.-J.; Sakagami, M.; Vanbever, R.; Ehrhardt, C. The Particle has Landed—Characterizing the Fate of Inhaled Pharmaceuticals. *J. Aerosol. Med. Pulm. Drug Deliv.* **2010**, *23*, S-71–S-87. [CrossRef]
15. Eedara, B.B. *Slow Dissolving Inhalable Dry Powders for Treatment of Pulmonary Tuberculosis*; University of Otago: Dunedin, New Zealand, 2019.
16. Smyth, H.D.C.; Hickey, A.J. *Controlled Pulmonary Drug Delivery*, 1st ed.; Springer: New York, NY, USA, 2011.
17. El-Sherbiny, I.M.; Villanueva, D.G.; Herrera, D.; Smyth, H.D.C. Overcoming Lung Clearance Mechanisms for Controlled Release Drug Delivery. In *Controlled Pulmonary Drug Delivery*; Smyth, H.D.C., Hickey, A.J., Eds.; Springer: New York, NY, USA, 2011; pp. 101–126.
18. Eedara, B.B.; Tucker, I.G.; Zujovic, Z.D.; Rades, T.; Price, J.R.; Das, S.C. Crystalline adduct of moxifloxacin with trans-cinnamic acid to reduce the aqueous solubility and dissolution rate for improved residence time in the lungs. *Eur. J. Pharm. Sci.* **2019**, *136*, 104961. [CrossRef]
19. FDAU. *Guidance for Industry: Dissolution Testing of Immediate-Release Solid Oral Dosage Forms*; Food and Drug Administration: Silver Spring, MD, USA; Center for Drug Evaluation and Research (CDER): Silver Spring, MD, USA, 1997.
20. Arora, D.; Shah, K.A.; Halquist, M.S.; Sakagami, M. In Vitro Aqueous Fluid-Capacity-Limited Dissolution Testing of Respirable Aerosol Drug Particles Generated from Inhaler Products. *Pharm. Res.* **2010**, *27*, 786–795. [CrossRef]
21. Davies, N.M.; Feddah, M.R. A novel method for assessing dissolution of aerosol inhaler products. *Int. J. Pharm.* **2003**, *255*, 175–187. [CrossRef]
22. Franz, T.J. Percutaneous Absorption. On the Relevance of in Vitro Data. *J. Investig. Dermatol.* **1975**, *64*, 190–195. [CrossRef]
23. Gerde, P.; Malmlöf, M.; Havsborn, L.; Sjöberg, C.-O.; Ewing, P.; Eirefelt, S.; Ekelund, K. DissolvIt: An In Vitro Method for Simulating the Dissolution and Absorption of Inhaled Dry Powder Drugs in the Lungs. *ASSAY Drug Dev. Technol.* **2017**, *15*, 77–88. [CrossRef]
24. Gray, V.; Hickey, A.J.; Balmer, P.; Davies, N.; Dunbar, C.; Foster, T.S.; Olsson, B.L.; Sakagami, M.; Shah, V.P.; Smurthwaite, M.J.; et al. The Inhalation Ad Hoc Advisory Panel for the USP Performance Tests of Inhalation Dosage Forms. *Pharmacop. Forum* **2008**, *34*, 1068–1074.
25. May, S.; Jensen, B.; Wolkenhauer, M.; Schneider, M.; Lehr, C.M. Dissolution Techniques for In Vitro Testing of Dry Powders for Inhalation. *Pharm. Res.* **2012**, *29*, 2157–2166. [CrossRef]
26. Rohrschneider, M.; Bhagwat, S.; Krampe, R.; Michler, V.; Breitkreutz, J.; Hochhaus, G. Evaluation of the Transwell System for Characterization of Dissolution Behavior of Inhalation Drugs: Effects of Membrane and Surfactant. *Mol. Pharm.* **2015**, *12*, 2618–2624. [CrossRef]
27. Salama, R.O.; Traini, D.; Chan, H.-K.; Young, P.M. Preparation and characterisation of controlled release co-spray dried drug–polymer microparticles for inhalation 2: Evaluation of in vitro release profiling methodologies for controlled release respiratory aerosols. *Eur. J. Pharm. Biopharm.* **2008**, *70*, 145–152. [CrossRef] [PubMed]
28. Son, Y.-J.; McConville, J.T. Development of a standardized dissolution test method for inhaled pharmaceutical formulations. *Int. J. Pharm.* **2009**, *382*, 15–22. [CrossRef] [PubMed]
29. Jaafar-Maalej, C.; Andrieu, V.; Elaissari, A.; Fessi, H. Assessment methods of inhaled aerosols: Technical aspects and applications. *Expert Opin. Drug Deliv.* **2009**, *6*, 941–959. [CrossRef] [PubMed]
30. Bastola, R.; Young, P.M.; Das, S.C. Simulation of respiratory tract lining fluid for in vitro dissolution study. *Expert Opin. Drug Deliv.* **2021**, *18*, 1091–1100. [CrossRef] [PubMed]
31. Hastedt, J.E.; Bäckman, P.; Clark, A.R.; Doub, W.; Hickey, A.; Hochhaus, G.; Kuehl, P.J.; Lehr, C.-M.; Mauser, P.; McConville, J.; et al. Scope and relevance of a pulmonary biopharmaceutical classification system AAPS/FDA/USP Workshop 16–17 March 2015 in Baltimore, MD. *AAPS Open* **2016**, *2*, 1. [CrossRef]
32. Ochs, M.; Weibel, E.R. Functional design of the human lung for gas exchange. In *Fishman's Pulmonary Diseases and Disorders*, 5th ed.; Grippi, M.A., Elias, J.A., Fishman, J.A., Kotloff, R.M., Pack, A.L., Senior, R.M., Siegel, M.D., Eds.; McGraw Hill: New York, NY, USA, 2015; Volume 1, p. 7.

33. Haghi, M.; Ong, H.X.; Traini, D.; Young, P. Across the pulmonary epithelial barrier: Integration of physicochemical properties and human cell models to study pulmonary drug formulations. *Pharmacol. Ther.* **2014**, *144*, 235–252. [CrossRef]
34. Zhang, J.; Wu, L.; Chan, H.-K.; Watanabe, W. Formation, characterization, and fate of inhaled drug nanoparticles. *Adv. Drug Deliv. Rev.* **2011**, *63*, 441–455. [CrossRef]
35. Eedara, B.B.; Rangnekar, B.; Doyle, C.; Cavallaro, A.; Das, S.C. The influence of surface active l-leucine and 1,2-dipalmitoyl-sn-glycero-3-phosphatidylcholine (DPPC) in the improvement of aerosolization of pyrazinamide and moxifloxacin co-spray dried powders. *Int. J. Pharm.* **2018**, *542*, 72–81. [CrossRef]
36. Eedara, B.B.; Rangnekar, B.; Sinha, S.; Doyle, C.; Cavallaro, A.; Das, S.C. Development and characterization of high payload combination dry powders of anti-tubercular drugs for treating pulmonary tuberculosis. *Eur. J. Pharm. Sci.* **2018**, *118*, 216–226. [CrossRef]
37. Eedara, B.B.; Tucker, I.G.; Das, S.C. Phospholipid-based pyrazinamide spray-dried inhalable powders for treating tuberculosis. *Int. J. Pharm.* **2016**, *506*, 174–183. [CrossRef]
38. Rangnekar, B.; Momin, M.A.M.; Eedara, B.B.; Sinha, S.; Das, S.C. Bedaquiline containing triple combination powder for inhalation to treat drug-resistant tuberculosis. *Int. J. Pharm.* **2019**, *570*, 118689. [CrossRef]
39. Fröhlich, E. Toxicity of orally inhaled drug formulations at the alveolar barrier: Parameters for initial biological screening. *Drug Deliv.* **2017**, *24*, 891–905. [CrossRef]
40. Gerde, P.; Scholander, P. A mathematical model of the penetration of polycyclic aromatic hydrocarbons through the bronchial lining layer. *Environ. Res.* **1987**, *44*, 321–334. [CrossRef]
41. Patton, J.S.; Byron, P.R. Inhaling medicines: Delivering drugs to the body through the lungs. *Nat. Rev. Drug Discov.* **2007**, *6*, 67–74. [CrossRef]
42. Parra, E.; Pérez-Gil, J. Composition, structure and mechanical properties define performance of pulmonary surfactant membranes and films. *Chem. Phys. Lipids* **2015**, *185*, 153–175. [CrossRef]
43. Mason, R.J.; Dobbs, L.G. Alveolar Epithelium and Pulmonary Surfactant. In *Murray and Nadel's Textbook of Respiratory Medicine*; Broaddus, V.C., Mason, R.J., Ernst, J.D., King, T.E., Lazarus, S.C., Murray, J.F., Nadel, J.A., Slutsky, A.S., Gotway, M.B., Eds.; Elsevier: Amsterdam, The Netherlands, 2016; pp. 134–149.e5.
44. Carvalho, T.C.; Peters, J.I.; Williams, R.O. Influence of particle size on regional lung deposition—What evidence is there? *Int. J. Pharm.* **2011**, *406*, 1–10. [CrossRef]
45. Cipolla, D.; Shekunov, B.; Blanchard, J.; Hickey, A. Lipid-based carriers for pulmonary products: Preclinical development and case studies in humans. *Adv. Drug Deliv. Rev.* **2014**, *75*, 53–80. [CrossRef]
46. Driving Results in Inhaler Testing [Brochure]. 2020. Available online: https://www.copleyscientific.com/wp-content/uploads/2020/02/Copley-Inhaler-Testing-Brochure-LowRes-0720.pdf (accessed on 21 September 2022).
47. May, S.; Jensen, B.; Weiler, C.; Wolkenhauer, M.; Schneider, M.; Lehr, C.-M. Dissolution Testing of Powders for Inhalation: Influence of Particle Deposition and Modeling of Dissolution Profiles. *Pharm. Res.* **2014**, *31*, 3211–3224. [CrossRef]
48. May, S.; Kind, S.; Jensen, B.; Wolkenhauer, M.; Schneider, M.; Lehr, C.-M. Miniature in vitro dissolution testing of powders for inhalation. *Dissolution Technol.* **2015**, *22*, 40–51. [CrossRef]
49. Tay, J.Y.S.; Liew, C.V.; Heng, P.W.S. Dissolution of fine particle fraction from truncated Anderson cascade impactor with an enhancer cell. *Int. J. Pharm.* **2018**, *545*, 45–50. [CrossRef]
50. Son, Y.J.; Horng, M.; Copley, M.; McConville, J.T. Optimization of an in vitro dissolution test method for inhalation formulations. *Dissolution Technol.* **2010**, *17*, 6–13. [CrossRef]
51. Son, Y.-J.; McConville, J.T. Preparation of sustained release rifampicin microparticles for inhalation. *J. Pharm. Pharmacol.* **2012**, *64*, 1291–1302. [CrossRef] [PubMed]
52. Duret, C.; Wauthoz, N.; Sebti, T.; Vanderbist, F.; Amighi, K. Solid dispersions of itraconazole for inhalation with enhanced dissolution, solubility and dispersion properties. *Int. J. Pharm.* **2012**, *428*, 103–113. [CrossRef] [PubMed]
53. Pilcer, G.; Rosière, R.; Traina, K.; Sebti, T.; Vanderbist, F.; Amighi, K. New Co-Spray-Dried Tobramycin Nanoparticles-Clarithromycin Inhaled Powder Systems for Lung Infection Therapy in Cystic Fibrosis Patients. *J. Pharm. Sci.* **2013**, *102*, 1836–1846. [CrossRef] [PubMed]
54. Chan, J.G.Y.; Chan, H.-K.; Prestidge, C.A.; Denman, J.A.; Young, P.M.; Traini, D. A novel dry powder inhalable formulation incorporating three first-line anti-tubercular antibiotics. *Eur. J. Pharm. Biopharm.* **2013**, *83*, 285–292. [CrossRef]
55. Grainger, C.I.; Greenwell, L.L.; Martin, G.P.; Forbes, B. The permeability of large molecular weight solutes following particle delivery to air-interfaced cells that model the respiratory mucosa. *Eur. J. Pharm. Biopharm.* **2009**, *71*, 318–324. [CrossRef]
56. Grainger, C.I.; Saunders, M.; Buttini, F.; Telford, R.; Merolla, L.L.; Martin, G.P.; Jones, S.A.; Forbes, B. Critical Characteristics for Corticosteroid Solution Metered Dose Inhaler Bioequivalence. *Mol. Pharm.* **2012**, *9*, 563–569. [CrossRef]
57. Haghi, M.; Traini, D.; Bebawy, M.; Young, P.M. Deposition, Diffusion and Transport Mechanism of Dry Powder Microparticulate Salbutamol, at the Respiratory Epithelia. *Mol. Pharm.* **2012**, *9*, 1717–1726. [CrossRef]
58. Eedara, B.B.; Tucker, I.G.; Das, S.C. In vitro dissolution testing of respirable size anti-tubercular drug particles using a small volume dissolution apparatus. *Int. J. Pharm.* **2019**, *559*, 235–244. [CrossRef]
59. Börjel, M.; Sadler, R.; Gerde, P. (Eds.) The dissolvIt: An in vitro evaluation of the dissolution and absorption of three inhaled dry powder drugs in the lung. In *Respiratory Drug Delivery to the Lungs Conference, Poster Stockholm*; Karolinska Institutet: Stockholm, Sweden, 2014.

60. *British Pharmacopoeia*; TSO: London, UK, 2018.
61. Son, Y.-J.; McConville, J.T. A new respirable form of rifampicin. *Eur. J. Pharm. Biopharm.* **2011**, *78*, 366–376. [CrossRef]
62. Eedara, B.B.; Tucker, I.G.; Das, S.C. A STELLA simulation model for in vitro dissolution testing of respirable size particles. *Sci. Rep.* **2019**, *9*, 18522. [CrossRef]
63. Al ayoub, Y.; Buzgeia, A.; Almousawi, G.; Mazhar, H.R.A.; Alzouebi, B.; Gopalan, R.C.; Assi, K.H. In-Vitro In-Vivo Correlation (IVIVC) of Inhaled Products Using Twin Stage Impinger. *J. Pharm. Sci.* **2022**, *111*, 395–402. [CrossRef]
64. Gerde, P.; Ewing, P.; Låstbom, L.; Ryrfeldt, Å.; Waher, J.; Lidén, G. A Novel Method to Aerosolize Powder for Short Inhalation Exposures at High Concentrations: Isolated Rat Lungs Exposed to Respirable Diesel Soot. *Inhal. Toxicol.* **2004**, *16*, 45–52. [CrossRef]
65. Jaspart, S.; Bertholet, P.; Piel, G.; Dogné, J.-M.; Delattre, L.; Evrard, B. Solid lipid microparticles as a sustained release system for pulmonary drug delivery. *Eur. J. Pharm. Biopharm.* **2007**, *65*, 47–56. [CrossRef]
66. Ortiz, M.; Jornada, D.S.; Pohlmann, A.R.; Guterres, S.S. Development of Novel Chitosan Microcapsules for Pulmonary Delivery of Dapsone: Characterization, Aerosol Performance, and In Vivo Toxicity Evaluation. *AAPS PharmSciTech* **2015**, *16*, 1033–1040. [CrossRef]
67. Asada, M.; Takahashi, H.; Okamoto, H.; Tanino, H.; Danjo, K. Theophylline particle design using chitosan by the spray drying. *Int. J. Pharm.* **2004**, *270*, 167–174. [CrossRef]
68. Huang, Y.C.; Yeh, M.K.; Cheng, S.N.; Chiang, C.H. The characteristics of betamethasone-loaded chitosan microparticles by spray-drying method. *J. Microencapsul.* **2003**, *20*, 459–472. [CrossRef]
69. Learoyd, T.P.; Burrows, J.L.; French, E.; Seville, P.C. Chitosan-based spray-dried respirable powders for sustained delivery of terbutaline sulfate. *Eur. J. Pharm. Biopharm.* **2008**, *68*, 224–234. [CrossRef]
70. Depreter, F.; Burniat, A.; Blocklet, D.; Lacroix, S.; Cnop, M.; Fery, F.; Van Aelst, N.; Pilcer, G.; Deleers, M.; Goldman, S.; et al. Comparative pharmacoscintigraphic and pharmacokinetic evaluation of two new formulations of inhaled insulin in type 1 diabetic patients. *Eur. J. Pharm. Biopharm.* **2012**, *80*, 4–13. [CrossRef]
71. Parikh, R.; Dalwadi, S. Preparation and characterization of controlled release poly-ε-caprolactone microparticles of isoniazid for drug delivery through pulmonary route. *Powder Technol.* **2014**, *264*, 158–165. [CrossRef]
72. Arora, S.; Haghi, M.; Loo, C.-Y.; Traini, D.; Young, P.M.; Jain, S. Development of an Inhaled Controlled Release Voriconazole Dry Powder Formulation for the Treatment of Respiratory Fungal Infection. *Mol. Pharm.* **2015**, *12*, 2001–2009. [CrossRef] [PubMed]
73. Pai, R.V.; Jain, R.R.; Bannalikar, A.S.; Menon, M.D. Development and Evaluation of Chitosan Microparticles Based Dry Powder Inhalation Formulations of Rifampicin and Rifabutin. *J. Aerosol Med. Pulm. Drug Deliv.* **2016**, *29*, 179–195. [CrossRef] [PubMed]
74. Maretti, E.; Rustichelli, C.; Romagnoli, M.; Balducci, A.G.; Buttini, F.; Sacchetti, F.; Leo, E.; Iannuccelli, V. Solid Lipid Nanoparticle assemblies (SLNas) for an anti-TB inhalation treatment—A Design of Experiments approach to investigate the influence of pre-freezing conditions on the powder respirability. *Int. J. Pharm.* **2016**, *511*, 669–679. [CrossRef] [PubMed]
75. Kumaresan, C.; Sathishkumar, K. Development of an Inhaled Sustained Release Dry Powder Formulation of Salbutamol Sulphate, an Antiasthmatic Drug. *Indian J. Pharm. Sci.* **2016**, *78*, 136–142. [PubMed]
76. Taylor, M.K.; Hickey, A.J.; VanOort, M. Manufacture, Characterization, and Pharmacodynamic Evaluation of Engineered Ipratropium Bromide Particles. *Pharm. Dev. Technol.* **2006**, *11*, 321–336. [CrossRef]
77. Cook, R.O.; Pannu, R.K.; Kellaway, I.W. Novel sustained release microspheres for pulmonary drug delivery. *J. Control. Release* **2005**, *104*, 79–90. [CrossRef]
78. Adi, H.; Young, P.M.; Chan, H.-K.; Salama, R.; Traini, D. Controlled release antibiotics for dry powder lung delivery. *Drug Dev. Ind. Pharm.* **2010**, *36*, 119–126. [CrossRef]
79. Möbus, K.; Siepmann, J.; Bodmeier, R. Zinc–alginate microparticles for controlled pulmonary delivery of proteins prepared by spray-drying. *Eur. J. Pharm. Biopharm.* **2012**, *81*, 121–130. [CrossRef]
80. Scalia, S.; Salama, R.; Young, P.; Traini, D. Preparation and in vitro evaluation of salbutamol-loaded lipid microparticles for sustained release pulmonary therapy. *J. Microencapsul.* **2012**, *29*, 225–233. [CrossRef]
81. Buttini, F.; Miozzi, M.; Balducci, A.G.; Royall, P.G.; Brambilla, G.; Colombo, P.; Bettini, R.; Forbes, B. Differences in physical chemistry and dissolution rate of solid particle aerosols from solution pressurised inhalers. *Int. J. Pharm.* **2014**, *465*, 42–51. [CrossRef]
82. Balducci, A.G.; Steckel, H.; Guarneri, F.; Rossi, A.; Colombo, G.; Sonvico, F.; Cordts, E.; Bettini, R.; Colombo, P.; Buttini, F. High shear mixing of lactose and salmeterol xinafoate dry powder blends: Biopharmaceutic and aerodynamic performances. *J. Drug Deliv. Sci. Technol.* **2015**, *30*, 443–449. [CrossRef]
83. Langenbucher, F.; Benz, D.; Kürth, W.; Möller, H.; Otz, M. Standardized flow-cell method as an alternative to existing pharmacopoeial dissolution testing. *Pharm. Ind.* **1989**, *51*, 1276–1281.
84. Fotaki, N. Flow-through cell apparatus (USP apparatus 4): Operation and features. *Dissolut. Technol.* **2011**, *18*, 46–49. [CrossRef]
85. Kanapilly, G.M.; Raabe, O.G.; Goh, C.H.T.; Chimenti, R.A. Measurement of in Vitro Dissolution of Aerosol Particles for Comparison to in Vivo Dissolution in the Lower Respiratory Tract after Inhalation. *Health Phys.* **1973**, *24*, 497–507. [CrossRef]
86. Riley, T.C.D.; Arp, J.; Casazzza, A.; Colombani, A.; Cooper, A.; Dey, M.; Maas, J.; Mitchell, J.; Reiners, M.; Sigari, N.; et al. Challenges with developing in vitro dissolution tests for orally inhaled products (OIPs). *Aaps Pharmscitech* **2012**, *13*, 978–989. [CrossRef]

87. Hassoun, M.; Malmlöf, M.; Scheibelhofer, O.; Kumar, A.; Bansal, S.; Selg, E.; Nowenwik, M.; Gerde, P.; Radivojev, S.; Paudel, A.; et al. Use of PBPK modeling to evaluate the performance of dissolv it, a biorelevant dissolution assay for orally inhaled drug products. *Mol. Pharm.* **2019**, *16*, 1245–1254. [CrossRef]
88. Saha, T.; Sinha, S.; Harfoot, R.; Quiñones-Mateu, M.E.; Das, S.C. Manipulation of Spray-Drying Conditions to Develop an Inhalable Ivermectin Dry Powder. *Pharmaceutics* **2022**, *14*, 1432. [CrossRef]
89. Rojewska, M.; Smułek, W.; Kaczorek, E.; Prochaska, K. Langmuir Monolayer Techniques for the Investigation of Model Bacterial Membranes and Antibiotic Biodegradation Mechanisms. *Membranes* **2021**, *11*, 707. [CrossRef]
90. Cingolani, E.; Alqahtani, S.; Sadler, R.C.; Prime, D.; Stolnik, S.; Bosquillon, C. In vitro investigation on the impact of airway mucus on drug dissolution and absorption at the air-epithelium interface in the lungs. *Eur. J. Pharm. Biopharm.* **2019**, *141*, 210–220. [CrossRef]
91. Eriksson, J.; Thörn, H.; Sjögren, E.; Holmstén, L.; Rubin, K.; Lennernäs, H. Pulmonary dissolution of poorly soluble compounds studied in an ex vivo rat lung model. *Mol. Pharm.* **2019**, *16*, 3053–3064. [CrossRef]
92. Khadka, P.; Sinha, S.; Tucker, I.G.; Dummer, J.; Hill, P.C.; Katare, R.; Das, S.C. Pharmacokinetics of rifampicin after repeated intra-tracheal administration of amorphous and crystalline powder formulations to Sprague Dawley rats. *Eur. J. Pharm. Biopharm.* **2021**, *162*, 1–11. [CrossRef] [PubMed]
93. Garcia Contreras, L.; Sung, J.; Ibrahim, M.; Elbert, K.; Edwards, D.; Hickey, A. Pharmacokinetics of inhaled rifampicin porous particles for tuberculosis treatment: Insight into rifampicin absorption from the lungs of guinea pigs. *Mol. Pharm.* **2015**, *12*, 2642–2650. [CrossRef] [PubMed]
94. Bitonti, A.J.; Dumont, J.A.; Low, S.C.; Peters, R.T.; Kropp, K.E.; Palombella, V.J.; Stattel, J.M.; Lu, Y.; Tan, C.A.; Song, J.J.; et al. Pulmonary delivery of an erythropoietin Fc fusion protein in non-human primates through an immunoglobulin transport pathway. *Proc. Natl. Acad. Sci. USA* **2004**, *101*, 9763–9768. [CrossRef] [PubMed]
95. Ratjen, F.; Rietschel, E.; Kasel, D.; Schwiertz, R.; Starke, K.; Beier, H.; Van Koningsbruggen, S.; Grasemann, H. Pharmacokinetics of inhaled colistin in patients with cystic fibrosis. *J. Antimicrob. Chemother.* **2006**, *57*, 306–311. [CrossRef] [PubMed]
96. Sakagami, M. In vitro, ex vivo and in vivo methods of lung absorption for inhaled drugs. *Adv. Drug Deliv. Rev.* **2020**, *161–162*, 63–74. [CrossRef]
97. Sakagami, M. In vivo, in vitro and ex vivo models to assess pulmonary absorption and disposition of inhaled therapeutics for systemic delivery. *Adv. Drug Deliv. Rev.* **2006**, *58*, 1030–1060. [CrossRef]
98. Nahar, K.; Gupta, N.; Gauvin, R.; Absar, S.; Patel, B.; Gupta, V.; Khademhosseini, A.; Ahsan, F. In vitro, in vivo and ex vivo models for studying particle deposition and drug absorption of inhaled pharmaceuticals. *Eur. J. Pharm. Sci.* **2013**, *49*, 805–818. [CrossRef]
99. Radivojev, S.; Zellnitz, S.; Paudel, A.; Fröhlich, E. Searching for physiologically relevant in vitro dissolution techniques for orally inhaled drugs. *Int. J. Pharm.* **2019**, *556*, 45–56. [CrossRef]
100. Ibrahim, B.M.; Park, S.; Han, B.; Yeo, Y. A strategy to deliver genes to cystic fibrosis lungs: A battle with environment. *J. Control. Release* **2011**, *155*, 289–295. [CrossRef]

pharmaceutics

Review

Advancements in Skin Delivery of Natural Bioactive Products for Wound Management: A Brief Review of Two Decades

Cameron Ryall [1], Sanjukta Duarah [1], Shuo Chen [1,*], Haijun Yu [2] and Jingyuan Wen [1,*]

[1] School of Pharmacy, Faculty of Medical and Health Sciences, The University of Auckland, Auckland 1010, New Zealand; crya086@aucklanduni.ac.nz (C.R.); s.duarah@auckland.ac.nz (S.D.)
[2] Shanghai Institute of Materia Medica, Chinese Academy of Sciences, Shanghai 201203, China; hjyu@simm.ac.cn
* Correspondence: shuo.chen@auckland.ac.nz (S.C.); j.wen@auckland.ac.nz (J.W.); Tel.: +64-9-9232762 (J.W.)

Abstract: Application of modern delivery techniques to natural bioactive products improves their permeability, bioavailability, and therapeutic efficacy. Many natural products have desirable biological properties applicable to wound healing but are limited by their inability to cross the stratum corneum to access the wound. Over the past two decades, modern systems such as microneedles, lipid-based vesicles, hydrogels, composite dressings, and responsive formulations have been applied to natural products such as curcumin or aloe vera to improve their delivery and efficacy. This article reviews which natural products and techniques have been formulated together in the past two decades and the success of these applications for wound healing. Many cultures prefer natural-product-based traditional therapies which are often cheaper and more available than their synthetic counterparts. Improving natural products' effect can provide novel wound-healing therapies for those who trust traditional compounds over synthetic drugs to reduce medical inequalities.

Keywords: wound healing; natural products; advanced delivery; traditional medicine; alternative medicine

Citation: Ryall, C.; Duarah, S.; Chen, S.; Yu, H.; Wen, J. Advancements in Skin Delivery of Natural Bioactive Products for Wound Management: A Brief Review of Two Decades. *Pharmaceutics* **2022**, *14*, 1072. https://doi.org/10.3390/pharmaceutics14051072

Academic Editors: Marzia Cirri and Bozena B. Michniak-Kohn

Received: 31 March 2022
Accepted: 13 May 2022
Published: 17 May 2022

1. Introduction

The field of wound-healing medicine has been advanced with modern technologies and modern drugs despite traditionally used natural products' known effectiveness. Wounds affect both developed and developing nations, yet they are generally treated differently. The healing process can be painful, develop into an infection, or come across obstacles such as bacterial biofilms causing the wound to become chronic [1,2]. As a prevalent and visible condition, multiple traditional/alternative wound-healing medicines exist from historic medical communities [3,4].

The WHO defines traditional medicines as *'the sum total of the knowledge, skill, and practices based on the theories, beliefs, and experiences indigenous to different cultures, whether explicable or not, used in the maintenance of health as well as in the prevention, diagnosis, improvement or treatment of physical and mental illness'* [5]. In 2019, the World Health Assembly formed resolutions promoting traditional medicines, especially in primary healthcare [5]. This resolution arose from an ever-increasing interest and belief that traditional natural medicines are safer and more commonly available than conventional drugs [6]. Cultures such as China and Egypt with established traditional practices use traditional medicines the most; however, it is a worldwide phenomenon, with 60% of the world's population estimated to rely on traditional medicine [7]. Traditional medicines are often used more in developing nations due to cultural norms or superior accessibility. Natural products already culturally established in developing nations should be re-examined as medicines to provide unique solutions to medical inequalities. Low bioavailability and poor solubility because of limited membrane permeability restricts many natural compounds from their full potential [8]. An example is the anti-inflammatory escin from horse-chestnut, which is poorly lipid-soluble and has a bioavailability of 12.5% [9]. Traditional medicine has gained popularity due to growing distrust of conventional medicine, and as traditional medicine rises in popularity, research should go into its safety, efficacy and optimisation [10].

This review describes how natural wound-healing products are being reapplied with modern delivery strategies. Additionally, we describe how different kinds of wounds form and heal, and then how they are treated. We categorize compounds by their bioactive function and then discuss novel delivery strategies. Our aim is to provide a new perspective on the future of natural products and the problems the field may face.

2. Wound-Healing Physiology

A wound is either acute or develops into a chronic wound due to various factors such as systemic illnesses and repeated trauma. An acute wound is defined as an injury to tissue healing within 8–12 weeks [11]. Acute wounds are commonly caused by burns, lacerations, and abrasions and have a four-stage healing process: hemostasis, inflammation, proliferation, and maturation [11,12]. The four stages are diagrammatically presented in Figure 1. Chronic wounds differ from acute wounds in their timeframe; differently to acute wounds, chronic wounds are yet to heal after 12 weeks and often reoccur [13]. Pre-existing conditions such as diabetes or repeated damage are common causes of chronic wounds and can lead to ulcers or amputations [14].

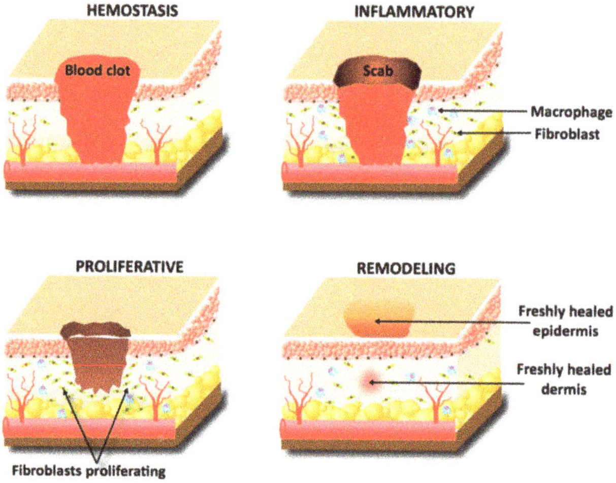

Figure 1. Wound self-healing process.

An acute injury's first phase of healing is hemostasis. This is clotting of the blood to prevent blood loss while also creating a temporary scaffold for future cells' use [2]. Immediately following the injury and during the hemostasis phase, cytokines recruit inflammatory cells to clear the wound area of foreign material and dead tissue [15]. With the wound now sealed and an immune response taking place, fibroblasts and keratinocytes migrate into the damaged area to begin the proliferation phase—some literature views this migration as a phase of healing itself [11]. Keratinocytes proliferate to cover the dermis and reform the epidermal barrier beneath the clot, while fibroblasts begin secreting collagen and extracellular matrix (ECM) to repair the dermis [15]. Capillary reformation responds to angiogenic growth factors such as vascular endothelial growth factor (VEGF) once the dermis has reformed enough to support vessel growth [2]. Finally, myofibroblasts contract the wound area while keratinocytes proliferate to reform its full epithelium, finishing the healing process [13].

Chronic wound healing is often stalled during the inflammation phase [2]. Prolonged inflammation causes imbalances in potent cytokines only meant to be present for a short time [16]. Such an imbalance can increase the degradation of ECM growth factors and receptors [16]. The degradation products of the breakdown require a continued immune response, beginning a cycle of non-healing and persistent inflammation [2,16]. The excess workload placed on immune cells impairs their function and allows bacteria to infiltrate the wound and form a multicellular plaque called a biofilm. This film is typical of staphylococcus aureus and other airborne bacteria; the film covers the topical surface of the wound and can block the delivery of healing pharmaceutics [1]. Breaking the cycle of inflammation and ECM breakdown and removing the biofilm layer are popular research areas aiming to treat the 6.5 million people diagnosed with chronic wounds each year [17].

3. Conventional Treatment

3.1. TIME and TWA: Deciding on a Treatment

A key focus in today's conventional treatment of wounds is managing the risk of a wound becoming chronic [18]. A wound should only require treatment if its natural healing is stalled or interrupted. The 'TIME' or 'TWA' processes are used to assess the wound and determine a treatment. No single treatment is applied to all wounds; hence, assessing wounds and making evidence-based decisions is emphasised [18,19]. Both TIME and TWA are acronyms. For TIME, T stands for 'tissue non-viable or deficient', I for 'infection or inflammation', M for 'moisture balance', and E for 'edge of wound—non-advancing or undermined' [18,20]. TWA stands for 'Triangle of Wound Assessment' [21,22]. TWA elaborates on TIME with a three-point 'triangle': wound bed, wound edge, and peri-wound skin [22]. TWA and TIME analysis provide a systematic way to analyse a wound and direct clinicians to the proper treatment.

3.2. Wound-Healing Dressings

The most common and historically present product for a wound is its dressing. The primary function of a dressing is to protect against foreign microbes and protect the skin from exudate [21,23]. It is often desirable for a dressing to be absorbent, particularly when a wound has too much exudate interfering with the patient's daily life or creating too friendly an environment for bacteria to colonise [20]. Absorbents can be fibrous, fabric, or a combination of the two: these forms are among the most accessible wound dressings around the world [19]. Modern technologies have added to this category with hydrofibres and impregnated gauzes, which are more bioactive than their fibre/fabric counterparts [23]. Such direct dressings can have the disadvantage of being painful when removed, hence the use of non-adherent dressings. Non-adherent dressings are often preferred for the contact layer dressing as they do not attach to the wound's tissue. Non-adherence allows the protection of granulation tissue and the epithelium at the expense of requiring a secondary dressing to secure the wound [19,22].

Water-based formations such as hydrogels and hydrocolloids are applied to wounds requiring a moist environment to heal. Hydrogels use hydrophilic polymers to attract water and create a three-dimensional network in the form of a gel. Hydrogels can be used to rehydrate a wound bed, rehydrate necrotic tissue, absorb excess exudate, or reduce pain [19,23,24]. Hydrogels can be loaded with bioactive compounds to deliver it directly to the wound area in a relatively painless manner. An available hydrogel is Curasol™ which is applied to an absorbent layer such as cotton or gauze and then taped, netted, or bandaged onto the wound. Hydrogel dressings often market themselves based on their pain relief and rehydrating abilities—one problem with these products is the complicated application that requires a healthcare professional [25]. Hydrogels are commonly applied to traditional medicine and are often fabricated using polymers derived from nature [26–28]. The polymers applied to hydrogels are becoming increasingly advanced; Yan et al. formulated a thermosensitive hydrogel that released a phage to combat bacterial infections. This hydrogel could be infected as a liquid but would form into a hydrogel dressing once exposed to the temperature of an inflamed wound bed [29]. Hydrocolloid dressings such as alginates have the advantage of requiring no secondary dressing. Hydrocolloid dressings are gel-forming agents that absorb and retain fluid to create a wound-moistening gel [24,30]. Hydrocolloids, like hydrogels, can be loaded with antiseptics or wound-healing drugs to make them bioactive. Hydrocolloid dressings derived from sodium alginate taken from brown seaweed are commonly used for wounds with excess exudate because of their absorptive properties. Other hydrocolloids such as Duoderm™ can be used for shallow acute wounds with little exudate present [24,31]. Hydrocolloids and hydrogels reduce pain sensation by keeping nerve endings moist and providing a provisional ECM to facilitate autolysis [24,30].

Semipermeable dressings such as foams and films can protect wounds from the external environment while allowing essential molecules to enter. Foams fabricated from polyurethane or silicone can protect against bacteria and moisten the wound bed while avoiding tissue damage when removed [32]. Foams are also used to encapsulate drugs and have been applied with natural products such as asiaticoside from *Centella asiatica* [33]. Recent advances in foams for wound care combine other technologies to create responsive/smart dressings. A multi-layer dressing made from an anti-microbial foam and an electrospun cellulose surface mesh was formulated by He et al. which changes colour in response to infection-caused pH changes [34]. Films are like foams by being semipermeable but are more often applied to epithelizing wounds with little exudate. Oxygen and carbon dioxide can pass through films but, similarly to foams, bacteria or pathogens are kept away. Koetse et al. and Babikian et al. have innovated different films for wound care which can record electrical signals in a wound [35,36]. Both devices aimed to capture a wide range of physiological parameters using impedance, current, and other parameters.

Another dressing that aids wound healing is bioadhesives. These adhere to the site of a wound to moisten, absorb exudate, and protect from external pathogens [37]. These can be injected as hydrogels which then adhere to the surface of a wound or be delivered as a patch placed similarly to a plaster [38]. Figure 2 shows how a bioadhesive can cover a wound bed. Bioadhesives must be biocompatible and biodegradable; thus, they are often derived from nature. One bioadhesive formulated by Ke et al. used two natural products in tannic acid and silk fibroin to help develop the ECM and protect against bacterial infection [39]. The full extent of advanced dressings used for wound care is beyond the scope of this review, but it is clearly a growing field expanding into dressings that are responsive or indicative of physiological parameters. Table 1 summarizes the many kinds of wound dressing. Many of these dressings are being made using natural compounds because of their biocompatibility and biodegradability; thus, it is a promising field for natural products in wound care [40].

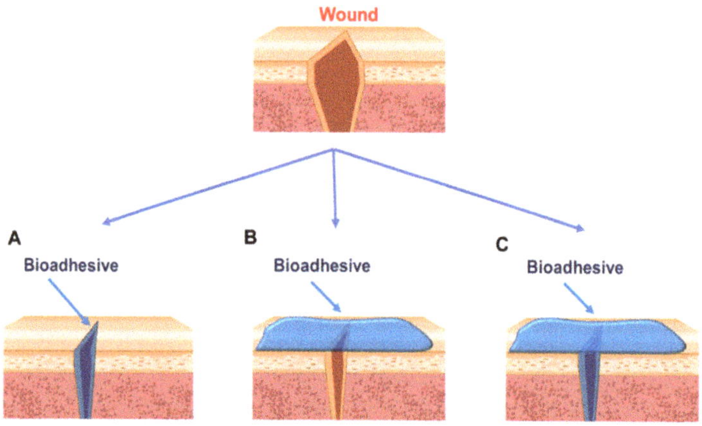

Figure 2. Strategies for bioadhesives used to close wounds. (**A**) Bioadhesives are applied between wound edges. (**B**) Bioadhesives are applied outside of the wounds. (**C**) Bioadhesives are applied between and outside the wounds. Reprinted with permission from Ref. [37].

Table 1. Characteristics of wound dressings.

Type of Wound Dressing	Features	Limitations	Product Name	References
Film dressings	Elastic, durable, comfortable, and conform well to body contours Waterproof and transparent Create a moist healing environment Bacterial and viral barrier Semi-permeable to water vapour and gas	Adhesive films might disrupt newly formed epithelium during dressing change Limited use for highly exuding wounds Might develop leakage channels	Tegaderm™ (3M™, UK Plc.) Opsite Films® (Smith and Nephew) Mepitel®Film (Mölnlycke Health Care Limited)	[32,34,41]
Foam dressings	Highly absorbent Easily removable Create a moist healing environment Bacterial and viral barrier Semi-permeable to water vapour and gas	Form an opaque layer, making wound monitoring difficult Limited use for dry wounds Poor stability	Flexsan Biopatch Biatain Cultinova Lyofoam Allevyn Unilene Tielle CuraSpon Kendall Hydrasorb	[33,42]
Hydrogel dressings	Create a moist healing environment Pain relief Self-applied or injectable Facilitate autolytic debridement Easily removed	Require a secondary dressing Lack of mechanical strength Inconsistent hydration properties Poor bacterial barrier	Suprasorb® AquaDerm™ Neoheal® Simpurity™ DermaGauze™ Restore	[43–45]
Bioadhesive dressings	Create a moist healing environment Self-injectable Adhesive	Unremovable Interference with other medical devices Might develop leakage channels	Ligate™	[37]

4. Natural Products

4.1. Modulators of Cellular Activity

The third stage of wound healing, proliferation, can be hastened by compounds promoting cellular growth and proliferation. While its uncommon for this stage to be stalled or force the development of a chronic wound, increasing the proliferation rate can heal a wound faster to remove physical and cosmetic discomfort to the patient [18,20]. Increasing cell proliferation also means a lesser likelihood of scarring—increased proliferation in fibroblasts mainly corresponds with increased collagen and, therefore, a better-developed wound bed [46]. Table 2 shows the natural products discussed in this review's mechanism of action for wound healing.

Table 2. Wound healing natural products are classified into their mechanism of action.

Mode of Action	Natural Products	References
Modulators of Cellular Activity	Turmeric, Honey, and *E. phaseoloides*	[46–56]
Modulators of Collagen Synthesis	Aloe vera, *A. boonei, C. asiatica*	[57–70]
Modulators of Angiogenesis	Honey, Aloe Vera, and *E. phaseoloides*	[59,63,71–76]
Modulators of the Extracellular Matrix	Honey	[57,77–81]
Modulators of Cytokines and Growth Factors	Essential Oils and Honey	[52,53,82–86]
Antibiotics and Antimicrobials	Garlic and Lavender	[87–90]
Modulators of Oxidant/Antioxidant Balance	Turmeric and Vanilla	[41,91–93]
Other	Vitamins A/B/C/D	[94]

Curcumin, an extract from turmeric, is known for its bioactivity as an antioxidant, anti-inflammatory agent, antibacterial, and as a promotor of collagen synthesis and cell proliferation [46–49]. For these reasons, curcumin has been used by many cultures as a wound-healing drug applied topically to a wound [50]. Curcumin's efficacy is limited by poor solubility in water and photosensitivity [46], hence its status as a traditional rather than conventional medicine [46].

Honey is another widespread medicine used traditionally for wound healing. The bioactive components of honey are a mixture of enzymes, pollen, and environment-specific molecules. However, some of honey's more basic characteristics act to modulate cellular activity to promote wound healing [51]. Honey's sugar content can provide nutrition to the cells fatigued from mass proliferation and inflammation to promote their survival and growth [52]. Honey's low pH has also been reported to create conditions ideal for fibroblasts activity, facilitating better collagen development and fibroblast migration to close the wound [52]. Studies by Ranzato et al. further tested honey's properties in an in vitro scratch wound healing model. They found honey to promote re-epithelisation and help close a wound in the final stages of its healing [53].

Another compound that promotes fibroblast proliferation and migration is tannin [54]. Tannin is a polyphenol that can be extracted from a myriad of plants and was traditionally used for tanning leather [55]. Alongside this purpose, plants such as *Entada phaseoloides* with high levels of tannins were used by South-East Asian cultures as a compound for wound healing. Su et al. studied the mechanism of action of tannin and found that it promotes fibroblast proliferation and migration. Increased cellular proliferation and migration quickens the wound-healing process and reduces the likelihood of scarring [54]. In this study, tannin acted similarly to the clinically used Bactroban with no significant difference between tannin from the *Entada* extract and Bactroban as a positive control [54]. Compounds such as honey, curcumin, and tannin used as traditional medicines have been analysed under modern pharmaceutical conventions to discover their modulation of cellular activity. A better understanding of this can allow future research to formulate such compounds into effective medicines [55,56].

4.2. Modulators of Collagen Synthesis

Synthesis of collagen returns structure and strength to the dermis after a wound [57]. Promoting collagen synthesis speeds up wound healing dramatically and reduces the risk of opening the wound again [20]. As well as the rate of collagen synthesis, the type of collagen being synthesised is important to promote non-scarred wound beds [58]. The importance of collagen in the wound-healing process has meant compounds that modulate the molecular mechanisms of collagen synthesis have been identified as wound-healing medicines.

Aloe vera is a natural compound still widely used and recognized in home, and clinical practices as a wound healing tool [59]. The most studied active ingredients of aloe vera are thought to be aloe-emodin, aloin, aloesin, emodin, and acemann [60]. While primarily known for reducing pain in burn wounds, aloe vera also increases the amount of collagen in wounds [61]. Beyond this, aloe vera affects collagen composition by promoting cross-linking; this develops greater three-dimensional structural integrity of the early granulation tissue and begins the return of the tissue to the regular dermis [62]. Aloe vera's common form is a gel that not only delivers the drug but moistens the wound to improve flexibility, acts as a barrier against foreign microbes, and bathes the nerves to reduce pain [63].

Alkaloids are a class of basic, natural compounds, which contain at least one nitrogen atom. Alkaloids are present in many plants, particularly in flowers such as nightshade, poppies, and buttercups [64]. A study by Fetse et al. on alkaloids from *A. boonei* showed an increase in wound healing which was attributed to the promotion of re-epithelisation, angiogenesis, and increased collagen deposition [65]. In the same paper, *A. boonei* extract was theorised to be involved in collagen maturation: early granulation tissue contains collagen type IV while fully healed tissue contains the stronger and more developed collagen type I [65]. This paper found alkaloids to contribute to many different stages and components of the complex wound-healing process.

Collagen synthesis in cultured fibroblasts is increased by asiatic acid. Asiatic acid comes from the popular medicinal plant *Centella asiatica*, which has a long history in sub-continental traditional medicine [66]. There are three bioactive compounds in *Centella*: madecassoside, asiatic acid, and asiaticoside. All three were tested by Bonte et al. and then Maquart et al., who found each compound had positive effects on collagen synthesis in vivo. Asiatic acid, however, showed the most significant efficacy in vitro [67,68]. *Centella* extract contains all three extracts; however, Nagoor-Meeran et al. identified asiatic acid as the best compound to isolate for pharmaceutical use [66]. All three compounds have other properties ranging from antioxidant, anti-inflammatory, or anti-cancerous. *Centella*'s widespread historical use is clearly justified and only requires improved solubility and stability in the biological environment [3,4,69,70].

4.3. Modulators of Angiogenesis

There is a wide range of natural products which modulate angiogenesis. Both anti-angiogenic and angiogenic compounds can be used at different stages of the wound-healing process. Angiogenesis is a natural part of the proliferation phase of acute wound healing but can become problematic in a chronically inflamed wound [71]. Plant extracts to be used in both applications are common and widely used.

Plants containing flavonoids act as anti-angiogenic agents. Flavonoids are phenolic compounds with a benzo-γ-prone structure [72]. These compounds are found widely in tea, cocoa, and red wine, of which tea, especially, has been used as a natural wound-healing medicine [73]. Green tea contains a significant amount of flavonoids and other phenol-based compounds, which alter mi-RNA expression to restrict angiogenesis controlled by the VEGF receptor family [74]. Green tea in its traditional oral form is not specific to a wound, and as a topical extract, it cannot penetrate the stratum corneum [74]. Without specificity, green tea is limited despite promising bioactive properties. Despite this, green tea is a common anti-angiogenic solution, as well as other options such as *Centella asiatica* [74,75].

Aloe vera is a widely applied natural medicine that contains the pro-angiogenic compound beta-sitosterol [76]. Aloe vera's pro-angiogenic activity makes it a candidate for promoting faster vessel growth and faster recovery in healing tissue. Beta-sitosterol works by stimulating vessel cell migration and enhancing the expression of angiogenesis-related proteins [76]. Aloe vera is widely available across the globe and is already used for other wound-healing properties, especially in burn wounds [59]. Aloe vera's high water content can reduce wound-related pain while stimulating collagen synthesis and cross-linking directly hastens a wound's natural healing process [63]. This, along with its pro-angiogenic properties, has made it a popular wound-healing drug across the world's traditional medicine and continues to be one of the most widely recognised natural wound-healing solutions [59].

4.4. Modulators of the Extracellular Matrix

The ECM is a complex structure in the dermis that contains countless proteins, enzymes, and inflammatory components influencing how the body reacts to a wound [58]. There are fewer ECM modulating compounds than the other categories described in this review; however, their efficacy and common usage justify their acknowledgement as a natural product modulating the wound-healing process.

Stingless bee honey is one of the few natural ECM modulators. Honey was traditionally applied on wounds primarily because of its antibacterial and hydrating qualities; however, a study by Malik et al. has uncovered honey's ECM modulating characteristics [57]. The unique mixture of enzymes, pollen, and other molecules in this honey down-regulated the MMP-1 gene, which encodes a protease protein, and up-regulated the gene for type I collagen, COL1A1 [57]. Reduced MMP activity and increased collagen will allow the development of collagen and extracellular proteins to recover the ECM earlier [77]. Malik et al. carried out this study in incubated human dermal fibroblasts and quantified gene expression using qRT-PCR [57]. Without an in vivo test, honey's use as a wound-healing drug cannot be confirmed; however, Malik et al.'s findings add further potential to a new formulation of honey that can regulate fibroblasts in direct contact beneath the epidermis.

Another compound belonging to bee honey, propolis, alters the expression and modification of ECM genes [78]. A notable protein altered by propolis is dermatan/heparan sulphate, a glycosaminoglycan which attracts water and cations to form most of the ECM's content [79]. Its induction and structural modification, allowing growth protein attachment by propolis, increases the amount of the glycosaminoglycan in the dermis to recover the ECM quickly [79,80]. Propolis was compared to the widely commercially used silver sulfadiazine, which out-performed it in its induction of key ECM proteins such as dermatan sulphate and hyaluronic acid [81]. This outperformance of the 'gold standard' for ECM modulation presents propolis as a promising natural medicine that demands further research.

4.5. Modulators of Cytokines and Growth Factors

Cytokines are proteins or glycoproteins which modulate inflammatory or immune responses [95]. Growth factors increase cell proliferation, growth, and differentiation. Both classes of compounds modulate the progression of the wound-healing stages and the inflammation cascade [96]. Changing the timing or levels of these important compounds can change the balance of the cocktail of compounds controlling the body's response to a wound. This critical role has meant a group of traditional medicines that alter the balance of cytokines and growth factors used specifically for wound healing [97].

Terpenoids are commonly found in essential oils and suppress cytokines to act as anti-inflammatories [82]. Marques et al. showed that terpenes reduced the pro-inflammatory cytokines TNF-α and IL-1α and increased production of IL-10. This had the net effect of suppressed inflammation to demonstrate its therapeutic potential [83]. In a systematic review, Barreto et al. found five preclinical terpenoids that showed potential as wound-healing drugs but were not well studied. Specifically, the mechanism of action requires better understanding to explain the clear evidence of anti-inflammatory activity [82]. The popularity of terpene products has risen with essential oils despite this poorly understood mechanism of action. The *B. morolensis* essential oil from Mexican folk medicine is an example of a terpene-containing essential oil that has been shown to promote wound healing [84].

Honey is a compound with many properties applicable to wound healing. One property is an effect on interleukins and MMPs. MMPs modulate the cleavage of cytokines controlling the inflammatory cascade and are a target enzyme to modulate cytokine levels [85]. Acacia and buckwheat honey especially showed this effect, while manuka, a more commonly known medicinal honey, showed a more minor modulatory effect [53,86]. Martinotti and Ranzato have also proposed a honey-based scaffold that can house growth factors to promote re-epithelisation [53]. This novel delivery system with honey, a known antibacterial and anti-inflammatory compound housing endogenous and modern synthetic growth factors, is a creative way to apply natural compounds to wound-healing medicine [52,86].

While not yet applied with natural compounds, cytokine modulators have been identified as novel therapeutic agents inhibiting fibrogenesis. Excess fibrogenesis often causes scarring and fibrosis of the skin; thus, modern cytokine modulators have become an active area of research [96]. Applying the modulatory effects of natural products such as terpenes and honey should be considered as another approach to prevent fibrosis. MMP modulators such as buckwheat and acacia honey should especially be considered as compounds preventing scarring and promoting re-epithelisation [53].

4.6. Natural Products Acting as Antibiotics or Antimicrobials

Antibiotic agents are important for the prevention and removal of bacteria from wounds. Bacterial invasion into a wound should be prevented at all measures as infection can form a chronic wound or develop into its own condition, such as gangrene or abscess [98]. Bacterial infections can become more complicated and severe than the wound itself hence the heavy emphasis in healthcare on antibiotic treatment of open wounds [77]. Products such as garlic, honey, and ginger have been used by ancient cultures as antibiotics to dress wounds and other bacterially inflicted conditions [5]. In the modern age of medicine, more efficient antibiotics such as penicillin have been developed; however, natural antibiotics continue to be commonly used worldwide [7].

Interestingly, many modern antibiotics are found in nature. Modern techniques have isolated active compounds from traditional antibiotics or antibiotics originating from fungi to achieve more refined and efficient use as pharmaceutics. An example of a traditional antibiotic is garlic. The compound responsible for its antibacterial activity is generally recognized as allicin, an organosulfur compound known to penetrate through the membranes of bacteria and interfere with essential enzymes [99]. Lu et al. investigated this in 2011 and had conclusive evidence of garlic concentrate's efficacy against bacterial growth [87]. Garlic has been described as a medicinal plant in literature as far back as 6 BC and was used by ancient Sumerian, Egyptian, Indian, Chinese, and Greek healers [100]. Garlic is applied as a traditional 'fix-all' medicine, it is used as an anti-inflammatory agent, an antibiotic, or an anti-tumour product, amongst others [88,99]. While traditional medicines' active compounds can inform the synthesis of novel antibiotic analogues, they should also be considered in modern applications, whether delivered traditionally or using modern pharmaceutical strategies. Petrovska et al. noted the value of garlic as an antibiotic even in the presence of the contemporary antibiotic, especially in an aged form [100]. Compounds trusted by many cultures such as garlic that have efficacy as antibiotics should continue to be researched to expand their natural potential.

Antimicrobials have been commercialised as an everyday supplement in the form of essential oils marketed as natural products curing all sorts of ailments ranging from anxiety to eczema [89,101]. A popular antimicrobial essential oil is lavender extract. Linalool, a chemical component of lavender, possesses antimicrobial activity [102]. Although essential oils are often designated as alternative medicine, the need for novel antimicrobial agents has directed research towards their efficacy [103]. Lavender oil has contradicting evidence for its efficacy; linalool was thought to increase bacterial cell wall permeability to increase another antimicrobial's efficacy [104]. Guo et al. further studied linalool's mechanism of antimicrobial action, finding that it not only ruptured cell walls but directly interacted with amino acid metabolism [90]. Other research has shown that linalool has little antimicrobial efficacy when used independently [105]. Predoi et al. found that linalool is not likely to prevent or improve microbial infections, contradicting Guo et al.'s growth curves showing linalool's anti-microbial activity [90,105]. Essential oils such as lavender remind us that while traditional medicine is used for a reason, modern pharmaceutical analysis is required to determine a compound's mechanism of action to formulate an effective delivery approach. Lavender has shown potential as an antimicrobial agent demanding further research and understanding to develop it into an effective therapy.

4.7. Modulators of the Oxidant–Antioxidant Balance of the Wound Microenvironment

Antioxidants have shown promise in their ability to hasten the wound-healing process [86]. Antioxidants work by reacting with highly reactive radical oxygen species (ROS) to stabilise the ROS without becoming reactive themselves [106]. Aerobic metabolism in the mitochondria creates ROS proportionally to the metabolic demands on the cells. The increased proliferation and migration occurring during wound healing elevate metabolic demand and ROS presence [86]. ROS serves essential functions in phagocytic and cell-signalling mechanisms but can also cause oxidative stress at high levels; therefore, their presence is tightly regulated [86]. Oxidative stress can degrade membranes, DNA, lipids, and protein in the skin, killing fibroblasts and tightening skin [107]. ROS and inflammation are tightly linked as they are elevated during inflammation but can also induce the process [46]. This forms a positive feedback loop and can contribute to a wound becoming chronically inflamed [108]. Antioxidants are released endogenously by the body's ROS regulatory mechanism but are also a popular diet supplement present in vegetables, berries, and other food groups [109]. Applying antioxidants systemically or locally can help balance ROS levels to reduce oxidative stress and enhance wound healing [106].

Curcumin has been used as an antioxidant in traditional medicine and is an example of a natural antioxidant requiring advanced delivery techniques. The active ingredient in turmeric, curcumin, possesses anti-inflammatory, anti-infective, and antioxidant properties [47]. Curcumin's use is limited by its low water solubility and stability, making effective delivery to the predominantly aqueous wound environment difficult [47,56,110]. Gopinath et al. proved curcumin's antioxidant ability by demonstrating a decrease in curcumin and the ROS oleic acid when combined using time-dependent studies. Results showed reduced absorption corresponding to decreased curcumin, indicating reactions between oleic acid and curcumin [41]. Curcumin's antioxidant activity was confirmed by analysing the expression of an endogenous antioxidant enzyme: superoxide dismutase (SoD). Curcumin's efficacy in stabilising ROS levels reduced the need for endogenous antioxidants; therefore, SoD's expression was reduced compared to control [41]. In multiple trials, Panahi et al. have also shown the effectiveness of curcumin as an antioxidant in humans using a dosage regime and blood testing [47]. On top of these experiments proving curcumin's antioxidant ability, Gopinath et al. and Zhao et al. have demonstrated curcumin's efficacy as a wound-healing drug [41,56]. These trials used a composite dressing and a collagen film, respectively, to improve the bioavailability of the drug and showed significant wound-healing ability of curcumin-loaded dressings/films [41,56]. Curcumin is an example of a traditional compound used by many different cultures which have antioxidant properties with the potential for better delivery [50].

Vanillin, a phenolic aldehyde found in olive oil and vanilla pods, is an antioxidant and an antimicrobial compound. This natural compound modifies oxidant balance by reacting with radicals in a self-dimerisation reaction to clear the wound bed of ROS [91]. When compared to ascorbic acid, vanillin showed superior anti-oxidising ability in ABTS(+), ORAC, and OxHLIA assays but no activity in the DPPH or galvinoxyl assays [91]. When applied in a dressing or hydrogel, vanillin has been shown to prevent ROS proliferation and bacterial infection in wounds [92,93]. Vanillin's bioactivity is a recent discovery; thus, it is a popular area of research.

4.8. Other Natural Products with Wound-Healing Properties

Although rarely seen as a treatment, monitoring intake of vitamins A, B, C, and D can impact the rate and extent to which a wound heals [111,112]. These vitamins are involved in collagen synthesis and inflammation and a deficit in vitamin levels during wound healing can lead to chronic wound development. Vitamin C is particularly well known as a common vitamin involved in wound healing which can cause scurvy if at low systemic levels [113]. Another notable compound is vitamin A and other associated retinoids. The efficacy of local retinoids is debated, and the mechanism of action is not fully understood [114]. Despite this, they are commonly used in dermatology as a topical ointment. Vitamin A is a compound whose delivery could be improved. Systemically, it is a detriment to wound healing, meaning delivery must be highly localised and separate from systemic circulation [94]. Vitamins are notable traditional medicines that are extensively researched and are at the forefront of many modern delivery adaptations [115].

There are countless herbs and plant extracts used in the many different cultures worldwide as wound-healing medicines. A more comprehensive list was compiled by Agyare et al., which lists many compounds less studied and not discussed in this review [97].

5. Advanced Delivery Strategies for Natural Wound-Healing Compounds

As our understanding of drugs have advanced, so has our ability to deliver them. As important as discovering novel drugs is discovering novel ways to deliver them. Older technologies such as dressings have been transformed into composite dressings which deliver a drug while still protecting the wound from the outside environment. This combination of drug and dressing adds functionality while maintaining the original purpose of a dressing. Similarly, hydrogels able to deliver a drug, moisten a wound, and protect it from the outside environment can remove the need for multiple wound treatments. Hydrogels are formed from water and polymers cross linked to form a gel with pores able to store a drug. Other techniques are the product of innovation, such as microneedles, lipid-based vesicles, and smart/responsive delivery. Microneedles are usually patches with tiny needles extending from their surface designed to penetrate the stratum corneum to access the dermis. Microneedles are painless and self-applicable and therefore are favoured over syringe-based applications. Lipid-based vesicles house drugs inside a bilayered sphere for transport through lipophilic membranes. These are often used for systemically applied drugs. Finally, smart/responsive delivery methods use environmental cues or remote control to release a drug at specific times and locations. This can be applied to most techniques and is able to release a drug at a specific moment in the temporally complex course of wound healing. Figure 3 graphically shows the different strategies and how they store and release a drug to the dermis.

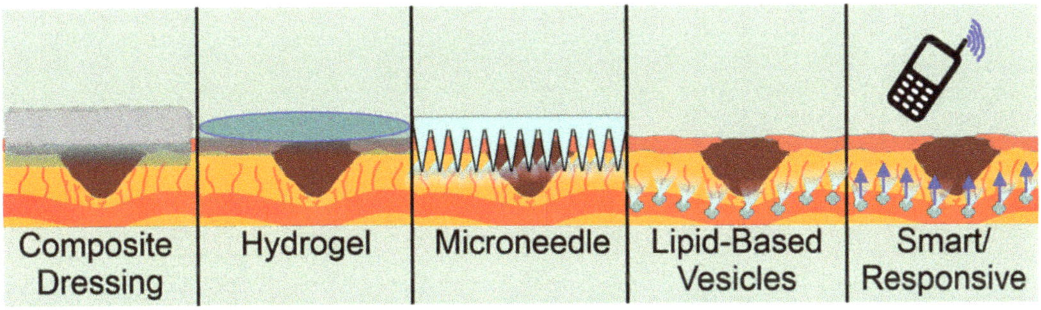

Figure 3. Modern delivery methods applied to natural products to improve their delivery and efficacy.

5.1. Composite Dressings

Composite dressings use the traditional dressing format but include a drug in the dressing itself. Dressings aim to allow oxygen exchange, maintain moisture, and protect the injury from infection [116]. Natural products which are biodegradable, versatile, and sustainable can be applied as biopolymer or biocomposite dressings. These can be more than just a dressing by promoting ECM regrowth, preventing scarring, or influencing inflammation [117]. Biodegradable dressings which produce no medical waste are of increasing interest as emissions and pollution are increasingly scrutinised [118].

A growing field is the delivery of growth factors by composite dressings. Modulating growth factors can speed up wound healing and promote an acute wound instead of a chronic wound [13]. Yao et al. developed a collagen sponge as a composite dressing to deliver endogenous growth factors to chronic ulcers and tested it in double-blinded controlled trial [119]. Their results showed an increased incidence of complete wound closure, a shortened healing time, and improved healing quality [119]. Using a dressing that delivers an endogenous therapeutic substance decreases the chance of an immune reaction or instability. Catanzano et al. discussed the potential of such systems, concluding that they will soon reach more widespread clinical use [120].

Composite dressings can contain natural products for delivery or be composed of a natural product itself [121]. An example of such a dressing was created by Gao et al., who used chitosan and diazo resin to create a hydrogel composite dressing [27]. Chitosan and diazo are both sourced from natural sources and are known antibacterial agents. Together with their antibacterial activity, the dressing showed an increased rate of wound healing [27]. Chitosan can be prone to lysosomal attack; thus, other combinations have been included with chitosan to improve composite dressings' efficacy. An alginate/ZnO_2 composite bandage formulated by Mohandas et al. showed desirable antibacterial effects against methicillin-resistant staphylococcus aureus and increased keratinocyte migration towards a wound area [122]. This formulation also included a chitosan hydrogel that worked with the ZnO_2 and alginate to achieve a therapeutic effect with less toxicity than a purely chitosan-derived gel [122]. The composite dressings formulated by Mohandas et al. and Gao et al. improve a traditional wound-healing structure; however, some researchers are innovating new forms of natural-product-based dressings altogether [123].

Electrospun nanofiber mats effectively deliver drugs topically while also acting as a wound dressing [124]. Many traditional wound-healing compounds such as curcumin from turmeric or thymol from thyme are lipophilic and are therefore challenging to localise when treating [125]. Nanofiber mats are created by charging droplets of a polymer and slowly releasing it across an electrical field to form a mat or sheet made up of long strands of tiny diameter—this creates space between fibers where a drug can be encapsulated [42,124]. Formulating a lipophilic drug this way allows the drug to be administered directly to the wound while the mat acts as a moistening dressing. Research reported that essential oil-loaded nanofiber mats showed more effective anti-inflammation/healing/antimicrobial activity (depending on the compound used) compared to essential oil itself [124,125]. Thymol was effective using this method—thymol's lipophilicity meant it could leave the mat and diffuse towards the wound quickly. In Garcia et al.'s study, thymol delivered by nanofiber mats showed similar anti-inflammatory properties to the commonly used drug dexamethasone, suggesting thymol as an effective natural alternative [125]. Electrospun nanofibrous structures could increase traditional medicine's efficacy, which was previously difficult to deliver due to their high lipophilicity locally.

Foams for wound healing are typically formed from synthetic polymers used as a replacement for gauze. Foams can be used to deliver drugs, moisturise wound beds, or manage exudate [126]. The release profile of foam dressings is typically rapid due to their free form; however, they usually require another bandage/dressing to prevent infection [33]. One such foam dressing was designed by Bai et al., which delivered a mix of silk fibroin protein, gastrodia elata, and tea tree oil [43]. Their foam dressing showed accelerated wound recovery by generating more abundant and thicker collagen in the dermis [43]. Foam dressings and other composite dressings are common ways of developing natural products historically and are now an area of active research. Technologies such as electrospun nano mats improve how natural products can be delivered while retaining the known benefits of dressing a wound.

5.2. Hydrogels

Hydrogels form a moistening barrier to the outside world at the surface of a wound to protect from foreign microbes while keeping the wound moist [125]. Therapeutic compounds are stored in the pores of hydrogels to be released onto the wound. When forming a hydrogel, a polymer with correctly sized pores is required to maximise drug release from the gel to the wound. Hydrogels delivering curcumin, aloe vera, and cordycepin have been designed successfully as novel delivery strategies [28,49,127,128]. Song et al.'s development of a cordycepin/chitosan complex hydrogel is an excellent example of a natural-product-based gel. This hydrogel showed desirable structural, swelling, and mechanical properties as well as a self-healing ability. The ability to self-heal allows the gel to mould itself to the status of the wound rather than require pre-moulding. Song et al. showed improved re-epithelisation and increased collagen deposition in wounds with the gel compared to a control [28].

More complex hydrogels such as curcumin/chitosan nanoemulsions have also been developed. The antibacterial chitosan stabilises curcumin in a hydrogel to create an antibacterial dressing that moistens the wound while delivering curcumin as an antioxidant [49]. Aloe vera has also been formulated into a nanohydrogel that polarises macrophages to modulate their activity during wound healing [128]. Nanohydrogels have much smaller pores than regular hydrogels, which allows 'smart' hydrogel development to alter their properties in response to external stimuli [128]. The nanohydrogel (made by aloe and chitosan) reported by Ashouri had shown significant changes in cytokines involved with macrophage polarisation when the cells became closer to an M1 subtype [128]. Future treatments responsive to changes in the wound environment can be designed to change their output to direct wounds away from becoming chronic and reduce the need for constant changing of dose and drugs [2].

Hydrogels not only deliver natural compounds but can also be fabricated from naturally occurring polymers. These polymers can be safer and more biocompatible than other synthetic polymers [26]. Zhi et al. created natural-product gels composed of self-assembling triterpenoids [129]. The triterpenoids were taken from Chinese medicinal herbs and used as a gel scaffold to deliver DOX-1 to treat murine tumours [129]. The gels showed an excellent network polymer structure and a sustained release profile comparable to other synthetic compounds [129]. Triterpenoids have antioxidant activity, which can complement the anti-tumour activity of DOX-1. Rather than giving both compounds in tandem, this study pioneered a system that could deliver DOX-1 with a triterpenoid-based structure. Another natural gel uses a decellularised ECM to create a hydrogel that replicates the (ECM when delivering a drug [44]. This helps the ECM return quickly while causing the least disruption possible to a wound. This hydrogel application promotes tissue remodelling and cell proliferation and can deliver a select drug to the application site. These novel hydrogel formulations show how hydrogels can deliver natural products and form the scaffold of the hydrogel.

Hydrogels allow drugs to be delivered locally to a wound without the need for a clinician. Combined with their ability to act as a dressing, hydrogels have become a popular prescription for clinicians and an emerging field for delivering traditional compounds [127,130].

5.3. Microneedles

With the turn of the century, microneedles have emerged as an exciting new method for transdermal drug delivery [2]. The traditional transdermal or subcutaneous delivery method of hypodermic needle injection results in medical waste, requires a clinician, and is traumatic. Microneedle technology is a relatively painless and frequently self-administered approach for drug delivery. Drugs with wound-healing ability are often formulated and tested in the microneedle format [131]. There are five classes of microneedles: solid, hollow, coated, dissolving, and hydrogel-forming [2]. Solid microneedles do not have drugs loaded onto the microneedles but disrupt the skin to create pores for a topically applied drug to enter the following microneedling. Hollow microneedles contain an internal pore that can hold a larger volume of drug to be released into the dermis [132]. Coated microneedles have a similar makeup to solid microneedles but are coated in the drug before application. Dissolving and hydrogel-forming microneedles differ from solid/coated microneedles by being left in the skin for an extended period. Dissolving microneedles have the drug incorporated into their own needles. When inserted into the dermis, the needles dissolve to release the drug. Hydrogel-forming microneedles can have the drug in the needles or in the patch supporting the microneedles and work by partially dissolving to create a liquid channel between the drug-loaded patch and the needles into the dermis [132]. As the field has advanced, so has the design of microneedles. 'Smart' microneedles can modulate their release of anti-inflammatory compounds according to inflammation-induced temperature changes [133]. Smart microneedles can reduce the need for clinical care of an inflamed wound and prevent the formation of a chronic wound in an inflammation loop [108]. Park and Frydman reported that the antibacterial, antioxidant, and wound-healing effects were significantly increased using microneedles loaded with manuka honey and green tea extracts, compared to traditional formulations such as cream or topical solutions [51,134].

Microneedles are not just used to bypass the stratum corneum but can also pierce the bacterial biofilm often present in chronic wounds. Biofilms are impermeable to most drugs and can be difficult to remove. The development of microneedles as an alternative to the painful and dangerous hypodermic needle has also introduced it as a new delivery strategy for the removal of biofilms [1,2,132]. Frydman and Chi both reported that the antibacterial-agent-loaded microneedle arrays could effectively remove or inhibit the growth of biofilms [51,133]. Biofilms are present in conditions other than wound healing and demand constant vigilance from healthcare workers to prevent their formation on medical equipment or open wounds. Antibacterial microneedle patches composed of manuka and chitosan have great potential to remove biofilms in wounds and other contexts, thus making antibacterial microneedles a hot topic in research [2].

5.4. Lipid-Based Vesicles/Nanotech

Molecules that are difficult to deliver can be encapsulated into lipid-based vesicles to improve their solubility and stability [135,136]. Most natural products are biologically unstable, insoluble in water, and poorly distributed to target sites. Lipid-based vesicles can improve their solubility and stability to improve their delivery [137].

Liposomes form double-chain phospholipids to form a bilayered sphere with a hydrophobic layer surrounded by a hydrophilic core and surface [135,136,138]. Compounds such as thymol and carvacrol from oregano which have poor solubility and stability can be encapsulated in liposomes to improve their bioavailability and delivery. Liolios et al. reported that both thyme and carvacrol showed better distribution and stability, resulting in greater efficacy [136]. Liolios et al. were not targeting wound healing with their study; however, others have used liposomes in this context. Given that thymol and carvacrol have proven efficacy in wound healing as antioxidants and antimicrobial agents, there is an opportunity to develop a liposomal formulation of the drugs aimed at wound healing [139]. Li et al. used madecassoside from *Centella asiatica* in biodegradable liposomes targeted at burn wounds in rats [140]. This formulation improved madecassoside's delivery by enhancing its stability and controlling its release. The significant findings in Li et al.'s study demand further research into the many other lipophilic natural compounds. Liposomes are useful vehicles for typically insoluble drugs and more studies on their efficacy in wound healing will hopefully be carried out.

Another lipid-based vesicle, which drugs can be encapsulated in, is a niosome. Niosomes are also bilayered spheres but differ from liposomes being formed from non-ionic single-chain surfactants and amphipathic compounds [135,141]. Niosomes are easier to fabricate and are more stable than liposomes. Niosomes are less expensive and do not require unique methods for handling and purification [135]. These favourable characteristics have brought niosomes to the forefront of lipid-based vesicle research—many consider niosomes to be the future of the field with widespread applications across medicine and nutrition [135,142]. Curcumin's solubility, stability, and efficacy against cancer cells were improved in a niosomal formulation compared to a dissolved curcumin solution [143]. Similarly to Akbarzadeh et al.'s study, Xu et al. applied a niosomal formulation to the long process of wound healing [144]. Xu et al.'s curcumin-loaded niosomal formulation displayed a controlled release profile reaching 80% release after 25 h and a significantly greater cellular uptake compared to free curcumin dissolved in solution [144]. Such characteristics and promising results suggest that niosomal formulation could be ideal for wound healing.

Exosomes are another lipid-bilayer spherical vesicle that can carry both hydrophilic and hydrophobic drugs. Exosomes differ from liposomes and niosomes in the complexity of their surface, which contains organotrophic proteins allowing directed transport inside and outside the cell [145,146]. Laborious production, safety issues, and low yield have slowed the development of exosomes, with only natural exosomes being viable to form [145]. These natural exosomes from fruit and dairy have not shown much advantage over liposomes other than increased safety and biocompatibility [147]. Sun et al. formulated curcumin into exosomes to protect the drug from biodegradation (over 2.5 h) and only a quarter amount of curcumin was degraded compared to curcumin dissolved in solution [148]. This paper focused on curcumin's anti-inflammatory activity, which can be easily applied to a wound-healing context. Some reviewers of lipid-based vesicles encourage mixing liposomes, exosomes, and niosomes to use together [137,145]. A suggested solution is to engineer the organotrophic proteins of exosomes onto niosomes or liposomes to create targeted easily produced vesicles. While lipid-based vesicles have been used in wound-healing applications to deliver natural compounds, only a few studies describe how natural compounds can be fabricated into vesicles and be delivered to wounds.

Nanocarriers can be used to control or optimise the delivery of drugs. As with microneedles and hydrogels, nanocarriers can be designed to be responsive to external stimuli, making them smart nanocarriers [149]. For drugs that struggle to bypass membranes or have undesirable pharmacokinetic characteristics, nanocarriers can help drugs diffuse across lipophilic membranes and optimise their release. Thymol extracted from oregano and thyme has been formulated into a chitosan/tragacanth gum nanocarrier by Sheorain [150]. Thyme was used by ancient Mediterranean cultures as an antioxidant and antimicrobial agent but was limited by low bioavailability and insolubility [151]. Sheorain's study improved both characteristics by encapsulating thymol into a chitosan/tragacanth gum nanocarrier that has antibacterial properties derived from chitosan. As a result, thymol displayed more significant antioxidant activity (as measured by ROS-scavenging activity) at multiple doses formulated in nanocarriers rather than its natural form [150]. Using such carriers can harness the effectiveness of traditional compounds such as thymol which need a better formulation to be delivered effectively.

Similarly to nanocarriers, porous microspheres encapsulate a drug and alter the drug's absorption and release profile. Porous microspheres act more as reservoirs than nanocarriers—they protect the drug avoiding inactivation from the external environment and prolonging the drug's absorption [152]. This technology was effectively applied to the traditional compound of asiaticoside by Zhang et al. [153]. Asiaticoside has a variety of favourable pharmacological characteristics as a wound-healing drug but is limited by its poor solubility and encapsulation inside a soluble microsphere successfully facilitated its entry into a wound and sustained its release over time to achieve a more favourable time/concentration relationship absorption [153].

5.5. Responsive and Smart Delivery

At the forefront of drug delivery innovation are smart/responsive delivery systems. A smart system can respond to endogenous or exogenous stimuli to alter drug release. These technologies aim to modulate drug release according to properties such as pH, glucose levels, and temperature as a gauge of a wound's status [154]. Identifying how these properties reflect changes in the wound has been the rate-limiting step in this field, meaning few examples currently exist [45]. Such devices show great potential for delivering natural products in a sustained and controlled fashion. This field is rapidly expanding and will continue to develop systems applicable to a wide variety of wound-healing drugs [155].

Inadequate oxygenation is a known cause of wounds becoming chronic; therefore, the oxygen content is a property commonly sensed by smart delivery systems. One such system was developed by Ochoa et al. as a biocompatible patch that can deliver oxygen to a wound bed when oxygenation decreases too far [156]. While not yet developed, a similar patch that senses perfusion could deliver natural antioxidant products to prevent ROS production when perfusion is fluctuating. Compounds such as curcumin, which can be loaded into nanofibers with smart-delivery potential, should be investigated for this purpose [157].

Smart devices can also respond to exogenous stimuli such as smartphone activation. Tamayol et al. produced nanofibrous textile platform that could respond to such external stimuli to release chitosan-based nanoparticles [158]. The platform included flexible heaters responsive to an external signal that triggers thermosensitive nanoparticles to release into a wound. Mostafalu et al. used the same system to deliver VEGF and antibiotics in a controlled and sustained manner [159]. Their system demonstrated efficacy and controlled drug release profiles, further showing that smart delivery systems should continue to add a new dimension to drug delivery.

6. Future Perspectives

Growing distrust of pharmaceutical companies and governments has raised public and private interest in traditional medicines over the past few decades [160,161]. Studying these compounds and improving their delivery can lead to quickly commercialised products. Some markets are likely to be more receptive to a wound-healing drug synthesised from thyme than a drug developed in silico or from a library [162]. The current work being carried out to improve the delivery of traditional compounds can improve drug efficacy and add academic legitimacy to the use of natural products.

85% of the world's population rely on plant products for their medicine, mostly in developing countries that have less access to modern synthetic drugs [163,164]. Table 3 further shows a correlation between the use of traditional medicine in developing nations and geographic location and income. Oyebode et al. showed that people of lower socioeconomic status that are unemployed, live in rural areas, and report a lower health status are more likely to use traditional medicine [165]. Medicine development aimed at developing countries should consider natural products already established in that country or culture to maximise accessibility. While growing, there are few pharmaceutical labs in developing countries that are able to create and apply such treatments [166,167], which is unlikely to change and is a critique of this approach. Another problem is maintaining the allure of natural products when delivered non-traditionally—such an approach may remove the appeal of natural products.

A potential concern is tarnishing a drug's appeal as a natural product by using complex pharmaceutical delivery techniques. For example, traditional medicines such as curcumin or manuka honey may not be culturally accepted if loaded into nanocarriers. This field's future is toeing the line of compounds that are accepted as natural while remaining effective in their delivery and method of action. Microneedles are a promising field with an increasing amount of research going into it. Microneedles formed of compounds such as chitosan or made from the active compound itself (such as Frydman's manuka microneedles) have the potential to be marketed as totally naturally based [51]. Nanocarriers, nanofibers, hydrogels, and microneedles also improve their encapsulated drugs' access to a wound while removing the need for systemic administration or subcutaneous injection [15]. All four of these technologies also have the potential to be 'smart,' where they can respond to stimuli such as ultrasound or temperature to change their physicochemical characteristics. Some of the most successful formulations of natural compounds have been vesicle-based smart delivery systems delivering catechin, thymol, curcumin, and madecassoside [138,168–172].

Modern nanotechnology has led to novel techniques such as 3D printing and lithography being applied to drug delivery. Lithography has been applied to microneedle formation and to survey endothelial cell migration in the field of wound healing [173,174]. The process of 3D printing using bio-inks has also been tested in the area with promising results: in vitro and in vivo animal studies of bio-ink engineering promote wound healing [175]. Indeed, the field of wound healing will keep expanding as technological advances do.

Table 3. Adjusted odds ratios and 95% confidence intervals of users of traditional healers by demographics in China, Ghana, and India. Adapted with permission from Ref. [165]. Copyright 2016, Oyebode.

	China	
	OR (CI)	***p*-Value**
Rural	6.9 (5.4–8.9)	<0.001
Income quintile	1.2 (1.1–1.2)	<0.001
	Ghana	
	OR (CI)	***p*-Value**
Rural	1.4 (1–2.2)	0.077
Income quintile	0.8 (0.7–0.9)	0.002
	India	
	OR (CI)	***p*-Value**
Rural	1.3 (0.9–2)	0.217
Income quintile	0.8 (0.7–0.9)	0.001

7. Conclusions

It is important to apply advanced delivery systems to natural products used traditionally. This benefits developing countries where traditional medicines are more accessible. Many traditional medicines have been shown to be efficacious and should no longer be considered an inferior approach to therapy. The delivery of traditional medicines is one of the most common problems with these drugs; thus, modern delivery techniques should be applied to maximise their natural potential. The authors believe that advanced drug delivery systems would improve the therapeutic efficacy of traditional wound-healing medicines, placing natural compounds such as curcumin and thymol at the forefront of the wound-healing field.

Author Contributions: Conceptualization, J.W.; writing—original draft preparation, C.R.; writing—review and editing, S.C., S.D. and H.Y.; visualization, C.R. and S.C.; supervision, J.W. All authors have read and agreed to the published version of the manuscript.

Funding: Faculty of Medical and Health Sciences Summer Scholarship funded by the University of Auckland.

Institutional Review Board Statement: Not applicable.

Informed Consent Statement: Not applicable.

Conflicts of Interest: The authors declare no conflict of interest. The funders had no role in the design of the study; in the collection, analyses, or interpretation of data; in the writing of the manuscript; or in the decision to publish the results.

References

1. Yi, X.; Yu, X.; Yuan, Z. A Novel Bacterial Biofilms Eradication Strategy Based on the Microneedles with Antibacterial Properties. *Procedia CIRP* **2020**, *89*, 159–163. [CrossRef]
2. Barnum, L.; Samandari, M.; Schmidt, T.A.; Tamayol, A. Microneedle Arrays for the Treatment of Chronic Wounds. *Exp. Opin. Drug Deliv.* **2020**, *17*, 1767–1780. [CrossRef] [PubMed]
3. Bahramsoltani, R.; Farzaei, M.H.; Rahimi, R. Medicinal Plants and their Natural Components as Future Drugs for the Treatment of Burn Wounds: An Integrative Review. *Arch. Dermatol. Res.* **2014**, *306*, 601–617. [CrossRef] [PubMed]
4. Hou, Q.; Li, M.; Lu, Y.; Liu, D.; Li, C. Burn Wound Healing Properties of Asiaticoside and Madecassoside. *Exp. Ther. Med.* **2016**, *12*, 1269–1274. [CrossRef] [PubMed]

5. World Health Assembly. *Traditional Medicine*; WHO: Geneva, Switzerland, 2014; Volume 9.1.
6. Liu, S.; Chuang, W.; Lam, W.; Jiang, Z.; Cheng, Y. Safety Surveillance of Traditional Chinese Medicine: Current and Future. *Drug Saf.* **2015**, *38*, 117–128. [CrossRef]
7. Ahmad Khan, M.S.; Ahmad, I. Chapter 1—Herbal Medicine: Current Trends and Future Prospects. In *New Look to Phytomedicine*; Ahmad Khan, M.S., Ahmad, I., Chattopadhyay, D., Eds.; Academic Press: Cambridge, MA, USA, 2019; pp. 3–13. [CrossRef]
8. Mukherjee, P.K.; Harwansh, R.K.; Bhattacharyya, S. Chapter 10—Bioavailability of Herbal Products: Approach toward Improved Pharmacokinetics. In *Evidence-Based Validation of Herbal Medicine*; Mukherjee, P.K., Ed.; Elsevier: Boston, MA, USA, 2015; pp. 217–245.
9. Lang, W.; Mennicke, W.H. Pharmacokinetic Studies on Triatiated Aescin in the Mouse and Rat. *Arzneimittelforschung* **1972**, *22*, 1928–1932.
10. Carey, B. When Trust in Doctors Erodes, Other Treatments Fill the Void. *The New York Times*, 3 February 2006; p. A-1.
11. Dai, C.; Shih, S.; Khachemoune, A. Skin Substitutes for Acute and Chronic Wound Healing: An Updated Review. *J. Dermatol. Treat.* **2020**, *31*, 639–648. [CrossRef]
12. Verma, N.; Kumari, U.; Mittal, S.; Mittal, A.K. Effect of Asiaticoside on the Healing of Skin Wounds in the Carp Cirrhinus Mrigala: An Immunohistochemical Investigation. *Tissue Cell* **2017**, *49*, 734–745. [CrossRef]
13. Boateng, J.S.; Matthews, K.H.; Stevens, H.N.E.; Eccleston, G.M. Wound Healing Dressings and Drug Delivery Systems: A Review. *J. Pharm. Sci.* **2008**, *97*, 2892–2923. [CrossRef]
14. Olsson, M.; Järbrink, K.; Divakar, U.; Bajpai, R.; Upton, Z.; Schmidtchen, A.; Car, J. The Humanistic and Economic Burden of Chronic Wounds: A Systematic Review. *Wound Repair Regen.* **2019**, *27*, 114–125. [CrossRef]
15. Lee, J.; Kim, H.; Lee, M.H.; Yuo, K.E.; Kwon, B.; Seo, H.J.; Park, J. Asiaticoside Enhances Normal Human Skin Cell Migration, Attachment and Growth in Vitro Wound Healing Model. *Phytomedicine* **2012**, *19*, 1223–1227. [CrossRef] [PubMed]
16. Xue, M.; Zhao, R.; Lin, H.; Jackson, C. Delivery Systems of Current Biologicals for the Treatment of Chronic Cutaneous Wounds and Severe Burns. *Adv. Drug Deliv. Rev.* **2018**, *129*, 219–241. [CrossRef] [PubMed]
17. Chouhan, D.; Dey, N.; Bhardwaj, N.; Mandal, B.B. Emerging and Innovative Approaches for Wound Healing and Skin Regeneration: Current Status and Advances. *Biomaterials* **2019**, *216*, 119267. [CrossRef] [PubMed]
18. Gray, K. *TIME Wounds Will Health*; Pharmac: Wellington, New Zealand, 2017.
19. Cockbill, S.M.E.; Turner, T.D. The development of wound management products. In *Chronic Wound Care: The Essentials E-Book*; Krasner, D.L., van Rijswijk, L., Eds.; HMP: Melvern, KS, USA, 2018; pp. 145–164.
20. Tottoli, E.M.; Dorati, R.; Genta, I.; Chiesa, E.; Pisani, S.; Conti, B. Skin Wound Healing Process and New Emerging Technologies for Skin Wound Care and Regeneration. *Pharmaceutics* **2020**, *12*, 735. [CrossRef] [PubMed]
21. Kim, H.S.; Sun, Z.; Lee, J.; Kim, H.; Fu, X.; Leong, K.W. Advanced Drug Delivery Systems and Artificial Skin Grafts for Skin Wound Healing. *Adv. Drug Deliv. Rev.* **2019**, *146*, 209–239. [CrossRef]
22. Romanelli, M.; Dowsett, C.; Doughty, D.; Senet, P.; Munter, C.; Martinez, J.L.L. *Advances in Wound Care: The Triangle of Wound Assessment*; World Union of Wound Healing Societies: London, UK, 2016.
23. Clements, D. *Skin and Wound Care Manual*; St. Clare's Mercy Hospital: St. John's, NL, Canada, 2008.
24. Hawkins, M. Volume D—Nursing Standards, Policies & Procedures. In *Wound Care*; Canterbury DHB: Christchurch, New Zealand, 2009; pp. 303–381.
25. DermNet, N.Z. *Wound Dressings*; New Zealand Dermatological Society Incorporated: Wellington, New Zealand, 2009; Volume 2021.
26. Cui, X.; Lee, J.J.L.; Chen, W.N. Eco-Friendly and Biodegradable Cellulose Hydrogels Produced from Low Cost Okara: Towards Non-Toxic Flexible Electronics. *Sci. Rep.* **2019**, *9*, 18166. [CrossRef]
27. Gao, L.; Zhang, H.; Yu, B.; Li, W.; Gao, F.; Zhang, K.; Zhang, H.; Shen, Y.; Cong, H. Chitosan Composite Hydrogels Cross-Linked by Multifunctional Diazo Resin as Antibacterial Dressings for Improved Wound Healing. *J. Biomed. Mater. Res. A* **2020**, *108*, 1890–1898. [CrossRef]
28. Song, R.; Zheng, J.; Liu, Y.; Tan, Y.; Yang, Z.; Song, X.; Yang, S.; Fan, R.; Zhang, Y.; Wang, Y. A Natural Cordycepin/Chitosan Complex Hydrogel with Outstanding Self-Healable and Wound Healing Properties. *Int. J. Biol. Macromol.* **2019**, *134*, 91–99. [CrossRef]
29. Yan, W.; Banerjee, P.; Liu, Y.; Mi, Z.; Bai, C.; Hu, H.; To, K.K.W.; Duong, H.T.T.; Leung, S.S.Y. Development of Thermosensitive Hydrogel Wound Dressing Containing Acinetobacter Baumannii Phage Against Wound Infections. *Int. J. Pharm.* **2021**, *602*, 120508. [CrossRef]
30. Weller, C. Interactive dressings and their role in moist wound management. In *Advanced Textiles for Wound Care*; Rajendran, S., Ed.; Woodhead Publishing: Cambridge, UK, 2009; pp. 97–112. [CrossRef]
31. Wietlisbach, C.M. 17—Wound Care. In *Cooper's Fundamentals of Hand Therapy*, 3rd ed.; Wietlisbach, C.M., Ed.; Mosby: St. Louis, MO, USA, 2020; pp. 154–166.
32. Shi, C.; Wang, C.; Liu, H.; Li, Q.; Li, R.; Zhang, Y.; Liu, Y.; Shao, Y.; Wang, J. Selection of Appropriate Wound Dressing for various Wounds. *Front. Bioeng. Biotechnol.* **2020**, *8*, 182. [CrossRef]
33. Namviriyachote, N.; Lipipun, V.; Akkhawattanangkul, Y.; Charoonrut, P.; Ritthidej, G.C. Development of Polyurethane Foam Dressing Containing Silver and Asiaticoside for Healing of Dermal Wound. *Asian J. Pharm. Sci.* **2019**, *14*, 63–77. [CrossRef]

34. He, M.; Ou, F.; Wu, Y.; Sun, X.; Chen, X.; Li, H.; Sun, D.; Zhang, L. Smart Multi-Layer PVA Foam/CMC Mesh Dressing with Integrated Multi-Functions for Wound Management and Infection Monitoring. *Mater. Des.* **2020**, *194*, 108913. [CrossRef]
35. Koetse, M.; Rensing, P.; van Heck, G.; Sharpe, R.; Allard, B.; Wieringa, F.; Kruijt, P.; Meulendijks, N.; Jansen, H.; Schoo, H. In Plane Optical Sensor Based on Organic Electronic Devices. In *Organic Field-Effect Transistors VII and Organic Semiconductors in Sensors and Bioelectronics*; SPIE: Bellingham, WA, USA, 2008; p. 70541I. [CrossRef]
36. Babikian, S.; Li, G.P.; Bachman, M. Integrated Bioflexible Electronic Device for Electrochemical Analysis of Blood. In Proceedings of the 2015 IEEE 65th Electronic Components and Technology Conference (ECTC), San Diego, CA, USA, 26–29 May 2015; pp. 685–690. [CrossRef]
37. Duan, W.; Bian, X.; Bu, Y. Applications of Bioadhesives: A Mini Review. *Front. Bioeng. Biotechnol.* **2021**, *9*, 716035. [CrossRef] [PubMed]
38. Li, J.; Yu, F.; Chen, G.; Liu, J.; Li, X.; Cheng, B.; Mo, X.; Chen, C.; Pan, J. Moist-Retaining, Self-Recoverable, Bioadhesive, and Transparent in Situ Forming Hydrogels to Accelerate Wound Healing. *ACS Appl. Mater. Interfaces* **2020**, *12*, 2023–2038. [CrossRef] [PubMed]
39. Ke, X.; Dong, Z.; Tang, S.; Chu, W.; Zheng, X.; Zhen, L.; Chen, X.; Ding, C.; Luo, J.; Li, J. A Natural Polymer Based Bioadhesive with Self-Healing Behavior and Improved Antibacterial Properties. *Biomater. Sci.* **2020**, *8*, 4346–4357. [CrossRef]
40. Barros Almeida, I.; Garcez Barretto Teixeira, L.; Oliveira de Carvalho, F.; Ramos Silva, É.; Santos Nunes, P.; Viana dos Santos Márcio, R.; de Souza Araújo, A.A. Smart Dressings for Wound Healing: A Review. *Adv. Skin Wound Care* **2021**, *34*, 1–8. [CrossRef]
41. Gopinath, D.; Ahmed, M.R.; Gomathi, K.; Chitra, K.; Sehgal, P.K.; Jayakumar, R. Dermal Wound Healing Processes with Curcumin Incorporated Collagen Films. *Biomaterials* **2004**, *25*, 1911–1917. [CrossRef]
42. İnal, M.; Mülazımoğlu, G. Production and Characterization of Bactericidal Wound Dressing Material Based on Gelatin Nanofiber. *Int. J. Biol. Macromol.* **2019**, *137*, 392–404. [CrossRef]
43. Bai, M.; Chen, M.; Yu, W.; Lin, J. Foam Dressing Incorporating Herbal Extract: An all-Natural Dressing for Potential use in Wound Healing. *J. Bioact. Compat. Polym.* **2017**, *32*, 293–308. [CrossRef]
44. Saldin, L.T.; Cramer, M.C.; Velankar, S.S.; White, L.J.; Badylak, S.F. Extracellular Matrix Hydrogels from Decellularized Tissues: Structure and Function. *Acta Biomater.* **2017**, *49*, 1–15. [CrossRef]
45. Saghazadeh, S.; Rinoldi, C.; Schot, M.; Kashaf, S.S.; Sharifi, F.; Jalilian, E.; Nuutila, K.; Giatsidis, G.; Mostafalu, P.; Derakhshandeh, H.; et al. Drug Delivery Systems and Materials for Wound Healing Applications. *Adv. Drug Deliv. Rev.* **2018**, *127*, 138–166. [CrossRef] [PubMed]
46. Panchatcharam, M.; Miriyala, S.; Gayathri, V.S.; Suguna, L. Curcumin Improves Wound Healingby Modulating Collagen and Decreasing Reactive Oxygen Species. *Mol. Cell. Biochem.* **2006**, *290*, 87–96. [CrossRef]
47. Panahi, Y.; Panahi, Y.; Khalili, N.; Khalili, N.; Sahebi, E.; Sahebi, E.; Namazi, S.; Namazi, S.; Karimian, M.; Karimian, M.; et al. Antioxidant Effects of Curcuminoids in Patients with Type 2 Diabetes Mellitus: A Randomized Controlled Trial. *Inflammopharmacology* **2017**, *25*, 25–31. [CrossRef]
48. Zhu, Y.; Luo, Q.; Zhang, H.; Cai, Q.; Li, X.; Shen, Z.; Zhu, W. A Shear-Thinning Electrostatic Hydrogel with Antibacterial Activity by Nanoengineering of Polyelectrolytes. *Biomater. Sci.* **2020**, *8*, 1394–1404. [CrossRef] [PubMed]
49. Thomas, L.; Zakir, F.; Mirza, M.A.; Anwer, M.K.; Ahmad, F.J.; Iqbal, Z. Development of Curcumin Loaded Chitosan Polymer Based Nanoemulsion Gel: In Vitro, Ex Vivo Evaluation and in Vivo Wound Healing Studies. *Int. J. Biol. Macromol.* **2017**, *101*, 569–579. [CrossRef]
50. Hatcher, H.; Planalp, R.; Cho, J.; Torti, F.M.; Torti, S.V. Curcumin: From Ancient Medicine to Current Clinical Trials. *Cell. Mol. Life Sci.* **2008**, *65*, 1631–1652. [CrossRef] [PubMed]
51. Frydman, G.H.; Olaleye, D.; Annamalai, D.; Layne, K.; Yang, I.; Kaafarani, H.M.A.; Fox, J.G. Manuka Honey Microneedles for Enhanced Wound Healing and the Prevention and/Or Treatment of Methicillin-Resistant Staphylococcus Aureus (MRSA) Surgical Site Infection. *Sci. Rep.* **2020**, *10*, 13229. [CrossRef] [PubMed]
52. Martinotti, S.; Ranzato, E. Honey, Wound Repair and Regenerative Medicine. *J. Funct. Biomater.* **2018**, *9*, 34. [CrossRef]
53. Ranzato, E.; Martinotti, S.; Burlando, B. Honey Exposure Stimulates Wound Repair of Human Dermal Fibroblasts. *Burn. Trauma* **2013**, *1*, 32–38. [CrossRef]
54. Su, X.; Liu, X.; Wang, S.; Li, B.; Pan, T.; Liu, D.; Wang, F.; Diao, Y.; Li, K. Wound-Healing Promoting Effect of Total Tannins from Entada Phaseoloides (L.) Merr. in Rats. *Burns* **2017**, *43*, 830–838. [CrossRef]
55. Pizzi, A. Tannins: Prospectives and Actual Industrial Applications. *Biomolecules* **2019**, *9*, 344. [CrossRef] [PubMed]
56. Zhao, Y.; Dai, C.; Wang, Z.; Chen, W.; Liu, J.; Zhuo, R.; Yu, A.; Huang, S. A Novel Curcumin-Loaded Composite Dressing Facilitates Wound Healing due to its Natural Antioxidant Effect. *Drug Des. Dev. Ther.* **2019**, *13*, 3269–3280. [CrossRef] [PubMed]
57. Malik, N.A.; Mohamed, M.; Mustafa, M.Z.; Zainuddin, A. In Vitro Modulation of Extracellular Matrix Genes by Stingless Bee Honey in Cellular Aging of Human Dermal Fibroblast Cells. *J. Food Biochem.* **2020**, *44*, e13098. [CrossRef]
58. Xue, M.; Jackson, C.J. Extracellular Matrix Reorganization during Wound Healing and its Impact on Abnormal Scarring. *Adv. Wound Care* **2015**, *4*, 119–136. [CrossRef] [PubMed]
59. Foster, M.; Hunter, D.; Samman, S. Evaluation of the Nutritional and Metabolic Effects of Aloe vera. In *Herbal Medicine: Biomolecular and Clinical Aspects*, 2nd ed.; Benzie, I.F.F., Wachtel-Galor, S., Eds.; CRC Press/Taylor & Francis: Boca Raton, FL, USA, 2011; Chapter 3.

60. Sánchez, M.; González-Burgos, E.; Iglesias, I.; Gómez-Serranillos, M.P. Pharmacological Update Properties of Aloe Vera and its Major Active Constituents. *Molecules* **2020**, *25*, 1324. [CrossRef]
61. Cho, S.; Lee, S.; Lee, M.; Lee, D.H.; Won, C.; Kim, S.M.; Chung, J.H. Dietary Aloe Vera Supplementation Improves Facial Wrinkles and Elasticity and it Increases the Type I Procollagen Gene Expression in Human Skin in Vivo. *Ann. Dermatol.* **2009**, *21*, 6–11. [CrossRef]
62. Boudreau, M.D.; Beland, F.A. An Evaluation of the Biological and Toxicological Properties of Aloe Barbadensis (Miller), Aloe Vera. *J. Environ. Sci. Health Part C* **2006**, *24*, 103–154. [CrossRef]
63. Hekmatpou, D.; Mehrabi, F.; Rahzani, K.; Aminiyan, A. The Effect of Aloe Vera Clinical Trials on Prevention and Healing of Skin Wound: A Systematic Review. *Iran. J. Med. Sci.* **2019**, *44*, 1–9.
64. Hussain, G.; Rasul, A.; Anwar, H.; Aziz, N.; Razzaq, A.; Wei, W.; Ali, M.; Li, J.; Li, X. Role of Plant Derived Alkaloids and their Mechanism in Neurodegenerative Disorders. *Int. J. Biol. Sci.* **2018**, *14*, 341–357. [CrossRef]
65. Fetse, J.P.; Kyekyeku, J.O.; Dueve, E.; Mensah, K.B. Wound Healing Activity of Total Alkaloidal Extract of the Root Bark of Alstonia Boonei (Apocynacea). *Br. J. Pharm. Res.* **2014**, *4*, 2642–2652. [CrossRef]
66. Nagoor Meeran, M.F.; Goyal, S.N.; Suchal, K.; Sharma, C.; Patil, C.R.; Ojha, S.K. Pharmacological Properties, Molecular Mechanisms, and Pharmaceutical Development of Asiatic Acid: A Pentacyclic Triterpenoid of Therapeutic Promise. *Front. Pharmacol.* **2018**, *9*, 892. [CrossRef] [PubMed]
67. Bonte, F.; Dumas, M.; Chaudagne, C.; Meybeck, A. Influence of Asiatic Acid, Madecassic Acid, and Asiaticoside on Human Collagen I Synthesis. *Planta Med.* **1994**, *60*, 133–135. [CrossRef]
68. Maquart, F.; Bellon, G.; Gillery, P.; Wegrowski, Y.; Borel, J. Stimulation of Collagen Synthesis in Fibroblast Cultures by a Triterpene Extracted from Centella Asiatica. *Connect. Tissue Res.* **1990**, *24*, 107–120. [CrossRef] [PubMed]
69. Gohil, K.J.; Patel, J.A.; Gajjar, A.K. Pharmacological Review on Centella Asiatica: A Potential Herbal Cure-All. *Indian J. Pharm. Sci.* **2010**, *72*, 546–556. [CrossRef] [PubMed]
70. Ahmed, A.S.; Taher, M.; Mandal, U.K.; Jaffri, J.M.; Susanti, D.; Mahmood, S.; Zakaria, Z.A. Pharmacological Properties of Centella Asiatica Hydrogel in Accelerating Wound Healing in Rabbits. *BMC Complementary Altern. Med.* **2019**, *19*, 213. [CrossRef]
71. Estrella-Mendoza, M.F.; Jiménez-Gómez, F.; López-Ornelas, A.; Pérez-Gutiérrez, R.M.; Flores-Estrada, J. Cucurbita Argyrosperma Seed Extracts Attenuate Angiogenesis in a Corneal Chemical Burn Model. *Nutrients* **2019**, *11*, 1184. [CrossRef] [PubMed]
72. Tsakiroglou, P.; VandenAkker, N.E.; Del Bo', C.; Riso, P.; Klimis-Zacas, D. Role of Berry Anthocyanins and Phenolic Acids on Cell Migration and Angiogenesis: An Updated Overview. *Nutrients* **2019**, *11*, 1075. [CrossRef]
73. Sun, Q.; Heilmann, J.; König, B. Natural Phenolic Metabolites with Anti-Angiogenic Properties—A Review from the Chemical Point of View. *Beilstein J. Org. Chem.* **2015**, *11*, 249–264. [CrossRef]
74. Rashidi, B.; Malekzadeh, M.; Goodarzi, M.; Masoudifar, A.; Mirzaei, H. Green Tea and its Anti-Angiogenesis Effects. *Biomed. Pharmacother.* **2017**, *89*, 949–956. [CrossRef]
75. Kusumo, W.D.; Mulyohadi, A.; Husnul, K.; Wibi, R.; Dianita, P.; Puspita, A.L.; Vanda, P. The Effect of Centella Asiatica to the Vascular Endothelial Growth Factor and Vascular Endothelial Growth Factor Receptor-2 on the Rotenone Induced Zebrafish Larvae (Danio Rerio) Stunting Model. *GSC Biol. Pharm. Sci.* **2018**, *5*, 88–95. [CrossRef]
76. Majewska, I.; Gendaszewska-Darmach, E. Proangiogenic Activity of Plant Extracts in Accelerating Wound Healing—A New Face of Old Phytomedicines. *Acta Biochim. Pol.* **2011**, *58*, 449–460. [CrossRef] [PubMed]
77. Hanna, J.R.; Giacopelli, J.A. A Review of Wound Healing and Wound Dressing Products. *J. Foot Ankle Surg.* **1997**, *36*, 2–14. [CrossRef]
78. Martinotti, S.; Ranzato, E. Propolis: A New Frontier for Wound Healing? *Burn. Trauma* **2015**, *3*, 9. [CrossRef] [PubMed]
79. Olczyk, P.; Mencner, Ł.; Komosinska-Vassev, K. The Role of the Extracellular Matrix Components in Cutaneous Wound Healing. *BioMed Res. Int.* **2014**, *2014*, 747584. [CrossRef] [PubMed]
80. Olczyk, P.; Komosinska-Vassev, K.; Winsz-Szczotka, K.; Stojko, J.; Klimek, K.; Kozma, E.M. Propolis Induces Chondroitin/Dermatan Sulphate and Hyaluronic Acid Accumulation in the Skin of Burned Wound. *Evid. Based Complementary Altern. Med.* **2013**, *2013*, 290675. [CrossRef]
81. Olczyk, P.; Komosińska-Vassev, K.; Winsz-Szczotka, K.; Koźma, E.M.; Wisowski, G.; Stojko, J.; Klimek, K.; Olczyk, K. Propolis Modulates Vitronectin, Laminin, and Heparan Sulfate/Heparin Expression during Experimental Burn Healing. *J. Zhejiang Univ. Sci. B* **2012**, *13*, 932–941. [CrossRef] [PubMed]
82. Barreto, R.S.S.; Albuquerque-Júnior, R.L.C.; Araújo, A.A.S.; Almeida Jackson, R.G.S.; Santos, M.R.V.; Barreto, A.S.; DeSantana, J.M.; Siqueira-Lima, P.; Quintans, J.S.S.; Quintans-Júnior, L.J. A Systematic Review of the Wound-Healing Effects of Monoterpenes and Iridoid Derivatives. *Molecules* **2014**, *19*, 846–862. [CrossRef]
83. Marques, F.M.; Figueira, M.M.; Schmitt, E.F.P.; Kondratyuk, T.P.; Endringer, D.C.; Scherer, R.; Fronza, M. In Vitro Anti-Inflammatory Activity of Terpenes via Suppression of Superoxide and Nitric Oxide Generation and the NF-κB Signalling Pathway. *Inflammopharmacology* **2019**, *27*, 281–289. [CrossRef]
84. Salas-Oropeza, J.; Jimenez-Estrada, M.; Perez-Torres, A.; Castell-Rodriguez, A.E.; Becerril- Millan, R.; Rodriguez-Monroy, M.A.; Jarquin-Yañez, K.; Canales-Martinez, M.M. Wound Healing Activity of A-Pinene and A-Phellandrene. *Molecules* **2021**, *26*, 2488. [CrossRef]
85. Deardorff, R.; Spinale, F.G. Cytokines and Matrix Metalloproteinases as Potential Biomarkers in Chronic Heart Failure. *Biomark. Med.* **2009**, *3*, 513–523. [CrossRef]

86. Fitzmaurice, S.D.; Sivamani, R.K.; Isseroff, R.R. Antioxidant Therapies for Wound Healing: A Clinical Guide to Currently Commercially Available Products. *Ski. Pharmacol. Physiol.* **2011**, *24*, 113–126. [CrossRef] [PubMed]
87. Lu, X.; Rasco, B.A.; Jabal, J.M.F.; Aston, D.E.; Lin, M.; Konkel, M.E. Investigating Antibacterial Effects of Garlic (Allium Sativum) Concentrate and Garlic-Derived Organosulfur Compounds on Campylobacter Jejuni by using Fourier Transform Infrared Spectroscopy, Raman Spectroscopy, and Electron Microscopy. *Appl. Environ. Microbiol.* **2011**, *77*, 5257–5269. [CrossRef] [PubMed]
88. Jang, H.; Lee, H.; Yoon, D.; Ji, D.; Kim, J.; Lee, C. Antioxidant and Antimicrobial Activities of Fresh Garlic and Aged Garlic by-Products Extracted with Different Solvents. *Food Sci. Biotechnol.* **2018**, *27*, 219–225. [CrossRef] [PubMed]
89. Malcolm, B.J.; Tallian, K. Essential Oil of Lavender in Anxiety Disorders: Ready for Prime Time? *Ment. Health Clin.* **2017**, *7*, 147–155. [CrossRef] [PubMed]
90. Guo, F.; Liang, Q.; Zhang, M.; Chen, W.; Chen, H.; Yun, Y.; Zhong, Q.; Chen, W. Antibacterial Activity and Mechanism of Linalool against Shewanella Putrefaciens. *Molecules* **2021**, *26*, 245. [CrossRef] [PubMed]
91. Tai, A.; Sawano, T.; Yazama, F.; Ito, H. Evaluation of Antioxidant Activity of Vanillin by using Multiple Antioxidant Assays. *Biochim. Biophys. Acta* **2011**, *1810*, 170–177. [CrossRef]
92. Arya, S.; Rookes, J.; Cahill, D.; Lenka, S. Vanillin: A Review on the Therapeutic Prospects of a Popular Flavouring Molecule. *Adv. Trad Med.* **2021**, *21*, 1. [CrossRef]
93. Zhou, G.; Ruhan, A.; Ge, H.; Wang, L.; Liu, M.; Wang, B.; Su, H.; Yan, M.; Xi, Y.; Fan, Y. Research on a Novel Poly (Vinyl Alcohol)/Lysine/Vanillin Wound Dressing: Biocompatibility, Bioactivity and Antimicrobial Activity. *Burns* **2014**, *40*, 1668–1678. [CrossRef]
94. Abdelmalek, M.; Spencer, J. Retinoids and Wound Healing. *Dermatol. Surg.* **2006**, *32*, 1219–1230. [CrossRef]
95. Raber-Durlacher, J.; von Bültzingslöwen, I.; Logan, R.M.; Bowen, J.; Al-Azri, A.; Everaus, H.; Gerber, E.; Gomez, J.G.; Pettersson, B.G.; Soga, Y.; et al. Systematic Review of Cytokines and Growth Factors for the Management of Oral Mucositis in Cancer Patients. *Support. Care Cancer* **2013**, *21*, 343–355. [CrossRef]
96. Gharaee-Kermani, M.; Phan, S.H. Role of Cytokines and Cytokine Therapy in Wound Healing and Fibrotic Diseases. *Curr. Pharm. Des.* **2001**, *7*, 1083–1103. [CrossRef] [PubMed]
97. Agyare, C.; Bekoe, E.O.; Boakye, Y.D.; Dapaah, S.O.; Appiah, T.; Bekoe, O.S. Medicinal Plants and Natural Products with Demonstrated Wound Healing Properties. In *Wound Healing—New Insights into Ancient Challenges*; Alexandrescu, V.A., Ed.; IntechOpen: London, UK, 2016. [CrossRef]
98. Al Wahbi, A. Autoamputation of Diabetic Toe with Dry Gangrene: A Myth or a Fact? *Diabetes Metab. Syndr. Obes.* **2018**, *11*, 255–264. [CrossRef] [PubMed]
99. Bayan, L.; Koulivand, P.H.; Gorji, A. Garlic: A Review of Potential Therapeutic Effects. *Avicenna J. Phytomed.* **2014**, *4*, 1–14. [PubMed]
100. Petrovska, B.B.; Cekovska, S. Extracts from the History and Medical Properties of Garlic. *Pharmacogn. Rev.* **2010**, *4*, 106–110. [CrossRef] [PubMed]
101. Anderson, C.; Lis-Balchin, M.; Kirk-Smith, M. Evaluation of Massage with Essential Oils on Childhood Atopic Eczema. *Phytother. Res.* **2000**, *14*, 452–456. [CrossRef]
102. Kwiatkowski, P.; Łopusiewicz, Ł.; Kostek, M.; Drozłowska, E.; Pruss, A.; Wojciuk, B.; Sienkiewicz, M.; Zielińska-Bliźniewska, H.; Dołęgowska, B. The Antibacterial Activity of Lavender Essential Oil Alone and in Combination with Octenidine Dihydrochloride Against MRSA Strains. *Molecules* **2019**, *25*, 95. [CrossRef]
103. Peterson, L.R. Currently Available Antimicrobial Agents and their Potential for use as Monotherapy. *Clin. Microbiol. Infect.* **2008**, *14*, 30–45. [CrossRef]
104. Liu, X.; Cai, J.; Chen, H.; Zhong, Q.; Hou, Y.; Chen, W.; Chen, W. Antibacterial Activity and Mechanism of Linalool Against Pseudomonas Aeruginosa. *Microb. Pathog.* **2020**, *141*, 103980. [CrossRef]
105. Predoi, D.; Iconaru, S.L.; Buton, N.; Badea, M.L.; Marutescu, L. Antimicrobial Activity of New Materials Based on Lavender and Basil Essential Oils and Hydroxyapatite. *Nanomaterials* **2018**, *8*, 291. [CrossRef]
106. Pham-Huy, L.A.; He, H.; Pham-Huy, C. Free Radicals, Antioxidants in Disease and Health. *Int. J. Biomed. Sci.* **2008**, *4*, 89–96.
107. Sarkar, P.; Arockiaraj, J.; Stefi, R.; Pasupuleti, M.; Paray, B.; Al-Sadoon, M.A. Antioxidant Molecular Mechanism Of adenosyl Homocysteinase From cyanobacteria and its Wound Healing Process in Fibroblast Cells. *Mol. Biol. Rep.* **2020**, *47*, 1821–1834. [CrossRef] [PubMed]
108. Shroff, A.; Mamalis, A.; Jagdeo, J. Oxidative Stress and Skin Fibrosis. *Curr. Pathobiol. Rep.* **2014**, *2*, 257–267. [CrossRef] [PubMed]
109. Carlsen, M.H.; Halvorsen, B.L.; Holte, K.; Bøhn, S.K.; Dragland, S.; Senoo, H.; Umezono, Y.; Sanada, C.; Barikmo, I.; Berhe, N.; et al. The Total Antioxidant Content of More than 3100 Foods, Beverages, Spices, Herbs and Supplements used Worldwide. *Nutr. J.* **2010**, *9*, 3. [CrossRef] [PubMed]
110. Fereydouni, N.; Darroudi, M.; Movaffagh, J.; Shahroodi, A.; Butler, A.E.; Ganjali, S.; Sahebkar, A. Curcumin Nanofibers for the Purpose of Wound Healing. *J. Cell. Physiol.* **2019**, *234*, 5537–5554. [CrossRef]
111. Barchitta, M.; Maugeri, A.; Favara, G.; Magnano San Lio, R.; Evola, G.; Agodi, A.; Basile, G. Nutrition and Wound Healing: An Overview Focusing on the Beneficial Effects of Curcumin. *Int. J. Mol. Sci.* **2019**, *20*, 1119. [CrossRef]
112. Palmieri, B.; Vadalà, M.; Laurino, C. Nutrition in Wound Healing: Investigation of the Molecular Mechanisms, a Narrative Review. *J. Wound Care* **2019**, *28*, 683–693. [CrossRef]
113. Callus, C.A.; Vella, S.; Ferry, P. Scurvy is Back. *Nutr. Metab. Insights* **2018**, *11*, 1178638818809097. [CrossRef]

114. Gunes Bilgili, S.; Calka, O.; Akdeniz, N.; Bayram, I.; Metin, A. The Effects of Retinoids on Secondary Wound Healing: Biometrical and Histopathological Study in Rats. *J. Dermatol. Treat.* **2013**, *24*, 283–289. [CrossRef]
115. Shekhar, C. An Innovative Technique in Local Antibiotic Delivery Method in Open Infected Wounds of the Musculoskeletal System. *Int. J. Low Extrem. Wounds* **2019**, *18*, 153–160. [CrossRef]
116. Gaspar-Pintiliescu, A.; Stanciuc, A.; Craciunescu, O. Natural Composite Dressings Based on Collagen, Gelatin and Plant Bioactive Compounds for Wound Healing: A Review. *Int. J. Biol. Macromol.* **2019**, *138*, 854–865. [CrossRef]
117. Suarato, G.; Bertorelli, R.; Athanassiou, A. Borrowing from Nature: Biopolymers and Biocomposites as Smart Wound Care Materials. *Front. Bioeng. Biotechnol.* **2018**, *6*, 137. [CrossRef] [PubMed]
118. Zakaria, A.; Labib, O. Evaluation of Emissions from Medical Waste Incinerators in Alexandria. *J. Egypt Public Health Assoc.* **2003**, *78*, 225–244.
119. Yao, C.; Yao, P.; Wu, H.; Zha, Z. Acceleration of Wound Healing in Traumatic Ulcers by Absorbable Collagen Sponge Containing Recombinant Basic Fibroblast Growth Factor. *Biomed. Mater.* **2006**, *1*, 33–37. [CrossRef] [PubMed]
120. Catanzano, O.; Quaglia, F.; Boateng, J.S. Wound Dressings as Growth Factor Delivery Platforms for Chronic Wound Healing. *Expert Opin. Drug Deliv.* **2021**, *18*, 737–759. [CrossRef] [PubMed]
121. Vivcharenko, V.; Przekora, A. Modifications of Wound Dressings with Bioactive Agents to Achieve Improved Pro-Healing Properties. *Appl. Sci.* **2021**, *11*, 4114. [CrossRef]
122. Mohandas, A.; PT, S.K.; Raja, B.; Lakshmanan, V.; Jayakumar, R. Exploration of Alginate Hydrogel/Nano Zinc Oxide Composite Bandages for Infected Wounds. *Int. J. Nanomed.* **2015**, *10*, 53–66. [CrossRef]
123. Pachuau, L. Recent Developments in Novel Drug Delivery Systems for Wound Healing. *Exp. Opin. Drug Deliv.* **2015**, *12*, 1895–1909. [CrossRef]
124. Ardekani, N.T.; Khorrama, M.; Zomorodian, K.; Yazdanpanah, S.; Veisi, H.; Veisi, H. Evaluation of Electrospun Poly (Vinyl Alcohol)-Based Nanofiber Mats Incorporated with Zataria Multiflora Essential Oil as Potential Wound Dressing. *Int. J. Biol. Macromol.* **2019**, *125*, 743–750. [CrossRef]
125. Garcia-Salinas, S.; Evangelopoulos, M.; Gamez-Herrera, E.; Arrueboa, M.; Irusta, S.; Taraballi, F.; Mendoza, G.; Tasciotti, E. Electrospun Anti-Inflammatory Patch Loaded with Essential Oils for Wound Healing. *Int. J. Pharm.* **2020**, *577*, 119067. [CrossRef]
126. Bullough, L.; Johnson, S.; Forder, R. Evaluation of a Foam Dressing for Acute and Chronic Wound Exudate Management. *Br. J. Community Nurs.* **2015**, *20*, S17–S24. [CrossRef]
127. Li, J.; Mooney, D.J. Designing Hydrogels for Controlled Drug Delivery. *Nat. Rev. Mater.* **2016**, *1*, 16071. [CrossRef]
128. Ashouri, F.; Beyranvand, F.; Beigi Boroujeni, N.; Tavafi, M.; Sheikhian, A.; Mohammad Varzi, A.; Shahrokhi, S. Macrophage Polarization in Wound Healing: Role of Aloe Vera/Chitosan Nanohydrogel. *Drug Deliv. Transl. Res.* **2019**, *9*, 1027–1042. [CrossRef] [PubMed]
129. Zhi, K.; Wang, J.; Zhao, H.; Yang, X. Self-Assembled Small Molecule Natural Product Gel for Drug Delivery: A Breakthrough in New Application of Small Molecule Natural Products. *Acta Pharm. Sin. B* **2020**, *10*, 913–927. [CrossRef] [PubMed]
130. Buwalda, S.J.; Vermonden, T.; Hennink, W.E. Hydrogels for Therapeutic Delivery: Current Developments and Future Directions. *Biomacromolecules* **2017**, *18*, 316–330. [CrossRef] [PubMed]
131. Lutton, R.E.M.; Moore, J.; Larrañeta, E.; Donnelly, R.F. Microneedle Characterisation: The Need for Universal Acceptance Criteria and GMP Specifications when Moving Towards Commercialisation. *Drug Deliv. Transl. Res.* **2016**, *5*, 313–331. [CrossRef] [PubMed]
132. Duarah, S.; Sharma, M.; Wen, J. Recent Advances in Microneedle-Based Drug Delivery: Special Emphasis on its use in Paediatric Population. *Eur. J. Pharm. Biopharm.* **2019**, *136*, 48–69. [CrossRef] [PubMed]
133. Chi, J.; Zhang, X.; Chen, C.; Shao, C.; Zhao, Y.; Wang, Y. Antibacterial and Angiogenic Chitosan Microneedle Array Patch for Promoting Wound Healing. *Bioact. Mater.* **2020**, *5*, 253–259. [CrossRef]
134. Park, S.Y.; Lee, H.U.; Lee, Y.; Kim, G.H.; Park, E.C.; Han, S.H.; Lee, J.G.; Choi, S.; Heo, N.S.; Kim, D.L.; et al. Wound Healing Potential of Antibacterial Microneedles Loaded with Green Tea Extracts. *Mater. Sci. Eng. C* **2014**, *42*, 757–762. [CrossRef]
135. Gharbavi, M.; Amani, J.; Kheiri-Manjili, H.; Danafar, H.; Sharafi, A. Niosome: A Promising Nanocarrier for Natural Drug Delivery through Blood-Brain Barrier. *Adv. Pharmacol. Sci.* **2018**, *2018*, e6847971. [CrossRef]
136. Liolios, C.C.; Gortzi, O.; Lalas, S.; Tsaknis, J.; Chinou, I. Liposomal Incorporation of Carvacrol and Thymol Isolated from the Essential Oil of Origanum Dictamnus, L. and in Vitro Antimicrobial Activity. *Food Chem.* **2009**, *112*, 77–83. [CrossRef]
137. Shoji, Y.; Nakashima, H. Nutraceutics and Delivery Systems. *J. Drug Target.* **2004**, *12*, 385–391. [CrossRef] [PubMed]
138. De Figueiredo-Rinhel, A.S.G.; de Andrade, M.F.; Landi-Librandi, A.P.; Azzolini, A.E.C.S.; Kabeya, L.M.; Bastos, J.K.; Lucisano-Valim, Y.M. Incorporation of Baccharis Dracunculifolia DC (Asteraceae) Leaf Extract into Phosphatidylcholine-Cholesterol Liposomes Improves its Anti-Inflammatory Effect in Vivo. *Nat. Prod. Res.* **2019**, *33*, 2521–2525. [CrossRef]
139. Roesken, F.; Uhl, E.; Curri, S.B.; Menger, M.D.; Messmer, K. Acceleration of Wound Healing by Topical Drug Delivery Via Liposomes. *Langenbecks Arch. Surg.* **2000**, *385*, 42–49. [CrossRef] [PubMed]
140. Li, Z.; Liu, M.; Wang, H.; Du, S. Increased Cutaneous Wound Healing Effect of Biodegradable Liposomes Containing Madecassoside: Preparation Optimization, in Vitro Dermal Permeation, and in Vivo Bioevaluation. *Int. J. Nanomed.* **2016**, *11*, 2995–3007. [CrossRef] [PubMed]
141. Bartelds, R.; Nematollahi, M.H.; Pols, T.; Stuart, M.C.A.; Pardakhty, A.; Asadikaram, G.; Poolman, B. Niosomes, an Alternative for Liposomal Delivery. *PLoS ONE* **2018**, *13*, e0194179. [CrossRef] [PubMed]

142. Kazi, K.M.; Mandal, A.S.; Biswas, N.; Guha, A.; Chatterjee, S.; Behera, M.; Kuotsu, K. Niosome: A Future of Targeted Drug Delivery Systems. *J. Adv. Pharm. Technol. Res.* **2010**, *1*, 374–380. [CrossRef]
143. Akbarzadeh, I.; Shayan, M.; Bourbour, M.; Moghtaderi, M.; Noorbazargan, H.; Eshrati Yeganeh, F.; Saffar, S.; Tahriri, M. Preparation, Optimization and in-Vitro Evaluation of Curcumin-Loaded Niosome@calcium Alginate Nanocarrier as a New Approach for Breast Cancer Treatment. *Biology* **2021**, *10*, 173. [CrossRef]
144. Xu, Y.; Chen, W.; Tsosie, J.K.; Xie, X.; Li, P.; Wan, J.; He, C.; Chen, M. Niosome Encapsulation of Curcumin: Characterization and Cytotoxic Effect on Ovarian Cancer Cells. *J. Nanomater.* **2016**, *2016*, e6365295. [CrossRef]
145. Antimisiaris, S.G.; Mourtas, S.; Marazioti, A. Exosomes and Exosome-Inspired Vesicles for Targeted Drug Delivery. *Pharmaceutics* **2018**, *10*, 218. [CrossRef]
146. Goodarzi, P.; Larijani, B.; Alavi-Moghadam, S.; Tayanloo-Beik, A.; Mohamadi-Jahani, F.; Ranjbaran, N.; Payab, M.; Falahzadeh, K.; Mousavi, M.; Arjmand, B. Mesenchymal Stem Cells-Derived Exosomes for Wound Regeneration. In *Cell Biology and Translational Medicine*; Turksen, K., Ed.; Springer: Cham, Switzerland, 2018; Volume 4, pp. 119–131.
147. Akuma, P.; Okagu, O.D.; Udenigwe, C.C. Naturally Occurring Exosome Vesicles as Potential Delivery Vehicle for Bioactive Compounds. *Front. Sustain. Food Syst.* **2019**, *3*, 23. [CrossRef]
148. Sun, D.; Zhuang, X.; Xiang, X.; Liu, Y.; Zhang, S.; Liu, C.; Barnes, S.; Grizzle, W.; Miller, D.; Zhang, H. A Novel Nanoparticle Drug Delivery System: The Anti-Inflammatory Activity of Curcumin is Enhanced when Encapsulated in Exosomes. *Mol. Ther.* **2010**, *18*, 1606–1614. [CrossRef] [PubMed]
149. Hossen, S.; Hossain, M.K.; Basher, M.K.; Mia, M.N.H.; Rahman, M.T.; Uddin, M.J. Smart Nanocarrier-Based Drug Delivery Systems for Cancer Therapy and Toxicity Studies: A Review. *J. Adv. Res.* **2019**, *15*, 1–18. [CrossRef]
150. Sheorain, J.; Mehra, M.; Thakur, R.; Grewal, S.; Kumari, S. In Vitro Anti-Inflammatory and Antioxidant Potential of Thymol Loaded Bipolymeric (Tragacanth Gum/Chitosan) Nanocarrier. *Int. J. Biol. Macromol.* **2019**, *125*, 1069–1074. [CrossRef] [PubMed]
151. Ocaña, A.; Reglero, G. Effects of Thyme Extract Oils (from Thymus Vulgaris, Thymus Zygis, and Thymus Hyemalis) on Cytokine Production and Gene Expression of oxLDL-Stimulated THP-1-Macrophages. *J. Obes.* **2012**, *2012*, 104706. [CrossRef] [PubMed]
152. Ghosh Dastidar, D.; Saha, S.; Chowdhury, M. Porous Microspheres: Synthesis, Characterisation and Applications in Pharmaceutical & Medical Fields. *Int. J. Pharm.* **2018**, *548*, 34–48. [CrossRef] [PubMed]
153. Zhang, C.; Niu, J.; Chong, Y.; Huang, Y.; Chu, Y.; Xie, S.; Jiang, Z.; Peng, L. Porous Microspheres as Promising Vehicles for the Topical Delivery of Poorly Soluble Asiaticoside Accelerate Wound Healing and Inhibit Scar Formation in Vitro & in Vivo. *Eur. J. Pharm. Biopharm.* **2016**, *109*, 1–13. [CrossRef]
154. Wang, Y.; Guo, M.; He, B.; Gao, B. Intelligent Patches for Wound Management: In Situ Sensing and Treatment. *Anal. Chem.* **2021**, *93*, 4687–4696. [CrossRef]
155. Stan, D.; Tanase, C.; Avram, M.; Apetrei, R.; Mincu, N.; Mateescu, A.L.; Stan, D. Wound Healing Applications of Creams and "smart" Hydrogels. *Exp. Dermatol.* **2021**, *30*, 1218–1232. [CrossRef]
156. Ochoa, M.; Rahimi, R.; Zhou, J.; Jiang, H.; Yoon, C.K.; Maddipatla, D.; Narakathu, B.B.; Jain, V.; Oscai, M.M.; Morken, T.J.; et al. Integrated Sensing and Delivery of Oxygen for Next-Generation Smart Wound Dressings. *Microsyst. Nanoeng.* **2020**, *6*, 1–16. [CrossRef]
157. Andreu, V.; Mendoza, G.; Arruebo, M.; Irusta, S. Smart Dressings Based on Nanostructured Fibers Containing Natural Origin Antimicrobial, Anti-Inflammatory, and Regenerative Compounds. *Materials* **2015**, *8*, 5154–5193. [CrossRef]
158. Tamayol, A.; Hassani Najafabadi, A.; Mostafalu, P.; Yetisen, A.K.; Commotto, M.; Aldhahri, M.; Abdel-wahab, M.S.; Najafabadi, Z.I.; Latifi, S.; Akbari, M.; et al. Biodegradable Elastic Nanofibrous Platforms with Integrated Flexible Heaters for on-Demand Drug Delivery. *Sci. Rep.* **2017**, *7*, 9220. [CrossRef] [PubMed]
159. Mostafalu, P.; Kiaee, G.; Giatsidis, G.; Khalilpour, A.; Nabavinia, M.; Dokmeci, M.R.; Sonkusale, S.; Orgill, D.P.; Tamayol, A.; Khademhosseini, A. A Textile Dressing for Temporal and Dosage Controlled Drug Delivery. *Adv. Funct. Mater.* **2017**, *27*, 1702399. [CrossRef]
160. Cordier, C.; Morton, D.; Murrison, S.; Nelson, A.; O'Leary-Steele, C. Natural Products as an Inspiration in the Diversity-Oriented Synthesis of Bioactive Compound Libraries. *Nat. Prod. Rep.* **2008**, *25*, 719–737. [CrossRef]
161. Meier, B.P.; Lappas, C.M. The Influence of Safety, Efficacy, and Medical Condition Severity on Natural Versus Synthetic Drug Preference. *Med. Decis. Mak.* **2016**, *36*, 1011–1019. [CrossRef] [PubMed]
162. Chambers, E.; Chambers, E.; Castro, M. What is "Natural"? Consumer Responses to Selected Ingredients. *Foods* **2018**, *7*, 65. [CrossRef] [PubMed]
163. Pevsic, M. Development of Natural Product Drugs in a Sustainable Manner. In *Brief for GSDR*; United Nations: San Francisco, CA, USA, 2015.
164. Choudhary, I. Back to Nature. *Nature* **2008**, *456*, 41. [CrossRef]
165. Oyebode, O.; Kandala, N.; Chilton, P.J.; Lilford, R.J. Use of Traditional Medicine in Middle-Income Countries: A WHO-SAGE Study. *Health Policy Plan.* **2016**, *31*, 984–991. [CrossRef]
166. McNerney, R. Diagnostics for Developing Countries. *Diagnostics* **2015**, *5*, 200–209. [CrossRef]
167. Harris, E. Building Scientific Capacity in Developing Countries. *EMBO Rep.* **2004**, *5*, 7–11. [CrossRef]
168. Li, D.; Martini, N.; Liu, M.; Falconer, J.R.; Locke, M.; Wu, Z.; Wen, J. Non-Ionic Surfactant Vesicles as a Carrier System for Dermal Delivery of (+)-Catechin and their Antioxidant Effects. *J. Drug Target.* **2021**, *29*, 310–322. [CrossRef]

169. Engel, J.B.; Heckler, C.; Tondo, E.C.; Daroit, D.J.; da Silva Malheiros, P. Antimicrobial Activity of Free and Liposome-Encapsulated Thymol and Carvacrol Against Salmonella and Staphylococcus Aureus Adhered to Stainless Steel. *Int. J. Food Microbiol.* **2017**, *252*, 18–23. [CrossRef]
170. Herrmann, I.K.; Wood, M.J.A.; Fuhrmann, G. Extracellular Vesicles as a Next-Generation Drug Delivery Platform. *Nat. Nanotechnol.* **2021**, *16*, 748–759. [CrossRef]
171. Kim, M.W.; Kwon, S.; Choi, J.H.; Lee, A. A Promising Biocompatible Platform: Lipid-Based and Bio-Inspired Smart Drug Delivery Systems for Cancer Therapy. *Int. J. Mol. Sci.* **2018**, *19*, 3859. [CrossRef]
172. Sinjari, B.; Pizzicannella, J.; D'Aurora, M.; Zappacosta, R.; Gatta, V.; Fontana, A.; Trubiani, O.; Diomede, F. Curcumin/Liposome Nanotechnology as Delivery Platform for Anti-Inflammatory Activities Via NFkB/ERK/pERK Pathway in Human Dental Pulp Treated with 2-HydroxyEthyl MethAcrylate (HEMA). *Front. Physiol.* **2019**, *10*, 633. [CrossRef] [PubMed]
173. Chen, Z.; Ye, R.; Yang, J.; Lin, Y.; Lee, W.; Li, J.; Ren, L.; Liu, B.; Jiang, L. Rapidly Fabricated Microneedle Arrays using Magnetorheological Drawing Lithography for Transdermal Drug Delivery. *ACS Biomater. Sci. Eng.* **2019**, *5*, 5506–5513. [CrossRef] [PubMed]
174. Yang, Y.; Wong, P.K. A Plasma Lithography Microengineered Assay for Studying Architecture Dependent Wound Healing of Endothelial Cells. In Proceedings of the 15th International Conference on Miniaturized Systems for Chemistry and Life Sciences 2011 MicroTAS, Seattle, WA, USA, 2–6 October 2011; pp. 326–328.
175. Smandri, A.; Nordin, A.; Hwei, N.M.; Chin, K.; Abd Aziz, I.; Fauzi, M.B. Natural 3D-Printed Bioinks for Skin Regeneration and Wound Healing: A Systematic Review. *Polymers* **2020**, *12*, 1782. [CrossRef] [PubMed]

pharmaceutics

Review

Application of CRISPR-Cas9 System to Study Biological Barriers to Drug Delivery

Ji He [1], Riya Biswas [1], Piyush Bugde [1], Jiawei Li [1], Dong-Xu Liu [1,2] and Yan Li [1,2,3,*]

1 School of Science, Auckland University of Technology, Auckland 1010, New Zealand; ji.he@aut.ac.nz (J.H.); riya.biswas@aut.ac.nz (R.B.); piyushbugde@gmail.com (P.B.); jiawei.li@aut.ac.nz (J.L.); dong-xu.liu@aut.ac.nz (D.-X.L.)
2 The Centre for Biomedical and Chemical Sciences, School of Science, Faculty of Health and Environmental Sciences, Auckland University of Technology, Auckland 1010, New Zealand
3 School of Interprofessional Health Studies, Auckland University of Technology, Auckland 1010, New Zealand
* Correspondence: yan.li@aut.ac.nz; Tel.: +64-9921-9999 (ext. 7109)

Abstract: In recent years, sequence-specific clustered regularly interspaced short palindromic repeats (CRISPR)-CRISPR-associated (Cas) systems have been widely used in genome editing of various cell types and organisms. The most developed and broadly used CRISPR-Cas system, CRISPR-Cas9, has benefited from the proof-of-principle studies for a better understanding of the function of genes associated with drug absorption and disposition. Genome-scale CRISPR-Cas9 knockout (KO) screen study also facilitates the identification of novel genes in which loss alters drug permeability across biological membranes and thus modulates the efficacy and safety of drugs. Compared with conventional heterogeneous expression models or other genome editing technologies, CRISPR-Cas9 gene manipulation techniques possess significant advantages, including ease of design, cost-effectiveness, greater on-target DNA cleavage activity and multiplexing capabilities, which makes it possible to study the interactions between membrane proteins and drugs more accurately and efficiently. However, many mechanistic questions and challenges regarding CRISPR-Cas9 gene editing are yet to be addressed, ranging from off-target effects to large-scale genetic alterations. In this review, an overview of the mechanisms of CRISPR-Cas9 in mammalian genome editing will be introduced, as well as the application of CRISPR-Cas9 in studying the barriers to drug delivery.

Keywords: CRISPR-Cas9; blood-brain barrier; intestinal epithelial barrier; drug permeability

Citation: He, J.; Biswas, R.; Bugde, P.; Li, J.; Liu, D.-X.; Li, Y. Application of CRISPR-Cas9 System to Study Biological Barriers to Drug Delivery. *Pharmaceutics* **2022**, *14*, 894. https://doi.org/10.3390/pharmaceutics14050894

Academic Editor: Tomáš Etrych

Received: 23 February 2022
Accepted: 19 April 2022
Published: 20 April 2022

1. Introduction

Accumulating evidence has suggested membrane transporter proteins play pivotal roles in drug permeability across biological membranes and thus determine the efficacy and safety of drugs [1–6]. Two major transporter superfamilies, namely the ATP-binding cassette (ABC) and the solute carrier (SLC) transporters, have been identified to modulate the drug absorption and disposition. The human ABC transporter family contains 48 members with 7 subfamilies, including several important drug transporters, such as P-gp (ABCB1), MRP2 (ABCC2) and BCRP (ABCG2). They are widely distributed in various tissues, functioning to actively extrude pharmacologically diverse substrate drugs out of cells against the concentration and chemical-potential gradients by using energy derived from ATP hydrolysis. The SLC transporters include 298 influx transporters responsible for nutrient intake and drug disposition into various organs. Certain ABC and SLC transporters are co-localised in a specific tissue and play in concert with selective permeability to specific drugs, excluding circulating drugs and toxic agents but allowing essential nutrients and other drugs into the tissue. Using endogenous transport pathways may lead to more effective drug delivery into the pharmacological sanctuaries. However, the contribution of the transporter(s) to overall drug permeability across a biological membrane is often unknown or cannot be accurately measured. Although the heterogeneous expression systems have been used as valuable tools, the interpretation of results could be complicated by the presence of endogenous transporters and species differences. With the development of CRISPR-Cas9 genome editing techniques, it is now possible to efficiently study the functional consequences of genetic mutations and delineate the interactions between membrane proteins and drugs.

This review elaborates on the principles and application of CRISPR-Cas9 genome editing techniques with a special focus on drug permeability-related membrane proteins.

2. CRISPR-Cas9 System

The CRISPR-Cas adaptive immune systems are a natural defence mechanism of bacteria against foreign genetic elements [7]. Some types of these CRISPR-Cas systems have been repurposed to facilitate precise genome engineering in eukaryotic cells [8,9]. Generally, CRISPR-Cas systems are categorised into two classes (1 and 2), which are further subdivided into six types (I–VI) based on the structure and function of Cas protein [10,11]. Class 1 CRISPR-Cas systems (type I, III and IV) recruit multi-subunit effectors, in contrast to the single effector of class 2 (type II, V and VI) [10,11]. CRISPR-Cas9 comprises three major components, Cas9 nuclease, CRISPR RNA (crRNA) and trans-activating crRNA (tracrRNA).

The type II CRISPR-SpyCas9 derived from *Streptococcus pyogenes* is one of the best developed and broadly used systems in site-specific genetic engineering of human cells [8,12,13]. SpyCas9 has a bi-lobed architecture formed by a recognition (REC) lobe and a nuclease (NUC) lobe (Figure 1) [14]. An arginine-rich (R-rich) Bridge helix (BH) connects these two lobes [15]. In the case of genetic engineering of human cells using the CRISPR-SpyCas9 system, either the hybridised crRNA-tracrRNA duplex combining a 42-nt crRNA and an 80-nt tracrRNA or a modified single 102-nt guide RNA (sgRNA, crRNA fused to tracrRNA) is loaded onto SpyCas9 to form ribonucleoprotein (RNP) and direct RNP to the target site bearing a 5′-NGG-3′ PAM (N = A/T/G/C) [14–18]. Notably, the 10-nt PAM-proximal seed region is critical for the SpyCas9-catalysed DNA cleavage. Some mismatches may be tolerated in the rest of the gRNA sequence [15].

The NUC lobe of SpyCas9 contains the HNH and RuvC nuclease domains, which cleave the target and non-target strands of the target DNA through the single-metal and two-metal mechanisms, respectively [14,15,19–21]. SpyCas9 nuclease thus stimulates a DSB at the target locus, i.e., normally 3-nt upstream PAM. These DSBs are mainly re-ligated by one of the two major DNA repair pathways, the error-prone non-homologous end joining (NHEJ) and the high-fidelity homology-directed repair (HDR) in mammalian cells [22]. NHEJ mediates gene knockouts (KOs) through the formation of indel (nucleotides insertion/deletion) known to facilitate frameshift mutations and premature stop codons [23]. Dual-gRNA-induced multiple DSBs can additionally facilitate more extensive excisions in the genome [24]. By contrast, the activation of HDR is contingent on the cell type and state, since it is normally active in dividing cells [25]. HDR can typically knock in a predesigned repair template to the open reading frame (ORF) to terminate the transcription of the target gene. The integrated constructs may comprise genes encoding biomarkers for screening and probing purposes, such as antibiotic-resistant genes and genes encoding fluorescent probes.

Aside from the canonical SpyCas9 from *Streptococcus pyogenes*, many other Cas9 orthologs and the type V CRISPR-Cas12 systems have been uncovered and used for mammalian genome editing, as summarised in Table 1 [16,26–40].

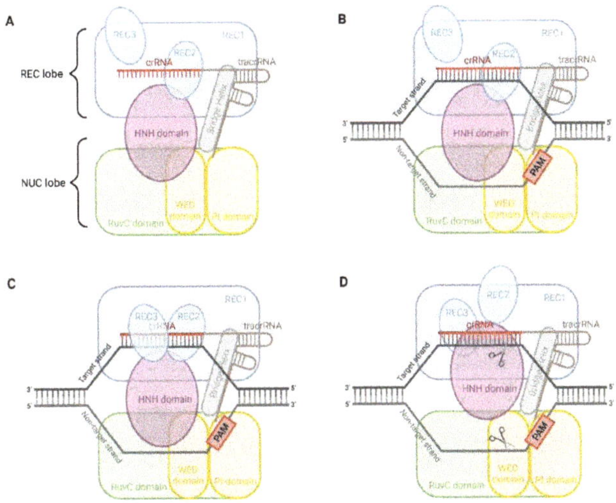

Figure 1. Schematic illustration of DNA recognition and cleavage by CRISPR-SpyCas9. (**A**) RNA duplex is loaded onto SpyCas9 to form ribonucleoprotein (RNP). (**B**) The PAM-interacting (PI) domain of the NUC lobe recognises 5′-NGG-3′ PAM and facilitates the binding of crRNA to the target DNA to form R-loop. (**C**) The REC3 domain of the REC lobe and Bridge helix (BH) sense mismatches. (**D**) The REC2 domain of the REC lobe undergoes a large outward rotation, leading to the conformational transition of the HNH domain into an active state. The HNH and RuvC domain of the NUC lobe then cleaves the target and non-target strands of the target DNA, respectively. The cleavage site is always located at 3- to 4-nt upstream of PAM. *Created with BioRender.com.*

Table 1. Summary of CRISPR-Cas systems used for genome editing of mammalian cells.

Class 2	Subtype	Effector Nuclease	Size (aa)	Target	TracrRNA Requirement	Seed Sequence Requirement	PAM Sequence	Cleavage Product
Type II	A	SpyCas9	1368	dsDNA (or ssDNA/ssRNA with PAMmers)	Yes	Yes	NGG	DSB (blunt end)/SSB
	A	St1Cas9	1121	dsDNA	Yes	Yes	NNRGAA	DSB (blunt end)
	A	St3Cas9	1388	dsDNA	Yes	Yes	NGGNG	DSB (blunt end)
	A	SauCas9	1053	dsDNA/ssRNA	Yes	Yes	NNAGAAW/-	DSB (blunt end)/SSB
	B	FnoCas9	1629	dsDNA/ssRNA	Yes	Yes	NGG/-	DSB (blunt end)/SSB
	C	CjeCas9	984	dsDNA/ssRNA	Yes	Yes	NNNVRYM/-	DSB (blunt end)/SSB
	C	NmeCas9	1082	dsDNA/ssDNA	Yes/No	Yes	NNNNGATT/-	DSB (blunt end)/SSB
Type V	A	Cas12a	1200–1500	dsDNA/ssDNA	No	Yes	Optimal 5′ T-rich and suboptimal C-containing PAMs/-	DSB (sticky end with 5-nt 5′-overhang)/SSB
	B	Cas12b	1100–1300	dsDNA/ssDNA	Yes	Yes	Optimal 5′ T-rich and suboptimal C-containing PAMs/-	DSB (sticky end with 6-nt 5′-overhang)/SSB
	E	Cas12e	<1000	dsDNA	Yes	Unknown	5′ T-rich PAMs	DSB (sticky end with 10-nt 5′-overhang)
	F	Cas12f	400–600	dsDNA/ssDNA	Yes	Unknown	5′ T-rich PAMs/-	DSB (sticky end with 5′-overhang)

N represents A, T, G and C; V represents A, C, and G; M represents A and C; R represents A and G; W represents A and T; Y represents C and T.

The common negative effects of CRISPR-Cas9 include the endonuclease activity-induced cell damage and the off-target effect. The recently developed techniques, such as base editing and prime editing, may help minimise the off-target effect of CRISPR-Cas9 [41–43]. The cleavage efficiency of CRISPR-Cas9 could be influenced by factors in terms of designing sgRNA and Cas9 constructs (e.g., construction and composition of sgRNA and Cas9 protein) [33,44], the GC content, secondary structure and nucleotide preference of sgRNA [44,45], and the primary target sequence [46]. However, emerging evidence suggests that some more complicated matters may also impact CRISPR-Cas9's editing efficiency, such as different chromatin states (i.e., euchromatin and heterochromatin) [47], the location of target DNA in the nucleosome [25,47,48], truncated protein isoforms [47,49], induction of DNA damage responses (e.g., *p53* and *KRAS*) [50–52], and large-scale gene rearrangements [23].

Chromatin states can affect both Cas9 binding and the repair pathway choice. The relatively unpacked euchromatin is more accessible to Cas9 protein over heterochromatin [47]. It was also reported that the frequencies of long double-stranded donor-based HDR were higher at heterochromatin compared to euchromatin. In contrast, NHEJ frequencies were higher in euchromatin [25]. Furthermore, Smits, Ziebell [49] reported that residual protein expression was found in about one third out of 193 KOs at variable levels from low to original. These truncated protein isoforms could remain with their original cellular functions and presumably involve other unknown roles [53].

Moreover, the Cas9-induced DSBs were found to cause p53-dependent cellular toxicity and eventually reduce cellular viability [50,52]. Similar to p53, the wild-type *KRAS* gene might hamper the growth of KO cells [51]. These findings support the involvement of *p53* and *KRAS* in CRISPR-Cas9-induced DNA damage response (DDR) activation, leading to the selective advantage of the *p53*- and *KRAS*-mutant cells. In addition, large-scale gene rearrangements, chromosomal translocations, gene inversions or large insertions/deletions were reported in a comprehensive study of Cas9-induced mutagenesis [23]. Similarly, chromosome structural alterations, such as micronuclei and chromosome bridges, were observed in mouse embryos after CRISPR-Cas9 genome editing [54]. These genomic alterations may induce ectopic expression of other genes.

Despite the potential drawbacks that the CRISPR-Cas9 system has, it is superior to other genome editing technologies, such as zinc-finger nucleases (ZFNs) and transcription activator-like effector nucleases (TALENs), considering its ease of design, cost-effectiveness, greater on-target DNA cleavage activity, multiplexing capabilities, and wide suitability for diverse cell types and organisms [8,55]. Moreover, as compared to gene knockdown technologies, such as RNAi (i.e., siRNA and shRNA), CRISPR-Cas9 is thought to present advantages, including lower off-target activity, stable and heritable complete elimination of the target gene expression and multiple genome editing potentials [56,57]. These advantages make CRISPR-Cas9 a reliable and versatile gene-editing approach and enable advances in molecular biology research for a variety of applications.

3. Application of CRISPR-Cas9 in Drug Delivery Barrier Studies

3.1. Intestinal Barriers to Drug Delivery

In order for orally administered drugs to exert their beneficial effects (other than on the GI tract itself), they must be delivered to their target organ(s) and tissues by systemic circulation. Adequate concentrations at the site(s) of action are only achieved by overcoming several absorption and metabolism barriers, both in the intestine and in the liver. Atypical absorption kinetics of many drugs suggest their intestinal absorption cannot be simply predicted from their physicochemical properties, and their interactions with intestinal ABC and SLC transporters may lead to limited or nonlinear intestinal permeability and absorption of drugs, resulting in extensive variability in their oral bioavailability and inadequate plasma concentrations and lack of pharmacological effect.

P-gp (MDR1/ABCB1) is a 170-KDa efflux transporter located on the plasma membrane in many tissues, such as the intestine, liver, kidney and brain. It exerts a critical barrier role in the intestinal absorption of lipophilic and amphipathic drugs with diverse pharmacological actions. Indeed, the oral bioavailability of its substrate talinolol in humans can be increased by 34% when co-administered with the P-gp inhibitor, erythromycin [58]. Similarly, coadministration of oral Cys A enhanced the human oral bioavailability of paclitaxel and docetaxel by 7- and 10-fold, respectively, and reduced interpatient variability in the systemic exposure of docetaxel to that seen in intravenous administration [59,60]. CRISPR-Cas9 gene editing in cell culture and animal models for drug transport has mainly focused on *ABCB1*.

3.1.1. Knockout of Abcb1 in MDCK Cells by CRISPR-Cas9

The main in vitro models of intestinal absorption include subcellular fractions, cell cultures, isolated tissues and membrane vesicles. In recent years, cultured cells, such as Caco-2 or Madin-Darby canine kidney (MDCK) cells, have been increasingly used to study drug absorption.

Madin-Darby canine kidney II cells (MDCK) heterogeneously expressing single or multiple human transport proteins are commonly used models to study polarised drug transport and identify substrates. However, endogenous canine transporters such as canine Mdr1/P-glycoprotein (Abcb1) and canine Mrp2 (Abcc2) transport various drugs and complicate the interpretation of directional transport studies [61]. Complete KO of endogenous canine *Abcb1* (*cAbcb1*) (homozygous disruption) (2) resulted in indistinguishable differences in directional transport of model human ABCB1 substrates, such as digoxin, labetalol and quinidine [61,62]. Similarly, a comparison of efflux ratios (ER) between MDCKI wild-type and gMDCKI (KO of endogenous cAbcb1) showed that out of 135 compounds tested, 38% showed efflux activity in MDCKI wt, while no significant efflux was observed in gMDCKI cells [63]. Further overexpression of human ABCB1 (MDR1) in those *cAbcb1*-KO MDCK cells generated less complicated drug transport models, which enabled substrate identification and removed the interference from cAbcb1 (Figure 2) [62,63]. The *cAbcb1*-KO MDCK cells human overexpressing BCRP (ABCG2) were also generated and used to accurately identify human BCRP substrates, which may be potentially transported by cAbcb1 (Figure 2) [64]. The expression of BCRP and MRP2 transcripts and proteins in the human small intestine is similar to that of MDR1 [65,66], suggesting these two efflux transporters also play important roles in regulating the oral absorption of their substrates.

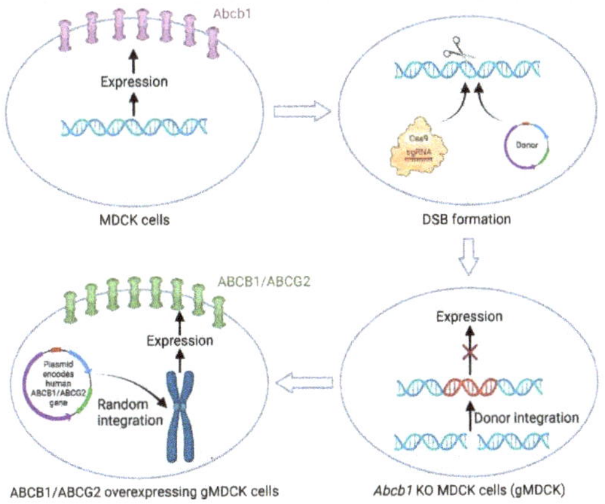

Figure 2. Schematic illustration of generating *Abcb1* KO MDCK (gMDCK) cells and ABCB1/ABCG2 overexpressing gMDCK cells. After transfection, the target sequence is recognised and cleaved by the sgRNA-Cas9 complex, followed by the integration of the donor template through the HDR repair pathway. The expression of *Abcb1* is thus disrupted in *Abcb1* KO MDCK (gMDCK) cells. To generate ABCB1/ABCG2 overexpressing gMDCK cells, plasmids encoding human *ABCB1* or *ABCG2* genes are delivered into gMDCK cells and randomly integrated into the genome, leading to constant overexpression of ABCB1 or ABCG2 protein. *Created with BioRender.com.*

3.1.2. Mdr1a/b Double-Knockout Rat Models

Drug permeability across the intestine can be easily extrapolated across mammalian species due to the similar composition of the epithelial cell membranes. Laboratory animals are commonly used to predict oral drug absorption in humans by determining absolute bioavailability with the comparison of area under the plasma concentration-time curve (AUC) after intravenous and oral administration. They are also used for the prediction of potential absorption-based drug interactions by comparing oral bioavailability values with and without coadministration of another drug. With the manipulations in embryonic stem cells commonly used to create mouse knockouts, transgenic mice have provided an appropriate model to investigate the roles of specific drug transporter(s) or metabolising enzyme(s). For example, intestinal P-gp limits the bioavailability of a wide range of drugs, including paclitaxel, digoxin, aliskiren, betrixaban, celiprolol, fexofenadine and talinolol, as shown in P-gp knockout mice [65–67]. However, species differences exist in gastrointestinal pH, intestinal flora mobility, transit time, and activity and expression level of transporters and metabolism enzymes. Although rats are empirically superior to mice as models for intestinal drug absorption, the generation of transgenic rat models was difficult, as rat genes are much more difficult to manipulate using embryonic stem cells. A novel MDR1 (Mdr1a/b) double-knockout (KO) rat model was generated by the CRISPR/Cas9 system without any off-target effect detected for compensatory mechanisms (e.g., CYP3A subfamily and transporter-related genes) [68]. The rate and extent of oral absorption of digoxin, a typical MDR1 substrate, was significantly increased in *Mdr1a/b* (-/-) rats compared with WT. With the high efficient KI and KO via CRISPR genome editing technologies, more useful in vivo tools (e.g., humanised animal models) would be generated for studying drug absorption barriers.

3.2. Biological Barriers to Anticancer Drugs

Many anticancer drugs are targeting intracellular DNA or proteins and thereby cause DNA damage or inhibition of DNA synthesis and inhibition of cell division. The intracellular concentration of some anticancer drugs is vital, and it has been suggested that the intracellular concentration of a drug is the product of a competition between its passive or active uptake rate and either an active efflux rate or metabolic rate. However, the mechanisms whereby some anticancer drugs enter cancer cells and overcome the biological barriers remain poorly understood. The CRISPR-Cas9 system has provided extra tools to unfold the underlying mechanisms at the genome-scale and simplified the interpretation of results.

3.2.1. Knockout and Regulation of ABC Transporter Genes in Cancer Cells by CRISPR-Cas9

Although the clinical relevance between ABC transporters and multidrug-resistance (MDR) phenotype is controversial and unclear, extensive in vitro studies strongly support their potential roles in the cellular pharmacokinetics of substrate drugs [53,69]. The CRISPR-Cas9 gene manipulation technique has been used to reverse ABC transporter-related MDR and restore non-malignant phenotype in many types of cancer cell models. It was reported that KO of *ABCB1* significantly enhanced the sensitivity to doxorubicin (aka., Adriamycin (ADR)) in the ADR-resistant ovarian cancer cell line A2780/ADR [70], breast cancer cell line MCF7/ADR [71], osteosarcoma cell line KHOSR2 and U-2OSR2 [72]. Similarly, KO of *ABCB1* in two ABCB1-overexpressing multidrug-resistance (MDR) cell lines, KBV_{200} and HCT-8/V, remarkedly improved the sensitivity and accumulation of ABCB1 substrate drugs, such as vincristine and doxorubicin. Furthermore, the sensitivity of carfilzomib (CFZ)-resistant myeloma cell line AMO-CFZ [73] and acute lymphoblastic leukaemia (ALL) cell line HALO1 [74] to CFZ was recovered after knocking out *ABCB1* using the CRISPR-Cas9 system.

In addition, a CRISPR/Cas9 KO of BEN domain-containing protein 3 (BEND3) upregulated efflux transporter breast cancer resistance protein (BCRP; ABCG2) and reduced the intracellular levels of TAK-243 and induced resistance in acute myeloid leukaemia (AML) cells [75]. Similarly, silencing ubiquitin-editing enzymes A20 by CRISPR/Cas9 modulated brentuximab vedotin sensitivity (BV, a drug-conjugated anti-CD30 antibody) in Hodgkin lymphoma line L428, occurred through NF-kappaB-mediated ABCB1 expression [76]. Targeting NF-kappaB activity synergised well with BV in killing Hodgkin lymphoma cell lines, augmented BV sensitivity, and overcame BV resistance in vitro and in Hodgkin lymphoma xenograft mouse models.

Therefore, CRISPR-Cas9-mediated modulation of ABC transporter genes or their regulator(s) may represent a promising in vitro cancer cell model for substrate identification and molecular pathology research that potentially contributes to uncovering novel therapeutic biomarkers.

3.2.2. Genome-Wide CRISPR-Cas9 Knockout Screen

Historically, genome-wide loss-of-function screening in mammalian cells has employed the RNA interference (RNAi) gene knockdown technology. However, this method is limited by incomplete protein depletion and off-target effects-induced false positives [77]. The application of CRISPR-Cas9 in genome-scale functional screening may overcome these drawbacks of RNAi and simplify the interpretation of the loss of gene function. GeCKO is the first library of sgRNAs targeting 5′ constitutive exons of 18,080 genes in the human genome with an average coverage of 3–4 sgRNAs per gene, which was applied to both negative and positive selection screens in human cells models [78]. The optimised sgRNA libraries, for the human and mouse genomes, named Brunello and Brie, respectively, have been created by maximising on-target activity and minimising off-target effects to enable more effective and efficient genetic screens [79]. Genome-wide CRISPR screens reveal that expression of the multidrug-resistant gene *ABCC1* and the lysosomal transporter SLC46A3 differentially impact tumour cell sensitivity to PCA062, a P-cadherin targeting antibody-drug (DM1, a maytansine-derived potent microtubule-inhibiting agent) conjugate for the treatment of multiple cancer types, including basal-like breast cancer [80]. ABCC1 confers antibody maytansine conjugate resistance [81], and SLC46A3 transports catabolite of antibody maytansine conjugate from lysosome to cytoplasm [82,83]. Silencing ABCC1 could lead to cytoplasmic accumulation of the warhead, while KO SLC46A3 cause lysosomal accumulation (Figure 3).

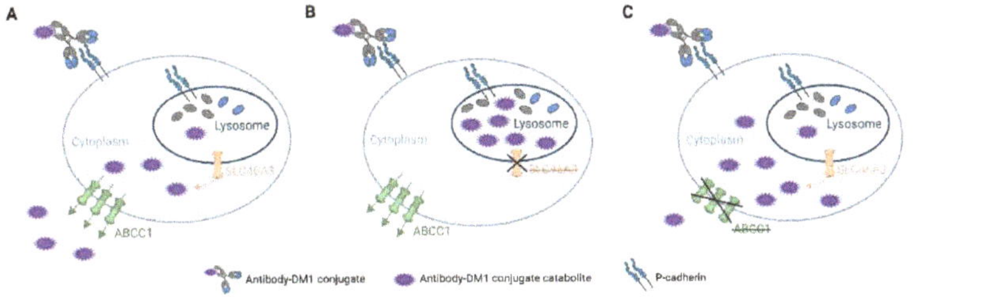

Figure 3. Proposed mechanisms of cellular distribution of catabolite of antibody maytansine conjugate in wild-type (**A**), SLC46A3-KO (**B**) and ABCC1-KO (**C**) cancer cells. *Created with BioRender.com.*

A genome-wide CRISPR/Cas9 knockout screen identified that SLC1A3 confers L-asparaginase resistance in human prostate cancer PC3 cells [84]. L-asparaginase serves as a crucial medicine for adolescent acute lymphoblastic leukaemia but is frequently associated with solid tumour resistance. ASNase stimulates aspartate and glutamate consumption and decreases their intracellular concentrations. SLC1A3 is an aspartate and glutamate transporter, and overexpression of SLC1A3 may promote cancer cell proliferation via "enhanced permeability" of aspartate and glutamate and fueling aspartate, glutamate and glutamine metabolisms. SLC1A3 inhibition caused cell cycle arrest or apoptosis and myriads of metabolic vulnerabilities in the tricarboxylic acid cycle, urea cycle, nucleotides biosynthesis, energy production, redox homeostasis and lipid biosynthesis.

3.2.3. Novel Mechanisms of Platinum Accumulation in Cancer Cells

The platinum-containing drugs such as cisplatin, carboplatin and oxaliplatin have been widely integrated into the standard and preferred regimens for various solid cancers. Several SLC transporters, such as CTR1 (SLC31A1) and CTR2 (SLC31A2), have been reported to participate in cisplatin influx in several heterogeneous expression systems (e.g., yeast and mouse embryonic fibroblast models) [85]. However, complete KO of either *CTR1* or *CTR2* in ovarian carcinoma OVCAR8 cells showed indistinguishable differences in cisplatin sensitivity compared to wild-type cells [86]. A study using CRISPR-Cas9-mediated gene deletion suggests volume-regulated anion channels (VRACs), configured as leucine-rich repeat-containing 8 (LRRC8) heteromers, significantly contribute to cisplatin and carboplatin accumulation in human cells, accounting for 50–70% of total platinum accumulation under isotonic conditions [87]. Loss of LRRC8D causes resistance to carboplatin and cisplatin, but not to oxaliplatin in KBM-7 leukaemia cells [87]. To put this into perspective, silencing LRRC8D also confers cisplatin resistance in *BRCA1*-mutated ovarian cancer cells in a genome-scale CRISPR-Cas9 knockout screen study [88], and a retrospective analysis of two small cohorts of ovarian cancer patients that received platinum drugs reveals that lower expression levels of LRRC8D were correlated with lower survival rates [87]. Further research is warranted to establish greater confidence in supporting experimental and clinical correlative data and address key gaps in current knowledge.

3.3. *Blood-Brain Barriers*

Endothelial cells that line the microvasculature of the central nervous system (CNS) constitute the blood-brain barrier (BBB), selectively excluding circulating drugs and toxic agents from entering the majority of the central nervous system but allowing essential nutrients, hormones and certain drugs into the brain. Drug permeability across BBB is mainly determined by the interactions between their physicochemical characteristics and the specialised BBB features, including tight intercellular junctions that markedly limit paracellular permeability, plus a unique expression of ABC and SLC transporters that determine the transcellular permeability. The two most abundant ABC transporters in the human BBB are ABCB1 (MDR1) and ABCG2 (BCRP) [89], which function as pivotal rate-limiting barriers to drug distribution or access to the brain [90]. Moreover, one attractive approach to brain drug delivery is to utilise SLC transporters as an efficient vehicle to circumvent BBB [91]. CRISPR-Cas9 allows cost-effective gene manipulation at more physiologically relevant levels and readily expands our knowledge of the novel territories.

Solute carrier family 35, member F2 (SLC35F2), is highly expressed in the BBB and is localised exclusively on the apical membrane of brain microvascular endothelial cells (BMECs), differentiated from human induced pluripotent stem cells (hiPS-BMECs). Silencing SLC35F2, by CRISPR/Cas9 mediated knockout, diminished the apical-to-basolateral transport and intracellular accumulation of its substrate drug YM155 in hiPS-BMECs [92]. By contrast, in studies using an in situ brain perfusion in mice, neither CRISPR/Cas9 KO of Slc35f2 nor pharmacological perturbation reduced brain uptake of YM155. YM155 is a substrate of human and mouse SLC35F2 [92], and SLC35F2 is a major determinant of YM155 antitumour efficacy in xenografted models, comparing the effects of YM155 on tumour growth between wild-type and SLC35F2 KO SW480 cells [93]. It is suggested that the limited role of slc35f2 in the distribution of YM155 in mouse brain was due to a substantial uptake mediated by organic anion transporting polypeptide oatp1a4 [92].

OATP1A2 (SLC21A3) is abundantly expressed in the apical (blood) side of the human BBB [94–96] and facilitates the transport of analgesic opioids (e.g., [D-penicillamine2,5] encephalin, deltorphin II), antimigraine triptans (e.g., sumatriptan), levofloxacin and methotrexate [4]. A mouse line humanised for human OATP1A2 was established by CRISPR-Cas9 mediated knock-in of the coding region downstream of the mouse *Oatp1a4* promoter [97]. Such a humanised mouse model would be an invaluable tool for studying the transcellular transport of drug substrates across the blood-brain barrier (BBB). OATP1A2 mRNA in the brain was increased, corresponding to the disappearance of Oatp1a4, and OATP1A2 was localised on both the luminal and abluminal sides of the BBB. However, incomplete translation or posttranslational modification of OATP1A2 occurred in the BBB, as evidenced by the peptide-dependent quantitative levels of OATP1A2, leading to the lack of functional transport of model substrates across BBB. These examples highlight the fact that we are still a long way from being able to generate clinic-relevant BBB transporter models.

3.4. Regulation of Transporter Genes

The CRISPR/Cas9 system has been applied to edit non-transcribed DNA sequences, including DNA methylation tags. DNA methylation, occurring at the 5-carbon position of cytosine residues located in dinucleotide CpG sites and regions of high CpG density, called CpG islands (CGIs), has been observed in the promoter regions of 60–70% of genes in mammals, which are involved in the epigenetic regulation of genes [98]. ABCC3 is highly expressed in human skin tissues, with its mRNA accounting for 20% of the total mean transporter mRNA content [99]. The expression of ABCC3 mRNA showed large interindividual variability (9.5-fold) but cannot be explained by single nucleotide polymorphisms. In human skin HaCaT cells, the disruption of the region surrounding a CGI, located approximately 10 kb upstream of the ABCC3 gene, by CRISPR/Cas9 led to significantly decreased ABCC3 mRNA levels [99]. Consistently, ABCC3 mRNA was upregulated in HaCaT cells by the demethylating agent 5-aza-2′-deoxycytidine. A better understanding of epigenetic regulation of skin transporter genes is important for the design of drug delivery across this essential barrier.

Multidrug and toxin extrusion protein 1 (MATE1), which is encoded by solute carrier 47A1 (SLC47A1), functions as the final excretion step of drugs/toxins into bile and urine. Its substrates include vitamin thiamine, cimetidine, metformin, guanidine, procainamide, antiviral agents (e.g., acyclovir and ganciclovir) and antibiotics (e.g., cephalexin and cephradine) as well as an endogenous substrate creatinine [4]. Some differences in the pharmacokinetics of MATE1 substrate drugs cannot be explained by genetic variations in humans. MATE1 mRNA expression levels negatively correlated with methylation levels of the CpG island in the 27 kb upstream of *SLC47A1*. The CRISPR-Cas9-induced deletions in this CpG area significantly lower *SLC47A1/MATE1* mRNA expression in HepG2 cells. This study highlights the importance of epigenetic regulation in pharmacokinetics and the application of CRISPR/Cas9 for editing non-transcribed DNA targets in human cells.

4. Conclusions

The breathtaking CRISPR-Cas9-based gene-editing technology is undoubtedly an excellent genetic manipulation method for pharmacology and molecular biology studies. It provides researchers with a convenient tool to identify gene functions with significant advantages, including ease of design, cost-effectiveness, greater on-target DNA cleavage activity, and multiplexing capabilities. The exploitation of CRISPR-Cas9 techniques has expanded the tools to study biological barriers to drug delivery and generated novel insights in the field and may lead to the development of promising strategies to overcome therapeutic failures and minimise drug toxicity. The genome-scale CRISPR-Cas9 KO screen study also facilitates the identification of novel genes in which loss alters drug permeability across the biological membrane and thus, modulates the efficacy and safety of drugs. With the new strategies to enhance KI and KO efficiency via CRISPR genome editing technologies, more interpretable in vitro and in vivo tools are expected for studying barriers to drug delivery.

Author Contributions: Conceptualisation, Y.L. and D.-X.L.; methodology, J.H., R.B., P.B. and J.L.; software, J.H.; investigation, J.H., R.B., P.B., J.L. and Y.L.; resources, Y.L.; writing—original draft preparation, J.H. and Y.L.; writing—review and editing, J.H., Y.L. and D.-X.L.; visualisation, J.H.; supervision, Y.L. and D.-X.L.; project administration, Y.L.; funding acquisition, Y.L. All authors have read and agreed to the published version of the manuscript.

Funding: No external funding was received for this work.

Institutional Review Board Statement: Not applicable.

Informed Consent Statement: Not applicable.

Data Availability Statement: Not applicable.

Acknowledgments: Ji He is a recipient of the Auckland University of Technology Vice-Chancellor PhD Scholarship.

Conflicts of Interest: The authors declare no conflict of interest.

References

1. International Transporter Consortium; Giacomini, K.M.; Huang, S.M.; Tweedie, D.J.; Benet, L.Z.; Brouwer, K.L.; Chu, X.; Dahlin, A.; Evers, R.; Fischer, V.; et al. Membrane transporters in drug development. *Nat. Rev. Drug Discov.* **2010**, *9*, 215–236. [CrossRef] [PubMed]
2. Zamek-Gliszczynski, M.J.; Taub, M.E.; Chothe, P.P.; Chu, X.; Giacomini, K.M.; Kim, R.B.; Ray, A.S.; Stocker, S.L.; Unadkat, J.D.; Wittwer, M.B.; et al. Transporters in Drug Development: 2018 ITC Recommendations for Transporters of Emerging Clinical Importance. *Clin. Pharmacol. Ther.* **2018**, *104*, 890–899. [CrossRef] [PubMed]
3. Evers, R.; Piquette-Miller, M.; Polli, J.W.; Russel, F.G.M.; Sprowl, J.A.; Tohyama, K.; Ware, J.A.; de Wildt, S.N.; Xie, W.; Brouwer, K.L.R.; et al. Disease-Associated Changes in Drug Transporters May Impact the Pharmacokinetics and/or Toxicity of Drugs: A White Paper From the International Transporter Consortium. *Clin. Pharmacol. Ther.* **2018**, *104*, 900–915. [CrossRef] [PubMed]
4. Li, Y.; Revalde, J.; Paxton, J.W. The effects of dietary and herbal phytochemicals on drug transporters. *Adv. Drug Deliv. Rev.* **2017**, *116*, 45–62. [CrossRef]
5. Mao, Q.; Lai, Y.; Wang, J. Drug Transporters in Xenobiotic Disposition and Pharmacokinetic Prediction. *Drug Metab. Dispos.* **2018**, *46*, 561–566. [CrossRef]
6. Nakanishi, T.; Tamai, I. Interaction of Drug or Food with Drug Transporters in Intestine and Liver. *Curr. Drug Metab.* **2015**, *16*, 753–764. [CrossRef]
7. Jansen, R.; Embden, J.D.; Gaastra, W.; Schouls, L.M. Identification of genes that are associated with DNA repeats in prokaryotes. *Mol. Microbiol.* **2002**, *43*, 1565–1575. [CrossRef]
8. Ran, F.A.; Hsu, P.D.; Wright, J.; Agarwala, V.; Scott, D.A.; Zhang, F. Genome engineering using the CRISPR-Cas9 system. *Nat. Protoc.* **2013**, *8*, 2281–2308. [CrossRef]
9. Jinek, M.; Chylinski, K.; Fonfara, I.; Hauer, M.; Doudna, J.A.; Charpentier, E. A programmable dual-RNA-guided DNA endonuclease in adaptive bacterial immunity. *Science* **2012**, *337*, 816–821. [CrossRef]
10. Koonin, E.V.; Makarova, K.S.; Zhang, F. Diversity, classification and evolution of CRISPR-Cas systems. *Curr. Opin. Microbiol.* **2017**, *37*, 67–78. [CrossRef]
11. Liu, Z.; Dong, H.; Cui, Y.; Cong, L.; Zhang, D. Application of different types of CRISPR/Cas-based systems in bacteria. *Microb. Cell Fact.* **2020**, *19*, 172. [CrossRef] [PubMed]
12. Shmakov, S.; Smargon, A.; Scott, D.; Cox, D.; Pyzocha, N.; Yan, W.; Abudayyeh, O.O.; Gootenberg, J.S.; Makarova, K.S.; Wolf, Y.I.; et al. Diversity and evolution of class 2 CRISPR-Cas systems. *Nat. Rev. Microbiol.* **2017**, *15*, 169–182. [CrossRef]
13. Wang, X.; Huang, X.; Fang, X.; Zhang, Y.; Wang, W. CRISPR-Cas9 System as a Versatile Tool for Genome Engineering in Human Cells. *Mol. Ther. Nucleic. Acids* **2016**, *5*, e388. [CrossRef] [PubMed]
14. Nishimasu, H.; Ran, F.A.; Hsu, P.D.; Konermann, S.; Shehata, S.I.; Dohmae, N.; Ishitani, R.; Zhang, F.; Nureki, O. Crystal structure of Cas9 in complex with guide RNA and target DNA. *Cell* **2014**, *156*, 935–949. [CrossRef] [PubMed]
15. Bratovic, M.; Fonfara, I.; Chylinski, K.; Galvez, E.J.C.; Sullivan, T.J.; Boerno, S.; Timmermann, B.; Boettcher, M.; Charpentier, E. Bridge helix arginines play a critical role in Cas9 sensitivity to mismatches. *Nat. Chem. Biol.* **2020**, *16*, 587–595. [CrossRef] [PubMed]
16. Hirano, H.; Gootenberg, J.S.; Horii, T.; Abudayyeh, O.O.; Kimura, M.; Hsu, P.D.; Nakane, T.; Ishitani, R.; Hatada, I.; Zhang, F.; et al. Structure and Engineering of Francisella novicida Cas9. *Cell* **2016**, *164*, 950–961. [CrossRef] [PubMed]
17. Deltcheva, E.; Chylinski, K.; Sharma, C.M.; Gonzales, K.; Chao, Y.; Pirzada, Z.A.; Eckert, M.R.; Vogel, J.; Charpentier, E. CRISPR RNA maturation by trans-encoded small RNA and host factor RNase III. *Nature* **2011**, *471*, 602–607. [CrossRef]
18. Szczelkun, M.D.; Tikhomirova, M.S.; Sinkunas, T.; Gasiunas, G.; Karvelis, T.; Pschera, P.; Siksnys, V.; Seidel, R. Direct observation of R-loop formation by single RNA-guided Cas9 and Cascade effector complexes. *Proc. Natl. Acad. Sci. USA* **2014**, *111*, 9798–9803. [CrossRef]

19. Chen, J.S.; Dagdas, Y.S.; Kleinstiver, B.P.; Welch, M.M.; Sousa, A.A.; Harrington, L.B.; Sternberg, S.H.; Joung, J.K.; Yildiz, A.; Doudna, J.A. Enhanced proofreading governs CRISPR-Cas9 targeting accuracy. *Nature* **2017**, *550*, 407–410. [CrossRef]
20. Palermo, G.; Miao, Y.; Walker, R.C.; Jinek, M.; Mc Cammon, J.A. CRISPR-Cas9 conformational activation as elucidated from enhanced molecular simulations. *Proc. Natl. Acad. Sci. USA* **2017**, *114*, 7260–7265. [CrossRef]
21. Dagdas, Y.S.; Chen, J.S.; Sternberg, S.H.; Doudna, J.A.; Yildiz, A. A conformational checkpoint between DNA binding and cleavage by CRISPR-Cas9. *Sci. Adv.* **2017**, *3*, eaao0027. [CrossRef] [PubMed]
22. Ceccaldi, R.; Rondinelli, B.; D'Andrea, A.D. Repair Pathway Choices and Consequences at the Double-Strand Break. *Trends Cell. Biol.* **2016**, *26*, 52–64. [CrossRef] [PubMed]
23. Kosicki, M.; Tomberg, K.; Bradley, A. Repair of double-strand breaks induced by CRISPR-Cas9 leads to large deletions and complex rearrangements. *Nat. Biotechnol.* **2018**, *36*, 765–771. [CrossRef] [PubMed]
24. Binda, C.S.; Klaver, B.; Berkhout, B.; Das, A.T. CRISPR-Cas9 Dual-gRNA Attack Causes Mutation, Excision and Inversion of the HIV-1 Proviral DNA. *Viruses* **2020**, *12*, 330. [CrossRef]
25. Janssen, J.M.; Chen, X.; Liu, J.; Goncalves, M. The Chromatin Structure of CRISPR-Cas9 Target DNA Controls the Balance between Mutagenic and Homology-Directed Gene-Editing Events. *Mol. Ther. Nucleic. Acids* **2019**, *16*, 141–154. [CrossRef]
26. Xu, Y.; Li, Z. CRISPR-Cas systems: Overview, innovations and applications in human disease research and gene therapy. *Comput. Struct. Biotechnol. J.* **2020**, *18*, 2401–2415. [CrossRef]
27. Yamano, T.; Zetsche, B.; Ishitani, R.; Zhang, F.; Nishimasu, H.; Nureki, O. Structural Basis for the Canonical and Non-canonical PAM Recognition by CRISPR-Cpf1. *Mol. Cell* **2017**, *67*, 633–645.e3. [CrossRef]
28. Zetsche, B.; Gootenberg, J.S.; Abudayyeh, O.O.; Slaymaker, I.M.; Makarova, K.S.; Essletzbichler, P.; Volz, S.E.; Joung, J.; van der Oost, J.; Regev, A.; et al. Cpf1 is a single RNA-guided endonuclease of a class 2 CRISPR-Cas system. *Cell* **2015**, *163*, 759–771. [CrossRef]
29. Strecker, J.; Jones, S.; Koopal, B.; Schmid-Burgk, J.; Zetsche, B.; Gao, L.; Makarova, K.S.; Koonin, E.V.; Zhang, F. Engineering of CRISPR-Cas12b for human genome editing. *Nat. Commun.* **2019**, *10*, 212. [CrossRef]
30. Teng, F.; Cui, T.; Feng, G.; Guo, L.; Xu, K.; Gao, Q.; Li, T.; Li, J.; Zhou, Q.; Li, W. Repurposing CRISPR-Cas12b for mammalian genome engineering. *Cell Discov.* **2018**, *4*, 63. [CrossRef]
31. Bigelyte, G.; Young, J.K.; Karvelis, T.; Budre, K.; Zedaveinyte, R.; Djukanovic, V.; Van Ginkel, E.; Paulraj, S.; Gasior, S.; Jones, S.; et al. Miniature type V-F CRISPR-Cas nucleases enable targeted DNA modification in cells. *Nat. Commun.* **2021**, *12*, 6191. [CrossRef] [PubMed]
32. Liu, J.J.; Orlova, N.; Oakes, B.L.; Ma, E.; Spinner, H.B.; Baney, K.L.M.; Chuck, J.; Tan, D.; Knott, G.J.; Harrington, L.B.; et al. CasX enzymes comprise a distinct family of RNA-guided genome editors. *Nature* **2019**, *566*, 218–223. [CrossRef]
33. Ran, F.A.; Cong, L.; Yan, W.X.; Scott, D.A.; Gootenberg, J.S.; Kriz, A.J.; Zetsche, B.; Shalem, O.; Wu, X.; Makarova, K.S.; et al. In vivo genome editing using Staphylococcus aureus Cas9. *Nature* **2015**, *520*, 186–191. [CrossRef] [PubMed]
34. Kim, E.; Koo, T.; Park, S.W.; Kim, D.; Kim, K.; Cho, H.Y.; Song, D.W.; Lee, K.J.; Jung, M.H.; Kim, S.; et al. In vivo genome editing with a small Cas9 orthologue derived from Campylobacter jejuni. *Nat. Commun.* **2017**, *8*, 14500. [CrossRef] [PubMed]
35. Esvelt, K.M.; Mali, P.; Braff, J.L.; Moosburner, M.; Yaung, S.J.; Church, G.M. Orthogonal Cas9 proteins for RNA-guided gene regulation and editing. *Nat. Methods* **2013**, *10*, 1116–1121. [CrossRef] [PubMed]
36. Dugar, G.; Leenay, R.T.; Eisenbart, S.K.; Bischler, T.; Aul, B.U.; Beisel, C.L.; Sharma, C.M. CRISPR RNA-Dependent Binding and Cleavage of Endogenous RNAs by the Campylobacter jejuni Cas9. *Mol. Cell* **2018**, *69*, 893–905.e7. [CrossRef]
37. Ma, E.; Harrington, L.B.; O'Connell, M.R.; Zhou, K.; Doudna, J.A. Single-Stranded DNA Cleavage by Divergent CRISPR-Cas9 Enzymes. *Mol. Cell* **2015**, *60*, 398–407. [CrossRef]
38. Muller, M.; Lee, C.M.; Gasiunas, G.; Davis, T.H.; Cradick, T.J.; Siksnys, V.; Bao, G.; Cathomen, T.; Mussolino, C. Streptococcus thermophilus CRISPR-Cas9 Systems Enable Specific Editing of the Human Genome. *Mol. Ther.* **2016**, *24*, 636–644. [CrossRef]
39. Swiech, L.; Heidenreich, M.; Banerjee, A.; Habib, N.; Li, Y.; Trombetta, J.; Sur, M.; Zhang, F. In vivo interrogation of gene function in the mammalian brain using CRISPR-Cas9. *Nat. Biotechnol.* **2015**, *33*, 102–106. [CrossRef]
40. Agudelo, D.; Carter, S.; Velimirovic, M.; Duringer, A.; Rivest, J.F.; Levesque, S.; Loehr, J.; Mouchiroud, M.; Cyr, D.; Waters, P.J.; et al. Versatile and robust genome editing with Streptococcus thermophilus CRISPR1-Cas9. *Genome Res.* **2020**, *30*, 107–117. [CrossRef]
41. Komor, A.C.; Kim, Y.B.; Packer, M.S.; Zuris, J.A.; Liu, D.R. Programmable editing of a target base in genomic DNA without double-stranded DNA cleavage. *Nature* **2016**, *533*, 420–424. [CrossRef] [PubMed]
42. Chen, L.; Park, J.E.; Paa, P.; Rajakumar, P.D.; Prekop, H.T.; Chew, Y.T.; Manivannan, S.N.; Chew, W.L. Programmable C:G to G:C genome editing with CRISPR-Cas9-directed base excision repair proteins. *Nat. Commun.* **2021**, *12*, 1384. [CrossRef] [PubMed]
43. Anzalone, A.V.; Randolph, P.B.; Davis, J.R.; Sousa, A.A.; Koblan, L.W.; Levy, J.M.; Chen, P.J.; Wilson, C.; Newby, G.A.; Raguram, A.; et al. Search-and-replace genome editing without double-strand breaks or donor DNA. *Nature* **2019**, *576*, 149–157. [CrossRef] [PubMed]
44. Liu, X.; Homma, A.; Sayadi, J.; Yang, S.; Ohashi, J.; Takumi, T. Sequence features associated with the cleavage efficiency of CRISPR/Cas9 system. *Sci. Rep.* **2016**, *6*, 19675. [CrossRef] [PubMed]
45. Rahdar, M.; McMahon, M.A.; Prakash, T.P.; Swayze, E.E.; Bennett, C.F.; Cleveland, D.W. Synthetic CRISPR RNA-Cas9-guided genome editing in human cells. *Proc. Natl. Acad. Sci. USA* **2015**, *112*, E7110–E7117. [CrossRef] [PubMed]
46. Hsu, P.D.; Scott, D.A.; Weinstein, J.A.; Ran, F.A.; Konermann, S.; Agarwala, V.; Li, Y.; Fine, E.J.; Wu, X.; Shalem, O.; et al. DNA targeting specificity of RNA-guided Cas9 nucleases. *Nat. Biotechnol.* **2013**, *31*, 827–832. [CrossRef]

47. Verkuijl, S.A.; Rots, M.G. The influence of eukaryotic chromatin state on CRISPR-Cas9 editing efficiencies. *Curr. Opin. Biotechnol.* **2019**, *55*, 68–73. [CrossRef]
48. Daer, R.M.; Cutts, J.P.; Brafman, D.A.; Haynes, K.A. The Impact of Chromatin Dynamics on Cas9-Mediated Genome Editing in Human Cells. *ACS Synth. Biol.* **2017**, *6*, 428–438. [CrossRef]
49. Smits, A.H.; Ziebell, F.; Joberty, G.; Zinn, N.; Mueller, W.F.; Clauder-Munster, S.; Eberhard, D.; Falth Savitski, M.; Grandi, P.; Jakob, P.; et al. Biological plasticity rescues target activity in CRISPR knock outs. *Nat. Methods* **2019**, *16*, 1087–1093. [CrossRef]
50. Conti, A.; Di Micco, R. p53 activation: A checkpoint for precision genome editing? *Genome Med.* **2018**, *10*, 66. [CrossRef]
51. Sinha, S.; Barbosa, K.; Cheng, K.; Leiserson, M.D.M.; Jain, P.; Deshpande, A.; Wilson, D.M., 3rd; Ryan, B.M.; Luo, J.; Ronai, Z.A.; et al. A systematic genome-wide mapping of oncogenic mutation selection during CRISPR-Cas9 genome editing. *Nat. Commun.* **2021**, *12*, 6512. [CrossRef] [PubMed]
52. Mirgayazova, R.; Khadiullina, R.; Chasov, V.; Mingaleeva, R.; Miftakhova, R.; Rizvanov, A.; Bulatov, E. Therapeutic Editing of the TP53 Gene: Is CRISPR/Cas9 an Option? *Genes* **2020**, *11*, 704. [CrossRef] [PubMed]
53. He, J.; Fortunati, E.; Liu, D.X.; Li, Y. Pleiotropic Roles of ABC Transporters in Breast Cancer. *Int. J. Mol. Sci.* **2021**, *22*, 3199. [CrossRef] [PubMed]
54. Papathanasiou, S.; Markoulaki, S.; Blaine, L.J.; Leibowitz, M.L.; Zhang, C.Z.; Jaenisch, R.; Pellman, D. Whole chromosome loss and genomic instability in mouse embryos after CRISPR-Cas9 genome editing. *Nat. Commun.* **2021**, *12*, 5855. [CrossRef]
55. Doudna, J.A.; Charpentier, E. Genome editing. The new frontier of genome engineering with CRISPR-Cas9. *Science* **2014**, *346*, 1258096. [CrossRef]
56. Moreira, D.; Pereira, A.M.; Lopes, A.L.; Coimbra, S. The best CRISPR/Cas9 versus RNA interference approaches for Arabinogalactan proteins' study. *Mol. Biol. Rep.* **2020**, *47*, 2315–2325. [CrossRef]
57. Boettcher, M.; McManus, M.T. Choosing the Right Tool for the Job: RNAi, TALEN, or CRISPR. *Mol. Cell* **2015**, *58*, 575–585. [CrossRef]
58. Schwarz, U.I.; Gramatte, T.; Krappweis, J.; Oertel, R.; Kirch, W. P-glycoprotein inhibitor erythromycin increases oral bioavailability of talinolol in humans. *Int. J. Clin. Pharmacol. Ther.* **2000**, *38*, 161–167. [CrossRef]
59. Meerum Terwogt, J.M.; Beijnen, J.H.; ten Bokkel Huinink, W.W.; Rosing, H.; Schellens, J.H. Co-administration of cyclosporin enables oral therapy with paclitaxel. *Lancet* **1998**, *352*, 285. [CrossRef]
60. Malingre, M.M.; Richel, D.J.; Beijnen, J.H.; Rosing, H.; Koopman, F.J.; Ten Bokkel Huinink, W.W.; Schot, M.E.; Schellens, J.H. Coadministration of cyclosporine strongly enhances the oral bioavailability of docetaxel. *J. Clin. Oncol.* **2001**, *19*, 1160–1166. [CrossRef]
61. Simoff, I.; Karlgren, M.; Backlund, M.; Lindstrom, A.C.; Gaugaz, F.Z.; Matsson, P.; Artursson, P. Complete Knockout of Endogenous Mdr1 (Abcb1) in MDCK Cells by CRISPR-Cas9. *J. Pharm. Sci.* **2016**, *105*, 1017–1021. [CrossRef]
62. Karlgren, M.; Simoff, I.; Backlund, M.; Wegler, C.; Keiser, M.; Handin, N.; Muller, J.; Lundquist, P.; Jareborg, A.C.; Oswald, S.; et al. A CRISPR-Cas9 Generated MDCK Cell Line Expressing Human MDR1 Without Endogenous Canine MDR1 (cABCB1): An Improved Tool for Drug Efflux Studies. *J. Pharm. Sci.* **2017**, *106*, 2909–2913. [CrossRef] [PubMed]
63. Chen, E.C.; Broccatelli, F.; Plise, E.; Chen, B.; Liu, L.; Cheong, J.; Zhang, S.; Jorski, J.; Gaffney, K.; Umemoto, K.K.; et al. Evaluating the Utility of Canine Mdr1 Knockout Madin-Darby Canine Kidney I Cells in Permeability Screening and Efflux Substrate Determination. *Mol. Pharm.* **2018**, *15*, 5103–5113. [CrossRef]
64. Wegler, C.; Gazit, M.; Issa, K.; Subramaniam, S.; Artursson, P.; Karlgren, M. Expanding the Efflux In Vitro Assay Toolbox: A CRISPR-Cas9 Edited MDCK Cell Line with Human BCRP and Completely Lacking Canine MDR1. *J. Pharm. Sci.* **2021**, *110*, 388–396. [CrossRef] [PubMed]
65. Sparreboom, A.; van Asperen, J.; Mayer, U.; Schinkel, A.H.; Smit, J.W.; Meijer, D.K.; Borst, P.; Nooijen, W.J.; Beijnen, J.H.; van Tellingen, O. Limited oral bioavailability and active epithelial excretion of paclitaxel (Taxol) caused by P-glycoprotein in the intestine. *Proc. Natl. Acad. Sci. USA* **1997**, *94*, 2031–2035. [CrossRef] [PubMed]
66. Mayer, U.; Wagenaar, E.; Beijnen, J.H.; Smit, J.W.; Meijer, D.K.; van Asperen, J.; Borst, P.; Schinkel, A.H. Substantial excretion of digoxin via the intestinal mucosa and prevention of long-term digoxin accumulation in the brain by the mdr 1a P-glycoprotein. *Br. J. Pharmacol.* **1996**, *119*, 1038–1044. [CrossRef] [PubMed]
67. Miyake, T.; Tsutsui, H.; Haraya, K.; Tachibana, T.; Morimoto, K.; Takehara, S.; Ayabe, M.; Kobayashi, K.; Kazuki, Y. Quantitative prediction of P-glycoprotein-mediated drug-drug interactions and intestinal absorption using humanized mice. *Br. J. Pharmacol.* **2021**, *178*, 4335–4351. [CrossRef]
68. Liang, C.; Zhao, J.; Lu, J.; Zhang, Y.; Ma, X.; Shang, X.; Li, Y.; Ma, X.; Liu, M.; Wang, X. Development and Characterization of MDR1 (Mdr1a/b) CRISPR/Cas9 Knockout Rat Model. *Drug Metab. Dispos.* **2019**, *47*, 71–79. [CrossRef]
69. Holohan, C.; Van Schaeybroeck, S.; Longley, D.B.; Johnston, P.G. Cancer drug resistance: An evolving paradigm. *Nat. Rev. Cancer* **2013**, *13*, 714–726. [CrossRef]
70. Norouzi-Barough, L.; Sarookhani, M.; Salehi, R.; Sharifi, M.; Moghbelinejad, S. CRISPR/Cas9, a new approach to successful knockdown of ABCB1/P-glycoprotein and reversal of chemosensitivity in human epithelial ovarian cancer cell line. *Iran. J. Basic. Med. Sci.* **2018**, *21*, 181–187. [CrossRef]
71. Ha, J.S.; Byun, J.; Ahn, D.R. Overcoming doxorubicin resistance of cancer cells by Cas9-mediated gene disruption. *Sci. Rep.* **2016**, *6*, 22847. [CrossRef]

72. Liu, T.; Li, Z.; Zhang, Q.; De Amorim Bernstein, K.; Lozano-Calderon, S.; Choy, E.; Hornicek, F.J.; Duan, Z. Targeting ABCB1 (MDR1) in multi-drug resistant osteosarcoma cells using the CRISPR-Cas9 system to reverse drug resistance. *Oncotarget* **2016**, *7*, 83502–83513. [CrossRef] [PubMed]
73. Yang, Y.; Qiu, J.G.; Li, Y.; Di, J.M.; Zhang, W.J.; Jiang, Q.W.; Zheng, D.W.; Chen, Y.; Wei, M.N.; Huang, J.R.; et al. Targeting ABCB1-mediated tumor multidrug resistance by CRISPR/Cas9-based genome editing. *Am. J. Transl. Res.* **2016**, *8*, 3986–3994.
74. Takahashi, K.; Inukai, T.; Imamura, T.; Yano, M.; Tomoyasu, C.; Lucas, D.M.; Nemoto, A.; Sato, H.; Huang, M.; Abe, M.; et al. Anti-leukemic activity of bortezomib and carfilzomib on B-cell precursor ALL cell lines. *PLoS ONE* **2017**, *12*, e0188680. [CrossRef] [PubMed]
75. Barghout, S.H.; Aman, A.; Nouri, K.; Blatman, Z.; Arevalo, K.; Thomas, G.E.; MacLean, N.; Hurren, R.; Ketela, T.; Saini, M.; et al. A genome-wide CRISPR/Cas9 screen in acute myeloid leukemia cells identifies regulators of TAK-243 sensitivity. *JCI Insight* **2021**, *6*, e141518. [CrossRef] [PubMed]
76. Wei, W.; Lin, Y.; Song, Z.; Xiao, W.; Chen, L.; Yin, J.; Zhou, Y.; Barta, S.K.; Petrus, M.; Waldmann, T.A.; et al. A20 and RBX1 Regulate Brentuximab Vedotin Sensitivity in Hodgkin Lymphoma Models. *Clin. Cancer. Res.* **2020**, *26*, 4093–4106. [CrossRef] [PubMed]
77. Yu, J.S.L.; Yusa, K. Genome-wide CRISPR-Cas9 screening in mammalian cells. *Methods* **2019**, *164*, 29–35. [CrossRef] [PubMed]
78. Shalem, O.; Sanjana, N.E.; Hartenian, E.; Shi, X.; Scott, D.A.; Mikkelson, T.; Heckl, D.; Ebert, B.L.; Root, D.E.; Doench, J.G.; et al. Genome-scale CRISPR-Cas9 knockout screening in human cells. *Science* **2014**, *343*, 84–87. [CrossRef]
79. Doench, J.G.; Fusi, N.; Sullender, M.; Hegde, M.; Vaimberg, E.W.; Donovan, K.F.; Smith, I.; Tothova, Z.; Wilen, C.; Orchard, R.; et al. Optimized sgRNA design to maximize activity and minimize off-target effects of CRISPR-Cas9. *Nat. Biotechnol.* **2016**, *34*, 184–191. [CrossRef]
80. Sheng, Q.; D'Alessio, J.A.; Menezes, D.L.; Karim, C.; Tang, Y.; Tam, A.; Clark, S.; Ying, C.; Connor, A.; Mansfield, K.G.; et al. PCA062, a P-cadherin Targeting Antibody-Drug Conjugate, Displays Potent Antitumor Activity Against P-cadherin-expressing Malignancies. *Mol. Cancer Ther.* **2021**, *20*, 1270–1282. [CrossRef]
81. Loganzo, F.; Tan, X.; Sung, M.; Jin, G.; Myers, J.S.; Melamud, E.; Wang, F.; Diesl, V.; Follettie, M.T.; Musto, S.; et al. Tumor cells chronically treated with a trastuzumab-maytansinoid antibody-drug conjugate develop varied resistance mechanisms but respond to alternate treatments. *Mol. Cancer Ther.* **2015**, *14*, 952–963. [CrossRef] [PubMed]
82. Hamblett, K.J.; Jacob, A.P.; Gurgel, J.L.; Tometsko, M.E.; Rock, B.M.; Patel, S.K.; Milburn, R.R.; Siu, S.; Ragan, S.P.; Rock, D.A.; et al. SLC46A3 Is Required to Transport Catabolites of Noncleavable Antibody Maytansine Conjugates from the Lysosome to the Cytoplasm. *Cancer Res.* **2015**, *75*, 5329–5340. [CrossRef] [PubMed]
83. Kinneer, K.; Meekin, J.; Tiberghien, A.C.; Tai, Y.T.; Phipps, S.; Kiefer, C.M.; Rebelatto, M.C.; Dimasi, N.; Moriarty, A.; Papadopoulos, K.P.; et al. SLC46A3 as a Potential Predictive Biomarker for Antibody-Drug Conjugates Bearing Noncleavable Linked Maytansinoid and Pyrrolobenzodiazepine Warheads. *Clin. Cancer Res.* **2018**, *24*, 6570–6582. [CrossRef] [PubMed]
84. Sun, J.; Nagel, R.; Zaal, E.A.; Ugalde, A.P.; Han, R.; Proost, N.; Song, J.Y.; Pataskar, A.; Burylo, A.; Fu, H.; et al. SLC1A3 contributes to L-asparaginase resistance in solid tumors. *EMBO J.* **2019**, *38*, e102147. [CrossRef] [PubMed]
85. Abada, P.; Howell, S.B. Regulation of Cisplatin cytotoxicity by cu influx transporters. *Met. Based Drugs* **2010**, *2010*, 317581. [CrossRef] [PubMed]
86. Bompiani, K.M.; Tsai, C.Y.; Achatz, F.P.; Liebig, J.K.; Howell, S.B. Copper transporters and chaperones CTR1, CTR2, ATOX1, and CCS as determinants of cisplatin sensitivity. *Metallomics* **2016**, *8*, 951–962. [CrossRef]
87. Planells-Cases, R.; Lutter, D.; Guyader, C.; Gerhards, N.M.; Ullrich, F.; Elger, D.A.; Kucukosmanoglu, A.; Xu, G.; Voss, F.K.; Reincke, S.M.; et al. Subunit composition of VRAC channels determines substrate specificity and cellular resistance to Pt-based anti-cancer drugs. *EMBO J.* **2015**, *34*, 2993–3008. [CrossRef]
88. He, Y.J.; Meghani, K.; Caron, M.C.; Yang, C.; Ronato, D.A.; Bian, J.; Sharma, A.; Moore, J.; Niraj, J.; Detappe, A.; et al. DYNLL1 binds to MRE11 to limit DNA end resection in BRCA1-deficient cells. *Nature* **2018**, *563*, 522–526. [CrossRef]
89. Al-Majdoub, Z.M.; Achour, B.; Couto, N.; Howard, M.; Elmorsi, Y.; Scotcher, D.; Alrubia, S.; El-Khateeb, E.; Vasilogianni, A.M.; Alohali, N.; et al. Mass spectrometry-based abundance atlas of ABC transporters in human liver, gut, kidney, brain and skin. *FEBS Lett.* **2020**, *594*, 4134–4150. [CrossRef]
90. Henderson, J.T.; Piquette-Miller, M. Blood-brain barrier: An impediment to neuropharmaceuticals. *Clin. Pharmacol. Ther.* **2015**, *97*, 308–313. [CrossRef]
91. Dong, X. Current Strategies for Brain Drug Delivery. *Theranostics* **2018**, *8*, 1481–1493. [CrossRef] [PubMed]
92. Mochizuki, T.; Mizuno, T.; Kurosawa, T.; Yamaguchi, T.; Higuchi, K.; Tega, Y.; Nozaki, Y.; Kawabata, K.; Deguchi, Y.; Kusuhara, H. Functional Investigation of Solute Carrier Family 35, Member F2, in Three Cellular Models of the Primate Blood-Brain Barrier. *Drug Metab. Dispos.* **2021**, *49*, 3–11. [CrossRef] [PubMed]
93. Winter, G.E.; Radic, B.; Mayor-Ruiz, C.; Blomen, V.A.; Trefzer, C.; Kandasamy, R.K.; Huber, K.V.M.; Gridling, M.; Chen, D.; Klampfl, T.; et al. The solute carrier SLC35F2 enables YM155-mediated DNA damage toxicity. *Nat. Chem. Biol.* **2014**, *10*, 768–773. [CrossRef] [PubMed]
94. Gao, B.; Hagenbuch, B.; Kullak-Ublick, G.A.; Benke, D.; Aguzzi, A.; Meier, P.J. Organic anion-transporting polypeptides mediate transport of opioid peptides across blood-brain barrier. *J. Pharmacol. Exp. Ther.* **2000**, *294*, 73–79.

95. Lee, W.; Glaeser, H.; Smith, L.H.; Roberts, R.L.; Moeckel, G.W.; Gervasini, G.; Leake, B.F.; Kim, R.B. Polymorphisms in human organic anion-transporting polypeptide 1A2 (OATP1A2): Implications for altered drug disposition and central nervous system drug entry. *J. Biol. Chem.* **2005**, *280*, 9610–9617. [CrossRef]
96. Bronger, H.; Konig, J.; Kopplow, K.; Steiner, H.H.; Ahmadi, R.; Herold-Mende, C.; Keppler, D.; Nies, A.T. ABCC drug efflux pumps and organic anion uptake transporters in human gliomas and the blood-tumor barrier. *Cancer Res.* **2005**, *65*, 11419–11428. [CrossRef]
97. Sano, Y.; Mizuno, T.; Mochizuki, T.; Uchida, Y.; Umetsu, M.; Terasaki, T.; Kusuhara, H. Evaluation of Organic Anion Transporter 1A2-knock-in Mice as a Model of Human Blood-brain Barrier. *Drug Metab. Dispos.* **2018**, *46*, 1767–1775. [CrossRef]
98. Saxonov, S.; Berg, P.; Brutlag, D.L. A genome-wide analysis of CpG dinucleotides in the human genome distinguishes two distinct classes of promoters. *Proc. Natl. Acad. Sci. USA* **2006**, *103*, 1412–1417. [CrossRef]
99. Takechi, T.; Hirota, T.; Sakai, T.; Maeda, N.; Kobayashi, D.; Ieiri, I. Interindividual Differences in the Expression of ATP-Binding Cassette and Solute Carrier Family Transporters in Human Skin: DNA Methylation Regulates Transcriptional Activity of the Human ABCC3 Gene. *Drug Metab. Dispos.* **2018**, *46*, 628–635. [CrossRef]

pharmaceutics

Review

Evaluation of Recent Intranasal Drug Delivery Systems to the Central Nervous System

Tyler P. Crowe [1] and Walter H. Hsu [2,*]

[1] Carver College of Medicine, University of Iowa, Iowa City, IA 52242, USA; tyler-crowe@uiowa.edu
[2] Department of Biomedical Sciences, Iowa State University, Ames, IA 50011, USA
* Correspondence: whsu@iastate.edu

Abstract: Neurological diseases continue to increase in prevalence worldwide. Combined with the lack of modifiable risk factors or strongly efficacious therapies, these disorders pose a significant and growing burden on healthcare systems and societies. The development of neuroprotective or curative therapies is limited by a variety of factors, but none more than the highly selective blood-brain barrier. Intranasal administration can bypass this barrier completely and allow direct access to brain tissues, enabling a large number of potential new therapies ranging from bioactive peptides to stem cells. Current research indicates that merely administering simple solutions is inefficient and may limit therapeutic success. While many therapies can be delivered to some degree without carrier molecules or significant modification, a growing body of research has indicated several methods of improving the safety and efficacy of this administration route, such as nasal permeability enhancers, gelling agents, or nanocarrier formulations. This review shall discuss promising delivery systems and their role in expanding the clinical efficacy of this novel administration route. Optimization of intranasal administration will be crucial as novel therapies continue to be studied in clinical trials and approved to meet the growing demand for the treatment of patients with neurological diseases.

Keywords: intranasal; nose-to-brain; CNS; drug delivery; nanocarriers

Citation: Crowe, T.P.; Hsu, W.H. Evaluation of Recent Intranasal Drug Delivery Systems to the Central Nervous System. *Pharmaceutics* **2022**, *14*, 629. https://doi.org/10.3390/pharmaceutics14030629

Academic Editors: Jingyuan Wen and Yuan Huang

Received: 9 February 2022
Accepted: 9 March 2022
Published: 12 March 2022

1. Introduction

Neurological diseases represent a significant and growing disease burden both in the U.S. and worldwide. Alzheimer's Disease (AD) currently affects nearly 5 million Americans, incurring an annual estimated societal cost of >USD 100 billion [1,2]. This places AD among the most expensive diseases in the U.S., with regards to both the financial and human toll. This is projected to only increase, with prevalence climbing up to nearly 14 million Americans by 2050.

Despite this massive and growing problem, our treatments for AD and other neurological diseases remain incredibly limited, largely due to the anatomy of the central nervous system (CNS) and the blood-brain barrier (BBB). The BBB helps maintain homeostasis by severely limiting access to the CNS compartment through a combination of endothelial cells, intercellular tight junctions, and transport proteins [3,4]. Though lipophilic molecules can still access the CNS via diffusion, the movement of hydrophilic molecules across the BBB is reduced by 98–100% [5]. This is shown in many treatments for neurodegenerative diseases, such as levodopa for Parkinson's Disease (PD), where <5% of the dose reaches the CNS. Low bioavailability in the CNS requires the use of larger doses, leading to increased adverse effects. Therefore, formulations which can improve CNS bioavailability will be increasingly important for medications to be effective.

Intranasal delivery directly to the CNS offers exciting potential to bypass the highly selective BBB and deliver a greater variety of therapeutic agents to the brain in greater concentrations. Intranasally administered bioactive peptides, e.g., insulin, glial-derived neurotrophic factor, or leptin have been shown to be delivered directly from the nose to the brain in rodent models [6]. Though not every study has included the endpoint, many have shown a response in the animal such as improved cognition with insulin or decreased feeding with leptin. These thrilling animal model data have not been replicated in humans, however. Although several studies have demonstrated intranasal delivery to the brain like the animal models, it appears that a relatively small fraction of the dose is reaching the CNS [7,8]. Recent studies, such as intranasal oxytocin for autism, have failed to replicate the effects in humans [9]. Many of these studies were simply using a saline solution to administer the drug to the nasal cavity, just like in the animal models. It is becoming more apparent that due to anatomic and physiological differences between rodents and humans, more optimization is needed for the nose-to-brain pathway to reach its full therapeutic potential.

The purpose of this review is to discuss the various formulations, additives, and devices being studied to improve intranasal delivery to the CNS and the evidence for their potential.

2. Pathways to the CNS and Advantages of Intranasal Drug Delivery

2.1. Nasal Cavity Anatomy and Histology

The nasal cavity presents the most cephalic portion of the respiratory system, and the normal functions are to condition air for the respiratory system and facilitate olfaction [10,11]. The most anterior portion of the cavity vestibular region is characterized by a large amount of hair and mucus production, as well as a robust squamous epithelial lining [12,13]. It emphasizes this region's role in protection from mechanical irritation, rather than secretory or sensory which is in the other regions of the cavity (Figure 1).

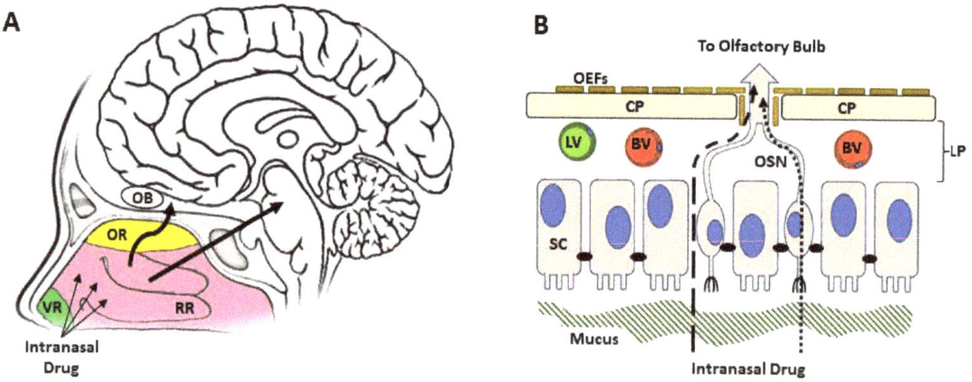

Figure 1. Anatomy and histology of the nasal cavity, epithelium, and transport pathway to the CNS. (**A**) Drugs administered to the nasal cavity cross the epithelium in either the superior olfactory region (OR) and move along the olfactory nerve (left arrow) to the olfactory bulb (OB), or the lateral respiratory regions (RR) and the trigeminal nerve (right arrow) to the pons. (**B**) From the lamina propria (LP), drugs are transported to the CNS along the olfactory sensory neuron (OSN, left arrow) p through the cribriform place (CP). A similar process occurs along the trigeminal nerve. Drugs can also be lost to systemic absorption via lymphatics (LV) or vasculature (BV). The anterior vestibular region (VR) is minimally involved in the intranasal route to the brain.

The cavity is bounded by the nasal floor (continuous with the roof of the mouth) below both the maxillary and ethmoid bones laterally. The conchae are found on the lateral wall and lined in respiratory epithelia, allowing them to play their role in filtering and humidifying inhaled air. This is collectively the respiratory region, and is lined with a single layer of pseudostratified, ciliated columnar epithelial cell also containing goblet cells. This allows for mucus production and removal, protecting the upper airway from inhaled irritants or dry air [14].

The most superior aspect of the nasal cavity is lined by olfactory epithelia, a pseudostratified layer of cells. Contrary to the respiratory epithelia of the rest of the cavity, olfactory epithelia contain olfactory neurons and Bowman's glands. Unlike the mucus-secreting and protective Goblet cells, this function is to wash away odor molecules from the nearby neurons. Deep and superior to this is the cribriform plate of the ethmoid bone, through which the olfactory neurons will project to the olfactory bulb and the rest of the CNS.

2.2. Nasal Cavity Vasculature and Innervation

The nasal cavity has a rich vascular supply full of anastomosis that is mostly centered in areas lined with respiratory epithelia on both the lateral walls and septum. Blood is supplied by branches of both the internal and external carotid arteries, including the anterior and posterior ethmoid arteries, the sphenopalatine, and greater palatine arteries. Small regions are supplied by the superior labial branch of the facial artery as well. Blood is returned via the facial vein for the anterior portions of the cavity and via the maxillary or sphenopalatine veins posteriorly into the pterygoid plexus. Lymphatics drain both anteriorly and posteriorly to the submandibular nodes.

The nasal cavity is innervated by the olfactory nerve (CN I) and trigeminal nerve (CN V). The olfactory nerve is found in the superior, olfactory region of the cavity and is comprised of bipolar neurons projecting through both the surrounding epithelia and cribriform plate. These axons synapse on the olfactory bulb in the ventral forebrain. These neurons and the spaces surrounding them are the primary route of intranasal transport to the CNS, as discussed in greater detail below. The trigeminal nerve innervates the larger remainder of the cavity via its ophthalmic (V1) and maxillary (V2) branches. General sensation is the primary function of these portions of the trigeminal nerve; the maxillary (V2) branch also contains parasympathetic fibers from the facial nerve (CN VII, greater petrosal) which controls glandular secretions in the cavity, as well as postganglionic sympathetic fibers.

Both the olfactory and trigeminal neurons are surrounded by pseudostratified epithelia in their respective regions of the nasal cavity. The trigeminal neuronal endings are only found within the lower regions of the epithelia, meaning they are not directly exposed to the nasal cavity. In stark contrast, for the olfactory neurons, cell bodies are within the epithelia and their cilia reach directly into the nasal cavity (Figure 2). This small difference is crucial for explaining why the smaller olfactory nerve plays a much larger role in intranasal transport, as detailed below. This point cannot be emphasized enough when considering how the histology ultimately informs the mechanism of intranasal delivery.

2.3. Mechanisms of Intranasal Transport to CNS

Understanding the various delivery systems used in intranasal-to-CNS therapies first requires a knowledge of the various routes and their respective mechanisms, since they dictate all factors from formulation and drug selection to safety and efficacy. Both the olfactory and trigeminal nerves have been shown to transport intranasally administered compounds to the CNS, but the olfactory nerve has been more thoroughly described in the literature. Recalling the different epithelia and vasculatures surrounding the nerves, the olfactory nerve provides better absorption and CNS transport with less systemic absorption. Additionally, due to the markedly shorter length of the nerve itself, the olfactory nerve is a significantly faster nerve than the trigeminal nerve. For the purposes of this article, the olfactory nerve will be discussed unless otherwise specified.

Several thorough and high-quality reviews are available which detail the exact mechanisms by which intranasal administered drugs reach the brain [6]. Broadly, routes can be considered either intracellular or extracellular with respect to the neuron and each contains several mechanisms. Most molecules are transported via a combination of mechanisms (Figure 3).

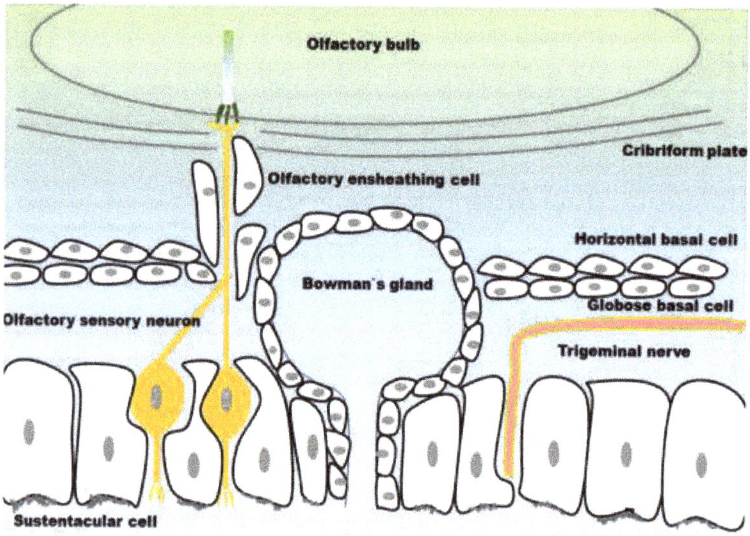

Figure 2. Comparison of olfactory (**left**) and respiratory epithelia (**right**), including location of the neurons within the sustentacular cell layers. The olfactory sensory neuron's exposure to the nasal cavity helps explain the olfactory nerve's larger role in intranasal delivery. Reprinted with permission from ref [15]. 2018 Stella Gänger.

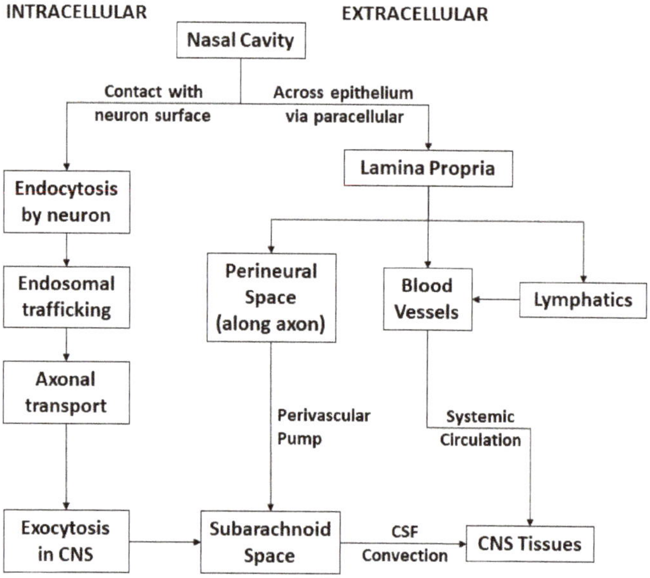

Figure 3. Schematic of intracellular and extracellular pathways for intranasal drug delivery.

2.3.1. Intracellular Transport Mechanism

The intracellular mechanism of intranasal transport involves internalization of the drug by the neuron at the site of the epithelium, transport along the axon, and exocytosis at the other end within the CNS. Intracellular transport of intranasally administered drugs or therapies to the CNS begins via endocytosis of the administered agent by olfactory (or trigeminal) neurons. This can occur via non-specific or receptor-mediated endocytosis, though the existing literature appears to indicate that non-specific binding and uptake is far more common [6]. Now bound within an endosome, the substance undergoes trafficking via the Golgi network and axonal transport to reach the synapse. This is either the olfactory bulb for the olfactory nerve, or within the pons for the trigeminal nerve. Intracellular trafficking rate is independent of size and takes 0.74–2.67 h or 3.69–13.33 h for the olfactory and trigeminal nerves, respectively [16]. Once exocytosed, the agent is moved around the CNS, via either reuptake or convectional transport. The intracellular transport occurs only across non-neuronal epithelial cells, transporting the compound from the nasal cavity to the lamina propria. This is referred to as transcellular transport and requires subsequent transportation to reach the CNS.

2.3.2. Extracellular Transport Mechanism

Extracellular transport can occur via a variety of mechanisms, which all share the basic principle of the drug moving through fluid in the spaces along which the neurons run. Notably this does not require binding and endocytosis by the neuron itself. First, the drug must cross the nasal epithelia from the nasal cavity. Although there are many tight junctions (TJs) between the epithelial cells, transient opening of the channels allows for the movement of molecules into the lamina propria. There are numerous methods of modifying the opening of TJs, which will be discussed in depth below. Additionally, olfactory neurons are not permanent like other neurons in the CNS, and they turnover every 30–60 days [17,18]. Between undergoing apoptosis and eventual replacement, this leaves a large opening among the surrounding sustentacular cells of the epithelium, which allows therapies access to the lamina propria.

From the lamina propria, intranasally administered drugs can be translocated to the brain via the perineural space. As the neurons which make up cranial nerves exit the CNS into the periphery, they take the layers of the mater ensheathing the nerve bundles [19]. This forms a perineural space with olfactory ensheathing fibroblasts (OEF) around the nerve filled with cerebrospinal fluid (CSF) that connects the subarachnoid space to the lamina propria. It is thought that drugs diffuse by bulk flow, pulsatile pressures created by concurrent arterioles, or to a lesser degree Brownian movement, to migrate into the CNS.

2.3.3. Kinetic Evidence for Mechanisms

Based on limited evidence in murine models, intranasally administered drugs reach the CNS as early as 5 min post-administration, and more distal regions of the brain by 30 min [20,21]. Peak concentrations of intranasally administered compounds vary by region of the brain. The olfactory bulb peaks as soon as 10 min post-administration, while deeper regions such as the striatum take up to 30 min. The most distal locations such as the midbrain or hypothalamus require 30 min to reach the peak concentration post-administration [19]. The average peak time for the whole brain has ranged from 30 min to 2 h, depending on the study [20,22]. Since this evidence is from different tracer molecules, formulations, and model organisms, it is difficult to extrapolate these values for clinical considerations in humans. Lastly, clearance from the CNS is completed by ~4 h, giving an early indication of duration of effect for intranasally administered therapies.

Taken together, this evidence indicates that the majority of transport to the CNS occurs via the extracellular pathway and should be the focus of optimization. Axonal transport alone via the intracellular pathway would take 0.74–2.67 h for the olfactory nerve and 3.69–13.33 h for the trigeminal nerve, based on studies of neuronal axonal transport rate [16,23]. This is without the complexities of internalization and endosomal trafficking. Simple diffusion is not too different, 0.73–2.3 h and 17–56 h for the olfactory and trigeminal nerves, respectively. Only the extracellular pathway in combination with the pulsatile movements of arteriole provides congruent transport times seen above [23,24]. As the arterioles expand in systole, they compress the fluid in the surrounding sheath and create a wave which moves at a rate of 214 μm/min in in vitro studies. This "perivascular pump" is a very efficient mode of transport, translating to 0.33 h and 1.7 h for the olfactory and trigeminal nerves, respectively. Though even these fall short of the in vivo evidence in the literature, it is reasonable to think the absence of skull bone around the channels allows for greater energy dissipation and slowing of the pathway in vitro. Still, this extracellular pathway powered by systolic pulsations is the most plausible mechanism with the in vivo and in vitro radiotracer evidence, and thus should be the primary consideration for therapeutic design.

2.4. Distribution within the CNS Compartment

Understanding the distribution within the CNS of intranasally administered therapies is crucial for the ability to produce effective, targeted interventions with minimal off-target effects. Although there can be distribution within the tissues of the brain via continued intracellular transport, this is likely not the primary mechanism based on kinetic evidence and the known inefficiencies of non-specific endocytosis at synapses. Instead, CNS-wide distribution occurs via a combination of the convective bulk flow and perivascular pump discussed above. This is supported by evidence in rodents which shows cardiac output is positively correlated to rate of distribution, providing intranasally-administered compounds reach regions of the brain adjacent to the origins of the olfactory and trigeminal nerves within 20 min of administration, including the olfactory bulb, striatum, and brainstem [25–28]. Other structures in the cortex of the forebrain and midbrain peak afterward. Discrete pathways are still unclear, though evidence in rodents shows the rostral migratory stream (RMS) is crucial for distribution beyond the olfactory bulb [29,30], where resection of the RMS reduces distribution by over 80%. The importance of the RMS in humans is unclear, as the development of the RMS or analogous structures is not well supported in the literature. Further research is needed to help elucidate pathways for targeting brain tissues, though it is clear that at least some portions of intranasal therapies reach all regions of the brain in some capacity.

The current evidence in the literature indicates that targeting drugs to sites of action within the brain is a problem that will require further attention. Nonetheless, the advantages are clear. The olfactory bulb, pons, and adjacent structures have been demonstrated to receive a markedly high dose of drug when administered intranasally, compared to intravenous (IV) administration which showed preference for the choroid and adjacent structure [26,31–33]. Furthermore, bypassing the BBB allows for a more expansive range of drug or therapy profiles, which will be further discussed ahead.

3. Factors Affecting Intranasal Drug Delivery

Understanding the anatomy of the nasal cavity, the extracellularly-based transport pathway along the cranial nerves, and how drugs will reach the target tissues of the brain is crucial when considering the factors salient to effective intranasal delivery (Table 1). We will now look at those factors more closely and within a more clinically practical context. Optimization of these factors will be absolutely crucial to the development of an effective therapy in humans. After all, almost all the evidence discussed so far comes from rodent model organisms using trained professionals to carefully and precisely administer the drug. Human anatomy is not a one-to-one comparison with rodents, and our healthcare system does not have this luxury for administration of widespread, frequently dosed therapies; especially in patients with limited transportation due to neurological decline.

Table 1. Description of factors affecting intranasal delivery.

Factor	Summary	References
Mucus	Negatively charged gel reduces movement of large, charged, and nonpolar molecules	[34–37]
Enzymatic degradation	Antimicrobial and other enzymes in mucus and epithelial cells degrade the drug	[36]
Ciliary clearance	Ciliary turnover of mucus will remove slowly diffusing drugs	[38]
Tight junctions	Apical proteins greatly restrict drug movement across epithelium between cells	[39–44]
Intrinsic drug characteristics	Molecule weight over 1 kDa, polarity, strong charge can affect absorption	[45–60]
Formulation factors	pH, buffer capacity, osmolarity, and volume are important for liquids. Solubility is additionally important for powders	[61–63]
Vasculature and Lymphatics drainage	Vasculature of lamina propria can drain away drug before transport into the CNS	[64]

3.1. Mucus

The first barrier any therapy will encounter is the mucus coating which protects the nasal epithelium beneath. Mucus is a gel-like compound composed primarily of mucins which are mostly bound to membranes in mammals [34–37]. In addition to physically protecting the epithelium from the dry, harsh air moving through the cavity, mucus contains other substances with antimicrobial and immunomodulatory effects. There are a variety of mucin types in the whole family, and these tend to vary in proportion between organisms and disease states.

Mucin uses a strongly negative net charge to dry in water when forming a gel. While this is neutralized somewhat by the presence of cations e.g., Ca^{2+} and H^{+}, this charge must be considered for formulation. Hydrophobic and charged hydrophilic molecules have been shown to diffuse poorly through mucus, whereas uncharged hydrophilic molecules are able to diffuse rapidly through the mesh of mucins nearly the speed of water for smaller molecules [65–69]. Drugs larger than 500 Da in size will be especially prone to poor mucus diffusion and becoming stuck, though most drugs will be smaller than 500 Da in size, thus it is not an important issue [15,70]. Additionally, the thickness of mucus can vary greatly depending on water content. Nasal mucus is one of the thinnest mucus types in the body; therefore, this is likely not a significant formulary consideration in most clinical cases [15]. Lastly, the rate of turnover of mucus (see below) must be considered. It appears that the addition of mucoadhesive coatings can increase absorption. Though this addition can be useful for increasing bioavailability, it may be limited since the nasal cavity produces a tremendous volume of mucus (20–40 mL per day) which is quickly turned over by ciliary propulsion (every 10–20 min) [38]. Even this rate varies in individuals' nasal passages, as the left and right passages alternate degrees of congestion throughout the day as a part of the well-described nasal cycle [71–73]. The olfactory epithelium lacks the motile cilia responsible for this movement, thus the rate of turnover is slower in the primary region of interest for intranasal nose-to-brain transport. However, an increase in expression of P-glycoprotein (P-gp) pumps in olfactory epithelia may negate this effect [74]. More research in this area will be required in the future to ultimately increase mucus permeation by intranasally administered therapies.

3.2. The Nasal Cavity Epithelium and Tight Junctions

Any intranasally administered drug must bind or cross the epithelial lining to reach the lamina propria before it can be transported further into the CNS. Recalling the mucus coating, presence of TJs and limited proportion of the total cavity this covers, optimizing a formulation to maximize crossing into the lamina propria will be crucial for any therapy.

This is especially true since the lamina propria also drains fluids back into either systemic circulation, local glands for excretion, or via lymphatics to the deep cervical chain of lymph nodes. It is actually a relatively small fraction which will be carried along the nerves and to the parenchyma of the brain, thus increasing the total amount arriving to the lamina propria is crucial for clinical efficacy.

TJs are a protein complex made of occludins, claudins, and more that connect epithelial cells at the apical surface and typically separate the basolateral sides of cells from the lumen or cavity. TJs can be modulated to increase or decrease permeability across the membrane primarily through phosphorylation signaling pathways on occludins. Several compounds have been used to transiently decrease nasal epithelial TJ tightness and increase intranasal delivery amounts, including papaverine, poly-L-arginine, 12-O-tetradecanotlophorbol-13-acetate (TPA), and bisindolylmaleimide [39–44]. Broadly, these compounds either directly dephosphorylate TJs or inhibit the function of various kinases (especially protein kinase C to reduce the function of the proteins and increase membrane permeability, ranging from two- to four-fold. Other options such as chitosan, a chitin derivative, have been shown to increase epithelial permeability by affecting TJs. When formulated as a cationic coating for nanostructured lipid carriers, researchers have observed increased delivery across a membrane and stronger pharmacological response [75–77]. Given the constrictions imposed by mucus on the types of drugs, this can provide a broad range of drugs access to this administration route.

Modulation of TJs may not even be absolutely required for effective intranasal delivery. Olfactory sensory neurons (OSNs), the functional unit of the olfactory nerve that binds to molecules to transduce the sense of smell, are relatively short lived by neuronal standards and turnover every 30–60 days [18]. New OSNs actually grow into the same spots in the olfactory epithelia, meaning there are cell-sized holes in the membrane at any given time. Since compounds as small as insulin (5.8 kDa) and as large as albumin (65 kDa) have been successfully delivered to the CNS intranasally in a simple saline solution, crossing these passages (a process known as persorption) may provide a floor for amounts delivered, even if most of the paracellular spaces are closed off by TJs [20,78–80]. It should be noted that this is only true for OSNs; the trigeminal nerve endings terminate in the transcellular space of the epithelia and do not reach into the nasal cavity.

3.3. *Size and Charge Matters*

Finally, the very biochemical nature of the drug itself has an impact on intranasal delivery bioavailability. Small, uncharged, hydrophilic molecules can move most freely through mucus and the matrix of mucins. For example, a small molecule such as dopamine (DA, 0.15 kDa) has a five-fold increase in CNS concentrations compared to the much larger nerve growth factor (NGF, 26.5 kDa) when administered at the same concentration [45,46]. Generally, 0.4 kDa is considered small enough to freely diffuse and pass through the nasal epithelia; it is only over 1 kDa that a drop off in diffusion is seen. This size limit is not entirely inhibiting though, as molecules as large as wheat germ agglutinin–horseradish peroxidase (80 kDa) and even whole stem cells have been transported to some degree [47–57].

Nonpolar compounds are thought to be transported poorly to the CNS intranasally, though there is a growly body of evidence that the proper microemulsion formulation can greatly increase the intranasal brain area under curve (AUC) compared to IV administration of the compound. Indeed, there is evidence that with some drugs *increasing* the hydrophobicity can increase delivery to the CNS [58,59]. It is known that hydrophobic compounds cross biological membranes such as the nasal epithelia, blood vessels, or BBB well. This shows that not only are hydrophobic drugs capable of being administered intranasally with the correct formulation, but this may be an advantage.

Similarly, nanocarriers and emulsions can be used to help increase the efficient delivery of highly charged compounds. Though there is existing evidence that strong cations such as Mn^{2+} and Co^{2+} or charged proteins and small molecules can be delivered without special formulation [60], achieving a desired therapeutic effect will likely require nanocarrier utilization, as chronic administration may lead to irritation and discomfort in human patients. Since many neurological diseases are chronic and without curative therapies currently, tolerance to preparations with nanocarriers is of the utmost concern.

3.4. Brief Comparative Anatomy and Translational Limits

When considering all of the evidence reviewed thus far, as well as that below, it is important to distinguish between research conducted on humans and that conducted on animal models. Both the conditions of the laboratory, with its highly trained workforce and controlled environment, and the anatomical differences between species play a significant role in the generalizability of the data. Often, researchers are administering doses as low as 25 μL but usually closer to 200 μL in size in these experiments; a size selected because this is the maximum volume of the nasal cavity in the model rodents [61,62]. In humans, the nasal cavity is 6–7 mL in volume, which is impractical at best [63]. Furthermore, 50% of the rodent nasal cavity is covered in olfactory epithelia, compared to <5% in humans [81]. This limitation in area will make delivery to the CNS less efficient and adds emphasis on making sure administered drugs reach the correct region of the nasal cavity. Animals are also positioned at a 90-degree angle or on their back, which can be difficult for elderly patients with limited mobility if dosing multiple times a day. Lastly, animals are typically anesthetized in these studies for administration, which slows the respiratory rate and drug clearance, leading to an increase in absorption which would not be seen in fully conscious patients. Evidence of this is limited and unclear, however, as few studies included unanesthetized control subjects/groups for comparison [82].

4. Types of Intranasal Strategy for Brain Drug Delivery

Strategies to improve intranasal delivery to the CNS include additives to the formulation, nanocarriers or particles which allow for molecules to cross the membrane (such as lipophilic compounds), or devices that increase the amount of drug that reaches the upper olfactory region of the cavity (Table 2). Each strategy has its own advantages and disadvantages. As this therapy transitions from trained professionals using model organisms in laboratories to everyday patients (many with a neurological disease), a combination of strategies will likely be required for therapeutic success. Based on the factors and limitations discussed before, it is seen in that <1% of intranasal administered compounds typically reach the brain [81]. To avoid irritation of the nasal epithelia, there will be a maximum tolerable dose, so additional strategies and preparations will be required.

Table 2. Notable additives and strategies for intranasal delivery systems.

Additive or Formulation	Summary	Examples	References
Simple solutions	Simplest strategy which has shown to be possible but likely insufficient	PBS or Saline solutions	[83–85]
Nasal Permeability enhancers	Broad category of agents which disrupt nasal epithelia to increase absorption	Cyclodextrans, Sodium Hyaluronate, Cremophor RH40, Chitosan, Cyclopentyladenosine	[58,86–90]
Enzyme Modulators	Disrupt the normal function of enzymes in the epithelium	P-glycoprotein inhibitors, CYP450 inhibitors, Acetazolamide	[91–96]
Vasoconstrictors	Reducing the rich vascular supply causes less drug to be absorbed into circulation	Phenylephrine	[64]
Mucoadhesives	Increase adherence to mucus and residence time in cavity for better absorption	Chitosan, Carbopol®, Carboxymethylcellulose	[15,97–99]
Ciliostatics	Impaired ciliary movement decreases mucus clearance increasing residence time	Chlorbutol, Hydroxybenzoate, Phenylmercuric acid, Thiomersal	[100]

Table 2. *Cont.*

Additive or Formulation	Summary	Examples	References
Biogels	Liquid that activates to gel in nasal cavity, increasing residence time and absorption	Pluronic/Carbopol gels, Cellulose derivatives/Paenol gels, Chitosan derivative gels	[101–107]
Devices	Devices target delivery of broader formulations to the olfactory region of the nasal cavity	ViaNase™, OptiNose™, Precision Olfactory Device®, Mechanical Spray bottles	[108–111]
US or Magnet guiding	Niche application of US or magnetic gradients to guide labeled drug delivery	Ultrasound and Magnetophoresis	[112,113]
Nanocarriers	Broad category of organic and inorganic nanoparticles that enhance absorption and delivery of bioactive drugs to brain	Chitosan, PGLA nanoparticles, Liposomes, Microemulsions, Solid-Lipid nanoparticles	[114–130]

5. Preparation and Evaluation of Intranasal Drug Delivery Systems

5.1. Solutions Alone

Though likely inadequate for clinically efficacious use, there is mixed evidence for intranasal administration of a drug in saline or phosphate-buffered saline (PBS) alone, which warrants discussion. Some studies in rodents have reported increased nose-to-brain delivery in these simple solutions, such as 5-fjuorouracil (104% increase compared to IV administration of the drug), remoxipride (50% increase in brain/plasma AUC, or morphine (30-fold higher brain/plasma AUC compared to IV administration of the drug) [83–85]. Still, others have found no difference between intranasal and IV administrations, such as a study using a 5-HT_{1A} receptor antagonist UH-301 in rats [86]. This variance in delivery may ultimately be a product of the chemical natures of the specific drugs, but this emphasizes the need for optimized formulations. Nonetheless, these results can be viewed as further proof of concept, as even the least effective intranasal formulation can deliver more to the CNS than the IV route. Thankfully, there is a broad range of types and specific formulations to overcome this phenomenon, which will be discussed below.

5.2. Additives to Increase Nasal Barrier Permeability

Though many studies involve administering a compound in a simple saline solution or even just water, the known poor delivery of these formulations (<1% of total dose reaching the CNS) will necessitate the addition of substances that increase intranasal absorption. In principle, most of these additives work to increase the amount of drug crossing the nasal epithelia into the lamina propria. Though this does not specifically work to increase the fraction moving along the nerves into the CNS from the lamina propria, it can improve the AUC in the brain and reduce the amount of dose that simply exits the nasal cavity or is degraded within mucus.

Permeability enhancers can be defined as any substance which increases the permeability of the nasal epithelial or membrane diffusion. This can take the form of additions which allowed for greater diffusion across membranes, e.g., surfactants, lipids, and cyclodextrans [58,87]. These permeability enhancers are especially useful for the transport of hydrophilic compounds or macromolecules. A significant disadvantage of these agents is that the mechanism involves disruption of the nasal epithelia, which can lead to potentially toxic irritation of the mucosae with time [88]. Such adverse reactions would greatly reduce the clinical potential for any drug requiring repeated dosing. Some agents, e.g., dextran, sodium hyaluronate, and Cremophor RH40 appear to be non-irritating and non-toxic. This list is far from comprehensive [89].

Another method to increase nasal membrane permeability is to modulate the function of TJs, which can be done via chitosan [90]. Indeed, early evidence shows administration of N-cyclopentyladenosine with chitosan microparticles resulted in a 10-fold increase in brain concentration following intranasal administration, compared to administration of N-cyclopentyladenosine with mannitol-lecithin [131]. Even transient opening of the TJs allows a larger and more hydrophilic drug to pass more readily through the paracellular space and to the lamina propria. Chitosans are also mucoadhesives allowing for more drug to be held in the nasal cavity adjacent to the membrane, resulting in increased retention time and absorption. Chitosans are also well-characterized and considered to be safe, non-irritating, and biodegradable; a strong perk for a chronically administered therapy [132].

Modulation or addition of enzymes has been used to increase permeability and intranasal delivery to the CNS. Several studies have shown that additions of matrix metalloproteinases (MMPs) can increase the intranasal delivery of compounds. Several studies have found fluorescently labelled dextran (10 kDa) to only reach the CNS when co-administered with an MMP [28,133]. Another study found that the addition of an MMP doubled the amount of biologically-active enzyme chloramphenicol acyltransferase (75 kDa) intranasally delivered to the brain [134]. Both authors acknowledged that destruction of the nasal extracellular matrix will likely be irritating with time, which greatly limits the application of this formulation in practice. More research will be needed to clarify the long-term safety of MMPs. Another example of enzymatic-focused options would be to block epithelial P-gp activity. Though not all drugs are P-gp substrates. The high expression of P-gp in the BBB, nasal membranes, and olfactory bulb will greatly limit the transport of drugs which are P-gp substrates. Several studies have shown that transport of verapamil, a P-gp substrate, to the brain can be increased by either the addition of a P-gp inhibitor, e.g., rifampin or cyclosporin A, or the use of P-gp-deficient mice [74,91–93]. For drugs which are substrates for P-gp, this evidence is very encouraging.

It is important to remember these additives must be tailored to specific medications. In some instances, these formulations can actually decrease the amount of drug transported to the brain. In one study, a chitosan nanoemulsion decreased the amount of pralidoxime delivered to the brain beyond the olfactory bulb compared to administration in a saline solution [135]. The authors thought this was due to loading efficiency issues. While this is an exception rather than the rule, it serves as a reminder that more is not always better.

5.3. Other Additives

Vasoconstrictors are other co-administered compounds which have been shown to significantly increase intranasal transport to the brain. One study used a vasoconstrictor phenylephrine and found that it increased the brain/plasma AUC ratio for several neuropeptides [64]. By reducing the vascular supply to the mucosa, it seems less drug in the lamina propria is lost via venous or lymphatic return to systemic circulation, allowing for more drug to reach the brain. Since the perivascular pump is a potentially significant contributor to the movement of drugs along the axons, modulation of the vascular system may decrease transport along both the trigeminal and olfactory nerves as well. Further research will be required for the mechanism of intranasal delivery to be fully understood. However, for drugs particularly prone to absorption into the systemic circulation, the use of a vasoconstrictor remains an option.

Inhibition of enzymes has also been shown to increase intranasal delivery. The nasal cavity possesses numerous enzymes capable of metabolizing drugs. This protective feature can greatly limit the intranasal pathway for drugs which are metabolized by these enzymes. Several studies have shown that inhibition of proteases or cytochrome P-450 enzyme in the nasal mucosa increases the amount of drug transported from the nasal cavity to the brain [81,94,95]. This same principle applies to the brain as well. Acetazolamide is a carbonic anhydrase inhibitor which decreases CSF production in the brain. Pretreatment with acetazolamide has shown to increase CSF concentration of intranasal drugs in several studies [83,96]. For drugs which require CSF convection to distribute to their site of action in the CNS, this presents an interesting option. It should be noted that this effect is only seen in pretreatment and not co-administration.

Though much of the evidence is preliminary and in rodent models, there are several promising additives which can potentially improve intranasal delivery to a level sufficient for clinical applications without causing adverse reactions that would exclude clinical use. Due to the design of these studies, few have the health of the animals' respiratory system as a measured endpoint. This will need to change before any of them can be thoroughly studied in humans. For that reason, chitosan in particular seems promising with its robust body of evidence and well-characterized safety profile, as do the other non-irritating or non-toxic permeability enhancers. However, intranasal delivery to the brain can be improved by altering the drug, not just the nasal mucosa.

5.4. Coatings

One major limitation of intranasal drug delivery is the mucus coating and its high rate of turnover due to the clearance by cilia, as described above. Several strategies have shown promise for improving the specific changes that muco-ciliary clearance poses. For large-size drugs which are significantly more prone to becoming stuck in the mucus, this is especially promising.

Mucoadhesives serve to improve the first step in intranasal transport by better adhering a drug to the mucus, allowing it to be absorbed. There is a broad category of generally positively-charged molecules, e.g., chitosan (and several derivatives), carboxymethylcellulose, polacrylic acid, etc. [15]. Functionally, they work by increasing the residence time of the drug to increase absorption. Since the olfactory region's cilia are non-motile, mucoadhesives may be effective for drugs especially targeting the olfactory nerve over the trigeminal nerve. The evidence for this method is mixed, with studies finding no significant difference in the clearance of small peptides [97]. However, this may not be the case with all types of drugs. Other research has shown that the brain AUC for buspirone in a mucoadhesive formulation was 2.5 times greater than a simple saline intranasal or IV formulation [98]. Similar results have been seen in other studies that lacked proper administration controls, thus comparison of results is difficult [86,98,99]. This strategy may be limited to certain drugs which have uniquely high clearance, such as buspirone (0.4 kDa).

Ciliostatics complement mucoadhesives by slowing the clearance time of mucus, further increasing the residence time of intranasal drugs. There is a long list of both reversible and irreversible ciliostatics and ciliotoxic drugs. Chlorbutol and several hydroxybenzoates are examples of reversible drugs, while chlorocresol edetate, phenylmercuric acetate, and thiomersal are irreversible examples [15]. Even chitosan has shown potential as a ciliostatics. This is far from an exhaustive list, there is limited but long-standing evidence that the irreversible benzalkonium chloride does not result in morphological changes to the nasal mucosa or the effective mucus clearance of the cavity [100]. Though this was used as a treatment for allergic rhinitis, long-term safety and tolerance will be crucial for any therapy treating neurological or psychiatric diseases. All the ciliostatics listed above are preservatives, which will be necessary for the stability of some formulations and can function in both roles.

Whether mucoadhesives and ciliostatics increase intranasal brain AUC by merely prolonging nasal residence time or some other mechanism is not clear. But more time in the cavity and mucus means more interaction with the network of intracellular and extracellular xenobiotic metabolism and proteases. Furthermore, if a patient develops a hypersensitivity to the drug, this will be less well tolerated. Optimization of these formulations will be dictated by this balance of absorption and in situ degradation.

5.5. Biogels

Biogels are another strategy for significantly increasing nasal retention time and absorption. Biogels are defined as solutions which can modulate or tune their viscosity in response to a physical or chemical stimulus. In intranasal drug administration, this means increasing loading dose efficiency and potentiation of release times; not unlike many mucoadhesives. Numerous polymers can serve as biogels, e.g., chitosan, poloxamer, derivatives of polyacrylic acid, or cellulose. This is far from an exhaustive list, and many more examples can be found depending on which trigger is desired.

Early evidence for biogels is promising. One study found the brain AUC of intranasal rufinamide to be doubled when administered in a xyloglucan-based, heat triggered biogel, as compared to a simpler suspension [101]. This particular example is an antiepileptic which when given orally has a poor bioavailability across the BBB, demonstrating the potential of intranasal administration. Additional studies have shown improved brain AUCs for other neurologic diseases too: pluronic acid and Carbopol® gels with rivastigmine for AD [102], poloxamer gels with rasagiline for PD [103], multiple gels with several drugs for treatment of depression [104–106], or even cellulose derivatives with paeonol for the treatment of ischemic and hemorrhagic brain injury [107]. While the clinical significance of these improved CNS bioavailabilities is unclear, biogels have a compelling and growing body of evidence suggesting that they are a promising strategy for intranasal drug administration and are worthy of studying in proper clinical trials.

5.6. Devices

Intranasal administration devices are another compelling strategy that will find a role in the clinical use of intranasal drugs. Recall that the olfactory region is <10% of the entire nasal cavity and located on the superior aspect as well as the rapid mucus clearance in the motile respiratory regions. Biology dictates that delivering the highest dose to the correct area is necessary to achieve meaningful clinical applications. Traditional spray pumps tend to only reach the anterior and lateral aspects of the nasal cavity, with <3% of the dose reaching the olfactory region [136] (Figure 4). Other alternatives such as nasal drops require the patients to precisely position their bodies, which is not suitable for many patients of all ages. The data listed so far have been conducted by trained professionals on model subjects positioned optimally in a controlled environment. The need to replicate this efficient delivery to the olfactory region in particular will be required to see results translate from labs into clinics. Fortunately, there are solutions for this challenge in the form of devices. Even these are not a magic solution. Most therapies require the patient to be conscious and cooperative with the procedure of inserting the device and triggering the release. While these devices will enable many more drugs to be clinically relevant, this approach will still pose a challenge for the very young and neurologically impaired alike.

Delivery devices all have the same goal of getting more of the dose to the olfactory region but do so by a variety of methods. While these methods will be detailed below, it is important to note that cross-comparisons are difficult as they use different formulations (liquids vs. powders) and measure different endpoints (or even different definitions of the same endpoint, such as the olfactory region itself). The advantages and disadvantages of each system provide an opportunity for optimal pairings, depending on each specific drug and disease in question.

Several types of devices have been produced and studied to date, though all in a preclinical context. First are electronic nebulizers, such as ViaNase™. This device has been used in studies to administer insulin for the treatment of AD, with significant improvement in cognition noted [108,109]. This is a great example of the untapped potential clinical improvements of the insulin administration route. These devices require additional research as there is limited evidence that they actually increase delivery to the olfactory region and do not release a substantial amount of dose into the lungs, where additional irritation or damage could occur [110]. There is a nitrogen-propelled version of this system, though these devices have yet to be studied in humans in a meaningful capacity.

Many powdered devices are available from a wide variety of pharmaceutical companies. Powdered formulations have the advantage of increased stability and in some cases improved nasal residence. One example of a powdered device designed for intranasal nose-to-brain delivery is the Opt-Powder™, made by the Optinose company [136]. This device also shows another advantage of powders, as more than six times the powder was delivered to the upper nasal cavity compared to liquids. This may just be that the device is more optimized for powders, there are devices that can deliver both powders and liquids effectively, such as the Precision Olfactory Delivery (POD®) device from Impel NeuroPharma [111]. Both these devices are powered by the patient simultaneously exhaling from their mouth. While this forces closure of the soft palate and lessens the dose accidentally arriving in the lungs, many patients with reduced pulmonary or cognitive function may struggle to use the device properly.

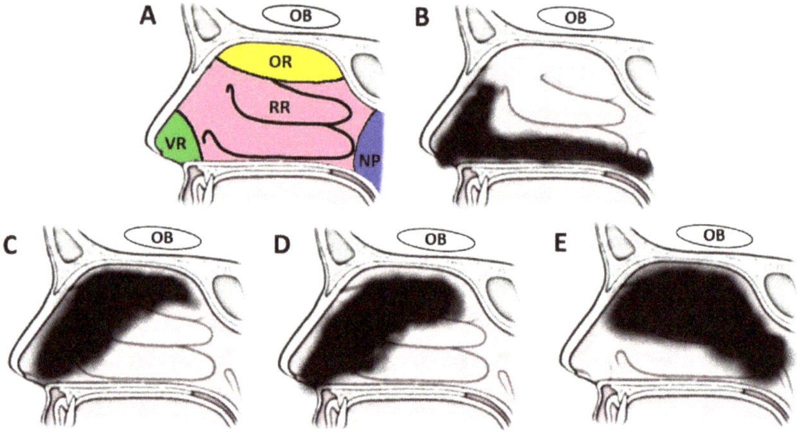

Figure 4. Estimation of deposition by nasal spray devices based on human in vivo studies. (**A**) regions of nasal cavity including the anterior vestibular (VR), superior olfactory (OR) and large respiratory regions (RR), as well as the posterior oropharynx (NP). The olfactory nerve is in the olfactory region and goes to the olfactory bulb (OB), while the trigeminal nerve is found in the respiratory regions and goes to the pons. (**B**) distribution of traditional nasal sprays is limited to vestibular and lower respiratory regions. (**C**–**E**) distributions of Vianase™ (**C**), Optinose Opt-Powder™ (**D**), and Impel POD® (**E**) all demonstrate significantly more dose reaching the olfactory region.

We have detailed the various additives, gels, nasal coatings, and devices that can be used to increase the brain AUC of intranasal administered drugs. Many appear to be capable of helping to overcome the obstacles inherent to the nasal cavity tissue and enabling this delivery route.

5.7. Ultrasound and Magnetophoresis

Though greatly limited in their application by the need of highly trained professionals, some preliminary research has examined other technologies to improve nose-to-brain delivery. First is magnetophoresis, whereby the drug is attached to a magnetic particle and directed to the olfactory region of the nasal cavity to improve the dose reaching the brain [112]. These authors reported an astounding 64-fold potential increase in delivery, with nearly a 50% delivery efficiency. In select settings this approach may prove to be a massively important tool, but not in any form of repeated or self-administered use. Other researchers have looked at using focused ultrasound sonication to increase localization of a drug within the CNS. While this method did significantly improve localization, it again requires trained operators and specialized equipment [113]. Nonetheless, both strategies provide interesting potential for singular and focused treatments. These strategies are illustrative of the absolute need for a device that increases the dose reaching the olfactory region of the nasal cavity. Further replication and research will be required of these preclinical potential therapies.

6. Nanocarriers in Brain Drug Delivery via the Intranasal Route

There are many nanocarriers that have been evaluated for their potential use in intranasal drug delivery, including both organic and inorganic compounds. The exact strategy used will depend on the specific drug properties. Hydrophobic, large, or strongly charged molecules have particular difficulty diffusing through the mucus [132]. The same can be said for drugs which are substrates of various enzymes found along the pathway while being transported to their target tissue in the brain. While biogels and mucoadhesives share some of the roles in enhancing drug transport, nanocarriers are unique in that they function as particulates. This section will explore some of the more common and well-characterized formulations, as well as the strengths and weaknesses of each formulation.

One important limitation to all types of nanoparticles is size. Particles of 100 nm in diameter or smaller have been shown to reach the brain, while those of 900 nm in diameter appear to be too large for any delivery. This upper limit in size will be crucial to the success of any individual strategy. The charge of the nanoparticle also has a significant role on the safety and efficacy of the carrier. Positively-charged molecules are more likely to be cytotoxic and induce lysis, which could result in increased irritation and nasal damage with time. Meanwhile, negatively-charged carriers are more likely to be phagocytosed, which would be removed from the nose-to-brain pathway or are transported by the much less efficient intracellular pathway [137–140]. Inorganic molecules have also been shown to be more cytotoxic than organics, making them less appealing candidates in the intranasal setting [137–139].

6.1. *Polymer Nanocarrier Formulations*

The first major class of nanocarriers are those derived from polymers. Chitosan and polymer-coupled chitosan derivatives have shown particular promise in recent years. One study found the use of chitosan nanoparticles allowed for the intranasal delivery of leucine-5-enkaphalin (LENK, an opioid receptor agonist) to the brain. When administered as a solution alone it resulted in no transport into the CNS [114]. Several other studies have replicated this result, showing as much as a five-fold increase in the delivery of drugs, e.g., rivastigmine, quetiapine, and pramipexole to the brain [115–117]. There is even evidence of the delivery of functioning siRNAs and plasmids to the brain using chitosan-derived nanoparticles [118,119,141]. One study using an siRNA targeting the chemotherapy-resistant gene for galectin-1 in mice demonstrated improved survival on temozolamide therapy, when given in a chitosan-tripolyphosphate carrier [142]. Not only can the nucleotides be delivered intact, but clinically significant doses appear possible even now in the early stages of research. As gene-based therapies continue to advance, this carrier has the potential to become particularly exciting in future research. Chitosan nanoparticles have successfully delivered lipid particles containing resveratrol to the CSF at six-fold greater concentrations than when the lipid particles were administered alone intranasally. No resveratrol lipid particles were transported to the CSF following IV administration [143]. For lipophilic drugs which would poorly penetrate the mucus layer otherwise, this particular evidence is exciting.

The exact mechanism by which these chitosan nanoparticles function is unknown, and will require additional research to fully elucidate. Though chitosan itself is known to be both a mucoadhesive and transiently open TJs, the nanoparticles do not always share this functionality. One derivative, *N*-palmitoyl-*N*-monomethyl-*N,N*-dimethyl-*N,N,N*-trimethyl-6-*O*-glycochitosan (or Nanomerics' molecular envelope technology) has been used to successfully deliver LENK as discussed in Section 6, but is known to not affect the function of TJs [144]. While the platform has exciting early evidence of viability, fuller characterization will be needed as it translates into human clinical settings.

Another nanoparticle which is known to be safe in humans and can transport either degradation-prone or hydrophobic drugs is poly(L-lactide-co-glycolide), or PGLA. PGLA nanoparticles have been shown to improve intranasal delivery of the small molecule olanzapine 10-fold over a simple solution alone, and further studies have demonstrated that this can cause seizure reduction in epileptic rats [120,121]. Though the preliminary evidence is as promising as chitosan, the mechanism is even less well-characterized; PGLA is not a known mucoadhesive or permeability enhancer like chitosan. PGLA can be conjugated with compounds to enhance delivery to target tissues. Various chitosan derivatives and lectins or ligands specific to the nasal epithelium have been successfully added to PGLA particles and shown to increase delivery efficiency [122–124]. The chitosan particles were again found to work the best, and even seemed to have an effect on rate of movement within the brain. No tissue-level deposition has been studied, so this potential example of targeting requires further evaluation. Even PLA nanoparticles alone (PGLA without the polyglycolic acid monomers) have been shown to improve intranasal transport 5.6–7.7-fold over solutions alone, as seen in wheat germ agglutinin-conjugated poly (ethene glycol)-poly (lactic acid) (WGA-PEG-PLA) coated coumarin [145].

This is far from an exhaustive list, and more polymer-based nanoparticles are being studied as the carriers listed above and novel ones are better characterized and developed.

6.2. Lipid Nanocarrier Formulations

Lipid-based nanoparticles have come a long way from their liposomal origin and now offer several solid lipid nanoparticle formulations which have shown promise for intranasal administration. Many lipid particles have the benefits of being more stable during storage and cheaper in mass production compared to their aqueous, polymer-based counterparts [125]. The composition of lipids must be carefully controlled. Phosphatidylcholine, phosphatidylserine, and phosphatidylethylamine are all known P-gp substrates, and their inclusion would lead to rapid clearance in an untreated nasal epithelium without reaching the CNS [126].

Microemulsions have been used to increase the delivery of hydrophobic drugs to the brain, such as the acetylcholinesterase inhibitor tacrine [127]. This formulation not only increased the brain AUC of tacrine compared to IV administration, but when a mucoadhesive was added to the emulsion the brain AUC was increased further. This result for mucoadhesive microemulsions has been repeated in rodents with several other drugs, e.g., risperidone, paliperidone, and olanzapine [15]. Interestingly, this mucoadhesive property may be required, as other studies using microemulsions alone found a lower brain AUC compared to IV administration for almost all regions of the brain. While this may be specific to the studied drug, nimopidine, the current evidence indicates that microemulsions are most effective with an increased content of mucoadhesive.

Solid lipid nanoparticles (SLNs) are an increasingly exciting lipid formulation strategy. Even more stable and cheaper to manufacture than microemulsions, SLNs also offer slower release and stability as a solid (which would be superior for powdered delivery devices) [125]. Though most research on SLNs is focused on delivery of anticancer therapies, several studies have shown promise for intranasal delivery to the CNS. One such study showed a 10-fold increase in delivery of the antipsychotic risperidone when carried by SLNs compared to a simple solution [128–130]. Should powder-based delivery devices prove more effective than liquids or mists, this nanocarrier strategy may be of particular interest. The added stability at room temperature in solid form could reduce the chances of spoilage or contamination. As objects as large as stem cells have been successfully delivered to the brain intranasally, the risk of CNS infection is far from trivial. Newer forms of SLNs are also called nanostructured lipid carriers (NLCs) in the literature, and though they have similar properties, they have not been studied in delivery models.

7. Recent Patents in Intranasal Drug Delivery Systems

Since Dr Frey's first patent in 1997, hundreds of patents for intranasal delivery ranging from drugs to nanoparticles to solvents have been filed for approval [6,146,147]. There are several excellent reviews on this subject, and to list every patent in detail here would be excessive in length; instead, this section will focus on the larger trends and popular types of patents. Of note, many FDA-approved intranasal drugs or therapies at the time of publication are actually for vaccines, which are absorbed well systemically via the rich vascular supply of the respiratory mucosa. Since these are not designed to target the brain, they will not be included in the discussion. Devices which enhance nose-to-brain administration follow a similar pattern. The Optinose™, ViaNase™, and POD™ devices discussed above have been specifically evaluated for delivery to the brain, though there are many other patented devices for delivery to the nasal cavity [147,148]. Nonetheless, their existence should be acknowledged.

More than 60 different drugs have been patented for intranasal delivery. These include the synthetic drugs, peptides, and hormones listed above, as well as nucleic acids and many more signaling molecules. These drugs are targeted for the treatment of neurodegenerative diseases, psychiatric disorders, headaches/migraines, and traumatic brain injuries as well as pain, obesity, sleep disturbances, and cancers. Truly this breadth speaks to the wide potential of this still novel administration route. If even a fraction of the patents make it to market, many patients will experience a benefit.

Well over 50 patents have been approved for solvents, including both hydrophilics such as water or glycerin as well as hydrophobics such as various organic oils or hexanes. Various alcohols, ketones, and fatty acid derivatives have been approved as well [147]. There are over 100 patents alone for surfactants, solubilizers, and gelling agents to add to these solvents. The candidates most likely to reach market have been mentioned by name in literature above, but many other options still exist. A similar number of nanoparticle and lipid coating formulations have been patented. Well-evaluated candidates such as 1-palmitoyl-2-linoleoyl-3-acetyl-rac-glycerol (PLAG), chitosan, and -polyethylene glycol (PEG) are all on the list, as well as many other polymeric compounds. These are examples of well-characterized, safe, and seemingly effective nanoparticles. Further research will be required to prove the superiority of other compounds, or to raise concerns over these leading candidates. There are several phospholipid, cholesterol, or fatty acid formulations patented for emulsions or lipid coatings, though the effectiveness of these formulations is unclear in comparison to SLNs or NLCs. Numerous chelating agents have been patented too, which would sequester Ca^{2+} and increase TJ permeability.

As shown across the various studies examined here, there is no one true formulation, carrier, or method that will work for all intranasal delivery to the brain. Given the variety of potential drugs, beyond the extensive list of those already patented, this will only be proven with time. However, the vast number of solvents, nanocarriers, and co-administered compounds which have been repeatedly shown to improve delivery also show that many of these drugs have potential for development. Further evaluation will be required to optimize these specific formulations, but the hope for success is there. Neurological diseases continue to affect greater numbers of patients every day. To date, our pharmacological tools to address this problem have been lacking, chiefly due to the restrictive BBB. The intranasal pathway offers an exciting chance to alleviate a tremendous load of disease burden in patients of all ages; these formulations may enable many CNS disorders.

8. Clinical Evidence of Intranasal Delivery to the Brain Therapies

Few trials have evaluated intranasal delivery in humans with endpoints assessing clinical efficacy. The evidence from them currently is insufficient to judge the entire delivery pathway. Nonetheless, we shall review two notable examples of intranasally administered drugs in humans and their efficacy.

8.1. Oxytocin

Oxytocin is a reproductive neuropeptide associated with increasing social behavior and memory in animals. When given to healthy humans, intranasal oxytocin has been shown to increase trusting behaviors, e.g., social affiliation, altruism, and empathy [11,148,149]. The hope was these findings would benefit patients with autism spectrum disorder (ASD), which is becoming increasingly prevalent and characterized by hallmark deficiencies in these and other behaviors. The results of initial studies were promising, as the intranasal oxytocin improved symptoms such as emotional recognition and communication skills in adolescent males with ASD [150,151]. These formulations were a simple aqueous solution of synthetic oxytocin (Syntocinon®), administered with standard nasal sprays. Subsequent studies have failed to replicate these results when randomized control groups were added and more complex and wholistic end points were used for analysis [11,152,153].

Intranasal oxytocin is a complicated case study where the failure is likely more a reflection of the difficulties in translating results from the laboratory to the clinic than an indication the administration pathway is not viable. ASD is a very heterogenous disease, with over 100 genes involved and most unrelated to oxytocin deficiency. It is possible that oxytocin therapy would only be efficacious for certain patients, which would require genetic screening to predict efficacy. Furthermore, no trial included concurrent behavioral therapy, which is well-recognized as an essential component to the treatment plan of any patient regardless of pharmacologic interventions. Nonetheless, the evidence for intranasal oxytocin having an effect exists in the early studies. Intranasal oxytocin may still have a future role as one of many treatments for disorders such as ASD, but the current body of evidence is clear that the drug treatment will likely not work alone.

8.2. Insulin

Intranasal insulin is perhaps the most storied potential application of intranasal delivery to the CNS. Insulin resistance in CNS tissues has been observed in patients with AD, as well as linked to elevated levels of hyperphosphorylated tau and β-amyloid deposition (both crucial to the pathogenesis of AD) [108,109]. Insulin receptors in the brain have been well described and implicated in functions beyond simply glucose metabolism [154]. Transport of insulin into the CNS is tightly regulated and saturated [155]. Insulin concentrations of CSF are dependent on serum concentration, rising only after an increase in serum concentration and peaking 30 min later [155]. Insulin concentrations of CSF will also be lower in magnitude. This shows the potential of intranasal delivery and bypassing the serum; insulin can be administered and achieve concentrations in the CSF that would otherwise be limited by massive peripheral effects when administered parenterally. Early studies showed intranasal insulin preserved cognition and enhanced cerebral glucose metabolism in patients with AD [109]. Notably, this study used the ViaNase™ device to optimize the insulin dose reaching the olfactory region of the nasal cavity and therefore the brain. When the researchers repeated the trial, adding multiple sites and many more patients, they were unable to replicate the results and instead found no significant difference in either outcome [156]. This study again started using the ViaNase™ device but switched to the POD® device early on due to repeated malfunction of the first device. Notably the subgroup patients in this study who used the same ViaNase™ device did again demonstrate the preservation of cognition after 12 months. It is possible that the ViaNase™ electric nebulization was crucial (POD® is a gas-driven atomizer), but this study was not designed for device comparisons. It is also impossible to assert if the difference is due to the different device use or the small sample size. It is not an unreasonable thought, since another study analyzing only the ViaNase™ patients did show a reduction in hippocampal white matter loss, compared to the placebo group using the device without insulin [157]. However, this reanalysis is further limited as neither study directly measured CSF insulin concentrations. Despite the immediate lack of results in the first phase 2/3 clinical trial, intranasal insulin still holds significant promise as a therapy for AD. A single early trial does not negate years of evidence in animal and human subjects. Instead, it is a potential reminder that not all devices or formulations are created equal; which one is used for a given drug should be considered.

There is also new evidence for insulin specifically that many of the nanocarriers described above can improve delivery to the brain, compared to native insulin alone [158]. SLNs, PGLAs and chitosan-coated formulations of both SLNs and PGLAs were tested and found to be superior for maintaining structural stability, improving nasal absorption, and prolonging insulin release [158]. This is all while only considering native insulin: there are several long-acting insulin preparations available that should theoretically function the same in the CNS. However, more studies will be needed to demonstrate this phenomenon in vivo. There is considerable evidence for intranasal insulin treating AD [21,25,79,108,109,154–157]. This evidence also points to the importance of maximizing the dose reaching the brain. Whether optimization is achieved by devices, nanoparticles, or a combination, future studies must include these technologies. They may well be the tools that finally move intranasal administration from the laboratory to patients in need.

9. Expert Opinion

Intranasal delivery is an exciting technique because it will allow for therapeutic concentrations of drugs in the CNS which previously could not be achieved without prohibitory peripheral side effects via conventional administration routes. Insulin exemplifies this concept well; a therapeutic dose for brain tissue given parenterally would cause unsafe blood concentrations before enough crossed the BBB. With intranasal administration one can bypass the peripheral blood and, therefore, many adverse effects. Clinical studies in humans have found mixed results so far. However, the broad body of evidence before makes this appear more of an issue of optimization than viability. The evidence discussed above demonstrates nanocarriers increase dose fraction delivered intranasally, and dosing will ultimately decide the viability of this delivery mechanism. Other drug classes, e.g., antipsychotics, antiepileptics, and chemotherapies could benefit greatly from bypassing the periphery as well. Nanocarriers will need to be carefully selected to achieve a stable brain AUC for these drugs to be viable in the clinical setting.

Bypassing the bloodstream can also improve drugs which would otherwise be degraded before reaching the brain. An example used today is levodopa, which requires coadministration with carbidopa to prevent metabolism. Intranasal delivery can allow for entirely new classes of drugs never before possible including peptides such as GDNF and nerve growth factor (NGF), or future siRNAs for gene therapies. Bypassing blood can mean bypassing pathology too, such as neuro-protective insulin for ischemic strokes. However, even these fragile peptides may need a nanocarrier that can protect them from nasal proteases.

Intranasal delivery means rapid, noninvasive access to the brain enabling numerous novel therapies. However, this is not a panacea, and careful optimization will be needed for any of these new treatments to reach patients. A major factor will be the formulations and devices described in this article. Early clinical applications will likely take the form of intranasally administering already FDA-approved drugs such as antipsychotic, seizure medications, or even insulin. Then as formulations are optimized with known therapies, more novel drugs will become available. The potential of intranasal delivery cannot be emphasized enough; these formulations are key to realizing this route.

10. Conclusions

Intranasal delivery directly to the brain is supported by robust evidence in rodents and humans that has been replicated for decades with all kinds of therapies. Recent studies have focused on translating these results from the laboratory into the clinic, but with mixed results. Undoubtedly, much of this is due to the complexities of treating any multifactorial disease. However, this technique and administration route is so new that almost nothing has been done in terms of optimization and efficiency of dosing. The formulations, additives, and devices reviewed here offer the promise of bridging the gap between trained technicians in a laboratory setting and ordinary patients in the clinical world. Many studies have demonstrated the correct nanocarrier can increase the dose reaching brain tissue by orders of magnitude. After all, even the best drugs cannot work if they do not reach their target. Future studies are warranted to implement and validate these advances, as they may be the key in bringing a novel therapy to market.

Author Contributions: Substantial contributions to the research and preparation of the manuscript and figures, T.P.C.; Substantial contribution to the conception, revision, and critical evaluation of the content, W.H.H. All authors have read and agreed to the published version of the manuscript.

Funding: This work was not supported by any funding.

Institutional Review Board Statement: Not applicable.

Informed Consent Statement: Not applicable.

Data Availability Statement: Not applicable.

Conflicts of Interest: The authors declare no conflict of interest.

Abbreviations

AD	Alzheimer's disease
ASD	autism spectrum disorder
AUC	area under curve
BBB	blood-brain barrier
CNS	central nervous system
CSF	cerebro-spinal fluid
IV	intravenous
LENK	leucine-5-enkaphalin
MMP	matrix metalloproteinase
NGF	nerve growth factor
NLC	nanostructured lipid carrier
OEF	olfactory ensheathing fibroblast
OSN	olfactory sensory neuron
PD	Parkinson's disease
PEG	polyethylene glycol
PGLA	poly(L-lactide-co-glycolide)
RMS	rostral migratory stream
TJ	tight junction

References

1. Hebert, L.E.; Weuve, J.; Scherr, P.A.; Evans, D.A. Alzheimer disease in the United States (2010–2050) estimated using the 2010 census. *Neurology* **2013**, *80*, 1778–1783. [CrossRef] [PubMed]
2. Meek, P.D.; McKeithan, K.; Schumock, G.T. Economic considerations in Alzheimer's disease. *Pharmacotherapy* **1998**, *18*, 68–73; Discussion 79–82; [CrossRef] [PubMed]
3. Ronaldson, P.T.; Davis, T.P. Targeting blood–brain barrier changes during inflammatory pain: An opportunity for optimizing CNS drug delivery. *Ther. Deliv.* **2011**, *2*, 1015–1041. [CrossRef] [PubMed]
4. Banks, W.A. Characteristics of compounds that cross the blood-brain barrier. *BMC Neurol.* **2009**, *9*, S3. [CrossRef]
5. Pardridge, W.M. The blood-brain barrier: Bottleneck in brain drug development. *NeuroRX* **2005**, *2*, 3–14. [CrossRef]
6. Crowe, T.P.; Greenlee, M.H.W.; Kanthasamy, A.G.; Hsu, W.H. Mechanism of intranasal drug delivery directly to the brain. *Life Sci.* **2018**, *195*, 44–52. [CrossRef]
7. Born, J.; Lange, T.; Kern, W.; McGregor, G.P.; Bickel, U.; Fehm, H.L. Sniffing neuropeptides: A transnasal approach to the human brain. *Nat. Neurosci.* **2002**, *5*, 514–516. [CrossRef]
8. Mischley, L.K.; Conley, K.E.; Shankland, E.G.; Kavanagh, T.J.; Rosenfeld, M.E.; Duda, J.E.; White, C.C.; Wilbur, T.K.; De La Torre, P.U.; Padowski, J.M. Central nervous system uptake of intranasal glutathione in Parkinson's disease. *NPJ Park. Dis.* **2016**, *2*, 16002. [CrossRef]
9. Sikich, L.; Kolevzon, A.; King, B.H.; McDougle, C.J.; Sanders, K.B.; Kim, S.-J.; Spanos, M.; Chandrasekhar, T.; Trelles, M.P.; Rockhill, C.M.; et al. Intranasal Oxytocin in Children and Adolescents with Autism Spectrum Disorder. *N. Engl. J. Med.* **2021**, *385*, 1462–1473. [CrossRef]
10. Chamanza, R.; Wright, J.A. A Review of the Comparative Anatomy, Histology, Physiology and Pathology of the Nasal Cavity of Rats, Mice, Dogs and Non-human Primates. Relevance to Inhalation Toxicology and Human Health Risk Assessment. *J. Comp. Pathol.* **2015**, *153*, 287–314. [CrossRef]
11. Cellina, M.; Gibelli, D.; Cappella, A.; Martinenghi, C.; Belloni, E.; Oliva, G. Nasal cavities and the nasal septum: Anatomical variants and assessment of features with computed tomography. *Neuroradiol. J.* **2020**, *33*, 340–347. [CrossRef] [PubMed]
12. Gizurarson, S. Anatomical and Histological Factors Affecting Intranasal Drug and Vaccine Delivery. *Curr. Drug Deliv.* **2012**, *9*, 566–582. [CrossRef] [PubMed]

13. Uraih, L.C.; Maronpot, R.R. Normal histology of the nasal cavity and application of special techniques. *Environ. Health Perspect.* **1990**, *85*, 187–208. [CrossRef] [PubMed]
14. Lai, S.K.; Wang, Y.-Y.; Hanes, J. Mucus-penetrating nanoparticles for drug and gene delivery to mucosal tissues. *Adv. Drug Deliv. Rev.* **2009**, *61*, 158–171. [CrossRef] [PubMed]
15. Gänger, S.; Schindowski, K. Tailoring Formulations for Intranasal Nose-to-Brain Delivery: A Review on Architecture, Physico-Chemical Characteristics and Mucociliary Clearance of the Nasal Olfactory Mucosa. *Pharmaceutics* **2018**, *10*, 116. [CrossRef]
16. Broadwell, R.D.; Balin, B.J. Endocytic and exocytic pathways of the neuronal secretory process and trans synaptic transfer of wheat germ agglutinin-horseradish peroxidase in vivo. *J. Comp. Neurol.* **1985**, *242*, 632–650. [CrossRef]
17. Farbman, A.I. Olfactory neurogenesis: Genetic or environmental controls? *Trends Neurosci.* **1990**, *13*, 362–365. [CrossRef]
18. Cowan, C.M.; Roskams, A.J. Apoptosis in the mature and developing olfactory neuroepithelium. *Microsc. Res. Tech.* **2002**, *58*, 204–215. [CrossRef]
19. Li, Y.; Field, P.M.; Raisman, G. Olfactory ensheathing cells and olfactory nerve fibroblasts maintain continuous open channels for regrowth of olfactory nerve fibres. *Glia* **2005**, *52*, 245–251. [CrossRef]
20. Falcone, J.A.; Salameh, T.S.; Yi, X.; Cordy, B.J.; Mortell, W.G.; Kabanov, A.V.; Banks, W.A. Intranasal Administration as a Route for Drug Delivery to the Brain: Evidence for a Unique Pathway for Albumin. *J. Pharmacol. Exp. Ther.* **2014**, *351*, 54–60. [CrossRef]
21. Salameh, T.S.; Bullock, K.M.; Hujoel, I.A.; Niehoff, M.L.; Wolden-Hanson, T.; Kim, J.; Morley, J.E.; Farr, S.A.; Banks, W.A. Central nervous system delivery of intranasal insulin: Mechanisms of uptake and effects on cognition. *J. Alzheimer's Dis.* **2015**, *47*, 715–728. [CrossRef] [PubMed]
22. Sipos, E.; Kurunczi, A.; Fehér, A.; Penke, Z.; Fülöp, L.; Kasza, Á.; Horváth, J.; Horvát, S.; Veszelka, S.; Balogh, G.; et al. Intranasal Delivery of Human β-Amyloid Peptide in Rats: Effective Brain Targeting. *Cell. Mol. Neurobiol.* **2009**, *30*, 405–413. [CrossRef] [PubMed]
23. Lochhead, J.J.; Thorne, R.G. Intranasal delivery of biologics to the central nervous system. *Adv. Drug Deliv. Rev.* **2012**, *64*, 614–628. [CrossRef] [PubMed]
24. Ichimura, T.; Fraser, P.A.; Cserr, H.F. Distribution of extracellular tracers in perivascular spaces of the rat brain. *Brain Res.* **1991**, *545*, 103–113. [CrossRef]
25. Renner, D.B.; Svitak, A.L.; Gallus, N.J.; Ericson, M.E.; Frey, W.H.; Hanson, L.R. Intranasal delivery of insulin via the olfactory nerve pathway. *J. Pharm. Pharmacol.* **2012**, *64*, 1709–1714. [CrossRef] [PubMed]
26. Thorne, R.G.; Pronk, G.J.; Padmanabhan, V.; Frey Ii, W.H. Delivery of insulin-like growth factor-I to the rat brain and spinal cord along olfactory and trigeminal pathways following intranasal administration. *Neuroscience* **2004**, *127*, 481–496. [CrossRef]
27. Hadaczek, P.; Yamashita, Y.; Mirek, H.; Tamas, L.; Bohn, M.C.; Noble, C.; Park, J.W.; Bankiewicz, K. The "Perivascular Pump" Driven by Arterial Pulsation Is a Powerful Mechanism for the Distribution of Therapeutic Molecules within the Brain. *Mol. Ther.* **2006**, *14*, 69–78. [CrossRef]
28. Lochhead, J.J.; Wolak, D.J.; Pizzo, M.E.; Thorne, R.G. Rapid Transport within Cerebral Perivascular Spaces Underlies Widespread Tracer Distribution in the Brain after Intranasal Administration. *J. Cereb. Blood Flow Metab.* **2015**, *35*, 371–381. [CrossRef]
29. Wang, C.; Liu, F.; Liu, Y.-Y.; Zhao, C.-H.; You, Y.; Wang, L.; Zhang, J.; Wei, B.; Ma, T.; Zhang, Q.; et al. Identification and characterization of neuroblasts in the subventricular zone and rostral migratory stream of the adult human brain. *Cell Res.* **2011**, *21*, 1534–1550. [CrossRef]
30. Scranton, R.A.; Fletcher, L.; Sprague, S.; Jimenez, D.F.; Digicaylioglu, M. The Rostral Migratory Stream Plays a Key Role in Intranasal Delivery of Drugs into the CNS. *PLoS ONE* **2011**, *6*, e18711. [CrossRef]
31. Vyas, T.K.; Babbar, A.K.; Sharma, R.K.; Singh, S.; Misra, A. Preliminary brain-targeting studies on intranasal mucoadhesive microemulsions of sumatriptan. *AAPS PharmSciTech* **2006**, *7*, E49–E57. [CrossRef] [PubMed]
32. Vyas, T.K.; Tiwari, S.B.; Amiji, M.M. Formulation and physiological factors influencing CNS delivery upon intranasal administration. *Crit. Rev. Ther. Drug Carr. Syst.* **2006**, *23*, 319–347. [CrossRef] [PubMed]
33. Wang, F.; Jiang, X.; Lu, W. Profiles of methotrexate in blood and CSF following intranasal and intravenous administration to rats. *Int. J. Pharm.* **2003**, *263*, 1–7. [CrossRef]
34. Williams, O.W.; Sharafkhaneh, A.; Kim, V.; Dickey, B.F.; Evans, C.M. Airway Mucus: From production to secretion. *Am. J. Respir. Cell Mol. Biol.* **2006**, *34*, 527–536. [CrossRef] [PubMed]
35. Williams, S.J.; Wreschner, D.H.; Tran, M.; Eyre, H.J.; Sutherland, G.R.; McGuckin, M.A. MUC13, a Novel Human Cell Surface Mucin Expressed by Epithelial and Hemopoietic Cells. *J. Biol. Chem.* **2001**, *276*, 18327–18336. [CrossRef]
36. Leal, J.; Smyth, H.D.C.; Ghosh, D. Physicochemical properties of mucus and their impact on transmucosal drug delivery. *Int. J. Pharm.* **2017**, *532*, 555–572. [CrossRef]
37. Shankar, V.; Gilmore, M.S.; Elkins, R.C.; Sachdev, G.P. A novel human airway mucin cDNA encodes a protein with unique tandem-repeat organization. *Biochem. J.* **1994**, *300*, 295–298. [CrossRef]
38. Schuhl, J.F. Nasal mucociliary clearance in perennial rhinitis. *J. Investig. Allergol. Clin. Immunol.* **1995**, *5*, 333–336.
39. Ohtake, K.; Maeno, T.; Ueda, H.; Ogihara, M.; Natsume, H.; Morimoto, Y. Poly-L-arginine enhances paracellular permeability via serine/threonine phosphorylation of ZO-1 and tyrosine dephosphorylation of occludin in rabbit nasal epithelium. *Pharm. Res.* **2003**, *20*, 1838–1845. [CrossRef]

40. Koizumi, J.-I.; Kojima, T.; Ogasawara, N.; Kamekura, R.; Kurose, M.; Go, M.; Harimaya, A.; Murata, M.; Osanai, M.; Chiba, H.; et al. Protein Kinase C Enhances Tight Junction Barrier Function of Human Nasal Epithelial Cells in Primary Culture by Transcriptional Regulation. *Mol. Pharmacol.* **2008**, *74*, 432–442. [CrossRef]
41. Ohtake, K.; Maeno, T.; Ueda, H.; Natsume, H.; Morimoto, Y. Poly-L-Arginine Predominantly Increases the Paracellular Permeability of Hydrophilic Macromolecules Across Rabbit Nasal Epithelium in Vitro. *Pharm. Res.* **2003**, *20*, 153–160. [CrossRef] [PubMed]
42. Krishan, M.; Gudelsky, G.A.; Desai, P.B.; Genter, M.B. Manipulation of olfactory tight junctions using papaverine to enhance intranasal delivery of gemcitabine to the brain. *Drug Deliv.* **2014**, *21*, 8–16. [CrossRef] [PubMed]
43. Tengamnuay, P.; Sahamethapat, A.; Sailasuta, A.; Mitra, A.K. Chitosans as nasal absorption enhancers of peptides: Comparison between free amine chitosans and soluble salts. *Int. J. Pharm.* **2000**, *197*, 53–67. [CrossRef]
44. Smith, J.; Wood, E.; Dornish, M. Effect of Chitosan on Epithelial Cell Tight Junctions. *Pharm. Res.* **2004**, *21*, 43–49. [CrossRef]
45. Pardeshi, C.V.; Rajput, P.V.; Belgamwar, V.S.; Tekade, A.R.; Surana, S.J. Novel surface modified solid lipid nanoparticles as intranasal carriers for ropinirole hydrochloride: Application of factorial design approach. *Drug Deliv.* **2013**, *20*, 47–56. [CrossRef] [PubMed]
46. Dahlin, M.; Jansson, B.; Björk, E. Levels of dopamine in blood and brain following nasal administration to rats. *Eur. J. Pharm. Sci.* **2001**, *14*, 75–80. [CrossRef]
47. Thorne, R.G.; Emory, C.R.; Ala, T.A.; Frey, W.H. Quantitative analysis of the olfactory pathway for drug delivery to the brain. *Brain Res.* **1995**, *692*, 278–282. [CrossRef]
48. Danielyan, L.; Schäfer, R.; von Ameln-Mayerhofer, A.; Buadze, M.; Geisler, J.; Klopfer, T.; Burkhardt, U.; Proksch, B.; Verleysdonk, S.; Ayturan, M.; et al. Intranasal delivery of cells to the brain. *Eur. J. Cell Biol.* **2009**, *88*, 315–324. [CrossRef]
49. Wu, S.; Li, K.; Yan, Y.; Gran, B.; Han, Y.; Zhou, F.; Guan, Y.T.; Rostami, A.; Zhang, G.X. Intranasal Delivery of Neural Stem Cells: A CNS-specific, Non-invasive Cell-based Therapy for Experimental Autoimmune Encephalomyelitis. *J. Clin. Cell. Immunol.* **2013**, *4*. [CrossRef]
50. Reitz, M.; Demestre, M.; Sedlacik, J.; Meissner, H.; Fiehler, J.; Kim, S.U.; Westphal, M.; Schmidt, N.O. Intranasal Delivery of Neural Stem/Progenitor Cells: A Noninvasive Passage to Target Intracerebral Glioma. *STEM CELLS Transl. Med.* **2012**, *1*, 866–873. [CrossRef]
51. Balyasnikova, I.V.; Prasol, M.S.; Ferguson, S.D.; Han, Y.; Ahmed, A.U.; Gutova, M.; Tobias, A.L.; Mustafi, D.; Rincón, E.; Zhang, L.; et al. Intranasal Delivery of Mesenchymal Stem Cells Significantly Extends Survival of Irradiated Mice with Experimental Brain Tumors. *Mol. Ther.* **2014**, *22*, 140–148. [CrossRef] [PubMed]
52. Danielyan, L.; Schäfer, R.; Von Ameln-Mayerhofer, A.; Bernhard, F.; Verleysdonk, S.; Buadze, M.; Lourhmati, A.; Klopfer, T.; Schaumann, F.; Schmid, B.; et al. Therapeutic Efficacy of Intranasally Delivered Mesenchymal Stem Cells in a Rat Model of Parkinson Disease. *Rejuvenation Res.* **2011**, *14*, 3–16. [CrossRef] [PubMed]
53. Van Velthoven, C.T.; Kavelaars, A.; Van Bel, F.; Heijnen, C.J. Nasal administration of stem cells: A promising novel route to treat neonatal ischemic brain damage. *Pediatr. Res.* **2010**, *68*, 419–422. [CrossRef] [PubMed]
54. Donega, V.; van Velthoven, C.T.J.; Nijboer, C.H.; van Bel, F.; Kas, M.J.H.; Kavelaars, A.; Heijnen, C.J. Intranasal Mesenchymal Stem Cell Treatment for Neonatal Brain Damage: Long-Term Cognitive and Sensorimotor Improvement. *PLoS ONE* **2013**, *8*, e51253. [CrossRef] [PubMed]
55. Wei, N.; Yu, S.P.; Gu, X.; Taylor, T.M.; Song, D.; Liu, X.-F.; Wei, L. Delayed Intranasal Delivery of Hypoxic-Preconditioned Bone Marrow Mesenchymal Stem Cells Enhanced Cell Homing and Therapeutic Benefits after Ischemic Stroke in Mice. *Cell Transplant.* **2013**, *22*, 977–991. [CrossRef] [PubMed]
56. Fransson, M.; Piras, E.; Burman, J.; Nilsson, B.; Essand, M.; Lu, B.; Harris, R.A.; Magnusson, P.U.; Brittebo, E.; I Loskog, A.S. CAR/FoxP3-engineered T regulatory cells target the CNS and suppress EAE upon intranasal delivery. *J. Neuroinflamm.* **2012**, *9*, 112. [CrossRef] [PubMed]
57. Ninomiya, K.; Iwatsuki, K.; Ohnishi, Y.-I.; Ohkawa, T.; Yoshimine, T. Intranasal delivery of bone marrow stromal cells to spinal cord lesions. *J. Neurosurg. Spine* **2015**, *23*, 111–119. [CrossRef]
58. Sakane, T.; Akizuki, M.; Yoshida, M.; Yamashita, S.; Nadai, T.; Hashida, M.; Sezaki, H. Transport of cephalexin to the cerebrospinal fluid directly from the nasal cavity. *J. Pharm. Pharmacol.* **1991**, *43*, 449–451. [CrossRef]
59. Jiang, F.; Lilge, L.; Logie, B.; Li, Y.; Chopp, M. Photodynamic Therapy of 9L Gliosarcoma with Liposome-Delivered Photofrin. *Photochem. Photobiol.* **1997**, *65*, 701–706. [CrossRef]
60. Warnken, Z.N.; Smyth, H.D.C.; Watts, A.B.; Weitman, S.; Kuhn, J.G.; Williams, R.O. Formulation and device design to increase nose to brain drug delivery. *J. Drug Deliv. Sci. Technol.* **2016**, *35*, 213–222. [CrossRef]
61. Illum, L. Is nose-to-brain transport of drugs in man a reality? *J. Pharm. Pharmacol.* **2004**, *56*, 3–17. [CrossRef] [PubMed]
62. Illum, L. Transport of drugs from the nasal cavity to the central nervous system. *Eur. J. Pharm. Sci.* **2000**, *11*, 1–18. [CrossRef]
63. Emirzeoglu, M.; Sahin, B.; Celebi, M.; Uzun, A.; Bilgic, S.; Tontus, H.O. Estimation of nasal cavity and conchae volumes by stereological method. *Folia Morphol.* **2012**, *71*, 105–108.
64. Dhuria, S.V.; Hanson, L.R.; Frey, W.H., 2nd. Intranasal delivery to the central nervous system: Mechanisms and experimental considerations. *J. Pharm. Sci.* **2010**, *99*, 1654–1673. [CrossRef] [PubMed]
65. Olmsted, S.S.; Padgett, J.L.; Yudin, A.I.; Whaley, K.J.; Moench, T.R.; Cone, R.A. Diffusion of Macromolecules and Virus-Like Particles in Human Cervical Mucus. *Biophys. J.* **2001**, *81*, 1930–1937. [CrossRef]

66. Lai, S.K.; O'Hanlon, D.E.; Harrold, S.; Man, S.T.; Wang, Y.-Y.; Cone, R.; Hanes, J. Rapid transport of large polymeric nanoparticles in fresh undiluted human mucus. *Proc. Natl. Acad. Sci. USA* **2007**, *104*, 1482–1487. [CrossRef] [PubMed]
67. Sigurdsson, H.H.; Kirch, J.; Lehr, C.-M. Mucus as a barrier to lipophilic drugs. *Int. J. Pharm.* **2013**, *453*, 56–64. [CrossRef] [PubMed]
68. Frey, A.; Giannasca, K.T.; Weltzin, R.; Giannasca, P.J.; Reggio, H.; Lencer, W.I.; Neutra, M.R. Role of the glycocalyx in regulating access of microparticles to apical plasma membranes of intestinal epithelial cells: Implications for microbial attachment and oral vaccine targeting. *J. Exp. Med.* **1996**, *184*, 1045–1059. [CrossRef]
69. Matsui, H.; Verghese, M.W.; Kesimer, M.; Schwab, U.E.; Randell, S.H.; Sheehan, J.K.; Grubb, B.R.; Boucher, R.C. Reduced Three-Dimensional Motility in Dehydrated Airway Mucus Prevents Neutrophil Capture and Killing Bacteria on Airway Epithelial Surfaces. *J. Immunol.* **2005**, *175*, 1090–1099. [CrossRef]
70. Pires, A.; Fortuna, A.; Alves, G.; Falcão, A. Intranasal Drug Delivery: How, Why and What for? *J. Pharm. Pharm. Sci.* **2009**, *12*, 288–311. [CrossRef]
71. Proetz, A.W. XLI Air Currents in the Upper Respiratory Tract and Their Clinical Importance. *Ann. Otol. Rhinol. Laryngol.* **1951**, *60*, 439–467. [CrossRef] [PubMed]
72. Baraniuk, J.N.; Merck, S.J. Nasal reflexes: Implications for exercise, breathing, and sex. *Curr. Allergy Asthma Rep.* **2008**, *8*, 147–153. [CrossRef]
73. Cole, P.; Haight, J.S.J.; Naito, K.; Kucharczyk, W. Magnetic Resonance Imaging of the Nasal Airways. *Am. J. Rhinol.* **1989**, *3*, 63–67. [CrossRef]
74. Graff, C.L.; Pollack, G.M. Functional Evidence for P-glycoprotein at the Nose-Brain Barrier. *Pharm. Res.* **2005**, *22*, 86–93. [CrossRef] [PubMed]
75. Gartziandia, O.; Herran, E.; Pedraz, J.L.; Carro, E.; Igartua, M.; Hernandez, R.M. Chitosan coated nanostructured lipid carriers for brain delivery of proteins by intranasal administration. *Colloids Surfaces B Biointerfaces* **2015**, *134*, 304–313. [CrossRef]
76. Gabal, Y.M.; Kamel, A.O.; Sammour, O.A.; Elshafeey, A.H. Effect of surface charge on the brain delivery of nanostructured lipid carriers in situ gels via the nasal route. *Int. J. Pharm.* **2014**, *473*, 442–457. [CrossRef]
77. Raj, P.M.; Raj, R.; Kaul, A.; Mishra, A.K.; Ram, A. Biodistribution and targeting potential assessment of mucoadhesive chitosan nanoparticles designed for ulcerative colitis via scintigraphy. *RSC Adv.* **2018**, *8*, 20809–20821. [CrossRef]
78. Bender, T.S.; Migliore, M.M.; Campbell, R.B.; John Gatley, S.J.; Waszczak, B.L. Intranasal administration of glial-derived neurotrophic factor (GDNF) rapidly and significantly increases whole-brain GDNF level in rats. *Neuroscience* **2015**, *303*, 569–576. [CrossRef]
79. Pang, Y.; Lin, S.; Wright, C.; Shen, J.; Carter, K.; Bhatt, A.; Fan, L.-W. Intranasal insulin protects against substantia nigra dopaminergic neuronal loss and alleviates motor deficits induced by 6-OHDA in rats. *Neuroscience* **2016**, *318*, 157–165. [CrossRef]
80. Lin, S.; Fan, L.-W.; Rhodes, P.G.; Cai, Z. Intranasal administration of IGF-1 attenuates hypoxic-ischemic brain injury in neonatal rats. *Exp. Neurol.* **2009**, *217*, 361–370. [CrossRef]
81. Wu, H.; Hu, K.; Jiang, X. From nose to brain: Understanding transport capacity and transport rate of drugs. *Expert Opin. Drug Deliv.* **2008**, *5*, 1159–1168. [CrossRef] [PubMed]
82. Hanson, L.R.; Fine, J.M.; Svitak, A.L.; Faltesek, K.A. Intranasal Administration of CNS Therapeutics to Awake Mice. *J. Vis. Exp.* **2013**, *8*, e4440. [CrossRef] [PubMed]
83. Shingaki, T.; Hidalgo, I.J.; Furubayashi, T.; Katsumi, H.; Sakane, T.; Yamamoto, A.; Yamashita, S. The transnasal delivery of 5-fluorouracil to the rat brain is enhanced by acetazolamide (the inhibitor of the secretion of cerebrospinal fluid). *Int. J. Pharm.* **2009**, *377*, 85–91. [CrossRef] [PubMed]
84. Stevens, J.; Ploeger, B.A.; Van Der Graaf, P.H.; Danhof, M.; de Lange, E.C. Systemic and Direct Nose-to-Brain Transport Pharmacokinetic Model for Remoxipride after Intravenous and Intranasal Administration. *Drug Metab. Dispos.* **2011**, *39*, 2275–2282. [CrossRef]
85. Westin, U.E.; Boström, E.; Gråsjö, J.; Hammarlund-Udenaes, M.; Björk, E. Direct Nose-to-Brain Transfer of Morphine After Nasal Administration to Rats. *Pharm. Res.* **2006**, *23*, 565–572. [CrossRef] [PubMed]
86. Dahlin, M.; Björk, E. Nasal absorption of (S)-UH-301 and its transport into the cerebrospinal fluid of rats. *Int. J. Pharm.* **2000**, *195*, 197–205. [CrossRef]
87. Sakane, T.; Akizuki, M.; Taki, Y.; Yamashita, S.; Sezaki, H.; Nadai, T. Direct Drug Transport from the Rat Nasal Cavity to the Cerebrospinal Fluid: The Relation to the Molecular Weight of Drugs. *J. Pharm. Pharmacol.* **1995**, *47*, 379–381. [CrossRef]
88. Illum, L. Nasal drug delivery—Recent developments and future prospects. *J. Control. Release* **2012**, *161*, 254–263. [CrossRef]
89. Horvát, S.; Fehér, A.; Wolburg, H.; Sipos, P.; Veszelka, S.; Tóth, A.; Kis, L.; Kurunczi, A.; Balogh, G.; Kürti, L.; et al. Sodium hyaluronate as a mucoadhesive component in nasal formulation enhances delivery of molecules to brain tissue. *Eur. J. Pharm. Biopharm.* **2009**, *72*, 252–259. [CrossRef]
90. Rassu, G.; Soddu, E.; Cossu, M.; Brundu, A.; Cerri, G.; Marchetti, N.; Ferraro, L.; Regan, R.F.; Giunchedi, P.; Gavini, E.; et al. Solid microparticles based on chitosan or methyl-β-cyclodextrin: A first formulative approach to increase the nose-to-brain transport of deferoxamine mesylate. *J. Control. Release* **2015**, *201*, 68–77. [CrossRef]
91. Graff, C.L.; Pollack, G.M. P-Glycoprotein Attenuates Brain Uptake of Substrates After Nasal Instillation. *Pharm. Res.* **2003**, *20*, 1225–1230. [CrossRef] [PubMed]
92. Graff, C.L.; Zhao, R.; Pollack, G.M. Pharmacokinetics of Substrate Uptake and Distribution in Murine Brain After Nasal Instillation. *Pharm. Res.* **2005**, *22*, 235–244. [CrossRef] [PubMed]

93. Hada, N.; Netzer, W.J.; Belhassan, F.; Wennogle, L.P.; Gizurarson, S. Nose-to-brain transport of imatinib mesylate: A pharmacokinetic evaluation. *Eur. J. Pharm. Sci.* **2017**, *102*, 46–54. [CrossRef] [PubMed]
94. Dimova, S.; Brewster, M.E.; Noppe, M.; Jorissen, M.; Augustijns, P. The use of human nasal in vitro cell systems during drug discovery and development. *Toxicol. Vitr.* **2005**, *19*, 107–122. [CrossRef]
95. Dhamankar, V.; Donovan, M.D. Modulating nasal mucosal permeation using metabolic saturation and enzyme inhibition techniques. *J. Pharm. Pharmacol.* **2017**, *69*, 1075–1083. [CrossRef]
96. Shingaki, T.; Inoue, D.; Furubayashi, T.; Sakane, T.; Katsumi, H.; Yamamoto, A.; Yamashita, S. Transnasal Delivery of Methotrexate to Brain Tumors in Rats: A New Strategy for Brain Tumor Chemotherapy. *Mol. Pharm.* **2010**, *7*, 1561–1568. [CrossRef]
97. Martins, P.P.; Smyth, H.D.C.; Cui, Z. Strategies to facilitate or block nose-to-brain drug delivery. *Int. J. Pharm.* **2019**, *570*, 118635. [CrossRef]
98. Patil, K.; Yeole, P.; Gaikwad, R.; Khan, S. Brain targeting studies on buspirone hydrochloride after intranasal administration of mucoadhesive formulation in rats. *J. Pharm. Pharmacol.* **2009**, *61*, 669–675. [CrossRef]
99. Bari, N.K.; Fazil, M.; Hassan, M.Q.; Haider, M.R.; Gaba, B.; Narang, J.K.; Baboota, S.; Ali, J. Brain delivery of buspirone hydrochloride chitosan nanoparticles for the treatment of general anxiety disorder. *Int. J. Biol. Macromol.* **2015**, *81*, 49–59. [CrossRef]
100. Rizzo, J.A.; Medeiros, D.; Silva, A.R.; Sarinho, E. Benzalkonium chloride and nasal mucociliary clearance: A randomized, placebo-controlled, crossover, double-blind trial. *Am. J. Rhinol.* **2006**, *20*, 243–247. [CrossRef]
101. Dalvi, A.; Ravi, P.R.; Uppuluri, C.T. Rufinamide-Loaded Chitosan Nanoparticles in Xyloglucan-Based Thermoresponsive In Situ Gel for Direct Nose to Brain Delivery. *Front. Pharmacol.* **2021**, *12*, 1274. [CrossRef] [PubMed]
102. Abouhussein, D.M.; Khattab, A.; Bayoumi, N.A.; Mahmoud, A.F.; Sakr, T.M. Brain targeted ri-vastigmine mucoadhesive thermosensitive In situ gel: Optimization, in vitro evaluation, radiolabeling, in vivo pharmacokinetics and biodistribution. *J. Drug Deliv. Sci. Technol.* **2018**, *43*, 129–140. [CrossRef]
103. Ravi, P.R.; Aditya, N.; Patil, S.; Cherian, L. Nasalin-situgels for delivery of rasagiline mesylate: Improvement in bioavailability and brain localization. *Drug Deliv.* **2015**, *22*, 903–910. [CrossRef] [PubMed]
104. Clevenger, S.S.; Malhotra, D.; Dang, J.; Vanle, B.; Ishak, W.W. The role of selective serotonin reuptake inhibitors in preventing relapse of major depressive disorder. *Ther. Adv. Psychopharmacol.* **2018**, *8*, 49–58. [CrossRef]
105. Thakkar, H.; Vaghela, D.; Patel, B.P. Brain targeted intranasal in-situ gelling spray of paroxetine: Formulation, characterization and in-vivo evaluation. *J. Drug Deliv. Sci. Technol.* **2021**, *62*, 102317. [CrossRef]
106. Bhandwalkar, M.J.; Avachat, A.M. Thermoreversible Nasal In situ Gel of Venlafaxine Hydrochloride: Formulation, Characterization, and Pharmacodynamic Evaluation. *AAPS PharmSciTech* **2013**, *14*, 101–110. [CrossRef]
107. Xie, H.; Li, L.; Sun, Y.; Wang, Y.; Gao, S.; Tian, Y.; Ma, X.; Guo, C.; Bo, F.; Zhang, L. An Available Strategy for Nasal Brain Transport of Nanocomposite Based on PAMAM Dendrimers via In Situ Gel. *Nanomaterials* **2019**, *9*, 147. [CrossRef]
108. Reger, M.A.; Watson, G.S.; Green, P.S.; Wilkinson, C.W.; Baker, L.D.; Cholerton, B.; Fishel, M.A.; Plymate, S.R.; Breitner, J.; DeGroodt, W.; et al. Intranasal insulin improves cognition and modulates β-amyloid in early AD. *Neurology* **2008**, *70*, 440–448. [CrossRef]
109. Craft, S.; Baker, L.D.; Montine, T.J.; Minoshima, S.; Watson, G.S.; Claxton, A.; Arbucklet, M.; Callaghan, M.; Tsai, E.; Plymate, S.R.; et al. Intranasal Insulin Therapy for Alzheimer Disease and Amnestic Mild Cognitive Impairment: A Pilot Clinical Trial. *Arch. Neurol.* **2012**, *69*, 29–38. [CrossRef]
110. Djupesland, P.G. Nasal drug delivery devices: Characteristics and performance in a clinical perspective—A review. *Drug Deliv. Transl. Res.* **2013**, *3*, 42–62. [CrossRef]
111. Hoekman, J.D.; Ho, R.J.Y. Enhanced Analgesic Responses after Preferential Delivery of Morphine and Fentanyl to the Olfactory Epithelium in Rats. *Anesthesia Analg.* **2011**, *113*, 641–651. [CrossRef] [PubMed]
112. Xi, J.; Zhang, Z.; Si, X.A. Improving intranasal delivery of neurological nanomedicine to the olfactory region using magnetophoretic guidance of microsphere carriers. *Int. J. Nanomed.* **2015**, *10*, 1211–1222. [CrossRef]
113. Chen, H.; Yang, G.Z.X.; Getachew, H.; Acosta, C.; Sierra Sánchez, C.S.; Konofagou, E.E. Focused ultrasound-enhanced intranasal brain delivery of brain-derived neurotrophic factor. *Sci. Rep.* **2016**, *6*, 28599. [CrossRef]
114. Godfrey, L.; Iannitelli, A.; Garrett, N.L.; Moger, J.; Imbert, I.; King, T.; Porreca, F.; Soundararajan, R.; Lalatsa, A.; Schätzlein, A.G.; et al. Nanoparticulate peptide delivery exclusively to the brain produces tolerance free analgesia. *J. Control. Release* **2018**, *270*, 135–144. [CrossRef] [PubMed]
115. Shah, B.; Khunt, D.; Misra, M.; Padh, H. Formulation and In-vivo Pharmacokinetic Consideration of Intranasal Microemulsion and Mucoadhesive Microemulsion of Rivastigmine for Brain Targeting. *Pharm. Res.* **2018**, *35*, 8. [CrossRef] [PubMed]
116. Shah, B.; Khunt, D.; Misra, M.; Padh, H. Non-invasive intranasal delivery of quetiapine fumarate loaded microemulsion for brain targeting: Formulation, physicochemical and pharmacokinetic consideration. *Eur. J. Pharm. Sci.* **2016**, *91*, 196–207. [CrossRef]
117. Raj, R.; Wairkar, S.; Sridhar, V.; Gaud, R. Pramipexole dihydrochloride loaded chitosan nanoparticles for nose to brain delivery: Development, characterization and in vivo anti-Parkinson activity. *Int. J. Biol. Macromol.* **2018**, *109*, 27–35. [CrossRef]
118. Sanchez-Ramos, J.; Song, S.; Kong, X.; Foroutan, P.; Martinez, G.; Dominguez-Viqueria, W.; Mohapatra, S.; Mohapatra, S.; Haraszti, R.A.; Khvorova, A.; et al. Chitosan-Mangafodipir nanoparticles designed for intranasal delivery of siRNA and DNA to brain. *J. Drug Deliv. Sci. Technol.* **2018**, *43*, 453–460. [CrossRef]

119. Carlos, M.I.S.; Zheng, K.; Garrett, N.; Arifin, N.; Workman, D.G.; Kubajewska, I.; Halwani, A.A.; Moger, J.; Zhang, Q.; Schätzlein, A.G.; et al. Limiting the level of tertiary amines on polyamines leads to biocompatible nucleic acid vectors. *Int. J. Pharm.* **2017**, *526*, 106–124. [CrossRef]
120. Seju, U.; Kumar, A.; Sawant, K.K. Development and evaluation of olanzapine-loaded PLGA nanoparticles for nose-to-brain delivery: In vitro and in vivo studies. *Acta Biomater.* **2011**, *7*, 4169–4176. [CrossRef]
121. Musumeci, T.; Serapide, M.F.; Pellitteri, R.; Dalpiaz, A.; Ferraro, L.; Dal Magro, R.; Bonaccorso, A.; Carbone, C.; Veiga, F.; Sancini, G.; et al. Oxcarbazepine free or loaded PLGA nanoparticles as effective intranasal approach to control epileptic seizures in rodents. *Eur. J. Pharm. Biopharm.* **2018**, *133*, 309–320. [CrossRef] [PubMed]
122. Bonaccorso, A.; Musumeci, T.; Serapide, M.F.; Pellitteri, R.; Uchegbu, I.F.; Puglisi, G. Nose to brain delivery in rats: Effect of surface charge of rhodamine B labeled nanocarriers on brain subregion localization. *Colloids B Biointerfaces* **2017**, *154*, 297–306. [CrossRef] [PubMed]
123. Zhang, C.; Chen, J.; Feng, C.; Shao, X.; Liu, Q.; Zhang, Q.; Pang, Z.; Jiang, X. Intranasal nanoparticles of basic fibroblast growth factor for brain delivery to treat Alzheimer's disease. *Int. J. Pharm.* **2014**, *461*, 192–202. [CrossRef] [PubMed]
124. Meng, Q.; Wang, A.; Hua, H.; Jiang, Y.; Wang, Y.; Mu, H.; Wu, Z.; Sun, K. Intranasal delivery of Huperzine A to the brain using lactoferrin-conjugated N-trimethylated chitosan surface-modified PLGA nanoparticles for treatment of Alzheimer's disease. *Int. J. Nanomed.* **2018**, *13*, 705–718. [CrossRef] [PubMed]
125. Tan, M.S.A.; Parekh, H.S.; Pandey, P.; Siskind, D.J.; Falconer, J.R. Nose-to-brain delivery of antipsychotics using nanotechnology: A review. *Expert Opin. Drug Deliv.* **2020**, *17*, 839–853. [CrossRef]
126. Borst, P.; Zelcer, N.; van Helvoort, A. ABC transporters in lipid transport. *Biochim. Biophys. Acta (BBA)-Mol. Cell Biol. Lipids* **2000**, *1486*, 128–144. [CrossRef]
127. Jogani, V.V.; Shah, P.J.; Mishra, P.; Mishra, A.K.; Misra, A.R. Intranasal Mucoadhesive Microemulsion of Tacrine to Improve Brain Targeting. *Alzheimer's Dis. Assoc. Disord.* **2008**, *22*, 116–124. [CrossRef]
128. Patel, S.; Chavhan, S.; Soni, H.; Babbar, A.K.; Mathur, R.; Mishra, A.K.; Sawant, K. Brain targeting of risperidone-loaded solid lipid nanoparticles by intranasal route. *J. Drug Target.* **2010**, *19*, 468–474. [CrossRef]
129. Müller, R.H.; Mäder, K.; Gohla, S. Solid lipid nanoparticles (SLN) for controlled drug delivery: A review of the state of the art. *Eur. J. Pharm. Biopharm.* **2000**, *50*, 161–177. [CrossRef]
130. Zara, G.P.; Cavalli, R.; Bargoni, A.; Fundarò, A.; Vighetto, D.; Gasco, M.R. Intravenous Administration to Rabbits of Non-stealth and Stealth Doxorubicin-loaded Solid Lipid Nanoparticles at Increasing Concentrations of Stealth Agent: Pharmacokinetics and Distribution of Doxorubicin in Brain and Other Tissues. *J. Drug Target.* **2002**, *10*, 327–335. [CrossRef]
131. Dalpiaz, A.; Gavini, E.; Colombo, G.; Russo, P.; Bortolotti, F.; Ferraro, L.; Tanganelli, S.; Scatturin, A.; Menegatti, E.; Giunchedi, P. Brain uptake of an anti-ischemic agent by nasal administration of microparticles. *J. Pharm. Sci.* **2008**, *97*, 4889–4903. [CrossRef] [PubMed]
132. Casettari, L.; Illum, L. Chitosan in nasal delivery systems for therapeutic drugs. *J. Control. Release* **2014**, *190*, 189–200. [CrossRef] [PubMed]
133. Wolak, D.J.; Pizzo, M.E.; Thorne, R.G. Probing the extracellular diffusion of antibodies in brain using in vivo integrative optical imaging and ex vivo fluorescence imaging. *J. Control. Release* **2014**, *197*, 78–86. [CrossRef] [PubMed]
134. Appu, A.P.; Arun, P.; Krishnan, J.K.S.; Moffett, J.R.; Namboodiri, A.M.A. Rapid intranasal delivery of chloramphenicol acetyl-transferase in the active form to different brain regions as a model for enzyme therapy in the CNS. *J. Neurosci. Methods* **2016**, *259*, 129–134. [CrossRef]
135. Krishnan, J.K.S.; Arun, P.; Appu, A.P.; Vijayakumar, N.; Figueiredo, T.H.; Braga, M.F.; Baskota, S.; Olsen, C.H.; Farkas, N.; Dagata, J.; et al. Intranasal delivery of obidoxime to the brain prevents mortality and CNS damage from organophosphate poisoning. *NeuroToxicology* **2016**, *53*, 64–73. [CrossRef]
136. Djupesland, P.G.; Skretting, A. Nasal Deposition and Clearance in Man: Comparison of a Bidirectional Powder Device and a Traditional Liquid Spray Pump. *J. Aerosol. Med. Pulm. Drug Deliv.* **2012**, *25*, 280–289. [CrossRef]
137. Salvador-Morales, C.; Zhang, L.; Langer, R.; Farokhzad, O.C. Immunocompatibility properties of lipid–polymer hybrid nanoparticles with heterogeneous surface functional groups. *Biomaterials* **2009**, *30*, 2231–2240. [CrossRef]
138. Fröhlich, E. The role of surface charge in cellular uptake and cytotoxicity of medical nanoparticles. *Int. J. Nanomed.* **2012**, *7*, 5577–5591. [CrossRef]
139. Li, H.; Chen, Y.; Deng, Y.; Wang, Y.; Ke, X.; Ci, T. Effects of surface charge of low molecular weight heparin-modified cationic liposomes on drug efficacy and toxicity. *Drug Dev. Ind. Pharm.* **2017**, *43*, 1163–1172. [CrossRef]
140. Clogston, J.D.; Patri, A.K. Zeta potential measurement. *Methods Mol. Biol.* **2011**, *697*, 63–70. [CrossRef]
141. Hathout, R.M.; Abdelhamid, S.G.; El-Housseiny, G.S.; Metwally, A.A. Comparing cefotaxime and ceftriaxone in combating meningitis through nose-to-brain delivery using bio/chemoinformatics tools. *Sci. Rep.* **2020**, *10*, 21250. [CrossRef] [PubMed]
142. Van Woensel, M.; Mathivet, T.; Wauthoz, N.; Rosière, R.; Garg, A.D.; Agostinis, P.; Mathieu, V.; Kiss, R.; Lefranc, F.; Boon, L.; et al. Sensitization of glioblastoma tumor micro-environment to chemo- and immunotherapy by Galectin-1 intranasal knock-down strategy. *Sci. Rep.* **2017**, *7*, 1217. [CrossRef] [PubMed]
143. Trotta, V.; Pavan, B.; Ferraro, L.; Beggiato, S.; Traini, D.; dos Reis, L.G.; Scalia, S.; Dalpiaz, A. Brain targeting of resveratrol by nasal administration of chitosan-coated lipid microparticles. *Eur. J. Pharm. Biopharm.* **2018**, *127*, 250–259. [CrossRef] [PubMed]

144. Siew, A.; Le, H.; Thiovolet, M.; Gellert, P.; Schatzlein, A.; Uchegbu, I. Enhanced Oral Absorption of Hydrophobic and Hydrophilic Drugs Using Quaternary Ammonium Palmitoyl Glycol Chitosan Nanoparticles. *Mol. Pharm.* **2012**, *9*, 14–28. [CrossRef] [PubMed]
145. Gao, X.; Tao, W.; Lu, W.; Zhang, Q.; Zhang, Y.; Jiang, X.; Fu, S. Lectin-conjugated PEG–PLA nanoparticles: Preparation and brain delivery after intranasal administration. *Biomaterials* **2006**, *27*, 3482–3490. [CrossRef] [PubMed]
146. Frey, W.H., II. Method of Administering Neurologic Agents to the Brain. U.S. Patent 5,624,898, 8 January 1997.
147. Singh, R.; Brumlik, C.; Vaidya, M.; Choudhury, A. A Patent Review on Nanotechnology-Based Nose-to-Brain Drug Delivery. *Recent Patents Nanotechnol.* **2020**, *14*, 174–192. [CrossRef] [PubMed]
148. Kosfeld, M.; Heinrichs, M.L.; Zak, P.J.; Fischbacher, U.; Fehr, E. Oxytocin increases trust in humans. *Nature* **2005**, *435*, 673–676. [CrossRef]
149. De Dreu, C.K.W.; Greer, L.L.; Handgraaf, M.J.J.; Shalvi, S.; Van Kleef, G.A.; Baas, M.; Ten Velden, F.S.; Van Dijk, E.; Feith, S.W. The Neuropeptide Oxytocin Regulates Parochial Altruism in Intergroup Conflict among Humans. *Science* **2010**, *328*, 1408–1411. [CrossRef]
150. Guastella, A.J.; Einfeld, S.L.; Gray, K.M.; Rinehart, N.J.; Tonge, B.J.; Lambert, T.J.; Hickie, I.B. Intranasal Oxytocin Improves Emotion Recognition for Youth with Autism Spectrum Disorders. *Biol. Psychiatry* **2010**, *67*, 692–694. [CrossRef]
151. Watanabe, T.; Abe, O.; Kuwabara, H.; Yahata, N.; Takano, Y.; Iwashiro, N.; Natsubori, T.; Aoki, Y.; Takao, H.; Kawakubo, Y.; et al. Mitigation of Sociocommunicational Deficits of Autism Through Oxytocin-Induced Recovery of Medial Prefrontal Activity: A randomized trial. *JAMA Psychiatry* **2014**, *71*, 166–175. [CrossRef]
152. Cai, Q.; Feng, L.; Yap, K.Z. Systematic review and meta-analysis of reported adverse events of long-term intranasal oxytocin treatment for autism spectrum disorder. *Psychiatry Clin. Neurosci.* **2018**, *72*, 140–151. [CrossRef] [PubMed]
153. Yamasue, H.; Okada, T.; Munesue, T.; Kuroda, M.; Fujioka, T.; Uno, Y.; Matsumoto, K.; Kuwabara, H.; Mori, D.; Okamoto, Y.; et al. Effect of intranasal oxytocin on the core social symptoms of autism spectrum disorder: A randomized clinical trial. *Mol. Psychiatry* **2020**, *25*, 1849–1858. [CrossRef] [PubMed]
154. Schulingkamp, R.J.; Pagano, T.C.; Hung, D.; Raffa, R.B. Insulin receptors and insulin action in the brain: Review and clinical implications. *Neurosci. Biobehav. Rev.* **2000**, *24*, 855–872. [CrossRef]
155. Rhea, E.M.; Rask-Madsen, C.; Banks, W.A. Insulin transport across the blood-brain barrier can occur independently of the insulin receptor. *J. Physiol.* **2018**, *596*, 4753–4765. [CrossRef] [PubMed]
156. Craft, S.; Raman, R.; Chow, T.W.; Rafii, M.S.; Sun, C.-K.; Rissman, R.A.; Donohue, M.C.; Brewer, J.B.; Jenkins, C.; Harless, K.; et al. Safety, Efficacy, and Feasibility of Intranasal Insulin for the Treatment of Mild Cognitive Impairment and Alzheimer Disease Dementia: A randomized clinical trial. *JAMA Neurol.* **2020**, *77*, 1099–1109. [CrossRef] [PubMed]
157. Kellar, D.; Lockhart, S.N.; Aisen, P.; Raman, R.; Rissman, R.A.; Brewer, J.; Craft, S. Intranasal Insulin Reduces White Matter Hyperintensity Progression in Association with Improvements in Cognition and CSF Biomarker Profiles in Mild Cognitive Impairment and Alzheimer's Disease. *J. Prev. Alzheimer's Dis.* **2021**, *8*, 1–9. [CrossRef]
158. Akel, H.; Csóka, I.; Ambrus, R.; Bocsik, A.; Gróf, I.; Mészáros, M.; Szecskó, A.; Kozma, G.; Veszelka, S.; Deli, M.A.; et al. In Vitro Comparative Study of Solid Lipid and PLGA Nanoparticles Designed to Facilitate Nose-to-Brain Delivery of Insulin. *Int. J. Mol. Sci.* **2021**, *22*, 13258. [CrossRef]

pharmaceutics

Review

Delivery of Oligonucleotides: Efficiency with Lipid Conjugation and Clinical Outcome

Phuc Tran [1], Tsigereda Weldemichael [1], Zhichao Liu [2] and Hong-yu Li [1,*]

1 Department of Pharmaceutical Sciences, College of Pharmacy, University of Arkansas for Medical Sciences, Little Rock, AR 72205, USA; PDTran@uams.edu (P.T.); TGWeldemichael@uams.edu (T.W.)
2 Division of Bioinformatics and Biostatistics, National Center for Toxicological Research, US Food and Drug Administration, Jefferson, AR 72079, USA; zhichao.liu@fda.hhs.gov
* Correspondence: HLi2@uams.edu

Abstract: Oligonucleotides have shifted drug discovery into a new paradigm due to their ability to silence the genes and inhibit protein translation. Importantly, they can drug the un-druggable targets from the conventional small-molecule perspective. Unfortunately, poor cellular permeability and susceptibility to nuclease degradation remain as major hurdles for the development of oligonucleotide therapeutic agents. Studies of safe and effective delivery technique with lipid bioconjugates gains attention to resolve these issues. Our review article summarizes the physicochemical effect of well-studied hydrophobic moieties to enhance the cellular entry of oligonucleotides. The structural impacts of fatty acids, cholesterol, tocopherol, and squalene on cellular internalization and membrane penetration in vitro and in vivo were discussed first. The crucial assays for delivery evaluation within this section were analyzed sequentially. Next, we provided a few successful examples of lipid-conjugated oligonucleotides advanced into clinical studies for treating patients with different medical backgrounds. Finally, we pinpointed current limitations and outlooks in this research field along with opportunities to explore new modifications and efficacy studies.

Keywords: oligonucleotide; lipid conjugates; LNP; delivery; cholesterol; fatty acid; tocopherol; squalene

Citation: Tran, P.; Weldemichael, T.; Liu, Z.; Li, H.-y. Delivery of Oligonucleotides: Efficiency with Lipid Conjugation and Clinical Outcome. *Pharmaceutics* **2022**, *14*, 342. https://doi.org/10.3390/pharmaceutics14020342

Academic Editor: David Brayden

Received: 29 December 2021
Accepted: 27 January 2022
Published: 1 February 2022

1. Introduction

1.1. Background of Oligonucleotide

Oligonucleotide (ON) is a short strand of nucleic acid polymers mostly comprising of thirteen to twenty-five nucleotides, which can hybridize to targeted DNA or RNA. They are categorized into classes including antisense oligonucleotides (ASOs), small interfering RNA (siRNA), microRNA (miRNAs), and aptamer. Watson–Crick base pairing is quintessential for ON mechanisms to act on targeted mRNA, which leads to the following consequences: (1) RNase H activity degradation, (2) inhibiting the formation of matured mRNA, and (3) conjuring steric blockage from ribosome interaction [1]. Therefore, ONs are preferable therapeutic strategies to prevent and treat various disorders via selective inhibition of deleterious gene expression. It is indeed shifting the era of drug discoveries into an exciting new field—oligonucleotide therapy. Comparatively, the ease of manufacturing, base-pairing specificity/sensitivity potential, and its long duration of action give higher preference than the conventional therapy. Longer duration of action which varies from weeks to months of post-administration outweighs the technical hitches of being only in an injectable formulation. Given the knowledge of genes and their role accessibility, incurable genetic disorders are made possible through this novel approach. Its application is not merely limited to drug discovery but also pertinent for investigations of the mechanism and stereochemistry of biochemical reactions, mapping of nucleic acid-protein interactions, and diagnostic applications [2]. ON therapy is well aligned to play a noteworthy role in speeding up drug discovery against traditionally undruggable targets. Figure 1 displays some pros and cons of oligonucleotide-based drugs versus conventional small molecules. Hence, ON has gained its deserved attention in research in a wide range of disease indications from oncology to anti-viral therapy. However, the biggest concern for ON is cellular membrane penetration. This hurdle is the result of ON's highly hydrophilic nucleoside combing of anionic phosphate backbone. Thus, passive transport is not an effective option, and conquering this issue is not a straightforward task.

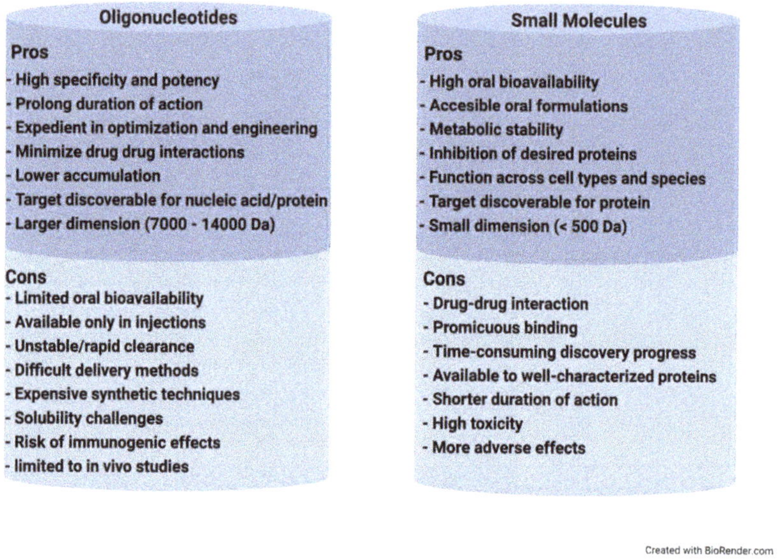

Figure 1. Pros and cons comparison of oligonucleotide versus small molecule drugs. Some highlighted advantages of oligonucleotide would be inhibitory specificity, expedient manufacture, and low in drug–drug interaction. Disadvantages of cost, stability, and formulation remained.

The assistance with external delivery systems such as liposomes, nanoparticles, or micelles were proposed and experimented thoroughly; however, toxicity was frequently reported due to the immunogenicity caused by polycationic material [3,4]. Alternatively, chemical conjugation to neutral lipid/hydrophobic moiety can overcome this backlash. Hypothetically, these naturally occurring biomolecules that are familiarized with the human system can reduce the risk of toxicity while enhancing cellular penetration and systemic stability. Different forms of lipid structures were incorporated and evaluated in vivo for improvement in pharmacokinetic and pharmacodynamic properties. In this review article, we will summarize the studies of characterizing hydrophobic moiety in the relationship of improving delivery efficacy. Additional discussion about potential therapeutic application and future outcomes of lipid-conjugated oligonucleotides will be highlighted.

1.2. Oligonucleotide-Based Drug Mechanism of Action

A comprehensive review composed by Crooke et al. has highlighted the fundamental aspects of ON mechanism of action. We would like to briefly summarize his work by discussing in two distinctive groups. Occupancy-only mechanism and occupancy-mediated degradation as illustrated in Figure 2.

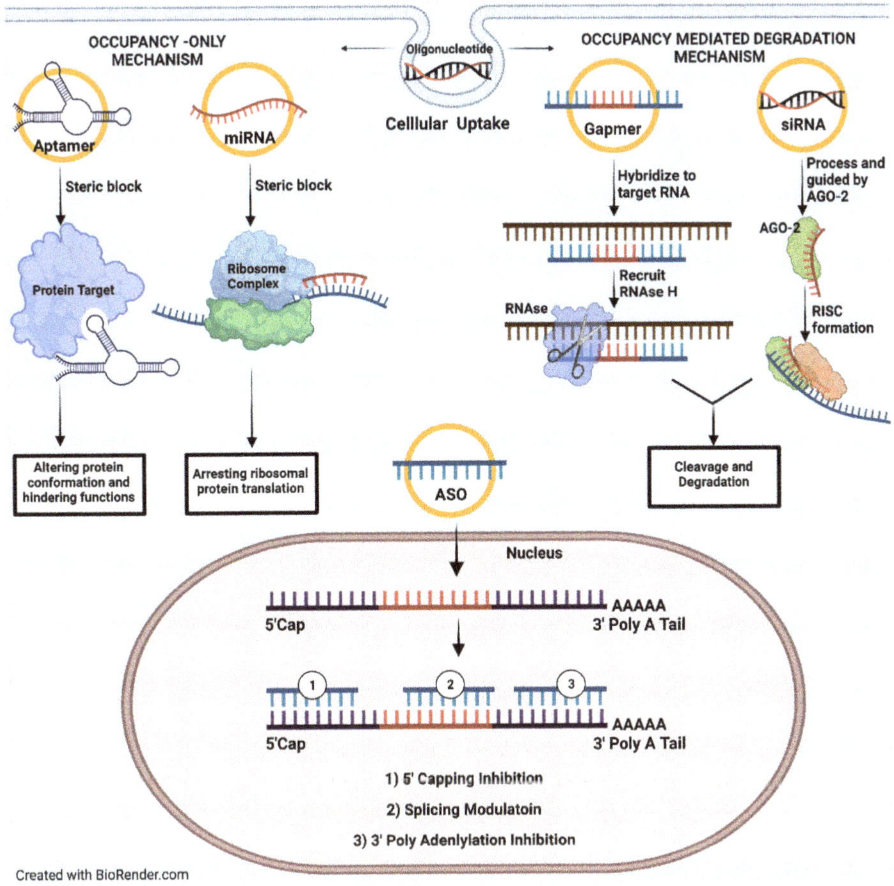

Figure 2. An illustration of main oligonucleotide mechanism of action as divided into two main groups: (1) Occupancy-only and (2) occupancy-mediated degradation. In occupancy only, oligonucleotide would act as steric blocker or inhibitor preventing any upcoming interaction with precedent targets. Meanwhile, occupancy-mediate degradation activates cleavage the targeted RNA via RNase or AGO-2.

In the occupancy-only approach or direct inhibition mechanism, ON will bind specifically to mRNA molecules via Watson–Crick base-pairing, which induces steric block from any followed-up interaction with proteins, nucleic acids, or transcription factors. In consequence, it can conjure either downregulation (translational arrest or cap inhibition) or upregulation (splicing modulation or RNA activation) processes. The most utilized, well studied, and therapeutically beneficial approach would be splicing inhibition. Once targeted mRNA hybridized with ON, a complex of small nuclear ribonucleoprotein (snRNP) would be sterically blocked from intron binding, thus halting the maturation of mRNA [2]. Splicing inhibition was successfully applied for Duchenne muscular dystrophy treatment, for which eteplirsen was approved by the FDA. Another plausible mechanism would be the disruption of RNA structural integrity following by ON hybridization. As result, abnormality in three-dimensional conformation interrupted its stability and halted sequential protein expression. Vickers et al. on disruption of HIV's TAR element would be a prime example. This research group implemented an ON to destabilize TAR's (trans-activating response sequence) stem loops, which followed by tarnishing HIV replication efficacy [5].

On the other hand, occupancy-mediated degradation was often emphasized with two major mechanisms: RNase or AGO-2 mediated degradation. Both mechanisms can result in deteriorating targeted mRNA but with slight differences in recruitment algorithms. For RNase, it is universally well documented as an enzyme responsible for degrading a single RNA strand, or RNA:DNA hybrid [6]. It has two isoforms (H1 and H2) which are identified in mammalian cells with expression in the cytoplasm and especially in the nucleus. RNase H1 participates more enthusiastically in cleavage than H2, though H2 is more abundant [7]. Recruitment of RNase is accompanied by a gapmer or even a short tetramer ON. Additionally, binding with an RNA metabolic protein such as P32 can enhance cleavage specificity which provided a good glimpse for optimizing chimera to accelerate RNase H1 activity. AGO-2 protein is one of the four argonaute family members, which facilitates endonuclease cleavage at the targeted RNAs and contains three domains. Mid and PIWI domains confer catalytic actions and perform simultaneously with Paz domain, which is responsible for small RNA binding. Being an indispensable component of the RISC, it operates with highly complementary at the translational or posttranscriptional level. Thus, it exerts RNA-based silencing mechanisms by altering protein synthesis and affecting RNA stability. Precise complementarity between guide RNA and the target is essential for the efficient cleavage of targets. Studies show that mismatches at the 5′ regions are less tolerated than the 3′region of guide RNA or cleavage site [8,9].

1.3. Biological Barriers That Challenged Druggability/Pharmacokinetic Profile of Oligonucleotide In Vivo

Dated back in 1998, oligonucleotide was an ultimate breakthrough in the discovery of a new drug modality. Significantly, Fomivirsen [10], a cytomegalovirus (CMV) retinitis ON-based treatment for AIDS immunocompromised patients, was recognized and approved by the FDA. Thus, marked the beginning of its massive emergence in the drug industry. Accounting in 2021, additional ON-based therapies were introduced into the market for non-cancerous indications as shown in Table 1; while there are still numerous entries examined in clinical trials for oncogenic targets [11]. Before approaching this height, the first unmodified ON was deemed expendable due to its high clearance rate after in vivo delivery. Agrawal et al. conducted the first report on the ON pharmacokinetic profile that showed unfavorable properties of unmodified ON after intravenous injection to a monkey with a dose of 30 mg/kg [12]. Quantification of polyacrylamide gel (PAGE) determined short systemic retention of approximately 15 min with a half-life of only 5 min. Structurally, the unmodified ON was identical with the endogenous mRNA in nature. Its highly polyanionic and hydrophilic characters still hampered the ability to penetrate the phospholipid membrane with the addition of high renal clearance.

From numerous pharmacokinetic data and mechanistic studies, scientists such as Juliano et al. [13] outlined four possible biological barriers that instigate unfavorable conditions for the efficacy of ON therapies as illustrated in Figure 3. We begin the discussion with the first barrier known as nuclease, especially 3′-exonuclease. It is an enzyme that is widely expressed in plasma and induces hydrolyzing reaction by cleaving phosphodiester bond at either at 3′ or 5′ ends. It can directly target ON indiscriminately and catalyze degradation reaction, which leads to complete loss of the therapeutic effect of ON before reaching the targeted site. The second barrier would be the reticuloendothelial system (RES) or mononuclear phagocyte system (MPS). It can easily be defined as a homogenous collection of phagocytotic cells that act as cellular securities to process and clear any form of alienated particles such as toxins, bacteria, or any xenobiotic. Therapeutic ONs are no exception as macrophages engulf ON, which endangers its survivability. Once these phagocytotic cells fused with the lysosome, therapeutic ON are considered dead. Consequently, long-term degradation of ON can lead to detrimental effects such as renal tube degradation, splenomegaly, and elevation of liver transaminase [14]. The third barrier is the thickness of endothelial tissue. The lining of endothelium must be sturdy to enclose safe blood flow; however, in the case of therapeutic ON (which is only administered via injection), the wall of the endothelium can prevent leakage of ON macromolecules. Thus, most therapeutic ON still lingers within circulation while an infinitesimal amount can escape from vascular lumen to interstitial fluid. The final barrier would be the cellular uptake mechanism in which scientists continued to manipulate for ON delivery. They studied the key concept of internalization mechanisms such as clathrin-based coated, caveolar, clathrin-independent carriers (CLIC), or micropinocytosis. As crucial as understanding the uptake mechanism, we beg a question: "How come the cellular uptake can be posed a challenge?" The answer lies in the late endosomal stage after ON is encapsulated in the cytoplasm. Late endosomes are usually fused with the lysosome to break down debris or recycle necessary material; hence, therapeutic ONs are victims of degradation and required to escape for maintaining a longer lifespan [15].

Table 1. List of FDA approved oligonucleotide drugs.

Name	Type	Modification	Mechanism	Indication/*Target*	FDA Approval
Fomivirsen	ASO	21 nt PS DNA	RNase H1	Cytomegalovirus retinitis/*CMV UL123*	Aug 1998
Pegaptanib	Aptamer	27 nt 2′-F/2′-OME PEGylated	Blocking binding	Neovascular age-related macular degeneration/*VEGF-165*	Dec 2004
Mipomersen	ASO Gapmer	20 nt PS 2′-MOE	RNase H1	Homozygous familial Hypercholesterolemia/*APOB*	Jan 2013
Defibrotide	ssDNA and dsDNA	Mixture of PO	Non single sequence dependent based mechanism	hepatic veno-occlusive disease	Mar 2016
Nusinersen	Steric block ASO	18 nt PS 2′-MOE	Splicing, intron 7	Spinal muscular atrophy/*SMN2 exon 7*	Dec 2016
Eteplirsen	Steric block ASO	30 nt PMO	Splicing, exon 51	Duchenne muscular dystrophy/*DMD exon 51*	Sep 2016
Milasen	ASO	22 nt PS 2′-MOE	Splicing	Batten disease/CLN7	Jan 2018
Patisiran	siRNA LNP formulation	19 + 2 nt 2′-OME	Ago2	Hereditary transthyretin amyloidosis, polyneuropathy-*TTR*	Aug 2018
Inotersen	Gapmer ASO	20 nt PS 2′-MOE	RNase H1	hereditary transthyretin amyloidosis, polyneuropathy/*TTR*	Oct 2018
Givosiran	Dicer substrate siRNA	21/23 nt- GalNAc conjugate	Ago2	Acute hepatic porphyria *ALAS1*	Nov 2019
Golodirsen	Steric block ASO	25 nt PMO	Splicing, exon 53	Duchenne muscular dystrophy/*DMD exon 53*	Dec 2019
Viltolarsen	ASO	21 nt-PMO	Splicing	Duchenne muscular dystrophy/*DMD exon 53*	Aug 2020
Casimersen	ASO	22-PMO	Splicing	Duchenne muscular dystrophy/DMD Exon 45	Feb 2021
Inclisiran	siRNA	21/23 nt- GalNAc conjugate	Ago2	Hypercholesterolaemia/PCSKK9	Dec 2021

As these hurdles tamper ON effectiveness, alternative solution such as direct nucleic acid modification was applied to overcome exonuclease cleavage. However, it was not adequate since these nucleic acid derivatives were continuously recognized by the immune systems to digest and excrete as foreign invaders. Nanoformulation and direct conjugation (with GalNac, lipid, or antibodies) were strongly recommended to mask ON and avoid from RES associating clearance. Additionally, both techniques could improve membrane penetration, which assist ON to permeate through endothelial lining. Enhancement of ON to escape late endosome-lysosomal degradation remained controversial and not understood clearly. Co-administration with chemical enhancers to disrupt encapsulating vesicle was suggested; however, it concurred with high risk of toxicity. Our Table 1 of FDA approved ON drugs also updated with the modificative modalities to achieve maximal clinical outcome and to bypass the mentioned challenges.

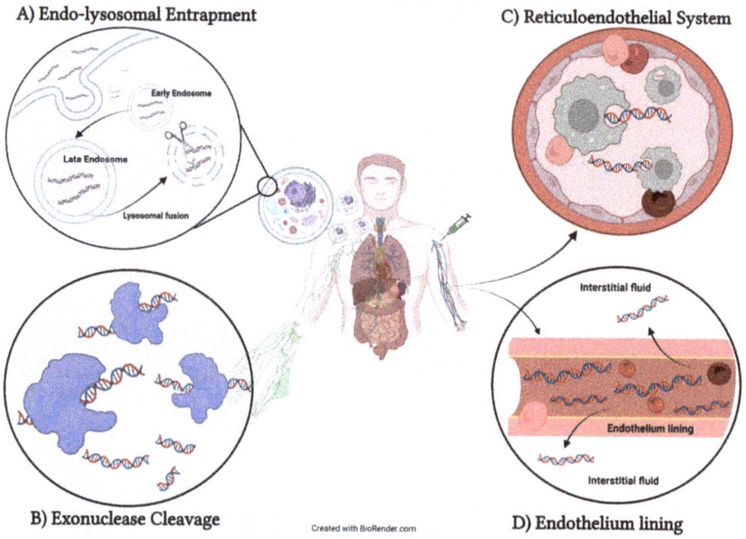

Figure 3. Four biological barriers preventing activity of therapeutic oligonucleotide. (**A**) Endo-lysosomal entrapment. ON required escape from late endosome before subjected to lysosomal degradation. (**B**) Exonuclease cleavage. Initiate hydrolysis of phosphodiester backbone, which deteriorate ON. (**C**) Reticuloendothelial system. Digestion of ON by macrophage can terminate its activity. (**D**) Endothelium lining. Blockage of transverse ON from vascular lumen to interstitial fluid.

1.4. Early Attempt of Oligonucleotide Chemical Modification

Direct chemical modification was conceptualized to battle the discussed biological barrier to safely deliver therapeutic ON to its site of action. The earliest attempt was sulfurization of phosphodiester backbone into phosphorothioate (PS), which altered its physiochemical properties. With the low electronegative element of sulfur, phosphorothioate would be less susceptible to be nucleophilic attacked by nuclease. Improvement from the first-generation phosphorothioate was documented with pharmacokinetic data showing extension of half-life up to 1 or 2 h. Moreover, the clearance rate was significantly decreased with less than 5% ON detected in urine or feces after murine dosing for 12 h [16,17]. This high systemic retention was accompanied by a high affinity to plasma protein with 95% bound. Even with phenomenal achievement, there is some evidence of relevant phosphorothioate potential flaws: (1) degradation still can occur via other mechanisms such as transesterification or pyrophosphatase [18] and (2) an excessive amount of phosphorothioate on ON can negatively impact the binding affinity of targeted RNA. This first-generation modification is still frequently applied in modern ON synthesis, but it is incorporated with the second-generation modification at 2′ribose.

For RNA, the 2′ hydroxyl group is a critical component for RNase to recognize and catalyze hydrolysis. Thus, protection of this group is necessary, which can perform via methoxylation. Moreover, 2′ ribose modification was reported to diminish unwanted immune stimulation [19]. Researchers explored this protection technique by starting with naturally occurring 2′-O-methyl (2′-OMe) RNA, which exudes the improvement of nuclease resistance and binding affinity. A bulkier group such as 2′-O-methoxylethyl (2′-MOE) emerged as the most prominent candidate, which can be confirmed via thermal shift assay revealing stronger binding affinity as ΔTm increased from 0.9 °C to 1.7 °C per modification counts. From these encouraging findings, the third generation was developed by introducing a constraint that hindered the nucleotide's conformational flexibility. The first attempt was bridging 2′-oxygen to 4′-carbon ribose to produce locked nucleic acid (LNA), which showed intense elevation of binding affinity (increasing of ΔTm from 4 °C to 8 °C per modification units binding to

RNA) [20]. Its derivatives with an additional methyl group, constrained ethyl (cET), were believed to conduct tighter binding. However, 2′ ribose modification caused therapeutic ON the incompetency to recruit and facilitate RNase cleavage mechanism due to inability to identify and covalently bind to 2′-hydroxyl group [21,22]. A clever solution to this drawback is implementing these second-generation to flank at both sides of the gapmer, an ON consisting of a central DNA region recruiting RNase H.

Moreover, ribose moiety can be completely substituted with less rotatable structures such as tricycle DNA (tcDNA) or cyclohexene nucleic acid (CeNA). A fully modified tcDNA, which is equipped with three extra carbons between C(5′) and C(3′), lifted the thermal stability up by 1.2 °C and 2.4 °C per modification while interacting with DNA and RNA, respectively [23]. Similarly, the replacement of a furanose ring with cyclohexene also restricts some flexibility while exhibiting superior serum stability from degradation and enhancing RNase recruitment capability [24]. Nonconventional nucleic acid modification is illustrated via phosphorodiamidate morpholino oligomer (PMO). The ribose moiety retains the traditional oxidative oxygen while being re-closed with an additional ammonia unit. The phosphodiester backbone is replaced with phosphorodiamidate linkage. This modification demonstrates exceptional degradative resistance either from protease, esterase, or 13 different hydrolases in serum and plasma. With the uncharged character, PMO prevents unwanted hybridization with surrounding protein, which exacerbated ON effectiveness [25]. Figure 4 illustrates the representative variation of ON modification segregated by their generation.

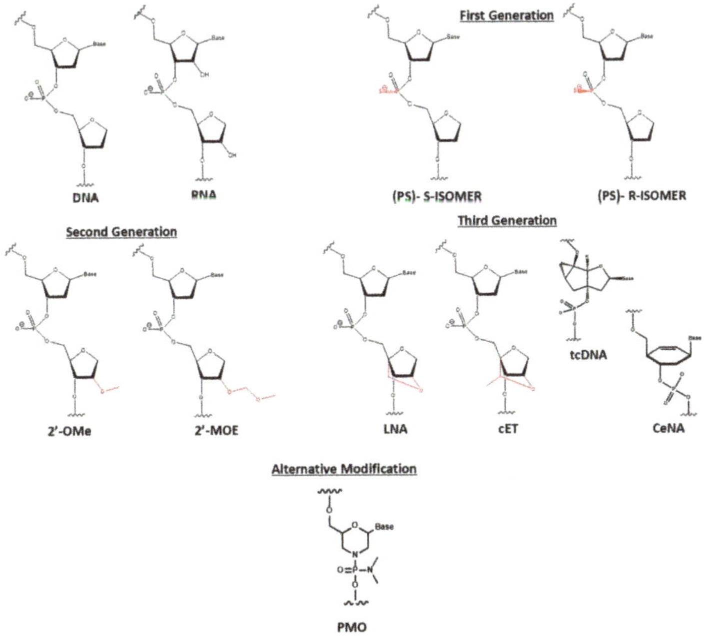

Figure 4. Three generations of common nucleic acid modifications. First generation replaced phosphodiester (PO) backbone to phosphorothioate (PS) to enhance degradative resistance. Second generation includes modification of 2′ ribose into 2′-O-methyl (2′-OMe) and 2′-O-Methoxyethyl (2′-MOE), which are popular in gapmer synthesis. Third generation restricts conformational flexibility by introducing a methyl bridge between 2′-O and 4′ of ribose. Locked nucleic acid (LNA) and constraint ethyl (cET). Ribose moiety would be completely replaced with tricyclic DNA (tcDNA) or cyclohexene (CeDNA). Alternative modification was phosphorodiamidate morpholino oligomer (PMO). This neutral nucleic acid was described with an additional amine accompanied with phosphorodiamidate backbone.

Despite these exciting discoveries, systemic toxicity inherited by nucleic acid modification plaque ON therapies as reported in vivo and significantly, clinical trials. For instance, P.S modification was known for enhancing protein plasma binding, however, excessive repetition of P.S in a single ON unit impacted the affinity to mRNA and promiscuously developed off-target toxicity after long-termed exposure [11,21,26]. The second-generation such as 2′-MOE, are encountered in vivo toxicity in mice reported by Zanardi et al. However, there were no significant increases in toxicity for longer treatment duration. cET was the candidate believed to reduce much toxicity compared to other 2′ ribose modifications [27]. Finally, the third generation cannot escape this trauma such as report in LNA with associating liver toxicity. Therefore, the modification must be considered with moderation to avoid unwanted adverse effects and needed additional sources of delivery.

1.5. Lipid-Conjugated Oligonucleotides: Method of Delivery and Example of Conjugation

1.5.1. Method of Enhanced Delivery and Lipid-Conjugated Structure

Finding the most optimal and efficient delivery method for therapeutic ON is still an ongoing campaign for the goal of achieving the maximal clinical outcome. Scientists usually implement one of the two following popular approaches: (1) external delivery capsules by utilizing nanoparticles and (2) covalent conjugation of endogenous biomolecules. Naturally occurring substances are preferable with some exceptions for artificial materials. Among these, hydrophobic or lipid moieties have gained much-wanted attention. It is abundant in biological systems and carries out essential functions such as executing signaling transportation. More importantly, it is a body of phospholipid bilayer that can help ON to mimic the hydrophobic properties.

The first exciting investigation of utilizing lipid nanoparticles as ON delivery was conducted by Felgner et al. He incorporated plasmid DNA with cationic lipid such as 1,2-O-octade-anyl-3-trimethylammonium propane (DOTMA) and dioleyl phosphatidyl ethanolamine (DOPE) to induce in vivo transfection into cells. This successful discovery leads to the use of LNP to be drug delivery carriers for small molecules as well. [28]. Significantly, there are eight LNP structures approved by the FDA. Patisiran is an example of ON carried by LNP approved in the market for the treatment of hereditary transthyretin amyloidosis. As by 2021, the most advanced LNP formulation was applied for delivery of two mRNA vaccines, BNT162b2/Comirnaty (Pfizer-BioNTech) and mRNA-1273 (Moderna) to counteract the global SARS-CoV-2 pandemic. For formulation of Comirnaty, ALC-0315 was the main component of this nanoformulation recipe. It was a synthetic lipid-like substance that has an ethanolamine headgroup along with two biodegradable branched ester tails. The LNP was formulated via mixture of ALC-0315/cholesterol/DSPC (Distearoylphosphatidylcholine)/PEG-lipid. In term of mRNA-1273, synthetic lipid SM-102 was selected as primary nanoparticles components. Its structure was similar to ALC-0315 containing an ethanolamine headgroup with difference of one mono and one branched degradable ester tails. mRNA-1273 was formulated strictly with SM-102/DSPC/cholesterol. Both synthetic lipids illustrated in Figure 5 were hypothesized to obtain cone-shaped structure from the branching tails, which boosted the strength of endosomal escape for mRNA molecules [29]. As advancing to clinical trials, Comirnaty was fully approved for individuals 16 years and older while mRNA-1273 is still in the third trial (approved for emergency use). They both encodes for stabilized full-length spike protein but their mRNA contents (100 µg and 30 µg for mRNA-1273 and BNT162b2, respectively). A review by Schoenmaker outlined the abridged and detailed information regarding of dosing and LNP components for both vaccines [30]. However, some ionizable lipids were feared to produce unwanted toxicity and in need of continuously monitoring due to the uncontrolled activation of cytokines after systemic administration [31].

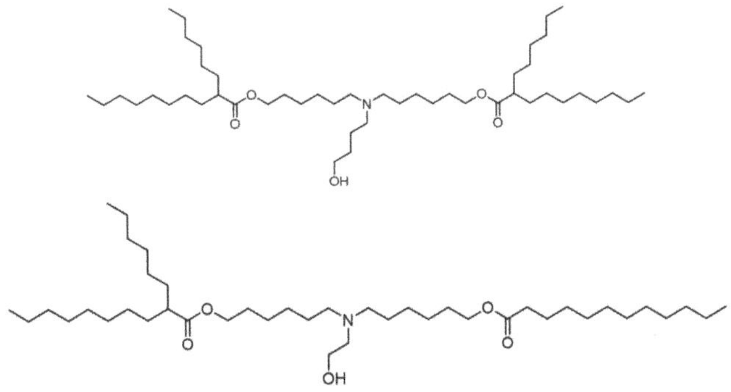

ALC-0315

SM-102

Figure 5. Chemical structure of two most advanced LNP that assisted in delivery of 2 mRNA COVID vaccines. ALC-0315 and SM-102 contains similar structure with ethanolamine head (one is shorter than others). ALC-0315 has two branched degradable ester tail, while SM-102 only has one branched ester tail.

Alternatively, the second approach by lipid conjugation is plausible. Scientific evidence suggests a unity of lipid conjugated oligonucleotide (LON) can reduce the risk of immunogenesis while can maintain tolerance with a high dose in vivo [32]. Similar to LNP, LON's hydrophobicity is enhanced and be more accessible to membrane permeability and higher rate of internalization. In contrast, LONs are relatively smaller than LNP, which contributes to a higher leakage rate from endothelial lining and perfuse to various tissue types. However, the majority of lipid derivatives are highly accumulated in primary excretory organs, liver and kidney. Administration route is a crucial concept when mentioning LON delivery because it dictates the targeted tissue. In vivo experiments, either intravenous or subcutaneous injections can result in LON migration to clearance organ and some miscellaneous (spleen, skeletal muscle, etc.); while intrathecal or direct cranial injection can occupy parts of the brain [33,34]. Therefore, optimizing delivery location is theoretically a balancing act of hydrophobicity adjustment and understanding the chemical nature of bioconjugates.

To achieve such a feat, an effective synthesis of LON is required. A fully functional LON consists of three distinct fragments as illustrated in Figure 6: (1) the designed ON (ssRNA, siRNA, aptamer, or any forms), (2) attaching linker, and (3) lipid derivatives. Synthetic LON was produced via either pre-synthetic or post-synthetic approach, which lipoid conjugate would be introduced in a different fashion. An articulate description of both LON's synthetic routes was reviewed by Raouane and Li et al. [2,35]. We would like to briefly compare two approaches and highlight vital conjugating procedures for lipoid species. When tackling LON with pre-synthetic approach, it provides more flexible lipid point of attachment options. Conjugation can occur either at 3′, 5′ or even between consecutive nucleotides. The most popular and convenient technique is attaching the hydrophilic group at the 5′ end as presynthesized phosphoramidite. However, 3′-lipoid attachment can be arduous because bioconjugation is required to be pre-tethered onto a solid support. For instance, Setsinger premade cholesteroyl solid support via oxidative phosphoramidation [36], while Nikan et al. built a solid support with a pre-formed amide bond with docosahexaenoic acid [37]. Some other example [38] using an alcoholic moiety attaching to a solid support via succinyl linker while bearing another hydroxyl group for cholesterol to attach. Ueno [39] selected glycerol to bridge lipophilic group and mRNA. Interchain bioconjugation was attempted through examples of Guzaev and Durand [40,41]. In contrast, the post-synthetic approach requires two completely independent entities of ON and lipoid conjugation with their complementary reactive group for coupling. Some available techniques could be the formation of triazole linkers resulting from click chemistry reaction between dibenzocycloctyne (DBCO) and azido-lipid conjugates [42]. Raoulane demonstrated the effectiveness of thiol-malamide bridge of RNA and squalene [43].

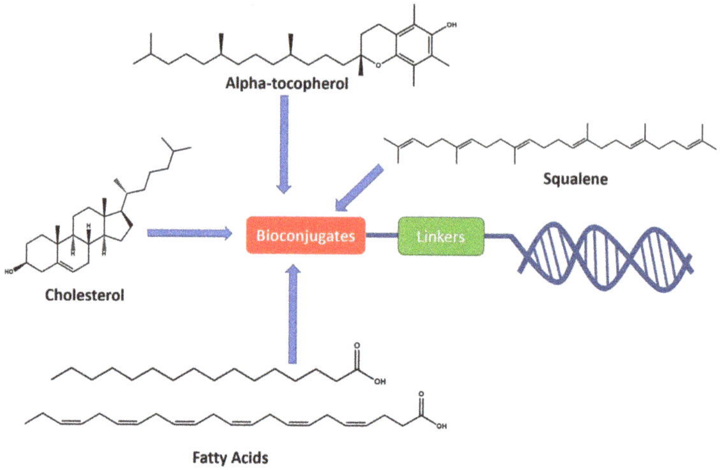

Figure 6. General molecular structure of conjugated oligonucleotides including: (1) synthetic oligonucleotide, (2) linkers, and (3) bioconjugates.

1.5.2. Example of Conjugations

A. Cholesterol Conjugates

Covalently attached cholesteryl moiety as non-vehicle delivery for oligonucleotides was conceptualized as early as the late 1990s [44]. Manoharan's group claimed 3′- cholesterol-conjugated ON produced the best silencing effect and continued in unfolding the delivery mechanism. They observed a 2-fold uptake increase in comparison to naked ON for silencing murine ICAM-1 and proposed liver uptake mechanism associated with scavenger receptors [45]. Later in the 2000s, scientists from Alnylam synthesized and examined a plethora of cholesteryl derivatives at two terminals of either sense or antisense strands [46,47], which confirmed better in vivo efficacy of 3′-cholesterol ON (3′-Chol ON). Wolfrum et al. expanded Manoharan's mechanistic notion and elucidated receptor-mediated endocytosis as a key for ON uptake. The cholesterol-conjugated ON was highly recognized and attached to either LDL (low-density lipoprotein) or HDL (high-density lipoprotein); thus, the resulting complex docked to scavenger receptors (SR-BI) and proceed to internalization [48]. At the same time, cholesterol conjugates enhanced the hydrophobicity of oligonucleotide, which ameliorated the drug-like properties. For researching a more feasible pharmacokinetic characterization technique, Godinho et al. attested 3′-Chol ON with rapid distribution phase ($t_{1/2\,\alpha}$ = 18–33 min) and slow elimination phase ($t_{1/2\,\beta}$ = 8–14 h) [49].

A complete pharmacokinetic parameter was summarized in Table 2 for intravenous administration. Nevertheless, it was noticeable that silencing capability can only reach near 50% efficacy even at a low dosage. It was believed that conjugated ON was sequestered during late endosome, which coiled the term endosomal entrapment [50]. Hence, chemical enhancers were used to damage vesicles along the endosomal system to promote escape [51,52]. Additionally, the delivery scope of cholesterol conjugated oligonucleotide was very limited to hepatic cells and to some extend pancreatic cells [53].

Table 2. Pharmacokinetic parameter of Chol-hsiRNA after intravenous injection adapted by Godinho et al.

Parameter (Units)	Chol-hsiRNA
$k(min^{-1})$	0.0013
$t_{1/2\ \alpha}$(min)	515.8
$t_{1/2\ \beta}$ (min)	33.2
C_{max} (μg/mL)	753.4
$AUC_{0\text{–}48\ h}$ (μg/mL·min)	54,532.5
$AUC_{0\text{-inf}}$ (μg/mL·min)	54,807.5
$MRT_{0\text{-inf}}$ (min)	156.9
Vz (mL)	6.8
Cl (mL/min)	0.0091

Most studies have demonstrated that cholesteryl conjugated ON was delivered effectively, and specifically to liver tissue. Hence, hepatic-related disorder would be its ideal target. For an instant, hypercholesterolemia is the excessive circulation of cholesterol in blood, which caused by either habitual diet or genetic condition. Antisense technology has provided a therapeutic platform through silencing of PCSK9 [54–56] or hepatic ApoB [57–60]; however, the unconjugated ASO treatments suffered mild to serious toxicity while giving questionable efficacy. Henceforth, studies from Wada and Nakajima demonstrated coupling ASO with cholesterol would enhance liver uptake while improving the degradation efficacy of PCSK9 (−50% silencing and 2 μmol/kg) [61] and ApoB (−85% silencing and 0.5 mg/kg) [62], respectively. Both research groups also pinpointed the cleavage of phosphodiester linkage as quintessential for liberating ASO, which showed a 3- to 5-fold increase in vivo potency [63]. Furthermore, the application of cholesterol conjugated ON is extended into the realm of cancer treatment. Liu et al. cholesterol-conjugated let-7a miRNA mimics could downregulate both transcriptional and translational levels of RAS in vitro, and minimize murine xenograft tumor in vivo [64]. Chernolovskaya group delved into silencing MDR1 (multidrug resistance protein), which overexpressed in oncogenic cells to efflux impending drug and amplify resistance [65,66]. 21-mer MDR1 targeting siRNA both as monomer and trimer (63-mer) were compared in vivo demonstrating monomeric siRNA obtained superior silencing efficacy while trimeric derivative accumulated highly in tumors [67,68]. Additional examples of other applicable disease would be including Huntington's disease [37,69,70], diabetes nephropathy [71], and herpes simplex virus-2 protection [72].

Some cholesterol conjugated ONs were successfully introduced to clinical trials. For example, ARC-520-HBV was the first RNA interference therapeutic for treatment against hepatitis B virus (HBV). ARC-520 injection consisted of a pair of synthetic cholesterol-conjugated siRNAs to augment its delivery to hepatocytes. It also contained polymer-based excipients such as dynamic polyconjugates that enable endosomal escape [73]. Mechanistically, it reduced all RNA transcripts from covalently closed circular DNA (cccDNA) leading to the diminishing of both viral antigen and DNA. ARC-520 was at phase II clinical studies with the promising pharmacokinetic profile in a single-dose study in healthy volunteers. The clinicians found out that IV injection with a dose of 3 mg/kg can increase the curative effect and reduce the viral antigen level by 81–96%. The dosage regimen was given 2 mg/kg once every 4 weeks for 3 total doses. As results, the degree of viral decline and duration of the effect was consistent with the previous animal experiments. Unfortunately, the inclusion of hepatocyte-targeted excipient ARC-EX1 melittin-derived peptide linked to *N*-acetylgalactosamine caused detrimental toxicity in nonhuman primates which rendered the trial to be terminated [74]. In another application, ARO-AAT (SEQUOIA) is currently in phase II/III of clinical trial for the treatment of Alpha-1 antitrypsin deficiency (ATTD)-associated liver disease. The subcutaneous dose of iRNA selectively degraded ATT mRNA caused by Pi*Z mutation. The trial was aimed to determine the safety, tolerability, and pharmacodynamic effect of the drug by gauging the level of plasma and intrahepatic Z-AAT levels. iRNA were given in incremental multiple doses and up to 300 mg in a single shot. It was well-tolerated and resulted in more than 91% serum reduction which was sustained for 6 weeks. To understand dosage window in practical term, this iRNA therapy could be administered four time a year or less to maintain desired silencing effect. The clinical trial is anticipated to be completed by July 2022 (ARO-AAT2001; NCT03945292).

Apart from this, the cholesterol conjugated ON is broadly used for connective tissue growth factor (CTGF) to battle against fibrotic disorders. For instance, Hwang et al. reported a novel application of this modified 2′-OMe phosphorothioate nucleic acid for antifibrotic skin therapeutics. The drug is composed of a cell-penetrating asymmetric interfering RNA (cp-asiRNA) known by OLX10010 as shown in Table 3 (cholesterol conjugate). This iRNA targets the expression of CTGF, and it is currently examined in an ongoing phase 2a clinical trial [75]. When compared to unconjugated siRNA, 1 mmol/L of cp-asiCTGF achieved more than 85% silencing knockdown of CTGF at mRNA level without the assistance of transfection media. The calculated IC_{50} was 0.315 nM in cell lines (the best efficiency was observed in keloid fibroblast cell). Hwang et al. also discussed in vivo studies on rat skin to demonstrate a significant gene-specific silencing capability with 1 mg intradermal injection of lipid modified siRNA after 72 h. Furthermore, the conjugated siRNA exhibited 10-fold lower in dosage efficacy as compared to the commercially available siRNA [73]. A recent study by Choe et al. suggested to co-administrate L-type calcium channel blockers to further facilitate cellular internalization. As result, silencing of cp-asiRNA was potentiated without significant adverse effect [76]. Likewise, RXI-109, a cholesterol conjugated siRNA discovered by RXi Pharmaceuticals', exhibited a reduction of CTGF during the course of wound healing followed by keloidectomy. This therapy was applicable for patients suffering from age-related macular degeneration with high risk of subretinal fibrosis (www.rxipharma.com/technology/rxi-109, accessed on 15 November 2021). Therefore, targeting CTGF with conjugated siRNA is a good direction for fibrotic disorders such as hypertrophic scars and keloids. Moreover, these ONs are anticipated to treat excess collagen from injury or after surgery which was conventionally treated with less effective silicon sheets with the application of pressure.

Table 3. A selective example of ON conjugated with lipoid moieties in corresponding with each bioconjugates section.

Sequences	Spacer	Conjugates (X)	Source
Passenger 5′-CUUACCGACUGGAAGA-3′-**X** Guide 3′-CCGGACGGGAGCGCCGAAUGGCUGACCUUCU-5	**N/A**	Cholesterol	Hwang et al.
X-5′-TAGGGTTAGACAA-3′	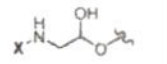	Palmitic acid (16C)	Herbert et al.
X-5′-TCAACAATAAATACCGAGG-3′	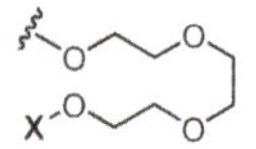	α-tocopherol	Østergaard et al.
Sense **X**-5′-GGAGGAACUCUCCUGAUGAAU-3′ Anti-sense 5′-UCAUCAGGAGAGUUCCUGCCG-3′	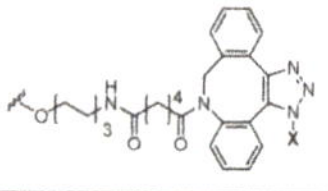	Squalene	Massaad-Massade et al.

Notation: red—2′MOE modification, green—cET modification, underline—PS backbone modification, and **X**—bioconjugates.

B. Fatty Acid Conjugates

Like cholesterol, fatty acid is an attractive entity for bioconjugation since it offered hydrophobicity customization and mimicked the uncanny composition of the phospholipid membrane. Currently, unbranched fatty acids were heavily delved such as the study conducted by Prakash et al. An array of fatty acid tethered to 16-mer-ASO through phosphodiester–linked hexaylamino spacer was synthesized. Two structure-activity relationship (SAR) studies were conducted and examined two revolving concepts: carbon length and degree of unsaturation. The first SAR involved with eight different fatty acids' lengths (C10 to C22) conjugated to ASO revealed two findings: (1) protein binding property with chain length shorter than 16-C was lower than their counterparts showed in Tables 3 and 4) Malat-1 expression was more significantly reduced by ASO with fatty.

Table 4. Adapted protein binding data from Prakash et al. displayed the trends depending on carbon lengths.

Sequence	Conjugates (X = 5′-end)	Albumin Ki (μM)	LDL Ki (μM)	HDL Ki (μM)
GCATTCTAATAGCAGC	None	24.00	N/A	N/A
X- GCATTCTAATAGCAGC	C8 (Octanoyl)	2.20	11.80	5.80
X- GCATTCTAATAGCAGC	C10 (Decanoyl)	4.99	3.20	1.70
X- GCATTCTAATAGCAGC	C12 (Dodecanoyl)	3.22	1.30	0.75
X- GCATTCTAATAGCAGC	C14 (Myristoyl)	1.97	0.36	0.79
X- GCATTCTAATAGCAGC	C16 (Palmitoyl)	0.92	0.13	0.79
X- GCATTCTAATAGCAGC	C18 (Stearoyl)	0.85	0.17	0.66
X- GCATTCTAATAGCAGC	C20 (Eicosanoyl)	0.91	0.22	1.26
X- GCATTCTAATAGCAGC	C22 (Docosanoyl)	0.97	0.31	1.30

Fatty acid chain longer than 12 in quadriceps while all remained similar in the heart [77]. Furthermore, the second SAR delved with 12 different unsaturated fatty acids. Protein binding to albumin, LDL, and HDL were slightly improved while there was no significant effect attributed to the double bond position. The activity of the representative unsaturated ASO displayed significant improvement compared to unconjugated ASO; however, there was no remarkable difference from their saturated counterparts. An interesting observation was none of the unsaturated moiety could outmatch palmitoyl's silencing activity. Hence, palmitoyl conjugated ASO was selected as to be the most efficacious and subjected for elucidating muscle uptake mechanism in rodent model. Chappel et al. examined the consequential efficacy of palmitoyl-ASO after injection to endocytosis receptor knockdown mice (CAV1-/-, FcRN-/- and Alb-/-) [78]. In CAV knockdown mice, ED_{50} of palmitoyl ASO in quadriceps decreased by four-fold compared to wild type (9.7 μmol/kg versus 2.4 μmol/kg). In FCRN -/- mice, attenuation of palmitoyl ASO's activity was observed compared to controlled groups with similar outcome (ED_{50} of 5.5 μmol/kg to 16 μmol/kg). A contrast was observed in Alb -/- mice with unchanged activity in quadriceps (0.73 μmol/kg in Alb -/- and 0.71 μmol/kg in controlled BL6). Thus, muscle uptake of palmitoyl-ASO was facilitated by caveolin-receptor-mediated endocytosis into endothelium cells once bound to albumin. Simultaneously, silencing FcRN could weaken the recycling of albumin into circulation thus impairing the albumin binding of ASO. However, Alb -/- mice contradicted the hypothesis, which would question if other proteins would be upregulated in compensation of drastic albumin reduction, and some would exist sufficient affinity for palmitoyl ASO binding.

Khvorova group compared the pharmacokinetic distribution property of diverse lipid moiety with emphasis on four fatty acids: myristic (Myr), docosahexaenoic (DHA), docosanoic (DCA), and eicosapentaenoic (EPA) acid. Length and degree of unsaturation constituted the hydrophobicity, which resulted in various in vivo distribution outcome. This study concluded with two premises: (1) more hydrophobic conjugates offered higher retention and (2) hydrophobicity instituted tissue accumulations [53]. Furthermore, shorter and less hydrophobic fatty acid such as myristic was synthesized and PK was analyzed as mono-, di-, or trimer. As discussed, the impact of hydrophobicity was profoundly shown in different behavior: (i) mono-lipid conjugates was quickly released with high kidney accumulation, (ii) di-lipid conjugates functioned as in-between showing preferential liver accumulation while flexibly distributed to other tissue (lung, heart, and fat), and (iii) tri-lipid conjugates resides at the injection site with no significant systemic exposure [79].

Table 5 summarized the pharmacokinetic parameter of three myristic variants. DCA-conjugated ON shared similar PK property as dimeric Myr and was able to silence the expression of myostatin (Mstn) in skeletal muscle after subcutaneous injection at 20 mg/kg dosage. Mstn, a growth factor expressed in skeletal muscles, negatively modulates muscle mass; hence, its inhibition was a potential therapeutic treatment against muscle wasting [80–82] or Duchenne muscular dystrophy (DMD) [83–85]. Interestingly, the toxicity profile of fatty acid conjugates was safer compared to cholesterol conjugates showing low activation of cytokine at high dose (100 mg/kg) [86].

Table 5. Pharmacokinetic parameters of three myristic variants after 7 days period injection adapted from Biscan et al.

Parameter (Units)	Monomeric Myr	Dimeric Myr	Trimeric Myr
k_{abs} (min^{-1})	0.0562	0.0213	0.0341
$t_{1/2\ abs}$ (min)	12.3	32.5	20.3
k_{β} (min^{-1})	0.0218	0.0050	0.0015
$t_{1/2\ \beta}$ (min)	54.1	139.0	465.3
T_{max} (min)	60	120	120
C_{max} (μg/mL)	21.4	6.1	0.9
AUC (μg/mL*min)	3768.1	3511.1	984.6
MRT (min)	644.7	1534.5	2009.6

Fatty acid would serve as an ideal conjugate to deliver therapeutic ON to muscle tissue. Currently, two ASO-splicing modulated therapy are approved by the FDA for muscle-related index such as eteplersen for Duchenne muscular dystrophy (DMD) [87] and nusinersen for spinal muscular atrophy [88]. Although eteplersen received such speedy approval with promising application, overall clinical efficacy [87,89] and renal toxicity from high dose [90] remained controversial. Thus, fatty acids can aspire to be a delivery platform to ameliorate both therapies for patients in need. Aside from muscular-related disorder, GRN163L (Imetelstat sodium) currently resides at phase III of clinical trials as a treatment for myelofibrosis as shown in Table 3 (fatty acid conjugate). It is a 13-mer phosphorothioate ASO with covalently attached palmitic acid at the 5′ terminal that exuded telomerase inhibitory activity. Observation of telomerase shortening was detected across multiple cancerous cells derived from glioblastoma [91], multiple myeloma [92], Barrett's esophageal adenocarcinoma [93], breast [94], lung [95], and liver [96]. From in vivo delivery perspective, IC_{50} values were seven-fold higher [97], and efficacy increased up to 56% compared to naked counterpart after 24 h followed by intravenous injection (50 mg/kg) [98]. In follow-up studies, a group of researchers managed to explore the effects of long-term GRN163L exposure on the maintenance of telomeres and lifespan of 10 pancreatic cancer cells. They summarized the study with IC_{50} value was ranged from 50 nM to 200 nM, and suggested continuous exposure of GRN163L eventually led a complete loss of viability after several doubling times. Conversely, telomerase reactivation and elongation were observed in the absence of GRN163L. This observation reinforced that GRN163L could target the RNA template region of telomerase and proven to produced outstanding inhibitory effect. Overall, these outcomes demonstrated that the lifespan of pancreatic tumor cells can be shortened by continuous exposure and can be used in patients in the future [99]. Additionally, co-administration of GRN163L with trastuzumab revealed to produce synergistic effect, which GRN163L reversed the resistance of HER 2 + metastatic breast cancer against trastuzumab.

The clinical application of fatty acid conjugate is extended to ameliorate antibacterial resistance and antibiotic treatment as well. The attachment of ketal bis C15 and cyanine to 25-mer oligonucleotide at 5′ or 3′ terminal proved the efficient strategies in cell delivery. It decreased the minimum inhibitory concentration (MIC) of laboratory and clinical resistant strains to cephalosporin drug (i.e., ceftriaxone) by 25-fold than the naked equivalence. The decrease of beta-lactamase activity was dose-dependent and 5μM was found to be efficacious. Furthermore, 3′ lipid modification was less efficient than 5′. The 3′-attachment could propel the destabilization of heteroduplex structure of mRNA-LON, which enhanced steric hinderance to prevent RNase cleavage rather than uptaking into the bacteria [100].

C. Vitamin E (α-tocopherol)

Vitamin E is a group of fat-soluble compounds consisting of either tocopherol or tocotrienols. Naturally occurring α-tocopherol is an essential dietary supplement so it would be a safe and interesting selection for chemical bioconjugation. Additionally, its structure is composed of hydroxyl chromane and a hydrophobic saturated side chain that potentially enhances ON membrane permeability. Nishina et al. synthesized a 17-mer gapmer targeting murine hepatic ApoB. Structurally, it consisted of a parent 13-mer gapmer flanked by two wings of LNA with additional 4-mer modified RNA as the second wing directly linked to α-tocopherol via a phosphodiester bond. In vivo efficacy examination, tocopherol 17-mer ON showed −70% ApoB mRNA silencing capability after murine injection at 0.75 mg/kg [101]. The mRNA silencing potency was heavily dependent on dosage level (drastic reduction of ApoB expression as dose increased to 1.5 and 3 mg/kg) and prolonged duration of exposure (maximum response occurs from day 3 to 14). A followed-up pharmacokinetic study using Alexa Fluor-647 tagged tocopherol 17-mer ON at 5′-end revealed more than 3.5-fold higher of accumulation in the liver compared to non-conjugated parent, while tocopherol 17-mer ON also possessed higher serum content (10,000 μg/L) than naked parent ON (>1000 μg/L) at 5 min after 5 mg/kg dose of injection. The pharmacokinetic parameter of tocopherol 17-mer ON was summarized in Table 6. Interestingly, western blot analysis suggested cleavage of full-length tocopherol 17-mer ON into naked 13-mer unit once arrived at the liver which hypothesized the second wing tagged tocopherol acting as a delivery enhancer and release the main frame of 13-mer to initiate RNase-H cleavage mechanism toward targeted ApoB mRNA.

Table 6. Pharmacokinetic parameter of Toc-17-mer ASO.

Parameter	Toc-17-mer ASO
AUC (∞) (ug/mL·min)	379 ± 14
CLtot (mL/min/g)	0.0079 ± 0.0005
MRT (min)	32 ± 1
Vdss (mL/g)	0.252 ± 0.023
K_α (min^{-1})	0.0571 ± 0.0041
K_β (min^{-1})	0.00272 ± 0.00137

AUC—area under the serum concentration time curve, CLtot—total body clearance, MRT—mean residence rate constant, K_α—initial elimination rate constant, K_β—terminal elimination rate constant, and Vdss—steady-state volume of distribution.

Another study conducted by Østergaard et al. comparing three different bioconjugates (cholesterol, tocopherol, and palmitate) ASO duplex targeting dystrophia myotonic protein kinase (DMPK), which caused myotic dystrophy (DM1) as the product of toxic repetition of nucleotide in the 3′- untranslated regions [102]. Structure of tocopherol-conjugated ON was illustrated in Table 3 (tocopherol conjugate). In vivo rat models, palmitate conjugated ASO responded with more improved silencing potency in skeletal muscle and heart compared to cholesterol and tocopherol after 10 mg/kg injection dose. However, in the monkey model, tocopherol conjugated-ASO came as more advantageous than the other two displaying a lower ED_{50} value of 7 mg/kg across three different DMPK expressed tissues (heart, quadriceps, and tibialis) [103]. Additionally, tocopherol moiety displayed tolerable high dose while cholesterol struggled with toxicity issues (in mice and unable to advance for primal testing). In plasma pharmacokinetics, tocopherol conjugates tended to co-elute with HDL and LDL, which displayed from size exclusion chromatography suggesting the essential of plasma protein binding was essential for receptor-mediated endocytosis. Benizri et al. disclosed additional pharmacokinetic data showing elevated liver accumulation after 6-h injection at a dose of 3 mg/kg (9–14 μg/g for tocopherol-ON versus 2–5 μg for naked-ON) [98]. However, tocopherol is remained understudied and required further preclinical investigation; thus, limited cases of human studies are often acquired.

D. Squalene

Squalene is a naturally occurring triterpene molecule that is frequently harvested from shark's liver and some variety of vegetable oil. It is an important precursor for human cholesterol synthesis. As hydrophobic moiety squalene is also a candidate for ON conjugation that can couple either at 3′ or 5′ terminal of the sense strand. Thiol-maleimide or DBCO via click chemistry are usually generated, and squalene-ON can spontaneously form nanoparticles. Due to the amphiphilic nature of squalene, these nanoparticles could assemble in different shapes. Raouane et al. synthesized a 5′ squalene attached mRNA duplex employing a thiol-maleimide linker. This spherical nanoparticle was characterized by a drastic increase in lipophilicity while maintaining exceptional stability in serum media as a negative suspension (zeta potential= −26 mV). Cytotoxicity MTT assay in BHP-10-3 cell lines demonstrated > 95% cell viability at 50 nM maximal concentration of squalene-ON nanoparticle, while qRT-PCR depicted −80% RET/PTC1 silencing capability in vitro. Mice implanted with tumor were intravenously administered with a dose of 2.5 mg/Kg in vivo also demonstrated approximately 80% silencing of RET/PTC1 through qRT-PCR. Tumor biopsy showed significant shrinkage compared to controlled naked mRNA duplex after 15 days of the injection [43]. In another oncogenic targeting study, Masaad et al. investigated the silencing outcome of 5′ squalene attached ON against TMPRSS2-ERG fusion oncogene. This group employed Cu-free click chemistry to functionalize reactive DBCO group tethering to the spacer of siRNA duplex to azido squalene. The structure was shown in Table 3 (squalene conjugate). Nanoformulation of 5′ end was characterized to be temperature sensitive and degradable at 37 °C, while its structure was constricted to be spherical and quite anionic (zeta = −37 mV). This formulation was subjected to in vitro inhibitory efficacy test with VCap cells. Wherein, 50 nM of 5′-squalene nanoparticle showed a similar silencing effect (−50%) as naked siRNA transfected by lipofectamine after 3 different time points. Additionally, xenografted mice with VCap tumors showed significant size growth inhibition by −60%. siRNA treated mice were sacrificed and collected with excretory organs to analyze biodistribution by detecting radioactive ^{32}P label. The majority of siRNA nanoparticles resided in either liver or kidney; however, it was interesting to see a significant accumulation directly at prostate tumors [42]. Hence, squalene conjugation was an exciting concept for ON's design. Nevertheless, squalene harvesting can be controversial due to the revolving of endangering the shark population.

2. Conclusions and Future Outcome

Hydrophobic modifications such as cholesterol, fatty acid, α-tocopherol, and squalene still have room to mature compared to medicinal nanoformulation such as micelle, lipoplex, or, even, LNP. Of course, the primary goal of bioconjugation is elevating hydrophobic profile of ON-based therapy but a deeper quantitative understanding of structure related to delivery efficacy is still underappreciated. As mentioned in Biscan et al., the hydrophobicity profile of three distinctive lipid conjugates (dimeric Myr, cholesterol, and tocopherol succinate) appear to be similar as quantified via HPLC (measured in retention time); however, the biodistribution pathways are concluded to be diverse. Countless observation of multiple lipoid conjugates is accumulated at large in the secretory organ (liver) but detection at other tissues includes the spleen, kidney, and, even, skeletal muscle tissue will pave the way to develop novel delivery techniques to extrahepatic tissues [53]. Some fatty acids, such as docosanoic acid, had the ability to penetrate to skeletal muscle and, even, in the brain, which required direct spinal injection (unfavorable for human application) [37]. Aimed with current understanding, additional structural explorations would lead to better optimization for highly stable and selective modified ON; thus, current drawbacks in pharmacokinetic and biodistribution can be properly addressed. Moreover, there were still potential and unexplored lipophilic moiety both naturally occurred and artificial that can be examined to potentiate the delivery of ON-based therapy. More so, the profound pharmacokinetic, efficacy, and toxicity data from the previous conjugation can be utilized to develop a learning-based artificial intelligence to predict of other lipid species or even fabricate novel artificial structures in the quest of advancing ON-based therapy in the new height.

In the future, the hope of better delivery of ON therapy can reduce the need of a large dose to patients which can significantly cut down the cost of treatment. Currently, the patient-affordable cost for ON therapy is astronomical for individuals in need. Eteplirsen, the current treatment for DMD, was marketed in 2017 with the price of $300,000/patient a year; while nusinersen charges patients up to $750,000 for the first year following with $350,000 for consecutive years [104]. Such skyscraper cost of therapy can associate to denial of coverage from insurance companies. Even with approval, the insurance coverage may increase annually, which will devastate other members within the same insurance network. Therefore, the work of uncovering the most optimized delivery is not only limited to certain method but it is a combination effort of both bioconjugation and nanoparticle formulation.

Author Contributions: Conceptualization, H.-y.L., P.T. and T.W.; writing—original draft preparation, P.T. and T.W.; writing—review and editing, P.T., Z.L. and H.-y.L.; visualization, P.T. and T.W.; supervision, H.-y.L.; project administration, H.-y.L.; funding acquisition, H.-y.L. All authors have read and agreed to the published version of the manuscript.

Funding: This research was supported by Helen Adams & Arkansas Research Alliance Endowed Chair Fund.

Institutional Review Board Statement: Not applicable.

Informed Consent Statement: Not applicable.

Conflicts of Interest: The authors declare no conflict of interest. This manuscript reflects the views of the authors and does not necessarily reflect those of the Food and Drug Administration. Any mention of commercial products is for clarification only and is not intended as approval, endorsement, or recommendation.

References

1. Crooke, S.T. Molecular Mechanisms of Antisense Oligonucleotides. *Nucleic Acid Ther.* **2017**, *27*, 70–77. [CrossRef] [PubMed]
2. Li, X.; Feng, K.; Li, L.; Yang, L.; Pan, X.; Yazd, H.S.; Cui, C.; Li, J., Moroz, L.; Sun, Y.; et al. Lipid Oligonucleotide Conjugates for Bioapplications. *Natl. Sci. Rev.* **2020**, *7*, 1933–1953. [CrossRef] [PubMed]
3. Lv, H.; Zhang, S.; Wang, B.; Cui, S.; Yan, J. Toxicity of Cationic Lipids and Cationic Polymers in Gene Delivery. *J. Control. Release* **2006**, *114*, 100–109. [CrossRef] [PubMed]
4. Monnery, B.D.; Wright, M.; Cavill, R.; Hoogenboom, R.; Shaunak, S.; Steinke, J.H.G.; Thanou, M. Cytotoxicity of Polycations: Relationship of Molecular Weight and the Hydrolytic Theory of the Mechanism of Toxicity. *Int. J. Pharm.* **2017**, *521*, 249–258. [CrossRef]
5. Vickers, T.; Baker, B.F.; Cook, P.D.; Zounes, M.; Buckheit, R.W.; Germany, J.; Ecker, D.J. Inhibition of HIV-LTR Gene Expression by Oligonucleotides Targeted to the TAR Element. *Nucl. Acids Res.* **1991**, *19*, 3359–3368. [CrossRef]
6. Donis-Keller, H. Site Specific Enzymatic Cleavage of RNA. *Nucl. Acids Res.* **1979**, *7*, 179–192. [CrossRef]
7. Casey, B.P.; Glazer, P.M. Gene Targeting via Triple-Helix Formation. In *Progress in Nucleic Acid Research and Molecular Biology*; Elsevier: Amsterdam, The Netherlands, 2001; Volume 67, pp. 163–192. ISBN 978-0-12-540067-1.
8. Rand, T.A.; Petersen, S.; Du, F.; Wang, X. Argonaute2 Cleaves the Anti-Guide Strand of SiRNA during RISC Activation. *Cell* **2005**, *123*, 621–629. [CrossRef]
9. Bumcrot, D.; Manoharan, M.; Koteliansky, V.; Sah, D.W.Y. RNAi Therapeutics: A Potential New Class of Pharmaceutical Drugs. *Nat. Chem. Biol.* **2006**, *2*, 711–719. [CrossRef]
10. De Smet, M.D.; Meenken, C.; van den Horn, G.J. Fomivirsen—a Phosphorothioate Oligonucleotide for the Treatment of CMV Retinitis. *Ocul. Immunol. Inflamm.* **1999**, *7*, 189–198. [CrossRef]
11. Xiong, H.; Veedu, R.N.; Diermeier, S.D. Recent Advances in Oligonucleotide Therapeutics in Oncology. *IJMS* **2021**, *22*, 3295. [CrossRef]
12. Agrawal, S.; Temsamani, J.; Galbraith, W.; Tang, J. Pharmacokinetics of Antisense Oligonucleotides. *Clin. Pharmacokinet.* **1995**, *28*, 7–16. [CrossRef] [PubMed]
13. Juliano, R.; Bauman, J.; Kang, H.; Ming, X. Biological Barriers to Therapy with Antisense and SiRNA Oligonucleotides. *Mol. Pharm.* **2009**, *6*, 686–695. [CrossRef] [PubMed]
14. Jason, T.L.H.; Koropatnick, J.; Berg, R.W. Toxicology of Antisense Therapeutics. *Toxicol. Appl. Pharmacol.* **2004**, *201*, 66–83. [CrossRef] [PubMed]
15. Crooke, S.T.; Wang, S.; Vickers, T.A.; Shen, W.; Liang, X. Cellular Uptake and Trafficking of Antisense Oligonucleotides. *Nat. Biotechnol.* **2017**, *35*, 230–237. [CrossRef] [PubMed]

16. Geary, R.S. Antisense Oligonucleotide Pharmacokinetics and Metabolism. *Expert Opin. Drug Metab. Toxicol.* **2009**, *5*, 381–391. [CrossRef]
17. Geary, R.S.; Norris, D.; Yu, R.; Bennett, C.F. Pharmacokinetics, Biodistribution and Cell Uptake of Antisense Oligonucleotides. *Adv. Drug Deliv. Rev.* **2015**, *87*, 46–51. [CrossRef]
18. Wójcik, M.; Cieślak, M.; Stec, W.J.; Goding, J.W.; Koziołkiewicz, M. Nucleotide Pyrophosphatase/Phosphodiesterase 1 Is Responsible for Degradation of Antisense Phosphorothioate Oligonucleotides. *Oligonucleotides* **2007**, *17*, 134–145. [CrossRef]
19. Khvorova, A.; Watts, J.K. The Chemical Evolution of Oligonucleotide Therapies of Clinical Utility. *Nat. Biotechnol.* **2017**, *35*, 238–248. [CrossRef]
20. Singh, S.K.; Koshkin, A.A.; Wengel, J.; Nielsen, P. LNA (Locked Nucleic Acids): Synthesis and High-Affinity Nucleic Acid Recognition. *Chem. Commun.* **1998**, 455–456. [CrossRef]
21. Agrawal, S.; Crooke, S.T. *Antisense Research and Application*; Springer: Berlin, Germany; New York, NY, USA, 1998; pp. 51–101. ISBN 978-3-642-58785-6.
22. Lima, W.F.; Crooke, S.T. Binding Affinity and Specificity of *Escherichia Coli* RNase H1: Impact on the Kinetics of Catalysis of Antisense Oligonucleotide−RNA Hybrids. *Biochemistry* **1997**, *36*, 390–398. [CrossRef]
23. Goyenvalle, A.; Leumann, C.; Garcia, L. Therapeutic Potential of Tricyclo-DNA Antisense Oligonucleotides. *J. Neuromuscular Dis.* **2016**, *3*, 157–167. [CrossRef] [PubMed]
24. Verbeure, B. RNase H Mediated Cleavage of RNA by Cyclohexene Nucleic Acid (CeNA). *Nucleic Acids Res.* **2001**, *29*, 4941–4947. [CrossRef] [PubMed]
25. Nan, Y.; Zhang, Y.-J. Antisense Phosphorodiamidate Morpholino Oligomers as Novel Antiviral Compounds. *Front. Microbiol.* **2018**, *9*, 750. [CrossRef] [PubMed]
26. Frazier, K.S. Antisense Oligonucleotide Therapies: The Promise and the Challenges from a Toxicologic Pathologist's Perspective. *Toxicol. Pathol.* **2015**, *43*, 78–89. [CrossRef] [PubMed]
27. Zanardi, T.A.; Kim, T.-W.; Shen, L.; Serota, D.; Papagiannis, C.; Park, S.-Y.; Kim, Y.; Henry, S.P. Chronic Toxicity Assessment of 2′-O -Methoxyethyl Antisense Oligonucleotides in Mice. *Nucleic Acid Ther.* **2018**, *28*, 233–241. [CrossRef] [PubMed]
28. Bozzer, S.; Bo, M.D.; Toffoli, G.; Macor, P.; Capolla, S. Nanoparticles-Based Oligonucleotides Delivery in Cancer: Role of Zebrafish as Animal Model. *Pharmaceutics* **2021**, *13*, 1106. [CrossRef]
29. Zhang, Y.; Sun, C.; Wang, C.; Jankovic, K.E.; Dong, Y. Lipids and Lipid Derivatives for RNA Delivery. *Chem. Rev.* **2021**, *121*, 12181–12277. [CrossRef] [PubMed]
30. Schoenmaker, L.; Witzigmann, D.; Kulkarni, J.A.; Verbeke, R.; Kersten, G.; Jiskoot, W.; Crommelin, D.J.A. MRNA-Lipid Nanoparticle COVID-19 Vaccines: Structure and Stability. *Int. J. Pharm.* **2021**, *601*, 120586. [CrossRef]
31. Moss, K.H.; Popova, P.; Hadrup, S.R.; Astakhova, K.; Taskova, M. Lipid Nanoparticles for Delivery of Therapeutic RNA Oligonucleotides. *Mol. Pharm.* **2019**, *16*, 2265–2277. [CrossRef]
32. Li, Z.; Rana, T.M. Therapeutic Targeting of MicroRNAs: Current Status and Future Challenges. *Nat. Rev. Drug Discov.* **2014**, *13*, 622–638. [CrossRef]
33. Osborn, M.F.; Coles, A.H.; Biscans, A.; Haraszti, R.A.; Roux, L.; Davis, S.; Ly, S.; Echeverria, D.; Hassler, M.R.; Godinho, B.M.D.C.; et al. Hydrophobicity Drives the Systemic Distribution of Lipid-Conjugated SiRNAs via Lipid Transport Pathways. *Nucleic Acids Res.* **2019**, *47*, 1070–1081. [CrossRef]
34. Hassler, M.R.; Turanov, A.A.; Alterman, J.F.; Haraszti, R.A.; Coles, A.H.; Osborn, M.F.; Echeverria, D.; Nikan, M.; Salomon, W.E.; Roux, L.; et al. Comparison of Partially and Fully Chemically-Modified SiRNA in Conjugate-Mediated Delivery in Vivo. *Nucleic Acids Res.* **2018**, *46*, 2185–2196. [CrossRef] [PubMed]
35. Raouane, M.; Desmaële, D.; Urbinati, G.; Massaad-Massade, L.; Couvreur, P. Lipid Conjugated Oligonucleotides: A Useful Strategy for Delivery. *Bioconjugate Chem.* **2012**, *23*, 1091–1104. [CrossRef] [PubMed]
36. Letsinger, R.L.; Zhang, G.R.; Sun, D.K.; Ikeuchi, T.; Sarin, P.S. Cholesteryl-Conjugated Oligonucleotides: Synthesis, Properties, and Activity as Inhibitors of Replication of Human Immunodeficiency Virus in Cell Culture. *Proc. Natl. Acad. Sci. USA* **1989**, *86*, 6553–6556. [CrossRef] [PubMed]
37. Nikan, M.; Osborn, M.F.; Coles, A.H.; Godinho, B.M.; Hall, L.M.; Haraszti, R.A.; Hassler, M.R.; Echeverria, D.; Aronin, N.; Khvorova, A. Docosahexaenoic Acid Conjugation Enhances Distribution and Safety of SiRNA upon Local Administration in Mouse Brain. *Mol. Ther. Nucleic Acids* **2016**, *5*, e344. [CrossRef] [PubMed]
38. Stetsenko, D.A.; Gait, M.J. A Convenient Solid-Phase Method for Synthesis of 3′-Conjugates of Oligonucleotides. *Bioconjugate Chem.* **2001**, *12*, 576–586. [CrossRef]
39. Ueno, Y.; Inoue, T.; Yoshida, M.; Yoshikawa, K.; Shibata, A.; Kitamura, Y.; Kitade, Y. Synthesis of Nuclease-Resistant SiRNAs Possessing Benzene-Phosphate Backbones in Their 3′-Overhang Regions. *Bioorganic Med. Chem. Lett.* **2008**, *18*, 5194–5196. [CrossRef]
40. Guzaev, A.; Lönnberg, H. Solid Support Synthesis of Ester Linked Hydrophobic Conjugates of Oligonucleotides. *Tetrahedron* **1999**, *55*, 9101–9116. [CrossRef]
41. Durand, A.; Brown, T. Synthesis And Properties Of Oligonucleotides Containing A Cholesterol Thymidine Monomer. *Nucleosides Nucleotides Nucleic Acids* **2007**, *26*, 785–794. [CrossRef]

42. Massaad-Massade, L.; Boutary, S.; Caillaud, M.; Gracia, C.; Parola, B.; Gnaouiya, S.B.; Stella, B.; Arpicco, S.; Buchy, E.; Desmaële, D.; et al. New Formulation for the Delivery of Oligonucleotides Using "Clickable" SiRNA-Polyisoprenoid-Conjugated Nanoparticles: Application to Cancers Harboring Fusion Oncogenes. *Bioconjugate Chem.* **2018**, *29*, 1961–1972. [CrossRef]
43. Raouane, M.; Desmaele, D.; Gilbert-Sirieix, M.; Gueutin, C.; Zouhiri, F.; Bourgaux, C.; Lepeltier, E.; Gref, R.; Ben Salah, R.; Clayman, G.; et al. Synthesis, Characterization, and in Vivo Delivery of SiRNA-Squalene Nanoparticles Targeting Fusion Oncogene in Papillary Thyroid Carcinoma. *J. Med. Chem.* **2011**, *54*, 4067–4076. [CrossRef] [PubMed]
44. Manoharan, M.; Tivel, K.L.; Andrade, L.K.; Mohan, V.; Condon, T.P.; Bennett, C.F.; Cook, P.D. Oligonucleotide Conjugates: Alteration of the Pharmacokinetic Properties of Antisense Agents. *Null* **1995**, *14*, 969–973. [CrossRef]
45. Bijsterbosch, M.K. Modulation of Plasma Protein Binding and in Vivo Liver Cell Uptake of Phosphorothioate Oligodeoxynucleotides by Cholesterol Conjugation. *Nucleic Acids Res.* **2000**, *28*, 2717–2725. [CrossRef]
46. Lorenz, C.; Hadwiger, P.; John, M.; Vornlocher, H.-P.; Unverzagt, C. Steroid and Lipid Conjugates of SiRNAs to Enhance Cellular Uptake and Gene Silencing in Liver Cells. *Bioorganic Med. Chem. Lett.* **2004**, *14*, 4975–4977. [CrossRef] [PubMed]
47. Soutschek, J.; Akinc, A.; Bramlage, B.; Charisse, K.; Constien, R.; Donoghue, M.; Elbashir, S.; Geick, A.; Hadwiger, P.; Harborth, J.; et al. Therapeutic Silencing of an Endogenous Gene by Systemic Administration of Modified SiRNAs. *Nature* **2004**, *432*, 173–178. [CrossRef] [PubMed]
48. Wolfrum, C.; Shi, S.; Jayaprakash, K.N.; Jayaraman, M.; Wang, G.; Pandey, R.K.; Rajeev, K.G.; Nakayama, T.; Charrise, K.; Ndungo, E.M.; et al. Mechanisms and Optimization of in Vivo Delivery of Lipophilic SiRNAs. *Nat. Biotechnol.* **2007**, *25*, 1149–1157. [CrossRef] [PubMed]
49. Godinho, B.M.D.C.; Gilbert, J.W.; Haraszti, R.A.; Coles, A.H.; Biscans, A.; Roux, L.; Nikan, M.; Echeverria, D.; Hassler, M.; Khvorova, A. Pharmacokinetic Profiling of Conjugated Therapeutic Oligonucleotides: A High-Throughput Method Based Upon Serial Blood Microsampling Coupled to Peptide Nucleic Acid Hybridization Assay. *Nucleic Acid Ther.* **2017**, *27*, 323–334. [CrossRef]
50. Pei, D.; Buyanova, M. Overcoming Endosomal Entrapment in Drug Delivery. *Bioconjugate Chem.* **2019**, *30*, 273–283. [CrossRef]
51. Zheng, Y.; Tai, W. Insight into the SiRNA Transmembrane Delivery—From Cholesterol Conjugating to Tagging. *WIREs Nanomed. Nanobiotechnol.* **2020**, *12*, e1606. [CrossRef]
52. Du Rietz, H.; Hedlund, H.; Wilhelmson, S.; Nordenfelt, P.; Wittrup, A. Imaging Small Molecule-Induced Endosomal Escape of SiRNA. *Nat. Commun.* **2020**, *11*, 1809. [CrossRef]
53. Biscans, A.; Coles, A.; Haraszti, R.; Echeverria, D.; Hassler, M.; Osborn, M.; Khvorova, A. Diverse Lipid Conjugates for Functional Extra-Hepatic SiRNA Delivery in vivo. *Nucleic Acids Res.* **2019**, *47*, 1082–1096. [CrossRef] [PubMed]
54. Lindholm, M.W. PCSK9 LNA Antisense Oligonucleotides Induce Sustained Reduction of LDL Cholesterol in Nonhuman Primates. *Cell Ther.* **2012**, *20*, 6. [CrossRef] [PubMed]
55. Rocha, C.S.J.; Wiklander, O.P.B.; Larsson, L.; Moreno, P.M.D.; Parini, P.; Lundin, K.E.; Smith, C.I.E. RNA Therapeutics Inactivate PCSK9 by Inducing a Unique Intracellular Retention Form. *J. Mol. Cell. Cardiol.* **2015**, *8*, 186–193. [CrossRef] [PubMed]
56. Poelgeest, E.P.; Hodges, M.R.; Moerland, M.; Tessier, Y.; Levin, A.A.; Persson, R.; Lindholm, M.W.; Erichsen, K.D.; Ørum, H.; Cohen, A.F.; et al. Antisense-Mediated Reduction of Proprotein Convertase Subtilisin/Kexin Type 9 (PCSK9): A First-in-Human Randomized, Placebo-Controlled Trial. *Br. J. Clin. Pharmacol.* **2015**, *80*, 1350–1361. [CrossRef]
57. Crooke, R.M. An Apolipoprotein B Antisense Oligonucleotide Lowers LDL Cholesterol in Hyperlipidemic Mice without Causing Hepatic Steatosis. *J. Lipid Res.* **2005**, *13*, 872–884. [CrossRef]
58. Mullick, A.E.; Fu, W.; Graham, M.J.; Lee, R.G.; Witchell, D.; Bell, T.A.; Whipple, C.P.; Crooke, R.M. Antisense Oligonucleotide Reduction of ApoB-Ameliorated Atherosclerosis in LDL Receptor-Deficient Mice. *J. Lipid Res.* **2011**, *52*, 885–896. [CrossRef]
59. Agarwala, A.; Jones, P.; Nambi, V. The Role of Antisense Oligonucleotide Therapy in Patients with Familial Hypercholesterolemia: Risks, Benefits, and Management Recommendations. *Curr. Atheroscler. Rep.* **2015**, *8*, 467. [CrossRef]
60. Santos, R.D.; Raal, F.J.; Catapano, A.L.; Witztum, J.L.; Steinhagen-Thiessen, E.; Tsimikas, S. Mipomersen, an Antisense Oligonucleotide to Apolipoprotein B-100, Reduces Lipoprotein(a) in Various Populations With Hypercholesterolemia. *Arterioscler. Thromb. Vasc. Biol.* **2015**, *11*, 689–699. [CrossRef]
61. Wada, S.; Yasuhara, H.; Wada, F.; Sawamura, M.; Waki, R.; Yamamoto, T.; Harada-Shiba, M.; Obika, S. Evaluation of the Effects of Chemically Different Linkers on Hepatic Accumulations, Cell Tropism and Gene Silencing Ability of Cholesterol-Conjugated Antisense Oligonucleotides. *J. Control. Release* **2016**, *226*, 57–65. [CrossRef]
62. Nakajima, M.; Kasuya, T.; Yokota, S.; Onishi, R.; Ikehara, T.; Kugimiya, A.; Watanabe, A. Gene Silencing Activity and Hepatic Accumulation of Antisense Oligonucleotides Bearing Cholesterol-Conjugated Thiono Triester at the Gap Region. *Nucleic Acid Ther.* **2017**, *27*, 232–237. [CrossRef]
63. Watanabe, A.; Nakajima, M.; Kasuya, T.; Onishi, R.; Kitade, N.; Mayumi, K.; Ikehara, T.; Kugimiya, A. Comparative Characterization of Hepatic Distribution and MRNA Reduction of Antisense Oligonucleotides Conjugated with Triantennary N-Acetyl Galactosamine and Lipophilic Ligands Targeting Apolipoprotein B. *J. Pharmacol. Exp. Ther.* **2016**, *357*, 320–330. [CrossRef] [PubMed]
64. Liu, Y.M.; Xia, Y.; Dai, W.; Han, H.Y.; Dong, Y.X.; Cai, J.; Zeng, X.; Luo, F.Y.; Yang, T.; Li, Y.Z.; et al. Cholesterol-Conjugated Let-7amimics: Antitumor Efficacy on Hepatocellular Carcinoma in Vitro and in a Preclinical Orthotopic Xenograft Model of Systemic Therapy. *BMC Cancer* **2014**, *14*, 889. [CrossRef] [PubMed]

65. Anthony, V.; Skach, W.R. Molecular Mechanism of P-Glycoprotein Assembly into Cellular Membranes. *Curr Protein Pept. Sci.* **2002**, *3*, 485–501. [CrossRef] [PubMed]
66. Yang, Z.; Wu, D.; Bui, T.; Ho, R.J.Y. A Novel Human Multidrug Resistance Gene *MDR1* Variant *G571A* (G191R) Modulates Cancer Drug Resistance and Efflux Transport. *J. Pharmacol. Exp. Ther.* **2008**, *327*, 474–481. [CrossRef] [PubMed]
67. Petrova, N.S.; Chernikov, I.V.; Meschaninova, M.I.; Dovydenko, I.S.; Venyaminova, A.G.; Zenkova, M.A.; Vlassov, V.V.; Chernolovskaya, E.L. Carrier-Free Cellular Uptake and the Gene-Silencing Activity of the Lipophilic SiRNAs Is Strongly Affected by the Length of the Linker between SiRNA and Lipophilic Group. *Nucleic Acids Res.* **2012**, *40*, 2330–2344. [CrossRef] [PubMed]
68. Chernikov, I.V.; Gladkikh, D.V.; Karelina, U.A.; Meschaninova, M.I.; Ven'yaminova, A.G.; Vlassov, V.V.; Chernolovskaya, E.L. Trimeric Small Interfering RNAs and Their Cholesterol-Containing Conjugates Exhibit Improved Accumulation in Tumors, but Dramatically Reduced Silencing Activity. *Molecules* **2020**, *25*, 1877. [CrossRef] [PubMed]
69. DiFiglia, M.; Sena-Esteves, M.; Chase, K.; Sapp, E.; Pfister, E.; Sass, M.; Yoder, J.; Reeves, P.; Pandey, R.K.; Rajeev, K.G.; et al. Therapeutic Silencing of Mutant Huntingtin with SiRNA Attenuates Striatal and Cortical Neuropathology and Behavioral Deficits. *Proc. Natl. Acad. Sci. USA* **2007**, *104*, 17204–17209. [CrossRef]
70. Alterman, J.F.; Hall, L.M.; Coles, A.H.; Hassler, M.R.; Didiot, M.-C.; Chase, K.; Abraham, J.; Sottosanti, E.; Johnson, E.; Sapp, E.; et al. Hydrophobically Modified SiRNAs Silence Huntingtin MRNA in Primary Neurons and Mouse Brain. *Mol. Ther.—Nucleic Acids* **2015**, *4*, e266. [CrossRef]
71. Yuan, H.; Lanting, L.; Xu, Z.-G.; Li, S.-L.; Swiderski, P.; Putta, S.; Jonnalagadda, M.; Kato, M.; Natarajan, R. Effects of Cholesterol-Tagged Small Interfering RNAs Targeting 12/15-Lipoxygenase on Parameters of Diabetic Nephropathy in a Mouse Model of Type 1 Diabetes. *Am. J. Physiol.—Ren. Physiol.* **2008**, *295*, F605–F617. [CrossRef]
72. Wu, Y.; Navarro, F.; Lal, A.; Basar, E.; Pandey, R.K.; Manoharan, M.; Feng, Y.; Lee, S.J.; Lieberman, J.; Palliser, D. Durable Protection from Herpes Simplex Virus-2 Transmission Following Intravaginal Application of SiRNAs Targeting Both a Viral and Host Gene. *Cell Host Microbe* **2009**, *5*, 84–94. [CrossRef]
73. Rozema, D.B.; Lewis, D.L.; Wakefield, D.H.; Wong, S.C.; Klein, J.J.; Roesch, P.L.; Bertin, S.L.; Reppen, T.W.; Chu, Q.; Blokhin, A.V.; et al. Dynamic PolyConjugates for Targeted in Vivo Delivery of SiRNA to Hepatocytes. *Proc. Natl. Acad. Sci. USA* **2007**, *104*, 12982–12987. [CrossRef] [PubMed]
74. Turner, A.M.; Stolk, J.; Bals, R.; Lickliter, J.D.; Hamilton, J.; Christianson, D.R.; Given, B.D.; Burdon, J.G.; Loomba, R.; Stoller, J.K.; et al. Hepatic-Targeted RNA Interference Provides Robust and Persistent Knockdown of Alpha-1 Antitrypsin Levels in ZZ Patients. *J. Hepatol.* **2018**, *69*, 378–384. [CrossRef] [PubMed]
75. Hwang, J.; Chang, C.; Kim, J.H.; Oh, C.T.; Lee, H.N.; Lee, C.; Oh, D.; Lee, C.; Kim, B.; Hong, S.W.; et al. Development of Cell-Penetrating Asymmetric Interfering RNA Targeting Connective Tissue Growth Factor. *J. Investig. Dermatol.* **2016**, *136*, 2305–2313. [CrossRef] [PubMed]
76. Choe, J.Y.; Son, D.S.; Kim, Y.; Lee, J.; Shin, H.; Kim, W.J.; Kang, Y.G.; Dua, P.; Hong, S.W.; Park, J.H.; et al. L-Type Calcium Channel Blocker Enhances Cellular Delivery and Gene Silencing Potency of Cell-Penetrating Asymmetric SiRNAs. *Mol. Pharm.* **2020**, *17*, 777–786. [CrossRef]
77. Prakash, T.P.; Mullick, A.E.; Lee, R.G.; Yu, J.; Yeh, S.T.; Low, A.; Chappell, A.E.; Østergaard, M.E.; Murray, S.; Gaus, H.J.; et al. Fatty Acid Conjugation Enhances Potency of Antisense Oligonucleotides in Muscle. *Nucleic Acids Res.* **2019**, *47*, 6029–6044. [CrossRef]
78. Chappell, A.E.; Gaus, H.J.; Berdeja, A.; Gupta, R.; Jo, M.; Prakash, T.P.; Oestergaard, M.; Swayze, E.E.; Seth, P.P. Mechanisms of Palmitic Acid-Conjugated Antisense Oligonucleotide Distribution in Mice. *Nucleic Acids Res.* **2020**, *48*, 4382–4395. [CrossRef]
79. Biscans, A.; Coles, A.; Echeverria, D.; Khvorova, A. The Valency of Fatty Acid Conjugates Impacts SiRNA Pharmacokinetics, Distribution, and Efficacy in Vivo. *J. Control. Release* **2019**, *302*, 116–125. [CrossRef]
80. Elkina, Y.; von Haehling, S.; Anker, S.D.; Springer, J. The Role of Myostatin in Muscle Wasting: An Overview. *J. Cachexia Sarcopenia Muscle* **2011**, *2*, 143–151. [CrossRef]
81. Pirruccello-Straub, M.; Jackson, J.; Wawersik, S.; Webster, M.T.; Salta, L.; Long, K.; McConaughy, W.; Capili, A.; Boston, C.; Carven, G.J.; et al. Blocking Extracellular Activation of Myostatin as a Strategy for Treating Muscle Wasting. *Sci. Rep.* **2018**, *8*, 2292. [CrossRef]
82. Kobayashi, M.; Kasamatsu, S.; Shinozaki, S.; Yasuhara, S.; Kaneki, M. Myostatin Deficiency Not Only Prevents Muscle Wasting but Also Improves Survival in Septic Mice. *Am. J. Physiol. -Endocrinol. Metab.* **2021**, *320*, E150–E159. [CrossRef]
83. St. Andre, M.; Johnson, M.; Bansal, P.N.; Wellen, J.; Robertson, A.; Opsahl, A.; Burch, P.M.; Bialek, P.; Morris, C.; Owens, J. A Mouse Anti-Myostatin Antibody Increases Muscle Mass and Improves Muscle Strength and Contractility in the Mdx Mouse Model of Duchenne Muscular Dystrophy and Its Humanized Equivalent, Domagrozumab (PF-06252616), Increases Muscle Volume in Cynomolgus Monkeys. *Skelet. Muscle* **2017**, *7*, 25. [CrossRef]
84. Wagner, K.R. The Elusive Promise of Myostatin Inhibition for Muscular Dystrophy. *Curr. Opin. Neurol.* **2020**, *33*, 621–628. [CrossRef] [PubMed]
85. Mariot, V.; Le Guiner, C.; Barthélémy, I.; Montus, M.; Blot, S.; Torelli, S.; Morgan, J.; Muntoni, F.; Voit, T.; Dumonceaux, J. Myostatin Is a Quantifiable Biomarker for Monitoring Pharmaco-Gene Therapy in Duchenne Muscular Dystrophy. *Mol. Ther.—Methods Clin. Dev.* **2020**, *18*, 415–421. [CrossRef] [PubMed]
86. Biscans, A.; Caiazzi, J.; McHugh, N.; Hariharan, V.; Muhuri, M.; Khvorova, A. Docosanoic Acid Conjugation to SiRNA Enables Functional and Safe Delivery to Skeletal and Cardiac Muscles. *Mol. Ther.* **2021**, *29*, 1382–1394. [CrossRef] [PubMed]

87. Lim, K.R.; Maruyama, R.; Yokota, T. Eteplirsen in the Treatment of Duchenne Muscular Dystrophy. *Drug Des. Dev. Ther.* **2017**, *11*, 533–545. [CrossRef] [PubMed]
88. Wurster, C.D.; Ludolph, A.C. Nusinersen for Spinal Muscular Atrophy. *Ther. Adv. Neurol. Disord.* **2018**, *11*, 1756285618754459. [CrossRef]
89. Scoto, M.; Finkel, R.; Mercuri, E.; Muntoni, F. Genetic Therapies for Inherited Neuromuscular Disorders. *Lancet Child Adolesc. Health* **2018**, *2*, 600–609. [CrossRef]
90. Carver, M.P.; Charleston, J.S.; Shanks, C.; Zhang, J.; Mense, M.; Sharma, A.K.; Kaur, H.; Sazani, P. Toxicological Characterization of Exon Skipping Phosphorodiamidate Morpholino Oligomers (PMOs) in Non-Human Primates. *J. Neuromuscul. Dis.* **2016**, *30*, 381–393. [CrossRef]
91. Marian, C.O.; Cho, S.K.; McEllin, B.M.; Maher, E.A.; Hatanpaa, K.J.; Madden, C.J.; Mickey, B.E.; Wright, W.E.; Shay, J.W.; Bachoo, R.M. The Telomerase Antagonist, Imetelstat, Efficiently Targets Glioblastoma Tumor-Initiating Cells Leading to Decreased Proliferation and Tumor Growth. *Clin. Cancer Res.* **2010**, *16*, 154–163. [CrossRef]
92. Shammas, M.A.; Koley, H.; Bertheau, R.C.; Neri, P.; Fulciniti, M.; Tassone, P.; Blotta, S.; Protopopov, A.; Mitsiades, C.; Batchu, R.B.; et al. Telomerase Inhibitor GRN163L Inhibits Myeloma Cell Growth in Vitro and in Vivo. *Leukemia* **2008**, *22*, 1410–1418. [CrossRef]
93. Shammas, M.A.; Qazi, A.; Batchu, R.B.; Bertheau, R.C.; Wong, J.Y.Y.; Rao, M.Y.; Prasad, M.; Chanda, D.; Ponnazhagan, S.; Anderson, K.C.; et al. Telomere Maintenance in Laser Capture Microdissection-Purified Barrett's Adenocarcinoma Cells and Effect of Telomerase Inhibition in Vivo. *Clin. Cancer Res.* **2008**, *14*, 4971–4980. [CrossRef] [PubMed]
94. Gellert, G.C.; Dikmen, Z.G.; Wright, W.E.; Gryaznov, S.; Shay, J.W. Effects of a Novel Telomerase Inhibitor, GRN163L, in Human Breast Cancer. *Breast Cancer Res. Treat.* **2006**, *96*, 73–81. [CrossRef] [PubMed]
95. Dikmen, Z.G.; Gellert, G.C.; Jackson, S.; Gryaznov, S.; Tressler, R.; Dogan, P.; Wright, W.E.; Shay, J.W. In Vivo Inhibition of Lung Cancer by GRN163L: A Novel Human Telomerase Inhibitor. *Cancer Res.* **2005**, *65*, 7866–7873. [CrossRef] [PubMed]
96. Djojosubroto, M.W.; Chin, A.C.; Go, N.; Schaetzlein, S.; Manns, M.P.; Gryaznov, S.; Harley, C.B.; Rudolph, K.L. Telomerase Antagonists GRN163 and GRN163L Inhibit Tumor Growth and Increase Chemosensitivity of Human Hepatoma. *Hepatology* **2005**, *42*, 1127–1136. [CrossRef]
97. Herbert, B.-S.; Gellert, G.C.; Hochreiter, A.; Pongracz, K.; Wright, W.E.; Zielinska, D.; Chin, A.C.; Harley, C.B.; Shay, J.W.; Gryaznov, S.M. Lipid Modification of GRN163, an N3′ → P5′ Thio-Phosphoramidate Oligonucleotide, Enhances the Potency of Telomerase Inhibition. *Oncogene* **2005**, *24*, 5262–5268. [CrossRef]
98. Benizri, S.; Gissot, A.; Martin, A.; Vialet, B.; Grinstaff, M.W.; Barthélémy, P. Bioconjugated Oligonucleotides: Recent Developments and Therapeutic Applications. *Bioconjugate Chem.* **2019**, *30*, 366–383. [CrossRef]
99. Burchett, K.M.; Yan, Y.; Ouellette, M.M. Telomerase Inhibitor Imetelstat (GRN163L) Limits the Lifespan of Human Pancreatic Cancer Cells. *PLoS ONE* **2014**, *9*, e85155. [CrossRef]
100. Kauss, T.; Arpin, C.; Bientz, L.; Vinh Nguyen, P.; Vialet, B.; Benizri, S.; Barthélémy, P. Lipid Oligonucleotides as a New Strategy for Tackling the Antibiotic Resistance. *Sci. Rep.* **2020**, *10*, 1054. [CrossRef]
101. Nishina, T.; Numata, J.; Nishina, K.; Yoshida-Tanaka, K.; Nitta, K.; Piao, W.; Iwata, R.; Ito, S.; Kuwahara, H.; Wada, T.; et al. Chimeric Antisense Oligonucleotide Conjugated to α-Tocopherol. *Mol. Ther.—Nucleic Acids* **2015**, *4*, e220. [CrossRef]
102. Orengo, J.P.; Chambon, P.; Metzger, D.; Mosier, D.R.; Snipes, G.J.; Cooper, T.A. Expanded CTG Repeats within the DMPK 3′ UTR Causes Severe Skeletal Muscle Wasting in an Inducible Mouse Model for Myotonic Dystrophy. *Proc. Natl. Acad. Sci. USA* **2008**, *105*, 2646–2651. [CrossRef]
103. Østergaard, M.E.; Jackson, M.; Low, A.; Chappell, A.E.; Lee, R.G.; Peralta, R.Q.; Yu, J.; Kinberger, G.A.; Dan, A.; Carty, R.; et al. Conjugation of Hydrophobic Moieties Enhances Potency of Antisense Oligonucleotides in the Muscle of Rodents and Non-Human Primates. *Nucleic Acids Res.* **2019**, *47*, 6045–6058. [CrossRef] [PubMed]
104. Stein, C.A.; Castanotto, D. FDA-Approved Oligonucleotide Therapies in 2017. *Mol. Ther.* **2017**, *25*, 1069–1075. [CrossRef] [PubMed]

pharmaceutics

MDPI

Review

Nanosystems, Drug Molecule Functionalization and Intranasal Delivery: An Update on the Most Promising Strategies for Increasing the Therapeutic Efficacy of Antidepressant and Anxiolytic Drugs

Jéssica L. Antunes [1], Joana Amado [1], Francisco Veiga [1,2], Ana Cláudia Paiva-Santos [1,2,*] and Patrícia C. Pires [1,2,3,*]

[1] Department of Pharmaceutical Technology, Faculty of Pharmacy, University of Coimbra, 3000-548 Coimbra, Portugal
[2] REQUIMTE/LAQV, Group of Pharmaceutical Technology, Faculty of Pharmacy, University of Coimbra, 3000-548 Coimbra, Portugal
[3] Health Sciences Research Centre (CICS-UBI), University of Beira Interior, Av. Infante D. Henrique, 6200-506 Covilhã, Portugal
* Correspondence: acsantos@ff.uc.pt (A.C.P.-S.); patriciapires93@gmail.com or patriciapires@ff.uc.pt (P.C.P.)

Abstract: Depression and anxiety are high incidence and debilitating psychiatric disorders, usually treated by antidepressant or anxiolytic drug administration, respectively. Nevertheless, treatment is usually given through the oral route, but the low permeability of the blood–brain barrier reduces the amount of drug that will be able to reach it, thus consequently reducing the therapeutic efficacy. Which is why it is imperative to find new solutions to make these treatments more effective, safer, and faster. To overcome this obstacle, three main strategies have been used to improve brain drug targeting: the intranasal route of administration, which allows the drug to be directly transported to the brain by neuronal pathways, bypassing the blood–brain barrier and avoiding the hepatic and gastrointestinal metabolism; the use of nanosystems for drug encapsulation, including polymeric and lipidic nanoparticles, nanometric emulsions, and nanogels; and drug molecule functionalization by ligand attachment, such as peptides and polymers. Pharmacokinetic and pharmacodynamic in vivo studies' results have shown that intranasal administration can be more efficient in brain targeting than other administration routes, and that the use of nanoformulations and drug functionalization can be quite advantageous in increasing brain–drug bioavailability. These strategies could be the key to future improved therapies for depressive and anxiety disorders.

Keywords: anxiety; blood–brain barrier; brain bioavailability; depression; drug molecule functionalization; intranasal; nanoemulsions; nanoparticles; nanosystems; nose-to-brain

Citation: Antunes, J.L.; Amado, J.; Veiga, F.; Paiva-Santos, A.C.; Pires, P.C. Nanosystems, Drug Molecule Functionalization and Intranasal Delivery: An Update on the Most Promising Strategies for Increasing the Therapeutic Efficacy of Antidepressant and Anxiolytic Drugs. *Pharmaceutics* **2023**, *15*, 998. https://doi.org/10.3390/pharmaceutics15030998

Academic Editor: Giuseppe De Rosa

Received: 25 February 2023
Revised: 9 March 2023
Accepted: 16 March 2023
Published: 20 March 2023

1. Introduction

1.1. Pathophysiology and Treatment of Depression and Anxiety Disorders: Current Aspects and Limitations

Anxiety is a central nervous system (CNS) disorder characterized by tension, restlessness, and increased effort to concentrate, with a persistent depressed mood and lack of interest in activities which pleasure was once taken from. We can consider the existence of several types of anxiety disorders, such as disorders related to separation, social anxiety, panic, specific phobias, and generalized anxiety disorder. These disorders generally begin in childhood, adolescence, or early adulthood. The general physiological mechanism by which these types of disorders arise is related to the γ-aminobutyric acid (GABA), which is inhibited and, hence, does not fulfill its role in the downregulation of neuronal excitability. It is estimated to affect millions of people worldwide, leading to a great loss in a person's quality of life [1–7].

In turn, depression is the biggest public health problem, making it a common mental disorder and one of the world's leading causes of disability. In 2020, this disease affected about 16% of the world's population [8]. The etiology of depression has been related to stress. It is usually manifested by a loss of interest, feelings of guilt, depressed mood, sleep disturbance, low energy, and suicidal thoughts and attempts. There are several theories around the origin of depression, but the most accepted is the monoamine theory, which is related to a decrease in serotonin, noradrenaline, and dopamine levels in the CNS. It is caused by decreased excitability on the dopaminergic and/or serotonergic pathway. The markers of oxidative stress may also indicate depression, such as low levels of glutathione (GSH) and other antioxidants, and high levels of thiobarbituric acid (TBARS), F2 isoprostanes, inflammatory cytokines, and reactive oxygen species. Depression has also been associated with low levels of catalase, an enzyme responsible for the degradation of hydrogen peroxide into water and oxygen. In depressive situations, this enzyme is in deficit and, therefore, there is an accumulation of reactive oxygen species and consequently oxidative stress [6,9–17].

Nowadays, oral and intravenous (IV) administrations are the most used in patients with depression or anxiety. However, for drugs whose target is the CNS, these routes have many disadvantages. The oral administration of central-acting drugs results in a low drug uptake by the brain and high drug distribution in the peripheral tissues. One of the main reasons for the failure of antidepressants and anxiolytics is the presence of the blood–brain barrier (BBB) and the existence of efflux pumps in the brain capillaries, endothelial cells, luminal membranes, and caveolae. As most antidepressant and anxiolytic drugs are substrates of these transporters, their brain bioavailability is limited, which causes a decrease in their effectiveness. Additionally, drugs that are administered orally can undergo chemical and metabolic degradation in the gastrointestinal tract, have drug–drug or food–drug interactions, have a slower therapeutic action which makes them non-adequate for emergency situations, and are only suitable for patients with the ability to swallow. On the other hand, the IV route is best in cases of emergency or when the patient is unable to swallow. However, it also has many disadvantages, such as invasiveness and the need for patient hospitalization, and difficulties in delivering the drug to the CNS due to the lack of penetration of the BBB [12,14,18–21].

The BBB is a physical and metabolic barrier that limits the transport of substances between the blood and the neuronal tissue and is responsible for maintaining the physiological stability of the brain and protecting the CNS from toxic agents and microorganisms. It is made of three layers, but it is the innermost layer that poses a greater problem for drug delivery to the CNS. The BBB is essentially made up of endothelial cells in the capillary walls and tight junctions that prevent the transport of drugs through the paracellular pathway between adjacent endothelial cells in the inner layer. The BBB also has a biochemical layer with high levels of efflux transport proteins, such as P-glycoprotein (P-gp) and multidrug-resistant protein-1, as well as the expression of many metabolic enzymes, which limit brain-drug uptake [22,23]. Despite all these limitations, small (molecular weight below 500 Da) and hydrophobic molecules, and some cells (such as monocytes, macrophages, and neutrophils) can be selectively transported to the brain [21–25].

Additionally, although currently a lot of different treatment strategies exist, including pharmacological treatments, psychotherapies, and brain stimulation techniques, less than half of patients achieve a complete remission with the first treatment [17,26,27]. For these reasons, several solutions have been studied to fight depression and anxiety in a more effective and safe way.

1.2. Potential Strategies for Enhancing Brain Drug Targeting and Bioavailability

1.2.1. Intranasal Administration

The nasal cavity has three main regions: the vestibular, respiratory, and olfactory regions. The vestibular region measures approximately 0.6 cm^2 and is located directly at the entrance of the nostrils. It contains nasal hairs (responsible for filtering inhaled particles), squamous epithelial cells, and some ciliated cells [28–31]. Next to it is the respiratory region (Figure 1), which corresponds to the largest nasal area, at 150 cm^2 [21,28]. It is the most vascularized region with the greatest variety of cells, containing goblet, ciliated, non-ciliated, and basal cells [28,31,32]. Goblet cells are responsible for secreting mucin, water, salts, a small group of proteins and lipids, and, together with some nasal glands, form the mucus layer. The mucus forms a layer in the respiratory epithelium and can trap inhaled molecules and send them to the pharynx, where they pass through to the gastrointestinal tract [21,28,29]. Basal cells are the key cells of the nasal cavity and have the ability to differentiate into another type of epithelial cell, if necessary. These cells also help to attach the ciliated and goblet cells to the lamina propria [21,29]. Ciliated cells, as the name suggests, have cilia that increase their surface area. They help to move the mucus toward the nasopharynx, resulting in mucociliary clearance [21,32]. Together with a high degree of vascularization, this makes the nasal respiratory region a site of high drug transport into the systemic circulation. However, the respiratory region is also innervated by the maxillary and ophthalmic branches of the trigeminal nerve (V1, V2), which originate in the brainstem fossa and have been suggested as a possible target for drug transport to the CNS [28,30].

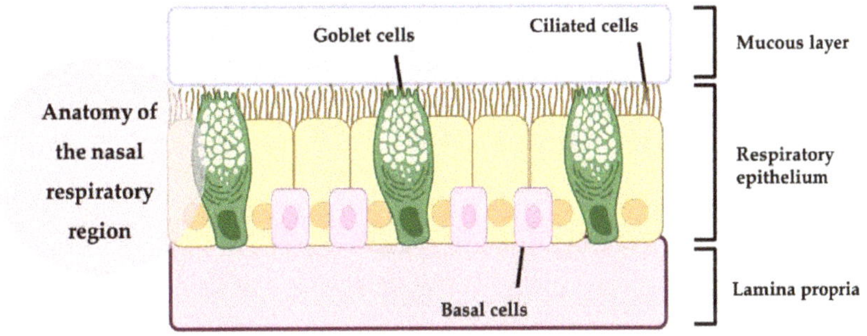

Figure 1. Anatomy of the nasal respiratory region (produced with BioRender).

In turn, the olfactory region is made up of olfactory receptors, the olfactory epithelium, and lamina propria (Figure 2). Olfactory receptors are unmyelinated neurons located in the nasal epithelium. In the lamina propria, each olfactory receptor forms thick bundles of axons that become olfactory nerves and innervate the cribriform plate, forming synaptic connections with the glomeruli of mitral cells in the olfactory bulb. There are two types of basal cells in this region: horizontal basal cells and spherical basal cells. In addition to horizontal basal cells, multipotent progenitor cells, and globular basal cells, this region also contains structural support cells that encase the olfactory receptors in the olfactory region, maintaining the structural integrity and ionization of the olfactory receptors. Drugs with small sizes can be transported through the axons, by the olfactory bulb, to the olfactory cortex, reaching the cerebellum [21,32,33].

Nasal secretions are composed of approximately 95% water, 2% mucin, 1% salts, 1% other proteins (albumin, immunoglobulins, lysozymes, and lactoferrin), and <1% lipids. They move through the nose at a rate of approximately 5 to 6 mm/min, resulting in particles being cleared from the nose every 15 to 20 min. In addition, enzymes such as isoforms of the cytochrome P450 (CYP1A, CYP2A, and CYP2E), carboxylesterases, and glutathione S-transferases can also be found in the nasal cavity Therefore, the residence time of the formulation (and, consequently, the drug) in the nasal cavity will also be affected by these enzymes' metabolism. To prolong the residence time of the formulation in the nasal cavity, and consequently increase the amount of drug that will be absorbed, biologically adhesive (mucoadhesive) excipients such as gelatin, chitosan, carbopol, and cellulose derivatives can be used [28,34].

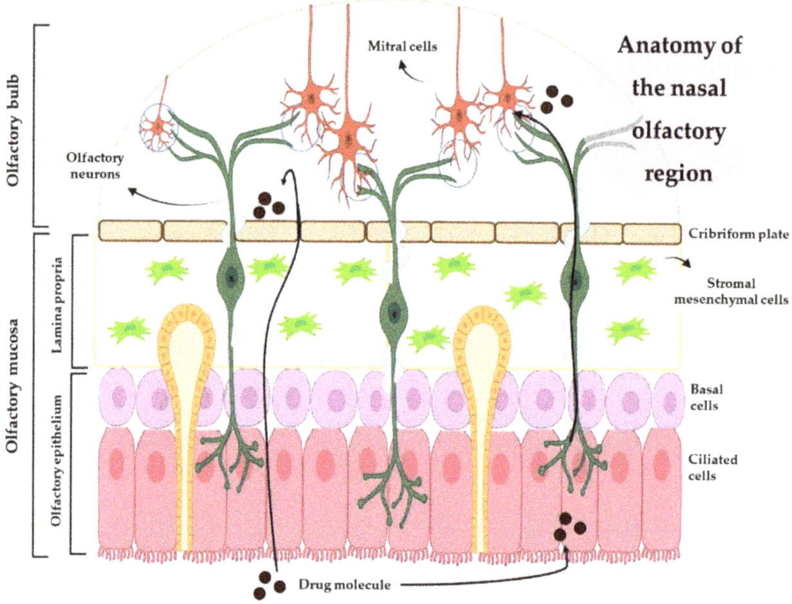

Figure 2. Anatomy of the nasal olfactory region (produced with BioRender).

IV drug delivery to the brain is largely influenced by the drug's plasma half-life, the extent of the metabolism, the degree of non-specific binding to plasma proteins, and the permeability of the compound across the BBB and into the peripheral tissues. Due to these issues, intranasal (IN) administration has been presented as a promising alternative to the IV route, having gained increasing interest over the past few years. After IN administration, the drug can take three different routes to the brain: one intracellular route and two extracellular routes (Figures 2 and 3). The intracellular route is activated after drug endocytosis by the olfactory sensory cells, and the drug is consequently transported through the neuronal axon to the synaptic clefts in the olfactory bulb, where it is released through exocytosis. Drugs are delivered by endocytosis to the olfactory sensory neurons and peripheral trigeminal neurons, and then transported intracellularly from the olfactory sensory nerve to the olfactory bulb, and from the trigeminal nerve to the brainstem. This is an extremely slow pathway and it can take hours for the drug to reach the olfactory bulb [28,33,35,36]. In the extracellular mechanism (Figure 3), the drug can follow two different routes: it can cross the gaps between the olfactory neurons and then be transported to the olfactory bulb, or it can be transported along the trigeminal nerve to avoid the BBB. Once the drug has reached the olfactory bulb or the trigeminal region, it can be transported to other areas of the brain by diffusion, which is facilitated by a perivascular pump that is activated by arterial pulsation [28,32,35].

1.2.2. Nanosystems

The currently marketed nasal preparations exist mainly in the form of solutions or suspensions, but labile, poorly soluble, poorly permeable, and/or less potent drugs may require a formulation that promotes drug bioavailability and, preferably, direct delivery to the brain. To this end, nanotechnology has emerged to fill the existing gaps. All nanosystems are characterized by their small size, which makes them suitable for transporting drugs to the target tissues and cells, where they are ideally released [20,37,38].

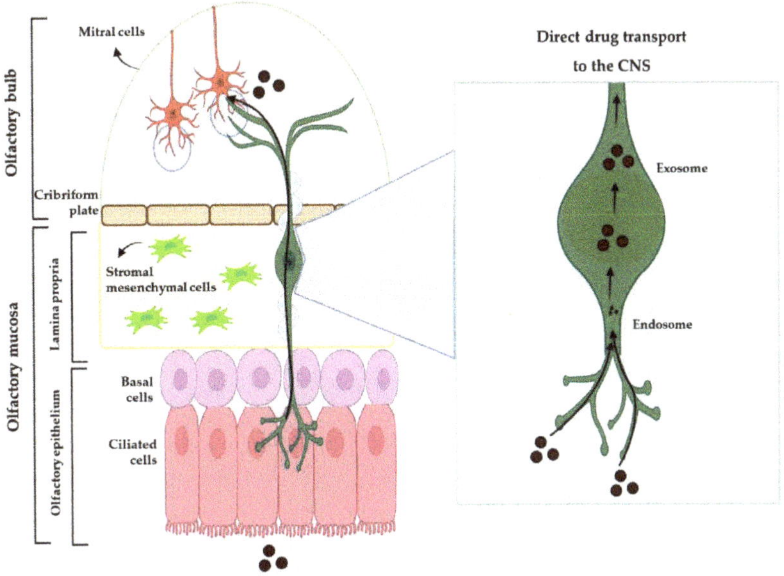

Figure 3. Extracellular mechanism of drug transport to the brain from the nasal cavity (produced with BioRender).

In terms of nanosystems that are meant to be administered by the IN route, these are designed to provide a longer residence time in the nasal cavity, overcome nasal mucociliary clearance, and facilitate rapid drug transport across the nasal mucosa. Independently of the intended administration route, there are several types of nanosystems (Figure 4), with the main being: polymeric nanoparticles (NP), which are divided into nanocapsules and nanospheres; lipid nanoparticles, namely solid lipid nanoparticles and nanostructured lipid carriers; liposomes; nanometric emulsions, such as nanoemulsions and microemulsions; and nanoemulgels [20,38–41].

Polymeric Nanoparticles

Polymeric nanoparticles are compact colloidal systems with a variable size range within the nanometric scale and can be composed of natural or synthetic polymers. They are composed of a dense core of polymeric matrix, suitable for encapsulating lipophilic drugs, and a hydrophilic crown that provides stability to the nanoparticles. The drug can be incorporated into the nanosystem in several ways: dissolved in the matrix, encapsulated within it, or adsorbed to it [20,39,42].

There are two main types of polymeric NP: nanocapsules (a reservoir system) and nanospheres (a matrix system). Nanocapsules consist of an oily core in which the drug is dissolved, surrounded by a polymeric shell that controls the drug release from the core. Nanospheres are based on a continuous polymeric network, and in these systems the drug is either retained inside the nanosphere or adsorbed onto its surface. Although NP can be presented in a variety of ways, they have common characteristics that make them advantageous formulations, such as biocompatibility, biodegradability, high drug loading, the possibility of controlled drug release, and stability during storage [43–45].

Several polymers can be used to produce NP for drug delivery. One of these is chitosan, a linear, natural, and biocompatible polysaccharide derived from the deacetylation of chitin from crustacean shells. It is a polymer that has some of the properties we need for effective and direct drug delivery to the brain, since it has the capacity to reduce mucociliary clearance and transiently opens tight junctions (protein kinase C pathway interaction), facilitating paracellular drug transport across the nasal mucosa to the brain [21,35,36,46].

Chitosan is insoluble at neutral and basic pH values, but forms salts with inorganic or organic acids, such as hydrochloric acid and glutamic acid, which are soluble in water up to about pH 6.3 (depending on the molecular weight and deacetylation degree and, therefore, pKa). To further improve the mucoadhesive properties of chitosan, derivatives with thiol groups have been developed. These groups provide enhanced ciliary mucoadhesion, by forming covalent bonds between the polymer and the mucus layer that are stronger than non-covalent bonds [21,35,47].

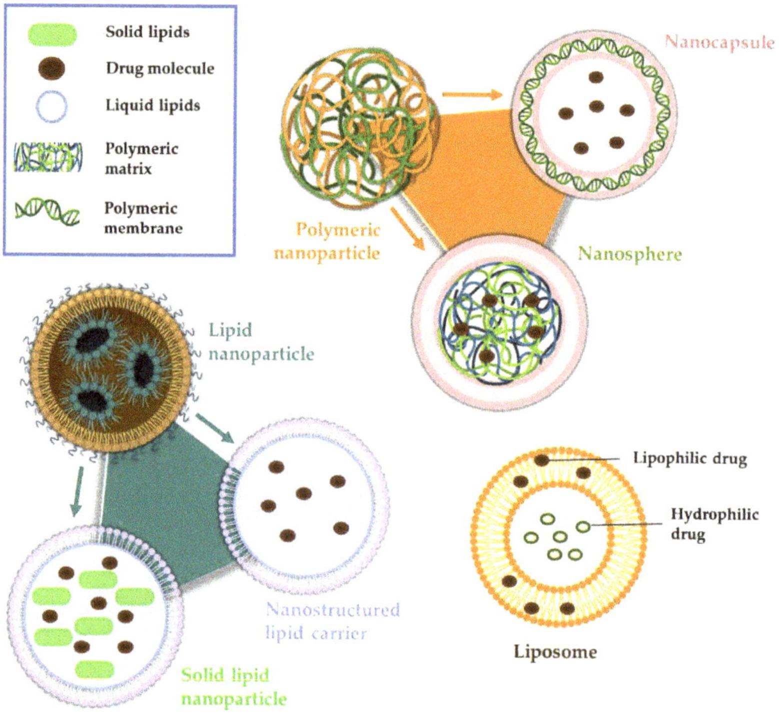

Figure 4. Main therapeutic nanosystem types (produced with BioRender).

Another polymer of interest is alginic acid, a natural polysaccharide found in the cell walls of brown algae. Alginate (AG) is a derivative of alginic acid, and it is usually used in formulations in salt form (sodium or calcium). It is a hydrophilic polymer that, when in the presence of divalent cations, forms a gel that allows a controlled drug release [21,46,48].

Poly lactic-co-glycolic acid (PLGA) is a synthetic polymer that is one of the most widely used polymers in controlled/directed drug delivery systems. This is due to its properties, such as biodegradability (hydrolysis to lactic acid and glycolic acid, which are metabolized by the body through the Krebs cycle), biocompatibility, and the ease of encapsulation of different types of drugs [21,49,50].

Lipid Nanoparticles

We can consider two categories of lipid nanoparticles: solid lipid nanoparticles (SLN) and nanostructured lipid carriers (NLC). SLN are matrix nanoparticles made of solid lipids dispersed in water or an aqueous surfactant solution. They have high physical stability, no organic solvents used in their manufacture, good biocompatibility and tolerability, and also allow a controlled drug release and prolong the nasal retention time due to their occlusive effect and adhesion to the mucosa. Despite these advantages, SLN have some drawbacks. These include a limited ability to solubilize hydrophilic molecules, low drug encapsulation efficiency (due to their crystalline structure), possible drug expulsion during storage due to the crystallization process, and an undesirable increase in particle size by agglomeration, which can lead to an immediate and unwanted drug release [33,36,42]. To improve some of these aspects, such as low stability, surfactants such as polyethylene glycol (PEG) can be used. PEG is a hydrophilic and biocompatible polymer that stabilizes nanoparticles and acts as a mucus penetration enhancer [21,51].

In turn, instead of having only solid lipids in their composition, NLC have a mixture of solid and liquid lipids that form an imperfect crystalline matrix into which drugs can be incorporated. This imperfect matrix increases the drug-loading capacity of the system and minimizes/avoids its immediate and undesired release during storage, thus overcoming these disadvantages of SLN. NLC are biodegradable and generally composed of physiological lipids, and therefore have low toxicity to the body and good tolerability. With this nanosystem, it is possible to achieve a higher drug encapsulation efficiency (compared to SLN), as hydrophobic molecules have a higher solubility in liquid lipids than in solid lipids. Nevertheless, the solubilization capacity of hydrophilic drugs is still low, which is a drawback of NLC [20,21,33].

Nanometric Emulsions

Regarding the nature of the external and internal phase(s), we can distinguish four types of nanometric emulsions: oil-in-water or water-in-oil (two phases) or oil-in-water-in-oil or water-in-oil-in-water (three phases). Oil-in-water nanometric emulsions, which are the most common, can solubilize and encapsulate hydrophobic drugs. A nanometric emulsion can improve drug stability and solubility and provide greater absorption due to the large surface area created by the small and numerous droplets [40,42,52].

Nanometric emulsions can also be classified according to other characteristics in microemulsions or nanoemulsions. Microemulsions (ME) are isotropic and thermodynamically stable colloidal dispersions. They are generally composed of oil, water, and surfactants, and have droplet sizes between 10 and 100 nm. The IN administration of an oil-in-water ME may allow direct transport to the brain due to its small droplet size and lipophilic nature. In turn, nanoemulsions are also colloidal systems of nanometric size, with droplet sizes between 20 and 200 nm, but they are thermodynamically unstable, which can lead to poor stability and drug release during storage. Similar to microemulsions, they also have an oil phase, an aqueous phase, and a surfactant. However, the latter is usually present in smaller quantities [21,38,41].

Nanogels

Nanogels are non-fluid colloidal or polymeric networks that increase their volume when in contact with a fluid, producing homogeneous solutions with low viscosity. These are defined as gel particles with a diameter of less than 100 nm. The use of nanogels is more effective than free drug administration (solution or other simple dispersion), since they have reported reduced toxicity, increased drug cellular uptake, high drug loading, and controlled drug release. This delivery system is effective for brain targeting as it leads to fast brain-drug absorption and has high biodegradability, biocompatibility, and hydrophilicity. It offers some advantages over other structures, such as the ability to encapsulate multiple molecules with different characteristics (both hydrophilic or hydrophobic) in the same formulation, leading to controlled drug release [53,54].

Liposomes

Liposomes are biocompatible and biodegradable vesicles composed of layers of phospholipids and cholesterol, enclosing one or more aqueous compartments. They may be unilamellar (smaller size) or multilamellar (larger size). Liposomes can transport hydrophilic and hydrophobic molecules due to their structural properties: hydrophilic drugs can be stored in the aqueous nucleus, whereas hydrophobic molecules can be dissolved in the lipid membrane. They have an overall good permeation capacity, including through the nasal mucosa, and can protect drugs from enzymatic degradation. Nevertheless, immunogenicity is a problem that needs to be solved, along with low encapsulation efficiency, to reduce the need for frequent administration. Compared to bigger liposomes, the smaller ones (generally neutral or positively charged) have a longer circulation time. Additionally, unmodified liposomes have a short circulation time and, therefore, are rapidly cleared, via systemic circulation, by the smooth endoplasmic reticulum cells [33,42,55].

Thus, to improve the circulation time of liposomes, modifications are made to their surface, such as coating them with PEG chains. In addition to PEG, it is common to use poloxamers, which are water-soluble, non-ionic polymers consisting of a triblock copolymer: a hydrophobic polypropylene glycol chain and two hydrophilic PEG chains. Suitable examples are poloxamer 407 and poloxamer 188, which have a high PEG content. Additionally, PEG reduces the viscosity of the nasal mucus and increases the penetration into the mucosa by interacting with lipid membranes and occlusion junctions, which is quite favorable for intranasal administration [21,42,54].

2. Successful Approaches to Increasing Brain Targeting and Bioavailability of Antidepressant and Anxiolytic Drugs

In general, the most common strategies for the increased brain targeting and bioavailability of antidepressant and anxiolytic drugs are: delivery via IN route; the use of several different types of nanosystems; and the complexation of drugs with compounds that allow them to be delivered more effectively to the desired site of action.

The most commonly studied classes of antidepressant drugs include selective serotonin reuptake inhibitors (SSRI), serotonin and noradrenaline reuptake inhibitors (SNRI), monoamine oxidase (MAO) inhibitors, and melatonin agonists. The effects of anxiolytic drugs, such as benzodiazepines, and natural products, antiepileptics, analgesics, and other drug classes on anxiety and depression have also been studied.

A summary of these molecules and their respective classifications is shown in Table 1, and a summary of the successful strategies that have been used to increase these drugs' brain targeting and bioavailability is present in Table 2.

Table 1. Summary of the drug molecules included in this review, including their approved drug classification and known action mechanism(s).

Drug Name	Drug Classification	Action Mechanism(s)	References
Agomelatine	Antidepressant	Melatonin MT1 and MT2 receptor agonist and a serotonin 5-HT2C receptor antagonist	[49]
Selegiline		MAO inhibitor	[56]
Buspirone	Anxiolytic	Serotonin 5-HT1A receptor agonist	[57–59]
Clobazam		Partial GABA receptor agonist	[60]
Venlafaxine	Antidepressant and anxiolytic	Serotonin and noradrenaline reuptake inhibitor	[61–64]
Duloxetine		Serotonin and noradrenaline reuptake inhibitor	[65]
Paroxetine		Selective serotonin reuptake inhibitor	[66]
Carbamazepine	Antiepileptic	Modulation of adenosine-mediated neurotransmitters	[67]
Tramadol	Analgesic	Opioid agonist and serotonin and noradrenaline reuptake inhibitor	[53]
Edaravone	Amyotrophic lateral sclerosis treatment	Free radical scavenger	[68]
Riluzole		Glutamate antagonist	[69]
Baicalein	Natural product	NA	[70]
Icariin		NA	[71]
Berberine		MAO inhibitor	[72]

NA—not available.

Table 2. Summary of the successful strategies that have been used to increase brain drug targeting and bioavailability in the treatment of depressive and anxiety disorders.

<table>
<tr><th>Drug Name</th><th>General Strategy</th><th>Nanosystem Type (When Applicable)</th><th>References</th></tr>
<tr><td>Agomelatine</td><td rowspan="4">Nanosystems and intranasal administration</td><td rowspan="3">Polymeric nanoparticles</td><td>[49]</td></tr>
<tr><td>Selegiline</td><td>[56]</td></tr>
<tr><td rowspan="3">Buspirone</td><td>[58]</td></tr>
<tr><td>Microemulsion</td><td>[59]</td></tr>
<tr><td>Intranasal administration</td><td>-</td><td>[57]</td></tr>
<tr><td>Clobazam</td><td>Nanosystems and intranasal administration</td><td>Microemulsion</td><td>[60]</td></tr>
<tr><td rowspan="4">Venlafaxine</td><td rowspan="3">Nanosystems and intranasal administration</td><td rowspan="3">Polymeric nanoparticles</td><td>[61]</td></tr>
<tr><td>[62]</td></tr>
<tr><td>[63]</td></tr>
<tr><td>Drug molecule functionalization</td><td>-</td><td>[64]</td></tr>
<tr><td>Duloxetine</td><td rowspan="2">Nanosystems and intranasal administration</td><td>Solid lipid nanoparticles</td><td>[65]</td></tr>
<tr><td>Paroxetine</td><td rowspan="2">Nanostructured lipid carriers</td><td>[66]</td></tr>
<tr><td>Carbamazepine</td><td>Nanosystems</td><td>[67]</td></tr>
<tr><td>Tramadol</td><td>Nanosystems and intranasal administration</td><td>Polymeric nanoparticles</td><td>[53]</td></tr>
<tr><td>Edaravone</td><td>Nanosystems</td><td>Liposomes</td><td>[68]</td></tr>
<tr><td>Riluzole</td><td>Nanosystems and intranasal administration</td><td>Polymeric nanoparticles</td><td>[69]</td></tr>
<tr><td>Baicalein</td><td>Nanosystems</td><td>Solid lipid nanoparticles</td><td>[70]</td></tr>
<tr><td>Icariin</td><td rowspan="2">Intranasal administration</td><td>-</td><td>[71]</td></tr>
<tr><td>Berberine</td><td>-</td><td>[72]</td></tr>
</table>

2.1. Antidepressant Drugs

2.1.1. Agomelatine

Agomelatine is a melatonin MT1 and MT2 receptor agonist and a serotonin 5-HT2C receptor antagonist. It has low oral bioavailability, a high first-pass effect, and a short elimination half-life (2–3 h) [49]. The study conducted by Jani et al. [49] aimed to circumvent these obstacles by producing a polymeric NP using PLGA and poloxamer 407. The PLGA NP had a size of 116 nm, a PDI of 0.057, and a zeta potential (ZP) of −22.7 mV. In ex vivo drug permeation studies (goat nasal mucosa), the developed formulation had the highest permeability, compared to an agomelatine suspension, probably due to its reduced particle size and high homogeneity. In vivo pharmacodynamic studies were conducted using forced swim tests. In these tests, it was demonstrated that rats induced with depression were immobile during the five minutes that they were in the water. In contrast, rats in which PLGA NP with agomelatine was administered (IN route) showed a significant reduction in immobility time. Hence, the PLGA NP proved to have therapeutic efficacy, effectively delivering the drug to the brain.

2.1.2. Selegiline

Selegiline is an MAO inhibitor and is a dose-dependent drug, which means that while a higher dose inhibits MAO-A and MAO-B, a lower dose only inhibits MAO-B. It has a high first-pass metabolism, low bioavailability, and a large number of adverse effects [56]. To overcome these problems, Singh et al. [56] developed thiolated chitosan NP (TCN) and unmodified chitosan NP (CNP) to enhance the intranasal delivery of selegiline. The particle size, PDI, and ZP of TCN were 215 nm, 0.057, and +17.06 mV, respectively. In terms of in vitro drug release, it was noted that at an early phase, within the first 2.5 h, the drug release from CNP was faster when compared to TCN. However, after 13 h, it was shown that the TCN had a cumulative release of 80%, whereas for the CNP this was only 68%, indicating an extended release by the TCN, but also a higher drug release at the end of the assay. In in vivo assays performed in rats, TCN significantly attenuated oxidative stress and restored mitochondrial complex activity. In addition, pharmacodynamic studies, which included immobility and locomotor activity tests, showed that, compared to CNP, which already resulted in more movement and less immobilized time, TCN had a more significant effect on improving the condition of the rats. Additionally, the sucrose preference test revealed that, at the beginning of the treatment, these rats had a decrease in water-with-sucrose intake, and an increase in intake at the end of the 14 days, during which the TCN were administered. Thus, the developed TCN seem to be promising candidates for IN administration in depression treatment.

2.2. *Anxiolytic Drugs*

2.2.1. Buspirone

Buspirone is a drug that has proven to be effective as an anxiolytic. Nevertheless, it undergoes extensive first-pass metabolism by the cytochrome P3A4 in the liver and intestine, resulting in low oral bioavailability (approximately 4%) and a short half-life (2–3 h). It is currently only available on the market as an oral tablet, and multiple daily doses are required because only a small amount of the drug reaches the intended therapeutic site of action [57–59].

Patil et al. [57] investigated whether the intranasal administration of buspirone could transport the drug directly to the brain, thereby increasing the cerebral bioavailability of the drug. Therefore, an intranasal buspirone solution was formulated with chitosan and β-cyclodextrins and compared with the intravenous administration of an aqueous solution of the drug. This study confirmed the increase in bioavailability and targeted delivery to the brain with the developed formulation IN delivery (DTP 76%), demonstrating the efficacy of the nasal route, as well as the incorporation of cyclodextrins and chitosan into the formulation, which increased not only drug solubility, but also its permeation and transport to the brain.

In turn, Bari et al. [58], developed TCN for the intranasal delivery of buspirone to the brain. Comparative studies were performed with CNP, and IN and IV drug solutions. In vitro drug release studies showed that while the percentage of buspirone release from the drug solution was almost complete after 2 h, the drug release in that same time from the CNP and TCN was only 51.8 and 46.6%, respectively. Hence, the developed nanosystems showed a controlled drug release. Furthermore, the ex vivo drug permeation study (porcine nasal mucosa) showed that TCN had a higher percentage of drug permeation across the nasal mucosa than all the other evaluated formulations. These results were probably due to the increased mucoadhesion capacity of the TCN, derived from the formation of a strong ionic bond between the amine groups of thiolated chitosan and the negatively charged sites on mucosal epithelial cell membranes, resulting in the transient opening of the tight junctions. In vivo behavioral studies were also carried out on rats to assess the formulation's anxiolytic activity, namely the maze test, in which part of the maze is exposed to light (open arm), and the other is not (closed arm). Characteristically, anxious animals tend to remain in the closed arm (as do anxious people, when they show a desire to be isolated and in dark places). This study concluded that rats treated with TCN spent more time in the open arm of the maze when compared to other groups, showing promising therapeutic efficacy. Furthermore, the brain maximum drug concentration (Cmax) of buspirone after the IN administration of TCN (797.46 ng/mL) was higher than that obtained with the IN and IV solution (417.77 ng/mL and 384.15 ng/mL, respectively). Additionally, the drug-targeting efficiency (DTE%) and direct transport percentage (DTP%) for the IN TCN were 79% and 96%, respectively, and hence brain drug transport was considered to be quite high, which further proved the developed formulation's potential.

In another study, by Bshara et al. [59], the aim was to develop a buspirone mucoadhesive ME for IN administration, to improve its bioavailability and deliver high drug concentrations to the brain. This ME was prepared using chitosan, hydroxypropyl cyclodextrin, isopropyl myristate, Tween® 80 (polysorbate derived from sorbitan esters), propylene glycol, and water. The results showed that mucoadhesive ME are suitable for IN administration, since the drug's brain bioavailability in in vivo studies was significantly increased compared to an IN solution, reaching peak plasma concentrations within 15 min. The DTE% and DTP% values obtained with the developed IN ME were 86.6% and 88%, respectively. From these results, it may be concluded that a buspirone mucoadhesive ME can contribute to a reduction in the dose and frequency of administration and possibly to an increase in the therapeutic effect in anxiety treatment.

2.2.2. Clobazam

Clobazam is a benzodiazepine derivative with an active metabolite, norclobazam. Both are partial GABA receptor agonists, meaning they bind allosterically to the GABA-A receptor. Clobazam is a lipophilic molecule and is highly bound to plasma proteins, which increases its systemic distribution in fat tissue, causing adverse effects such as gastrointestinal disturbances, muscle spasms, and an irregular heartbeat. The prolonged oral use of this drug leads to an accumulation of its active metabolite in the body (10 times higher) which can cause toxicity. Additionally, it can lead to dependence when used for prolonged periods of time [60]. Florence et al. [60] aimed to develop and characterize a mucoadhesive clobazam ME to assess the drug's transport to the brain, thereby decreasing the drug's systemic distribution and consequently its potential to cause adverse effects. The developed mucoadhesive ME consisted of Carbopol® 940P, Capmul® MCM (glyceryl mono and dicaprate), Acconan® CC6, Tween® 20 (polysorbate derived from sorbitan esters), and distilled water. Carbopol was used due to its capacity to increase paracellular transport by opening tight junctions in apical cells, resulting in higher drug absorption. The non-mucoadhesive microemulsion had a viscosity value of 7.73 cP, and the mucoadhesive microemulsion had a viscosity value of 25.8 cP, and hence the addition of Carbopol to the formulation led to a viscosity increase, which was expected, since, aside from being a mucoadhesive polymer, Carbopol also has viscosifying properties. The obtained droplet size was 20 nm, the PDI was 0.181, and the ZP was −15 mV. In the pharmacokinetic study in mice, the obtained brain/blood ratio was higher with IN administration of the mucoadhesive ME, with greater and longer drug retention at the site of action when compared to a clobazam non-mucoadhesive ME (same composition, but no Carbopol). In addition, the systemic distribution of the drug was generally lower with IN administration, and there was a higher accumulation in the brain, as intended. Hence, this study showed that the clobazam ME with the addition of a mucoadhesive agent delivered the drug rapidly and effectively to the mice's brains. This could provide an alternative to intravenous administration in the treatment of anxiety.

2.3. *Anxiolytic and Antidepressant Drugs*

2.3.1. Venlafaxine

Venlafaxine (VLF) belongs to the SNRI therapeutic class and has low oral bioavailability and a short half-life (4–5 h). It is also a P-glycoprotein substrate and is therefore pumped out of the brain, reducing its bioavailability in this organ. Its effectiveness also depends on its continuous presence at the site of action for a prolonged period of time [19,61,63].

To overcome these limitations, Haque et al. [61] investigated the usefulness of IN administration of VLF-loaded QT NP to improve their delivery to the brain, compared to IV infusion. The VLF nanoparticles were formulated using the ionic gelation technique, containing QT, tripolyphosphate (TPP), and acetic acid. The obtained particle size was 167 nm, with a PDI of 0.367 and a ZP of +23.83 mV. The VLF in vitro drug release from the developed NP showed two phases, with an initial burst release, corresponding to 44.3%, in the first 2 h, followed by a controlled release of the drug, over 24 h. An ex vivo permeation study, conducted on porcine nasal mucosa, showed that QT VLF NP were able to permeate the membrane three times more than a VLF solution. In vivo pharmacokinetic studies showed the effective brain drug targeting of the NP through the IN route (Figure 5A), when compared to the IV route (Figure 5B), reaching high DTE% (508.59%) and DTP% (80.34%) values. This proves that QT-NPs were highly efficient in delivering VLF to the brain when administered intranasally, which could be greatly due to their mucoadhesive properties. Additionally, in in vivo pharmacodynamic studies, QT NP significantly increased the total swimming and climbing time and decreased the immobility time of the mice (compared to the control groups), which further proved the nanosystem's therapeutic potential.

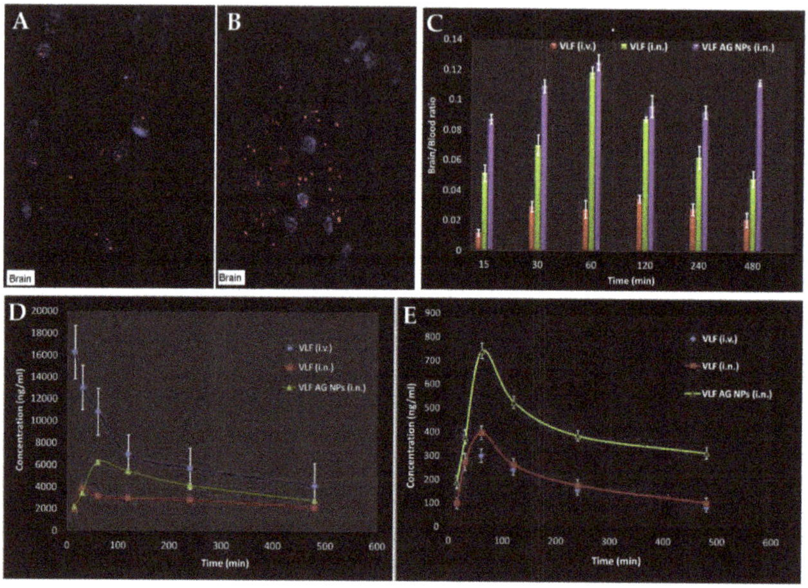

Figure 5. Confocal laser scanning microscopy rat brain images 120 min after IV administration (**A**) and IN administration (**B**) of the developed VLF QT NP, where blue fluorescence represents the brain cells and red fluorescence represents the drug (adapted from Haque et al. [61], reproduced with permission from Elsevier (license number 5495991231429)). Brain/blood ratios (**C**), plasma concentrations (**D**), and brain concentrations (**E**) of VLF after IV administration of a VLF solution (VLF (i.v.)), IN administration of a VLF solution (VLF (i.n.)), or IN administration of VLF AG NP (VLF AG NPs (i.n.)); adapted from Haque et al. [62], reproduced with permission from Elsevier (license number 5497041230698).

The same authors presented another study [62], where they also developed VLF-loaded NP for IN administration, but this time instead of QT they used AG. These NP had a particle size of 174 nm, a PDI of 0.391, a pH between 5.7 and 6.12, and a ZP of +37 mV. It was observed in pharmacokinetic in vivo studies that the drug concentration in the brain increased when the formulation was administered via IN when compared to the IV route. The brain/blood ratios (Figure 5C) obtained with the administration of the IN AG NP were generally higher than those obtained from the IV and IN drug solution, being equal to 0.1091, 0.0293, and 0.0700, respectively, at the final time point (480 min). The results also showed that the plasma concentration of VLF (Figure 5D) decreased when the drug was administered within the NP through IN delivery, showing the promise of higher safety, and that brain drug levels (Figure 5E) were also substantially higher with the IN NP when compared to the other groups, showing higher efficacy. The DTE% was almost double for the VLF AG NP when compared to the IN VLF solution. This proves that the mucoadhesive nanoparticulate delivery system enables an increased amount of drug to reach the brain. In vivo pharmacodynamic studies further demonstrated the efficacy of VLF AG NP delivered via the IN route to treat depression, since in forced swim tests there was a significantly reduced immobility time after IN NP administration, proving it to be more effective than all other groups.

Another study, by Cayero-Otero et al. [63], developed NP composed of PLGA and polyvinyl alcohol, with a particle size of 206 nm, a PDI of 0.041, and a ZP of −26.5 mV. These NP showed a higher capacity to reach the brain after IN administration than functionalized NP, with a specific transferrin receptor agonist peptide on their surface. This was explained by the fact that functionalized NP are transported to the brain by receptor-mediated endocytosis, which takes longer than simple NP, which are transported by facilitated transport.

In a different study, Zhao et al. [64] developed two solutions containing two different conjugates: venlafaxine-glucose (VLF-G) and thiamine disulfide system with venlafaxine-glucose conjugated (VLF-TDS-G). Type 1 glucose transporters (GLUT1) are responsible for transporting glucose to the brain and are present in the BBB. Therefore, this study aimed to investigate the binding of VLF to a glucose molecule in order to originate the drug's facilitated transport to the brain, through the BBB, after IV administration. A thiamine disulfide system was introduced into the VLF-G complex to prevent premature VLF release. In in vivo pharmacokinetics studies, the VLF-TDS-G conjugate significantly increased the brain VLF concentration, compared to the VLF-G conjugate, demonstrating good brain targeting. Thus, the VLF-TDS-G conjugate is promising for the brain delivery of intravenously administered drugs.

2.3.2. Duloxetine

Duloxetine is a drug that belongs to the SNRI class. It undergoes a high hepatic first-pass metabolism and has low oral bioavailability (only 50%) [65]. To overcome these problems, Alam et al. [65] developed duloxetine SLN for IN administration. The SLN were composed of glyceryl monostearate, Capryol® PGMC, bile salts (sodium taurocholate), Pluronic® F-68, and mannitol. The authors did not characterize the formulation, which at least raises questions about the homogeneity and particle size of the developed nanosystem, characteristics that can influence the absorption and bioavailability of the drug. Nevertheless, the SLN's performance was evaluated in in vivo studies. The IN administration of the developed SLN resulted in a six times higher concentration of duloxetine in the brain when compared to the IV administration of a drug solution. Hence, drug delivery to the brain was much lower with IV administration, with only small amounts of the drug being detected, due to loss in the systemic circulation and the hepatic first-pass effect. On the contrary, IN administration proved to be quite efficient in making the drug reach the brain, with the developed duloxetine SLN leading to high DTP (86.80%) and DTE (758%) values. The developed IN SLN also had a better brain targeting efficiency than an IN drug solution (DTP 65%, DTE 287%), which further proved the potential of the developed nanosystem for duloxetine IN brain delivery.

2.3.3. Paroxetine

Paroxetine belongs to the SSRI class, has low oral bioavailability (less than 50%), and undergoes an extensive first-pass effect. It also has a high potential for drug–drug interactions, especially when used in polytherapy [66]. To overcome some of these problems, Silva et al. [66] investigated the efficacy of the direct delivery of paroxetine to the brain in combination with another drug, borneol. Borneol is a natural compound that has already been shown to be effective in opening channels in the BBB. Therefore, researchers believe that borneol acts as a modulator of the ABC transporters by competitively inhibiting the P-gp and tight junction proteins, thereby reducing the efflux of drugs that are their substrates [46,66,73]. It is a reversible process characterized by transient and rapid BBB penetration. This co-administration of borneol with paroxetine works in a dose- and time-dependent manner. Thus, paroxetine was incorporated together with borneol into NLC containing Lauroglycol™ 90, Precirol® ATO 5, Tween® 80, and water. The developed nanosystem had a particle size of 160 nm, a PDI of 0.273, and a ZP of +11 mV. In vitro permeation studies in RPMI 2650 cells (human nasal cells) showed a 2.57-fold increase in drug permeation when the developed NLC was compared with a paroxetine suspension. The IN administration of borneol and paroxetine-loaded NLC to mice allowed the researchers to obtain a 63% higher brain exposure (as measured by the area under the concentration vs. time curve, AUC) than an IV injection. Additionally, the administration of a paroxetine IN solution only increased brain drug exposure by 49%, which further proves the superiority of the developed NLC. It was also observed that drug encapsulation reduced pulmonary exposure to the drug, which may contribute to a reduction in adverse effects. Thus, the developed NLC seem to be a good strategy to increase the IN delivery of lipophilic drugs, such as paroxetine, to the brain.

2.4. *Other Drug Classes*

2.4.1. Baicalein

Baicalein (BA) is the most therapeutically active natural flavonoid compound found in the dried roots of *Scutellaria baicalensis georgi*, with proven beneficial CNS and immunological effects [70]. Given these properties, Chen et al. [70] prepared SLN for baicalein encapsulation, composed of glyceryl monostearate, poloxamer 188, and 1,2-dipalmitoyl-sn-glycerol-3-phosphocholine. The developed nanosystems were additionally functionalized with the prolyl-glycyl-proline (PGP) peptide (PGP-BA-SLN) or without (BA-SLN) and had a ZP between −13 and −14 mV, and a pH of 5.5. The changes in lactate dehydrogenase (LDH) concentrations were studied in rats after the intraperitoneal administration of the developed formulations, as depression often involves hormonal changes leading to the negative regulation of LDH, resulting in the accumulation of lactate in the brain (from lactic acid fermentation). Both PGP-BA-SLN and BA-SLN enhanced the effect of BA in reducing LDH release compared to a drug solution. There was no statistically significant difference between the treatments. Pharmacodynamic tests were also carried out, and the results showed that both types of SLN reduced immobility time, increased climbing time, and increased swimming time in rats, with PGP-BA-SLN having a more significant effect than BA-SLN. Additionally, the brain drug distribution was determined, and the results showed that BA was found in higher concentrations in the basolateral amygdala after the administration of the developed SLN, a brain region associated with emotional and psychiatric disorders. All these results lead to the conclusion that modifying SLN with PGP may be beneficial in brain drug targeting, and hence producing effective antidepressant effects.

2.4.2. Icariin

Icariin is the main active constituent of the dried aerial parts of the *Epimedium brevicornum Maxim* plant. It has antitumor, cardiovascular, osteogenic, neuroprotective, and antidepressant effects. Nevertheless, it is poorly absorbed after oral administration [71]. To tackle these problems, Xu et al. [71] developed a thermosensitive nano-hydrogel (icariin-NGSTH) for the IN delivery of icariin, in order to enhance the antidepressant activity and bioavailability of this drug. A mixture of poloxamer 188 and poloxamer 407 was used to form an in situ thermosensitive hydrogel (Figure 6A), with the purpose of extending the drug's release time and therefore increasing its bioavailability, by giving it more time to be absorbed in the nasal cavity. The nano-hydrogel was also composed of Tween® 80 and Span® 80. The formulation had a particle size of 71 nm, a PDI of 0.50, and a ZP of −19 mV. Regarding pharmacokinetics, the in vivo distribution of the developed icariin nano-hydrogel in the brain of mice and rats was monitored after IN administration. The rats and mice treated with the developed IN nanosystem were compared to animals chronically treated with fluoxetine, an antidepressant of known effectiveness. After the IN administration of the icariin-NGSTH, fluorescence could be observed in the brain after 5 min, which became stronger after 30 min (Figure 6B). These results indicate that the drug reached the brain quickly, therefore producing a potentially fast therapeutic effect. This was further confirmed by the pharmacodynamic tests, since the IN administration of the developed formulation reduced the immobility time of the mice as well as other depressive behaviors. Moreover, the dose of icariin-NGSTH administered was only one-fifth of the dose of fluoxetine, and one-tenth of the dose of icariin administered in the form of a solution, demonstrating that the developed nanosystem indeed had promising antidepressant effects. Additionally, IL-6, a pro-inflammatory cytokine, is increased in depression because of neuroinflammatory processes. Hence, it was also observed that the icariin-NGSTH, at a lower dose, reduces the expression of IL-6 (Figure 6C), and also regulates the level of testosterone (Figure 6D).

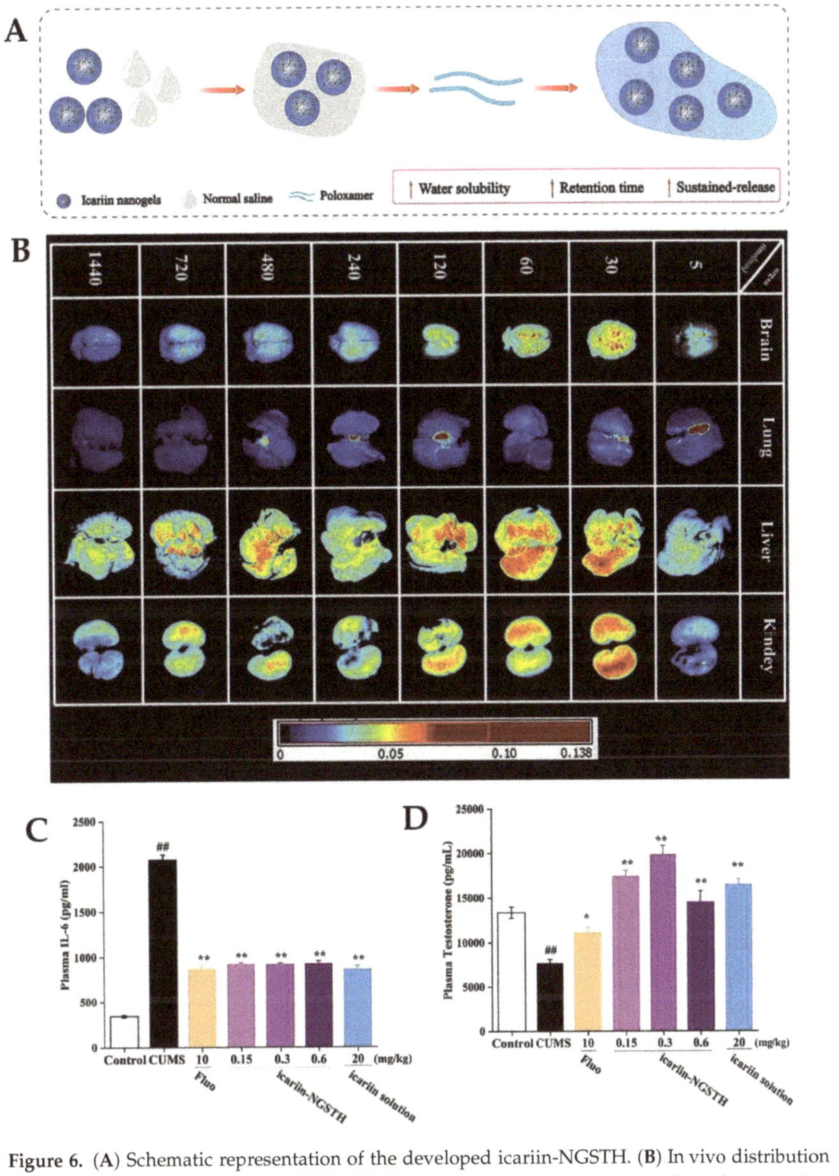

Figure 6. (**A**) Schematic representation of the developed icariin-NGSTH. (**B**) In vivo distribution of rhodamine B-labeled icariin-NGSTH. (**C**) IL-6 concentration in rat plasma after administration. (**D**) Testosterone concentration in rat plasma after administration. * $p < 0.05$, ## or ** $p < 0.01$; NGSTH—thermosensitive nano-hydrogel. Adapted from Xu et al. [71], reproduced with permission from Elsevier (license number 5496000528811).

2.4.3. Tramadol

Tramadol is a central analgesic with a low affinity for opioid receptors, but its active metabolite has a higher affinity for these receptors. It is also characterized by the inhibition of noradrenaline and serotonin receptors [53]. The study performed by Kaur et al. [53] aimed to evaluate the efficacy of tramadol NP administered through the IN route. The developed NP were composed of Pluronic® F-127 and TPP. The obtained particle size was 152 nm, with a PDI of 0.143 and a ZP of +31 mV. Pharmacodynamic tests were performed in rats, namely the forced swimming, locomotor activity, immobility, body weight variation, and glucose preference tests. The tests were conducted after the chronic administration of the developed formulations, and showed a significant decrease in immobility time and an increase in locomotor activity and body weight in the rats treated with the NP, compared to the control groups. Biochemical parameters were also measured in the animals' brains, and it was concluded that the developed NP could reduce nitrite and malondialdehyde levels more significantly than a drug solution. Additionally, GSH and catalase levels increased when the NP were administered.

2.4.4. Edaravone

Edaravone is a neuroprotective drug that scavenges free radicals and protects the neuronal membranes from oxidative damage. For this reason, it is used to treat amyotrophic lateral sclerosis. However, as oxidative processes also play a huge role in depression and anxiety, it has recently gained interest as a treatment for these pathologies [68]. Qin et al. [68] developed edaravone liposomes modified with the RGD peptide (arginine-glycine-aspartate), to be administered by intraperitoneal administration (Figure 7A). This peptide has the advantage of binding to leukocytes and thus penetrating the BBB in cases of neuroinflammation, which is present in depression. The cyclic RGD peptide (cRGD) has been shown to have an even higher affinity for the receptors expressed on the surface of leukocytes. In this study, a bacterial endotoxin (lipopolysaccharide, LPS) was administered to rats to impair their social behavior, since LPS leads to the production of inflammatory cytokines, such as IL-6, which causes neuropsychiatric disorders and depression. Three types of liposomes were prepared: functionalized edaravone liposomes composed of edaravone, cRGD, soy phosphatidylcholine, 1,2-dipalmitoyl-sn-glycero-3-phosphocholine, and cholesterol; non-functionalized edaravone liposomes consisting only of edaravone and cholesterol; and functionalized liposomes with no edaravone, composed of cRGD peptide, soy phosphatidylcholine, 1,2-dipalmitoyl-sn-glycero-3-phosphocholine, and cholesterol. The results showed that the functionalized edaravone liposomes were more effective than the other formulations in increasing the mobility of the rats in the forced swim test (Figure 7B). Notably, this formulation also significantly attenuated the levels and reduced the secretion of IL-1β (Figure 7C) and IL-6 (Figure 7D), suggesting that edaravone may suppress the production of pro-inflammatory cytokines by scavenging free radicals.

2.4.5. Carbamazepine

Carbamazepine (CBZ) is an antiepileptic and anxiolytic drug which exerts its anxiolytic activity by modulating the adenosine-mediated neurotransmitters to modify postsynaptic ionic currents. Its low aqueous solubility and extensive hepatic metabolism result in slow absorption after oral administration. Furthermore, the absorption is variable and depends on the drug's dissolution rate in the gastrointestinal fluids [67]. To improve CBZ's brain delivery, Khan et al. [67] investigated the potential of CBZ NLC by intraperitoneal administration. The optimized formulation had a particle size of 97.7 nm, a PDI of 0.27, and a ZP of −22 mV. The in vitro drug release assay showed that, when compared to a CBZ dispersion, the developed CBZ NLC exhibited a biphasic release profile, with a faster drug release in the first 4 h (Figure 8A). The achieved CBZ concentration after formulation administration was also assessed in mice, and the CBZ NLC significantly increased the AUC of CBZ (520.4 μg.h/mL) in the brain compared to the CBZ dispersion (244.9 μg.h/mL). Additionally, the administration of the CBZ NLC resulted in higher plasma (Figure 8B) and brain (Figure 8C) concentrations at each time point. Furthermore, at the same time points, the brain concentrations of CBZ-TLNs were higher than their plasma concentrations, which represents the potential for a favorable efficacy vs. safety profile. The anxiolytic effect of the CBZ NLC, assessed in in vivo pharmacodynamic studies, was demonstrated and proved to be higher than that produced with the CBZ dispersion (Figure 8D–F). Additionally, the CBZ NLC showed better results than diazepam treatment, which is a known effective anxiolytic drug.

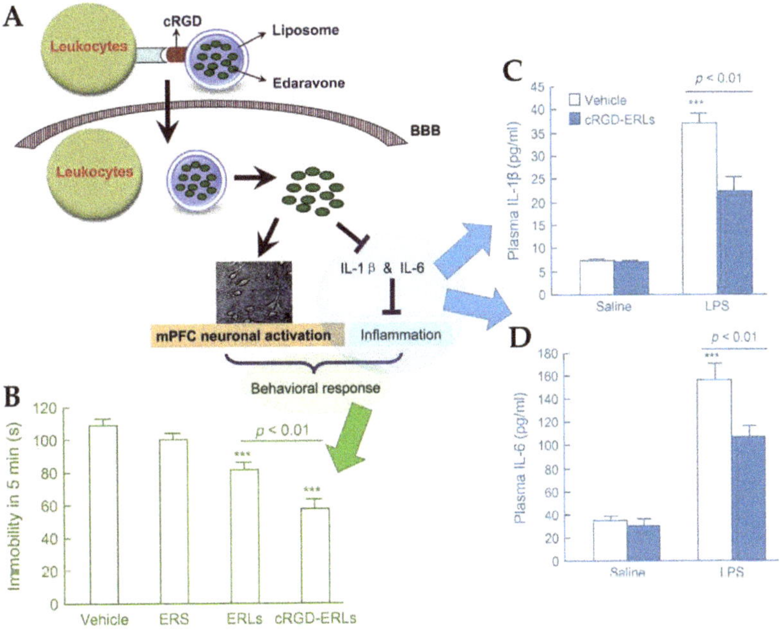

Figure 7. (**A**) Schematic representation of the developed functionalized edaravone liposomes. (**B**) Immobility time in the forced swim test after administration. Plasma IL-1β (**C**) and IL-6 (**D**) after administration. BBB—blood–brain barrier; cRGD—cyclic RGD (arginine-glycine-aspartate) peptide; cRGD-ERLs—functionalized edaravone liposomes; ER—edaravone; ERLs—non-functionalized edaravone liposomes; ERS—edaravone solution; IL—interleukin; LPS—lipopolysaccharide. Adapted from Qin et al. [68], reproduced with permission from Elsevier (license number 5496000926348).

2.4.6. Riluzole

Riluzole is a drug that works by reducing the release of glutamate in the synaptic cleft, making it difficult for glutamate receptors to be activated, thus protecting the dopaminergic neurons. It also helps to reduce oxidative stress and improve memory. All these factors are related to its potential anxiolytic activity. However, this drug undergoes extensive first-pass metabolism by CYP1A2, which hinders its clinical efficacy [69]. To circumvent these problems, Nabi et al. [69] developed chitosan NP, since it is a polymer that has been described as having the ability to enhance NP mucoadhesive strength and increase drug absorption, thereby improving drug delivery to the brain. Furthermore, as already mentioned, chitosan has the ability to facilitate the transient opening of tight junctions, as well as prevent the degradation of the encapsulated drug. The developed chitosan NP were also functionalized with transferrin, which allows them to cross the BBB by transcytosis. This happens because transferrin receptors are widely distributed on the brain capillary endothelial cells, which are involved in the transcytosis process. Therefore, transferrin can freely cross the unimpaired regions of the BBB. The developed NP were characterized and had a particle size of 207 nm and PDI of 0.406. In in vivo pharmacodynamic tests, haloperidol was administered to rats included in the study before the administration of any formulation, to induce anxiety symptoms, as haloperidol leads to neuronal degradation, which produces oxidative stress. The results showed that, compared to the control groups (treated with only haloperidol or with haloperidol plus a riluzole IN solution), the rats treated with IN administration of the developed NP showed a greater improvement in terms of neurological effects. Additionally, biochemically the group treated with haloperidol only showed decreased GSH levels and increased malondialdehyde, whereas the treatment group showed the reverse. In addition, the TBARS levels were found to be lower in the rats treated with the developed NP, with more significant effects than those provoked by the administration of a drug solution. Furthermore, in in vivo pharmacokinetic studies the developed NP led to a higher brain drug uptake by the IN route. The use of transferrin was shown to be an additional advantage, increasing the efficiency of drug delivery to the brain. Hence, the developed NP may have a high therapeutic potential for drug delivery via the IN route.

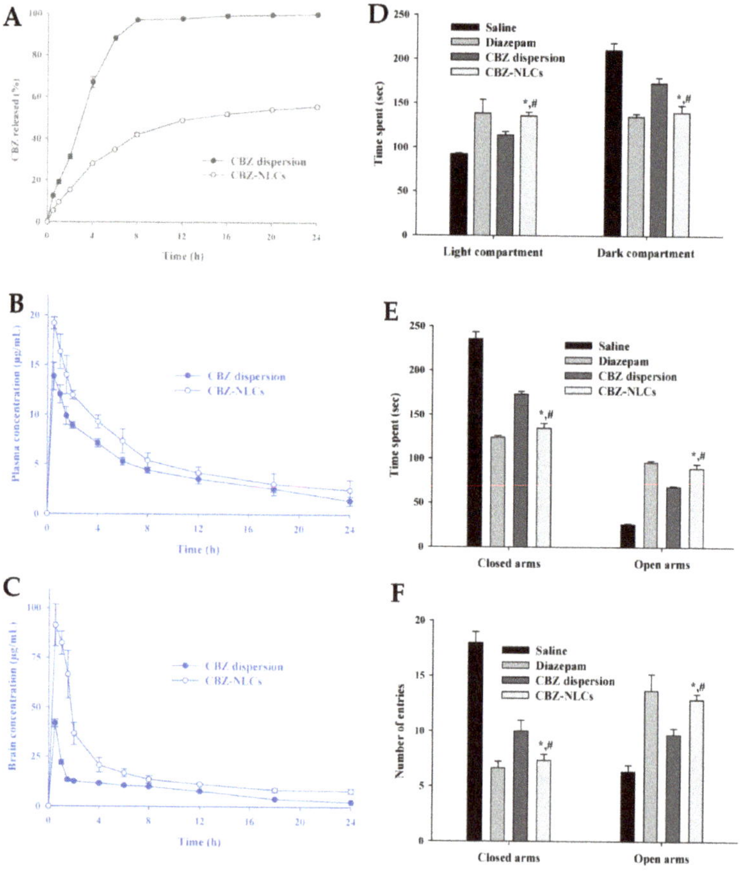

Figure 8. (**A**) In vitro drug release profile of a carbamazepine dispersion ("CBZ dispersion") and the developed NLC ("CBZ-NLCs"). CBZ plasma (**B**) and brain (**C**) concentration versus time curves after the intraperitoneal administration of a carbamazepine dispersion ("CBZ dispersion") and the developed NLC ("CBZ-NLCs"). (**D**) to (**E**) The results of the administration of several formulations in a light-dark box mice model (**D**) and elevated plus maze mice model (**E**,**F**). * and # $p < 0.01$. Adapted from Khan et al. [67], reproduced with permission from Elsevier (license number 5496001134122).

2.4.7. Berberine

Berberine is an alkaloid found in various medicinal plants, such as *Coptis Chinensis*, and is mainly isolated from its bark and roots. It has known medicinal properties, including antioxidant, anti-inflammatory, and hepatoprotective effects. Several studies show that berberine can inhibit MAO-A, the enzyme responsible for the degradation of noradrenaline and serotonin. Despite all these properties, it has low bioavailability [74–77]. Hence, Wang et al. [72] investigated the incorporation of berberine into a thermosensitive gel, to be administered through the IN route. This gel exhibited properties such as high fluid absorption and low surface tension, resulting in good biocompatibility and high drug incorporation capacity. These properties are due to the polymers included in its composition, namely poloxamers 407 and 188, non-ionic copolymers consisting of a hydrophobic polyoxypropylene chain and two hydrophilic polyoxyethylene chains. Before the preparation of the hydrogel system, the authors improved the solubility of berberine by using cyclodextrins. Hence, first a drug–cyclodextrin inclusion complex was prepared, and then this complex was incorporated into the hydrogel. The intermolecular interactions between the cyclodextrins and the poloxamers P407 and P188 resulted in the formation of a supramolecular matrix. This formulation was then evaluated in in vivo pharmacokinetic studies in rats: one group received the inclusion complex incorporated into a thermosensitive hydrogel through the IN route at a lower dose (0.15 mg/kg); and the other group received the inclusion complex in an aqueous dispersion (no incorporation into a gel) through the intragastric route at a higher dose (5 mg/kg). The inclusion complex incorporated into a thermosensitive hydrogel proved to be a more effective and faster treatment than the inclusion complex in an aqueous dispersion, even though it was administered at a dose three times lower (higher C_{max} and AUC values). Furthermore, in a study where reserpine was first administered to rats (reserpine is known to exhaust the monoamine neurotransmitters at the synapses, resulting in depression-like behavior), the IN administration of the hydrogel caused a significant increase in the levels of serotonin, noradrenaline, and dopamine in the rat hippocampus and striatum, showing superior efficacy compared to all the other groups.

2.5. General Analysis

2.5.1. Formulation Characteristics

Considering that most surveyed articles opted for drug incorporation into a nanosystem, it is necessary to make a general analysis of the reported formulation characteristics. These characteristics mostly included the particle size, PDI, ZP, pH, and viscosity.

Most of the articles mentioned the particle size, PDI, and ZP. These parameters are very important as they influence the absorption and consequently the bioavailability of the encapsulated drugs. The particle size must be in the nanometer range for more effective drug delivery. In addition, formulations with a smaller particle size are more likely to be able to penetrate the mucous membranes [21]. The PDI is directly related to the particle size, being defined as the standard deviation of the particle diameter distribution divided by the mean particle diameter [78]. It is usually used to estimate formulation homogeneity, which is very important in drug pharmacokinetics. A higher value means that the formulation is heterogeneous, which can lead to pharmacokinetic irregularities and variability in the therapeutic outcomes. It is usually recommended that the PDI must be less than 0.5, which was the case in all the articles that analyzed this parameter [20].

The nanosystem's surface charge can also affect the BBB and nasal mucosa penetration [46]. It is usually determined by ZP measurement. The nasal mucosa has a negative charge, so positively charged moieties are more likely to interact with the nasal mucosa through electrostatic forces, therefore increasing the residence time and the formulation's adhesion to the nasal epithelium. For this reason, many nanocarriers are positively charged. This will lead to a potential increase in the bioavailability of the delivered molecules [21]. Conventionally, nanosystems with a ZP between −10 and +10 mV are considered neutral, while nanoparticles with a ZP higher than +30 mV or less than −30 mV are considered strongly cationic or strongly anionic, respectively. In this review, only two articles presented formulations with a ZP above +30 mV or below −30 mV, which means that although most of the formulations were considered neutral, they still managed to permeate the membranes with some efficiency [79].

Most authors opted for IN administration of the developed formulations. Thus, these preparations had to meet certain conditions adapted to this specific administration route, namely a pH between 5.0 and 6.0 (nasal mucosa's pH) to avoid irritation or harm. The articles that reported pH values mentioned results between 4.62 and 7.00, which are appropriate for compatibility with the nasal mucosa's physiology. Viscosity is also a relevant factor in IN administration, since the higher a formulation's viscosity, the longer the formulation will remain in contact with the nasal mucosa, and hence the drug will have more time to undergo absorption [28]. Nevertheless, pH and viscosity were the two characteristics least mentioned in most articles, which may raise the question of the suitability of the preparations for IN administration.

2.5.2. In Vivo Pharmacokinetics and Pharmacodynamics

In vivo pharmacodynamic and/or pharmacokinetic studies were conducted to evaluate the performance of the developed formulations after administration. The used animal models were either rats or mice.

Pharmacokinetic studies were performed to quantify the drug that was delivered to the brain, and also the part that was not. Several different analytical methods were used to quantify the blood/plasma samples (representative of systemic distribution) and brain samples (representative of the desired site of action), namely: high-performance liquid chromatography, liquid chromatography coupled with mass spectrometry, gas chromatography coupled with mass spectrometry, scintigraphy, and fluorescence. C_{max}, which represents the maximum drug concentration that was reached during the study in a specific biological tissue, and AUC, which represents the change in drug concentration over time, are the main parameters that can be assessed in these types of study. From the brain and blood/plasma AUC values specific ratios can be calculated in order to assess the brain-targeting efficiency of the developed formulations: DTE% and DTP%. DTE% is a measure of brain drug transport via IN delivery versus IV delivery. DTE% values above 100% indicate that the drug is more efficiently transported to the brain by the IN route when compared to the IV route. It can be calculated as follows:

$$\text{DTE\%} = \frac{\left(\frac{\text{AUC brain}}{\text{AUC plasma}}\right)\text{IN}}{\left(\frac{\text{AUC brain}}{\text{AUC plasma}}\right)\text{IV}} \times 100$$

DTP% is a similar ratio, in the way that it also compares IN and IV administrations, but it represents the proportion of the drug that is transported directly to the brain. DTP% values above 0% indicate that the drug is transported by neuronal pathways (direct pathways). It can be calculated as follows:

$$\text{DTP\%} = \frac{B_{IN} - B_X}{B_{IN}} \times 100 \text{ where } B_X = \frac{B_{IV}}{P_{IV}} \times P_{IN}$$

Higher DTE% and DTP% values indicate that the drug's IN administration has better brain targeting efficiency than IV administration [20].

As for the performed pharmacodynamic tests, these included the forced swimming, locomotor activity, and sucrose preference tests. These are the main tests that are performed for the assessment of depression and/or anxiety. The forced swim test is one of the most commonly used tests to verify the immobility time of the animal. In general, the depressed animal has a longer immobility time than the healthy animal. After administering the various formulations to groups of animals in which depression was induced, a significant reduction in immobility time was obtained. This allows us to conclude that the administration of the developed formulations was successful in making the drugs reach the brain, and hence having an antidepressant effect. Another important test, reported in some of the articles included in this review, is the locomotor activity test. Depressed animals are more likely to show increased immobility compared to healthy ones, or those receiving antidepressant/anxiolytic treatment [53]. The third most reported test is the sucrose preference test, which evaluates sucrose consumption during treatment with antidepressants or anxiolytics compared to control groups. The results show that sucrose consumption does not change in treated animals but increases in untreated animals [80]. In general, all the analyzed studies showed a positive evolution in the animals' behavior, demonstrating that the developed treatment is more effective than other administration routes and/or formulations.

2.5.3. Overview and Future Prospects

After analyzing all the brain targeting strategies of different drugs, we can conclude that it is imperative to have as much information as possible to achieve a fast and effective brain drug delivery. In this way, we must know the nanosystem's characteristics, such as particle size, PDI, and ZP, as well as the characteristics of the final preparation, such as pH and viscosity. Among the analyzed articles, the most commonly used nanosystems were polymeric and lipid nanoparticles, which proved to be more effective in delivering the drug to the brain through the nasal cavity. Additionally, an IN formulation for the treatment of depression has already been developed and approved by the United States Food and Drug Administration in 2019. It is a nasal spray containing esketamine, with the brand name Spravato®. It is used for the treatment of major depression along with suicidal ideation when patients demonstrate resistance to oral antidepressants [81–83]. This can be an open door for the further development and approval of IN antidepressant and anxiolytic drugs. While there are currently no preparations containing nanosystems for the treatment of these diseases in the pharmaceutical market, multiple studies have now proven their efficacy. Hence, further studies still need to be performed in order to assess the true potential of nanosystems containing antidepressant and anxiolytic drugs for IN administration, especially regarding their efficacy and safety in clinical trials. Additionally, the scale-up difficulties that may arise from preparations containing nanosystems should be assessed and improved, so that one day the reported promising experimental results can originate a marketed formulation, and these preparations can be an option for improved depression and anxiety treatment.

3. Conclusions

Drug molecule functionalization has proven to be a promising alternative for antidepressant and/or anxiolytic drug modification when systemic administration is required, since with the right ligands it could lead to increased drug transport through the BBB, leading to higher brain drug concentrations. Nevertheless, the IN route has proven to be an excellent alternative to systemic routes, such as oral and intravenous administrations, as it can allow the drugs to be transported directly to the brain through neuronal transport without having to pass through the BBB. This administration route has proven to lead to higher efficacy (increased brain targeting and bioavailability) and safety (a reduction of systemic drug distribution). Furthermore, formulating drugs into nanosystems has proven to increase the therapeutic efficacy in animal models of these diseases, being especially relevant through IN administration. Hence, IN administration of antidepressant and anxiolytic drugs has been demonstrated to be a suitable alternative to the treatments currently available on the pharmaceutical market for the treatment of depressive and anxiety disorders. Hence, it is essential than in the future further studies are conducted, so that these formulations could one day reach the market and ensure an improvement in the quality of life of patients suffering from these pathologies.

Author Contributions: Conceptualization, P.C.P., A.C.P.-S. and F.V.; methodology, P.C.P.; formal analysis, J.L.A. and P.C.P.; investigation, J.L.A. and P.C.P.; writing—original draft preparation, J.L.A., P.C.P. and J.A.; writing—review and editing, P.C.P., A.C.P.-S. and F.V.; supervision, P.C.P., A.C.P.-S. and F.V. All authors have read and agreed to the published version of the manuscript.

Funding: This research received no external funding.

Institutional Review Board Statement: Not applicable.

Informed Consent Statement: Not applicable.

Data Availability Statement: Not applicable.

Conflicts of Interest: The authors declare no conflict of interest.

Abbreviations

AG—alginate; AUC—area under the concentration vs. time curve; BA—baicalein; BA-SLN—baicalein solid lipid nanoparticles; BBB—blood–brain barrier; BOR—borneol; CBZ—carbamazepine; C_{max}—maximum drug concentration; CNS—central nervous system; CNP—chitosan nanoparticles; cRGD—cyclic RGD peptide; CSF—cerebrospinal fluid; DTE%—drug targeting efficiency; DTP%—direct transport percentage; GLUT1—type 1 glucose transporters; GSH—glutathione; IN—intranasal; IV—intravenous; LDH—lactate dehydrogenase; LPS—lipopolysaccharide; MAO—monoamine oxidase; ME—microemulsion; NGSTH—thermosensitive nano-hydrogel; NLC—nanostructured lipid carriers; NP—polymeric nanoparticle; P-gp—P-glycoprotein; PDI—polydispersity index; PEG—polyethylene glycol; PGP—prolyl-glycyl-proline; PGP-BA-SLN—prolyl-glycyl-proline peptide functionalized baicalein solid lipid nanoparticles; PLGA—poly lactic-co-glycolic acid; RGD—arginine-glycine-aspartate peptide; SLN—solid lipid nanoparticles; SNRI—serotonin and noradrenaline reuptake inhibitors; SSRI—selective serotonin reuptake inhibitors; TBARS—thiobarbituric acid; TCN—thiolated chitosan nanoparticles; TPP—tripolyphosphate; VLF—venlafaxine; VLF-G—venlafaxine-glucose complex; VLF-TDS-G—thiamine disulfide system conjugated with venlafaxine-glucose complex; ZP—zeta potential.

References

1. Katzman, M.A.; Bleau, P.; Blier, P.; Chokka, P.; Kjernisted, K.; van Ameringen, M.; Antony, M.M.; Bouchard, S.; Brunet, A.; Flament, M.; et al. Canadian Clinical Practice Guidelines for the Management of Anxiety, Posttraumatic Stress and Obsessive-Compulsive Disorders. *BMC Psychiatry* **2014**, *14*, S1. [CrossRef] [PubMed]
2. Won, E.; Kim, Y.K. Neuroinflammation—Associated Alterations of the Brain as Potential Neural Biomarkers in Anxiety Disorders. *Int. J. Mol. Sci.* **2020**, *21*, 6546. [CrossRef] [PubMed]
3. Penninx, B.W.; Pine, D.S.; Holmes, E.A.; Reif, A. Anxiety Disorders. *Lancet* **2021**, *397*, 914–927. [CrossRef]
4. Nasir, M.; Trujillo, D.; Levine, J.; Dwyer, J.B.; Rupp, Z.W.; Bloch, M.H. Glutamate Systems in DSM-5 Anxiety Disorders: Their Role and a Review of Glutamate and GABA Psychopharmacology. *Front. Psychiatry* **2020**, *11*, 548505. [CrossRef]
5. Chesnut, M.; Harati, S.; Paredes, P.; Khan, Y.; Foudeh, A.; Kim, J.; Bao, Z.; Williams, L.M. Stress Markers for Mental States and Biotypes of Depression and Anxiety: A Scoping Review and Preliminary Illustrative Analysis. *Chronic Stress* **2021**, *5*, 1–17. [CrossRef]
6. James, S.L.; Abate, D.; Abate, K.H.; Abay, S.M.; Abbafati, C.; Abbasi, N.; Abbastabar, H.; Abd-Allah, F.; Abdela, J.; Abdelalim, A.; et al. GBD 2017 Disease and Injury Incidence and Prevalence Collaborators Global, Regional, and National Incidence, Prevalence, and Years Lived with Disability for 354 Diseases and Injuries for 195 Countries and Territories, 1990–2017: A Systematic Analysis for the Global Burden of Disease Study 2017. *Lancet* **2018**, *392*, 1789–1858. [CrossRef]
7. Hu, P.; Lu, Y.; Pan, B.-X.; Zhang, W.-H. New Insights into the Pivotal Role of the Amygdala in Inflammation-Related Depression and Anxiety Disorder. *Int. J. Mol. Sci.* **2022**, *23*, 11076. [CrossRef] [PubMed]
8. GBD 2019 Diseases and Injuries Collaborators. Global Burden of 369 Diseases and Injuries in 204 Countries and Territories, 1990–2019: A Systematic Analysis for the Global Burden of Disease Study 2019. *Lancet* **2020**, *396*, 1204–1222. [CrossRef]
9. American Psychological Association Clinical Practice Guideline for the Treatment of Depression across Three Age Cohorts. 2019. Available online: https://www.apa.org/depression-guideline/guideline.pdf. (accessed on 1 February 2023).
10. Zhao, Y.F.; Verkhratsky, A.; Tang, Y.; Illes, P. Astrocytes and Major Depression: The Purinergic Avenue. *Neuropharmacology* **2022**, *220*, 109252. [CrossRef]
11. Nemeroff, C.B. The State of Our Understanding of the Pathophysiology and Optimal Treatment of Depression: Glass Half Full or Half Empty? *Am. J. Psychiatry* **2020**, *177*, 671–685. [CrossRef]

12. Kircanski, K.; Joormann, J.; Gotlib, I.H. Cognitive Aspects of Depression. *Wiley Interdiscip. Rev. Cogn. Sci.* **2012**, *3*, 301–313. [CrossRef]
13. Gabriel, F.C.; de Melo, D.O.; Fraguas, R.; Leite-Santos, N.C.; da Silva, R.A.M.; Ribeiro, E. Pharmacological Treatment of Depression: A Systematic Review Comparing Clinical Practice Guideline Recommendations. *PLoS ONE* **2020**, *15*, 0231700. [CrossRef] [PubMed]
14. Nutt, D.J. Relationship of Neurotransmitters to the Symptoms of Major Depressive Disorder. *J. Clin. Psychiatry* **2008**, *69*, 4–7. [PubMed]
15. Skelin, I.; Kovaèević, T.; Diksic, M. Neurochemical and Behavioural Changes in Rat Models of Depression. *Croat. Chem. Acta* **2011**, *84*, 287–299. [CrossRef]
16. Camkurt, M.A.; Findikli, E.; Izci, F.; Kurutaş, E.B.; Tuman, T.C. Evaluation of Malondialdehyde, Superoxide Dismutase and Catalase Activity and Their Diagnostic Value in Drug Naïve, First Episode, Non-Smoker Major Depression Patients and Healthy Controls. *Psychiatry Res.* **2016**, *238*, 81–85. [CrossRef]
17. Elsayed, O.H.; Ercis, M.; Pahwa, M.; Singh, B. Treatment-Resistant Bipolar Depression: Therapeutic Trends, Challenges and Future Directions. *Neuropsychiatr. Dis. Treat* **2022**, *18*, 2927–2943. [CrossRef]
18. Lenox, R.H.; Frazer, A. Mechanism of Action of Antidepressants and Mood Stabilizers. In *Neuropsychopharmacology: The Fifth Generation of Progress*; ACNP: Brentwood, TN, USA, 2002; pp. 1139–1163. ISBN 9780781728379.
19. Kilts, C.D. Potential New Drug Delivery Systems for Antidepressants: An Overview. *J. Clin. Psychiatry* **2003**, *64*, 31–33.
20. Pires, P.C.; Santos, A.O. Nanosystems in Nose-to-Brain Drug Delivery: A Review of Non-Clinical Brain Targeting Studies. *J. Control. Release* **2018**, *270*, 89–100. [CrossRef]
21. Lee, D.; Minko, T. Nanotherapeutics for Nose-to-Brain Drug Delivery: An Approach to Bypass the Blood Brain Barrier. *Pharmaceutics* **2021**, *13*, 2049. [CrossRef]
22. Xie, J.; Shen, Z.; Anraku, Y.; Kataoka, K.; Chen, X. Nanomaterial-Based Blood-Brain-Barrier (BBB) Crossing Strategies. *Biomaterials* **2019**, *224*, 119491. [CrossRef]
23. Zhou, Y.; Peng, Z.; Seven, E.S.; Leblanc, R.M. Crossing the Blood-Brain Barrier with Nanoparticles. *J. Control. Release* **2018**, *270*, 290–303. [CrossRef] [PubMed]
24. Ulbrich, K.; Knobloch, T.; Kreuter, J. Targeting the Insulin Receptor: Nanoparticles for Drug Delivery across the Blood-Brain Barrier (BBB). *J. Drug Target.* **2011**, *19*, 125–132. [CrossRef]
25. Teixeira, M.I.; Lopes, C.M.; Amaral, M.H.; Costa, P.C. Surface-Modified Lipid Nanocarriers for Crossing the Blood-Brain Barrier (BBB): A Current Overview of Active Targeting in Brain Diseases. *Colloids Surf. B Biointerfaces* **2023**, *221*, 112999. [CrossRef] [PubMed]
26. Bhattaccharjee, S.A.; Murnane, K.S.; Banga, A.K. Transdermal Delivery of Breakthrough Therapeutics for the Management of Treatment-Resistant and Post-Partum Depression. *Int. J. Pharm.* **2020**, *591*, 120007. [CrossRef]
27. Akil, H.; Gordon, J.; Hen, R.; Javitch, J.; Mayberg, H.; McEwen, B.; Meaney, M.J.; Nestler, E.J. Treatment Resistant Depression: A Multi-Scale, Systems Biology Approach. *Neurosci. Biobehav. Rev.* **2018**, *84*, 272–288. [CrossRef] [PubMed]
28. Misra, A.; Kher, G. Drug Delivery Systems from Nose to Brain. *Curr. Pharm. Biotechnol.* **2012**, *13*, 2355–2379. [CrossRef] [PubMed]
29. Erdő, F.; Bors, L.A.; Farkas, D.; Bajza, Á.; Gizurarson, S. Evaluation of Intranasal Delivery Route of Drug Administration for Brain Targeting. *Brain Res. Bull.* **2018**, *143*, 155–170. [CrossRef]
30. Crowe, T.P.; Greenlee, M.H.W.; Kanthasamy, A.G.; Hsu, W.H. Mechanism of Intranasal Drug Delivery Directly to the Brain. *Life Sci.* **2018**, *195*, 44–52. [CrossRef] [PubMed]
31. Keller, L.-A.; Merkel, O.; Popp, A. Intranasal Drug Delivery: Opportunities and Toxicologic Challenges during Drug Development. *Drug Deliv. Transl. Res.* **2022**, *12*, 735–757. [CrossRef]
32. Aderibigbe, B.; Naki, T. Design and Efficacy of Nanogels Formulations for Intranasal Administration. *Molecules* **2018**, *23*, 1241. [CrossRef] [PubMed]
33. Zha, S.; Wong, K.; All, A.H. Intranasal Delivery of Functionalized Polymeric Nanomaterials to the Brain. *Adv. Healthc. Mater.* **2022**, *11*, 2102610. [CrossRef]
34. Rohrer, J.; Lupo, N.; Bernkop-Schnürch, A. Advanced Formulations for Intranasal Delivery of Biologics. *Int. J. Pharm.* **2018**, *553*, 8–20. [CrossRef] [PubMed]
35. Casettari, L.; Illum, L. Chitosan in Nasal Delivery Systems for Therapeutic Drugs. *J. Control. Release* **2014**, *190*, 189–200. [CrossRef]
36. Alavian, F.; Shams, N. Oral and Intra-Nasal Administration of Nanoparticles in the Cerebral Ischemia Treatment in Animal Experiments: Considering Its Advantages and Disadvantages. *Curr. Clin. Pharmacol.* **2020**, *15*, 20–29. [CrossRef]
37. Pires, P.C.; Melo, D.; Santos, A.O. Intranasal Delivery of Antiseizure Drugs. In *Drug Delivery Devices and Therapeutic Systems*; Academic Press: Cambridge, MA, USA, 2021; pp. 623–646. ISBN 978-0-12-819838-4.
38. Pires, P.C.; Rodrigues, M.; Alves, G.; Santos, A.O. Strategies to Improve Drug Strength in Nasal Preparations for Brain Delivery of Low Aqueous Solubility Drugs. *Pharmaceutics* **2022**, *14*, 588. [CrossRef] [PubMed]
39. Alberto, M.; Paiva-Santos, A.C.; Veiga, F.; Pires, P.C. Lipid and Polymeric Nanoparticles: Successful Strategies for Nose-to-Brain Drug Delivery in the Treatment of Depression and Anxiety Disorders. *Pharmaceutics* **2022**, *14*, 2742. [CrossRef] [PubMed]
40. Pires, P.C.; Paiva-Santos, A.C.; Veiga, F. Antipsychotics-Loaded Nanometric Emulsions for Brain Delivery. *Pharmaceutics* **2022**, *14*, 2174. [CrossRef]

41. Pires, P.C.; Paiva-Santos, A.C.; Veiga, F. Nano and Microemulsions for the Treatment of Depressive and Anxiety Disorders: An Efficient Approach to Improve Solubility, Brain Bioavailability and Therapeutic Efficacy. *Pharmaceutics* **2022**, *14*, 2825. [CrossRef]
42. Naqvi, S.; Panghal, A.; Flora, S.J.S. Nanotechnology: A Promising Approach for Delivery of Neuroprotective Drugs. *Front. Neurosci.* **2020**, *14*, 494. [CrossRef] [PubMed]
43. Zielińska, A.; Carreiró, F.; Oliveira, A.M.; Neves, A.; Pires, B.; Venkatesh, D.N.; Durazzo, A.; Lucarini, M.; Eder, P.; Silva, A.M.; et al. Polymeric Nanoparticles: Production, Characterization, Toxicology and Ecotoxicology. *Molecules* **2020**, *25*, 3731. [CrossRef]
44. Volpatti, L.R.; Matranga, M.A.; Cortinas, A.B.; Delcassian, D.; Daniel, K.B.; Langer, R.; Anderson, D.G. Glucose-Responsive Nanoparticles for Rapid and Extended Self-Regulated Insulin Delivery. *ACS Nano* **2020**, *14*, 488–497. [CrossRef] [PubMed]
45. Ferreira, M.D.; Duarte, J.; Veiga, F.; Paiva-Santos, A.C.; Pires, P.C. Nanosystems for Brain Targeting of Antipsychotic Drugs: An Update on the Most Promising Nanocarriers for Increased Bioavailability and Therapeutic Efficacy. *Pharmaceutics* **2023**, *15*, 678. [CrossRef] [PubMed]
46. Zhang, W.; Mehta, A.; Tong, Z.; Esser, L.; Voelcker, N.H. Development of Polymeric Nanoparticles for Blood–Brain Barrier Transfer—Strategies and Challenges. *Adv. Sci.* **2021**, *8*, 2003937. [CrossRef] [PubMed]
47. Racine, L.; Texier, I.; Auzély-Velty, R. Chitosan-Based Hydrogels: Recent Design Concepts to Tailor Properties and Functions. *Polym. Int.* **2017**, *66*, 981–998. [CrossRef]
48. Lee, K.Y.; Mooney, D.J. Alginate: Properties and Biomedical Applications. *Prog. Polym. Sci.* **2012**, *37*, 106–126. [CrossRef] [PubMed]
49. Jani, P.; Vanza, J.; Pandya, N.; Tandel, H. Formulation of Polymeric Nanoparticles of Antidepressant Drug for Intranasal Delivery. *Ther. Deliv.* **2019**, *10*, 683–696. [CrossRef]
50. Alsaab, H.O.; Alharbi, F.D.; Alhibs, A.S.; Alanazi, N.B.; Alshehri, B.Y.; Saleh, M.A.; Alshehri, F.S.; Algarni, M.A.; Almugaiteeb, T.; Uddin, M.N.; et al. PLGA-Based Nanomedicine: History of Advancement and Development in Clinical Applications of Multiple Diseases. *Pharmaceutics* **2022**, *14*, 2728. [CrossRef]
51. Ghasemiyeh, P.; Mohammadi-Samani, S. Solid Lipid Nanoparticles and Nanostructured Lipid Carriers as Novel Drug Delivery Systems: Applications, Advantages and Disadvantages. *Res. Pharm. Sci.* **2018**, *13*, 288. [CrossRef]
52. Bonferoni, M.; Rossi, S.; Sandri, G.; Ferrari, F.; Gavini, E.; Rassu, G.; Giunchedi, P. Nanoemulsions for "Nose-to-Brain" Drug Delivery. *Pharmaceutics* **2019**, *11*, 84. [CrossRef]
53. Kaur, P.; Garg, T.; Vaidya, B.; Prakash, A.; Rath, G.; Goyal, A.K. Brain Delivery of Intranasal in Situ Gel of Nanoparticulated Polymeric Carriers Containing Antidepressant Drug: Behavioral and Biochemical Assessment. *J. Drug Target.* **2015**, *23*, 275–286. [CrossRef]
54. Abdellatif, A.A.H.; Alsowinea, A.F. Approved and Marketed Nanoparticles for Disease Targeting and Applications in COVID-19. *Nanotechnol. Rev.* **2021**, *10*, 1941–1977. [CrossRef]
55. Bulbake, U.; Doppalapudi, S.; Kommineni, N.; Khan, W. Liposomal Formulations in Clinical Use: An Updated Review. *Pharmaceutics* **2017**, *9*, 12. [CrossRef]
56. Singh, D.; Rashid, M.; Hallan, S.S.; Mehra, N.K.; Prakash, A.; Mishra, N. Pharmacological Evaluation of Nasal Delivery of Selegiline Hydrochloride-Loaded Thiolated Chitosan Nanoparticles for the Treatment of Depression. *Artif. Cells Nanomed. Biotechnol.* **2016**, *44*, 865–877. [CrossRef] [PubMed]
57. Patil, K.; Yeole, P.; Gaikwad, R.; Khan, S. Brain Targeting Studies on Buspirone Hydrochloride after Intranasal Administration of Mucoadhesive Formulation in Rats. *J. Pharm. Pharmacol.* **2009**, *61*, 669–675. [CrossRef] [PubMed]
58. Bari, N.K.; Fazil, M.; Hassan, M.Q.; Haider, M.R.; Gaba, B.; Narang, J.K.; Baboota, S.; Ali, J. Brain Delivery of Buspirone Hydrochloride Chitosan Nanoparticles for the Treatment of General Anxiety Disorder. *Int. J. Biol. Macromol.* **2015**, *81*, 49–59. [CrossRef] [PubMed]
59. Bshara, H.; Osman, R.; Mansour, S.; El-Shamy, A.E.H.A. Chitosan and Cyclodextrin in Intranasal Microemulsion for Improved Brain Buspirone Hydrochloride Pharmacokinetics in Rats. *Carbohydr. Polym.* **2014**, *99*, 297–305. [CrossRef]
60. Florence, K.; Manisha, L.; Kumar, B.A.; Ankur, K.; Kumar, M.A.; Ambikanandan, M. Intranasal Clobazam Delivery in the Treatment of Status Epilepticus. *J. Pharm. Sci.* **2011**, *100*, 692–703. [CrossRef]
61. Haque, S.; Md, S.; Fazil, M.; Kumar, M.; Sahni, J.K.; Ali, J.; Baboota, S. Venlafaxine Loaded Chitosan NPs for Brain Targeting: Pharmacokinetic and Pharmacodynamic Evaluation. *Carbohydr. Polym.* **2012**, *89*, 72–79. [CrossRef]
62. Haque, S.; Md, S.; Sahni, J.K.; Ali, J.; Baboota, S. Development and Evaluation of Brain Targeted Intranasal Alginate Nanoparticles for Treatment of Depression. *J. Psychiatr. Res.* **2014**, *48*, 1–12. [CrossRef]
63. Cayero-Otero, M.D.; Gomes, M.J.; Martins, C.; Álvarez-Fuentes, J.; Fernández-Arévalo, M.; Sarmento, B.; Martín-Banderas, L. In Vivo Biodistribution of Venlafaxine-PLGA Nanoparticles for Brain Delivery: Plain vs. Functionalized Nanoparticles. *Expert Opin. Drug Deliv.* **2019**, *16*, 1413–1427. [CrossRef]
64. Zhao, Y.; Zhang, L.; Peng, Y.; Yue, Q.; Hai, L.; Guo, L.; Wang, Q.; Wu, Y. GLUT 1 -Mediated Venlafaxine-Thiamine Disulfide System-Glucose Conjugates with "Lock-in" Function for Central Nervous System Delivery. *Chem. Biol. Drug Des.* **2018**, *91*, 707–716. [CrossRef]
65. Alam, M.I.; Baboota, S.; Ahuja, A.; Ali, M.; Ali, J.; Sahni, J.K.; Bhatnagar, A. Pharmacoscintigraphic Evaluation of Potential of Lipid Nanocarriers for Nose-to-Brain Delivery of Antidepressant Drug. *Int. J. Pharm.* **2014**, *470*, 99–106. [CrossRef] [PubMed]

66. Silva, S.; Bicker, J.; Fonseca, C.; Ferreira, N.R.; Vitorino, C.; Alves, G.; Falcão, A.; Fortuna, A. Encapsulated Escitalopram and Paroxetine Intranasal Co-Administration: In Vitro/In Vivo Evaluation. *Front. Pharmacol.* **2021**, *12*, 751321. [CrossRef]
67. Khan, N.; Shah, F.A.; Rana, I.; Ansari, M.M.; ud Din, F.; Rizvi, S.Z.H.; Aman, W.; Lee, G.Y.; Lee, E.S.; Kim, J.K.; et al. Nanostructured Lipid Carriers-Mediated Brain Delivery of Carbamazepine for Improved in Vivo Anticonvulsant and Anxiolytic Activity. *Int. J. Pharm.* **2020**, *577*, 119033. [CrossRef] [PubMed]
68. Qin, J.; Zhang, R.X.; Li, J.L.; Wang, J.X.; Hou, J.; Yang, X.; Zhu, W.L.; Shi, J.; Lu, L. CRGD Mediated Liposomes Enhanced Antidepressant-like Effects of Edaravone in Rats. *Eur. J. Pharm. Sci.* **2014**, *58*, 63–71. [CrossRef]
69. Nabi, B.; Rehman, S.; Fazil, M.; Khan, S.; Baboota, S.; Ali, J. Riluzole-Loaded Nanoparticles to Alleviate the Symptoms of Neurological Disorders by Attenuating Oxidative Stress. *Drug Dev. Ind. Pharm.* **2020**, *46*, 471–483. [CrossRef] [PubMed]
70. Chen, B.; Luo, M.; Liang, J.; Zhang, C.; Gao, C.; Wang, J.; Wang, J.; Li, Y.; Xu, D.; Liu, L.; et al. Surface Modification of PGP for a Neutrophil–Nanoparticle Co-Vehicle to Enhance the Anti-Depressant Effect of Baicalein. *Acta Pharm. Sin. B* **2018**, *8*, 64–73. [CrossRef]
71. Xu, D.; Lu, Y.R.; Kou, N.; Hu, M.J.; Wang, Q.S.; Cui, Y.L. Intranasal Delivery of Icariin via a Nanogel-Thermoresponsive Hydrogel Compound System to Improve Its Antidepressant-like Activity. *Int. J. Pharm.* **2020**, *586*, 119550. [CrossRef] [PubMed]
72. Wang, Q.S.; Li, K.; Gao, L.N.; Zhang, Y.; Lin, K.M.; Cui, Y.L. Intranasal Delivery of Berberine: Via in Situ Thermoresponsive Hydrogels with Non-Invasive Therapy Exhibits Better Antidepressant-like Effects. *Biomater. Sci.* **2020**, *8*, 2853–2865. [CrossRef] [PubMed]
73. Zhang, Q.-L.; Fu, B.M.; Zhang, Z.-J. Borneol, a Novel Agent That Improves Central Nervous System Drug Delivery by Enhancing Blood–Brain Barrier Permeability. *Drug Deliv.* **2017**, *24*, 1037–1044. [CrossRef]
74. Jin, Y.; Khadka, D.B.; Cho, W.-J. Pharmacological Effects of Berberine and Its Derivatives: A Patent Update. *Expert Opin. Ther. Pat.* **2016**, *26*, 229–243. [CrossRef] [PubMed]
75. El-Sherbeni, A.A.; El-Kadi, A.O.S. Microsomal Cytochrome P450 as a Target for Drug Discovery and Repurposing. *Drug Metab. Rev.* **2017**, *49*, 1–17. [CrossRef] [PubMed]
76. Kulkarni, S.K.; Dhir, A. On the Mechanism of Antidepressant-like Action of Berberine Chloride. *Eur. J. Pharmacol.* **2008**, *589*, 163–172. [CrossRef] [PubMed]
77. Liu, Y.-M.; Niu, L.; Wang, L.-L.; Bai, L.; Fang, X.-Y.; Li, Y.-C.; Yi, L.-T. Berberine Attenuates Depressive-like Behaviors by Suppressing Neuro-Inflammation in Stressed Mice. *Brain Res. Bull.* **2017**, *134*, 220–227. [CrossRef] [PubMed]
78. Clayton, K.N.; Salameh, J.W.; Wereley, S.T.; Kinzer-Ursem, T.L. Physical Characterization of Nanoparticle Size and Surface Modification Using Particle Scattering Diffusometry. *Biomicrofluidics* **2016**, *10*, 054107. [CrossRef]
79. Clogston, J.D.; Patri, A.K. Zeta Potential Measurement. In *Characterization of Nanoparticles Intended for Drug Delivery*; Humana Press: Totowa, NJ, USA, 2011; pp. 63–70.
80. Belovicova, K.; Bogi, E.; Csatlosova, K.; Dubovicky, M. Animal Tests for Anxiety-like and Depression-like Behavior in Rats. *Interdiscip. Toxicol.* **2017**, *10*, 40–43. [CrossRef]
81. Salahudeen, M.S.; Wright, C.M.; Peterson, G.M. Esketamine: New Hope for the Treatment of Treatment-Resistant Depression? A Narrative Review. *Ther. Adv. Drug Saf.* **2020**, *11*, 204209862093789. [CrossRef]
82. Vasiliu, O. Esketamine for Treatment-resistant Depression: A Review of Clinical Evidence (Review). *Exp. Ther. Med.* **2023**, *25*, 111. [CrossRef]
83. Karkare, S.; Zhdanava, M.; Pilon, D.; Nash, A.I.; Morrison, L.; Shah, A.; Lefebvre, P.; Joshi, K. Characteristics of Real-World Commercially Insured Patients With Treatment-Resistant Depression Initiated on Esketamine Nasal Spray or Conventional Therapies in the United States. *Clin. Ther.* **2022**, *44*, 1432–1448. [CrossRef]

pharmaceutics

Review

Modulation of the Blood–Brain Barrier for Drug Delivery to Brain

Liang Han

Jiangsu Key Laboratory of Neuropsychiatric Diseases Research, College of Pharmaceutical Sciences, Soochow University, Suzhou 215123, China; hanliang@suda.edu.cn

Abstract: The blood–brain barrier (BBB) precisely controls brain microenvironment and neural activity by regulating substance transport into and out of the brain. However, it severely hinders drug entry into the brain, and the efficiency of various systemic therapies against brain diseases. Modulation of the BBB via opening tight junctions, inhibiting active efflux and/or enhancing transcytosis, possesses the potential to increase BBB permeability and improve intracranial drug concentrations and systemic therapeutic efficiency. Various strategies of BBB modulation have been reported and investigated preclinically and/or clinically. This review describes conventional and emerging BBB modulation strategies and related mechanisms, and safety issues according to BBB structures and functions, to try to give more promising directions for designing more reasonable preclinical and clinical studies.

Keywords: blood–brain barrier modulation; tight junction; active efflux; transcytosis; drug delivery

Citation: Han, L. Modulation of the Blood–Brain Barrier for Drug Delivery to Brain. *Pharmaceutics* **2021**, *13*, 2024. https://doi.org/10.3390/pharmaceutics13122024

Academic Editors: Yuan Huang, Jingyuan Wen and Ruggero Bettini

Received: 23 October 2021
Accepted: 25 November 2021
Published: 27 November 2021

1. Introduction

The blood–brain barrier (BBB) plays a crucial protective role in maintaining a highly precise brain microenvironment for neuronal activity by regulating material transport into and out of the brain. The structural bases of the BBB (Figure 1) are brain capillary endothelial cells with tight junctions, active efflux transporters, and major facilitator superfamily domain-containing protein 2a (Mfsd2a), which jointly endow the BBB with extremely low both paracellular permeability and transcellular permeability [1]. Tight junctions seal endothelial paracellular gaps, leading to high trans-endothelial electrical resistance and limited paracellular transport. Transmembrane tight junction proteins include claudins, occludin, and junctional adhesion molecules, which all attach to intracellular actin cytoskeleton by membrane-associated proteins (e.g., zonula occludins-1). Highly expressed active efflux transporters include P-glycoprotein (Pgp), breast cancer resistant protein (BCRP), and multidrug-resistance proteins (MRPs). Mfsd2a mediates unique BBB endothelial lipid composition via transporting lysophosphatidylcholine esterified docosahexaenoic acid to BBB endothelial cells, to limit formation of caveolae-mediated transcytotic vesicles [2–4]. In addition, endothelial cells, pericytes, and astrocytes jointly form the neurovascular unit (Figure 1), and regulate the development and function of the BBB microcirculation by interacting with each other via secreting several factors [5–7]. These above properties cause the BBB to be constantly and dynamically modulated by both physiological and pathological factors [8,9].

Despite its protective function, the BBB blocks the entry of therapeutic substances into the brain. Although various brain diseases can lead to BBB breakdown with impaired structure and increased permeability [8], BBB around lesion margins or after repairing (e.g., Pgp upregulation in epilepsy and brain tumor) can still block drug delivery to the brain [9–12]. Therefore, systemic drug therapy for brain diseases is severely limited by the BBB. BBB modulation contributes to an increased drug concentration in the brain, and thus increases the efficiency of various systemic therapies [13]. Crucial proteins and structures in formation and regulation of BBB and their changes in brain diseases have been selectively regulated to improve drug delivery for systemic therapies against various brain diseases.

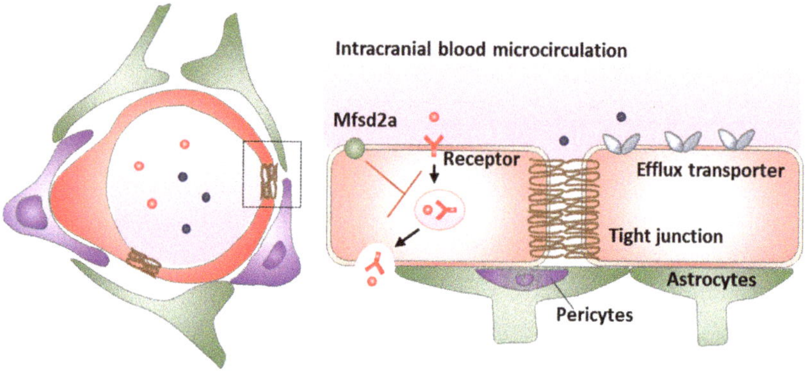

Figure 1. The neurovascular unit (**left**) and the mechanisms of transport inhibition by the BBB (**right**).

This review describes various conventional and emerging strategies for BBB modulation that increase both paracellular permeability and transcellular permeability of the BBB, and classifies these strategies according to BBB structures and functions including tight junctions, active efflux, and low transcytosis (Table 1). Furthermore, mechanisms responsible for increased BBB permeability and safe issues related to various strategies are also discussed, to try to give more promising directions for designing more reasonable preclinical and clinical studies.

Table 1. BBB regulation strategies and related advantages and disadvantages.

BBB Modulation Targets	Strategies	Advantages	Disadvantages
Tight junctions	Osmotic disruption	Transient and reversible	Nonselective, uncontrolled flow, invasive, anesthesia, and side effects
	Radiation-mediated disruption	Disease-specific	Unclear mechanisms and acute, subacute, and chronic dose-dependent toxicity
	Activating bradykinin B2 receptor	Disease-specific, rapid and transient	Limited application to only brain tumor and peripheral side effects
	Direct interference	Transient and reversible	Peripheral side effects
Active efflux	Direct Inhibition	Transient and reversible . . .	Tolerability concerns of the inhibitor, and side effects to both brain and peripheral tissues
	Targeting regulatory pathways	Disease-specific	Slow and side effects
Transcytosis	Upregulation of LRP1	Drug-specific	Slow and possible LRP1-associated side effects
	Inhibition of Mfsd2a	Transient and reversible	Possible Mfsd2a-associated side effects
	Upregulation of GLUT1	Efficient	Fasting-associated poor compliance

2. Modulation of Tight Junctions

Opening BBB tight junctions is supposed to increase paracellular BBB permeability and facilitate paracellular drug transport into the brain [14]. Ideally, tight junction opening should be transient and selective in a controlled manner to prevent unwanted accumulation (and toxicity) in the brain, and also avoid any short- or long-term peripheral side effects [15]. Various tight junction opening strategies have been reported with robust both preclinical and clinical performance (Figure 2). However, concerns of causing severe toxicity constantly exist, because the non-specific accumulation of neurotoxic blood components may induce neuronal degenerative changes and even cognitive impairments [16–18]. Various reported strategies are discussed here, which may help to promote the emergence of highly efficient approaches with minimal side effects.

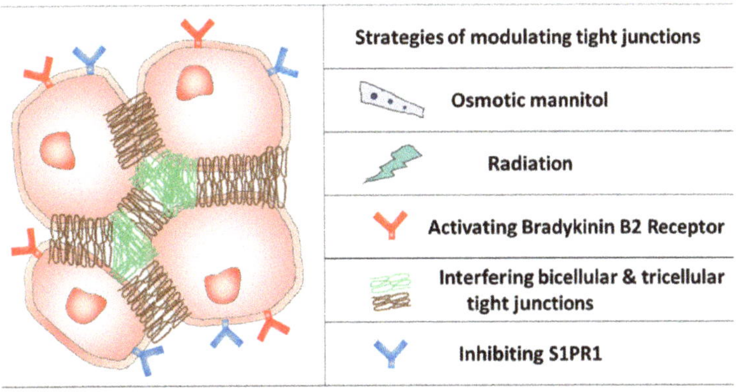

Figure 2. The BBB tight junctions and typical modulation strategies.

2.1. Osmotic BBB Disruption

Intra-arterial infusion of 25% hyperosmotic mannitol into the carotid or vertebral artery can induce vasodilation, endothelial cell shrinkage, and subsequent tight junction loosening and separation, leading to transient and reversible BBB disruption [15,19]. While conventional intra-arterial administration increases drug exposure of brain tumors 10-fold, osmotic BBB disruption can further increase drug exposure by up to 100-fold [20]. This strategy has been translated into the clinic to increase chemotherapy efficiency for brain tumors, and the tight junction opening window by osmotic BBB disruption can last for hours in humans [21]. Other hyperosmotic agents that transiently open tight junctions also include arabinose, lactamide, saline, urea, and radiographic contrast agents [15]. Osmotic BBB disruption is generally nonselective with uncontrolled flow into whole brain regions, such as neurotoxic blood components (e.g., albumin), leading to edema, neurological toxicity, epilepsy, aphasia, and hemiparesis [15,22–24]. In addition, the invasive nature and general anesthesia render the technique impractical for drug therapy against chronic brain diseases [14]. Therefore, the use of osmotic BBB disruption is confined to only clinical management of brain tumors.

2.2. Radiation-Mediated BBB Disruption

Radiation cannot only induce tumor cell apoptosis, but also disrupt the BBB [7,18,25–31]. Although the underlying mechanisms are still uncertain, BBB disruption induced by radiation leads to enhanced paracellular diffusion and transcellular transport [7]. Radiation therapy has been combined with systemic therapies to treat brain tumors. Although some study suggests that radiation failed to increase intracranial drug concentrations, increased gefitinib concentration in cerebrospinal fluid was shown with escalating radiation dose in patients with brain metastases in clinical trials [32,33]. Therefore, further research is needed to verify whether enhanced drug delivery to the brain can indeed occur after radiation and whether it is based on the effects on the BBB [34]. It has been reported that the disrupted BBB by radiation needs hours to years to recover [27]. Therefore, irradiation involves acute, subacute, and chronic dose-dependent toxicity [26,27]. For example, vasogenic edema from vascular damage causes early radiation toxicity syndrome including headache, nausea, or neurologic deficits [18]. Subacute side effects may appear around six months post radiation and progress into chronic dysfunction. Chronic side effects include radiation-induced necrosis, demyelination, leukoencephalopathy, cerebral atrophy, and neurocognitive deficits, and so on [35,36]. Stereotaxic radiosurgery may be an alternative approach to reduce radiation-related intracranial side effects and simultaneously maintain the BBB disrupting effects.

2.3. *Activating Bradykinin B2 Receptor*

Bradykinin B2 receptor is constitutively expressed on BBB endothelial cells. Its stimulation can rapidly and transiently disengage tight junctions and increase BBB permeability [37]. The expression of bradykinin B2 receptor is upregulated in the blood–tumor barrier (BTB) in brain tumors [38,39]. Therefore, activating the bradykinin B2 receptor may selectively modulate the BTB permeability and increase drug delivery to brain tumors. This strategy may be able to avoid side effects of osmotic BBB disruption towards the normal brain, owing to targeting effects on the BTB. Nonapeptide RMP-7 can selectively stimulate bradykinin B2 receptor and possesses longer blood circulation than endogenous bradykinin [37]. RMP-7 has been shown to be effective in opening BBB tight junctions and increasing intracranial drug concentrations in normal animal and in brain tumor animal models after intravenous infusion or intra-arterial injection [40–42].

Bradykinin B2 receptor is also expressed at numerous additional sites, and its activation at these sites can induce a wide variety of physiological responses including smooth muscle relaxation (e.g., vasculature) and contraction (e.g., intestine and uterus), inflammation modulation, pain mediation, and dose-limiting side effects (e.g., hypotension) [37]. The major side effects of intravenously administered tolerable RMP (up to 300 ng/kg over 10 min) were immediate and transient and included flushing, nausea, headache, and tachycardia [43–45]. At clinically approved dosage, the effects of intravenously infused RMP-7 weren't shown in Phase II clinical trials in patients with brain tumors [38,44–46]. Intracarotid injection rather intravenous infusion has the potential of concentrating RMP-7 to the brain and reducing effects on peripheral tissues. Except for transient decreases in arterial blood pressure, intra-arterial administration of RMP-7 wasn't shown to produce any other side effects, such as apparent cerebrovascular abnormalities and neurologic deficits in swine [47]. It is to be noted that bradykinin-increased BBB permeability may also be related with increased vesicular transport [48]. Considering the specific effect of RMP-7 on the BTB and the evidence demonstrated with the U87 glioma model that 7~100 nm pores in BTB are sufficient to allow the translocation of certain nanoparticles [49], the possibility of combining RMP-7 with targeting macromolecules or nanomedicine should be further evaluated.

2.4. *Direct Interference of Tight Junctions*

Claudins are major components of tight junctions, and claudin-5 dominates the BBB tight junctions by limiting paracellular penetration of small molecules [50–52]. Knockdown of BBB endothelial claudin-5 using specific siRNA was also shown to be able to transiently and reversibly increase BBB permeability to small molecules (MW up to 742) in mice [53]. The BBB opening and increased permeability after claudin-5 siRNA treatment were found to be size-selective and last for 72 h for small molecules with MW 443 and for 48 h for small molecules with MWs 562 and 742. It is also noteworthy that BBB opening after claudin-5 siRNA treatment also contributed to the clearance of water from the brain with cognitive improvement in mice with focal cerebral edema [54]. Anti-claudin-5 antibody can specifically recognize and bind with the extracellular loop domain of claudin-5, leading to impaired BBB tight junctions and increased BBB permeability to small molecules (e.g., sodium fluorescein with MW 376) [55–57]. The 3 mg/kg antibody didn't induce any liver and kidney injury, change of plasma biomarkers of inflammation, and behavior change in cynomolgus monkeys while vasodilation in liver, lung, and kidney, lung hemorrhage, and brain edema were shown with 6 mg/kg antibody [55]. The side effects of high dose of anti-claudin-5 antibody can be ascribed to the wide expression of claudin-5 in the vascular endothelium of peripheral tissues [52]. The narrow window between the tight junction opening and peripheral side effects should be considered and local delivery of anti-claudin-5 antibody may be able to prevent the above side effects. Peptide C5C2 can bind with the first extracellular loop of claudin-5 and was shown to internalize and downregulate claudin-5 [58]. However, in contrary to anti-claudin-5 antibody and claudin-5 siRNA, the transient and reversible BBB opening mediated by C5C2 was found to allow brain entry of molecules up to 40 kDa.

Angulin-1 and tricellulin constitute the functional BBB tricellular tight junctions, which blocking brain entry of macromolecules only [50,59,60]. Angubindin-1 is derived from the receptor-binding domain of *Clostridium perfringens* iota-toxin and can bind with angulin-1 of tricellular tight junctions and remove angulin-1 and tricellulin from tricellular tight junctions, leading to enhanced BBB permeability to macromolecules [61]. Intravenously injected angubindin-1 disrupted tricellular tight junctions without any overt adverse effect and increased BBB permeability for transient brain entry of macromolecules [60].

2.5. Other Potential Strategies

There also reported numerous other strategies for opening BBB tight junctions with enormous potential. For example, as a G protein-coupled receptor, sphingosine 1-phosphate receptor-1 (S1PR1) plays an important role in the barrier function of the BBB and peripheral vessels [17]. Knockout or downregulation of endothelial S1PR1 transiently and reversibly altered distribution of BBB tight junction proteins and allowed increased brain penetration of small molecules with MW less than 3000 in mice. The opening of BBB tight junctions by S1PR1 inhibition via FTY720 didn't show any signs of brain inflammation or injury. Controversially, FTY720 was also reported to reverse downregulation of S1P1 and S1P3 in retinas of diabetic rats and repair BBB by upregulating claudin-5 and downregulating VCAM-1 [62,63]. Therefore, further research is needed to verify whether FTY720 can indeed open BBB tight junctions and enhance paracellular drug delivery to the brain. The upregulation of astrocytic S1PR3 was linked to high permeability of brain metastases from breast cancer [64–66], suggesting contrary pathophysiological effects of S1PR3 to those of S1PR1. Further studies are also needed to elucidate the respective roles of S1PR1 and S1PR3 in the BBB.

Intracarotid injection of alkylglycerols was shown to transiently increase paracellular BBB permeability to small molecules and macromolecules with an efficiency comparable to that of osmotic BBB disruption and higher than that of intracarotid infusion of bradykinin [67–71]. Although intracarotid administration is an invasive procedure and the effects of alkylglycerols haven't been proven clinically, the strategy of alkylglycerol-mediated BBB opening didn't reveal any sign of toxicity at the animal level after long-term in vivo analyses [71]. In addition, intracarotid infusion of oleic acid or linoleic acid was also found to cause reversible BBB disruption and increase BBB permeability, but with brain edema, necrosis, and demyelination [72,73].

In theory, selectively disrupting the diseased BBB is more advantageous than nonspecific BBB disruption when systemic therapy of brain diseases is considered, owing to the absence of unwanted side effects to normal brain regions, e.g., the strategy of activating the bradykinin B2 receptor in 2.3. Pericytes derived from glioblastoma were reported to be directly associated with the BTB tight junctions and poor response of glioblastoma to chemotherapy [74]. Reducing pericyte coverage of the BTB was found to successfully increase paracellular BTB permeability and then improve chemotherapy efficiency against glioblastoma [75]. Ibrutinib with the ability of eliminating glioblastoma-derived pericytes by inhibiting BMX kinase was proven to be able to selectively impair the BTB tight junctions to enhance the therapeutic efficacy of drugs with poor BTB penetration [74].

Substance P is an important proinflammatory neuropeptide that functions as an immunoneuromodulator in the brain. Notably, substance P is also expressed by breast cancer and involves in chemoresistance and BBB crossing of breast cancer cells to form brain metastases [76]. Substance P secreted by breast cancer cells induces BBB endothelial cells to successively secret tumor necrosis factor alpha (TNFα) and angiopoietin-2 (Ang-2), which further activate their receptors to reorganize endothelial cytoskeleton and destabilize inter-endothelial adhesion complexes to alter distribution of tight junction proteins such as claudin-5 [76–79]. In addition, increased BBB permeability by secreted Ang-2 is also correlated with upregulated caveolin-1 and intensified caveolae-mediated vesicular transport [80]. Considering the substance P-mediated effects and corresponding specific expression of TNF receptors in the BTB (brain metastases), substance P, TNFα, Ang-2 and their derivatives can be used to open tight junctions in the BBB and tumor-associated BTB, respectively.

3. Modulation of Active Efflux

Active efflux transporters are selective gatekeepers at the BBB and cooperate with tight junctions to regulate substance transport into and out of the brain. Pathophysiological processes and pharmacological intervention further aggravate the efflux effect by intensifying expression and activity of these efflux transporters. Therefore, targeting regulatory pathways of BBB efflux transporters is supposed to be a feasible approach for efficient drug delivery to the brain [81,82]. BBB efflux transporters include Pgp, BCRP and MRPs. Although the role of other efflux transporters may be underestimated, Pgp with multiple binding domains for broad substrate spectrum is thought to be a predominant BBB efflux transporter [81,82]. Therefore, this section is focused on the modulation of Pgp. Typical strategies including direct inhibition and inhibiting transcriptional activation are introduced here. Notably, preserving and restoring their normal expression and activity after treatment is of specific importance, owing to the protective roles of active efflux. Many other modulating mechanisms of BBB Pgp expression and activity, such as posttranscriptional mechanisms, posttranslational mechanisms, and intracellular and intercellular trafficking, were not reviewed here, owing to the absence of reported pharmacological intervention [81].

3.1. *Direct Inhibition of Efflux Transporters*

Pgp activity can be directly inhibited using specific competitive inhibitors, such as verapamil (Figure 3) [83,84]. In vivo cerebral microdialysis can be used to directly measure the concentration of free drug in the brain to study possible drug–Pgp interactions [85]. For example, through brain microdialysis in rats, it has been shown that Pgp inhibition enhanced the brain concentration of Pgp substrates ceftriaxone and seliciclib [86,87]. Evaluated by intracerebral microdialysis on mice, topotecan penetration in gliomas was enhanced by modulating Pgp using gefitinib [88]. However, high dosed inhibitors are often used, owing to their low Pgp binding affinity and greater resistant Pgp inhibition at the BBB than peripheral Pgp [89], which may lead to tolerability concerns and side effects. In addition, Pgp inhibition at the BBB can enhance brain concentrations of unwanted substrates, which could lead to serious intracranial side effects from the unwanted compounds [85]. The second-generation inhibitors with improved tolerability, including valspodar, possess the shortcomings of inhibiting cytochrome P450 enzymes, leading to delayed drug clearance and prolonged systemic exposure of co-administered therapeutic drugs [82]. Thus, the effects on drug metabolism and pharmacodynamics limit the application of these two generation inhibitors. Third-generation inhibitors (e.g., elacridar) affect BBB efflux efficacy by inducing Pgp conformation changes.

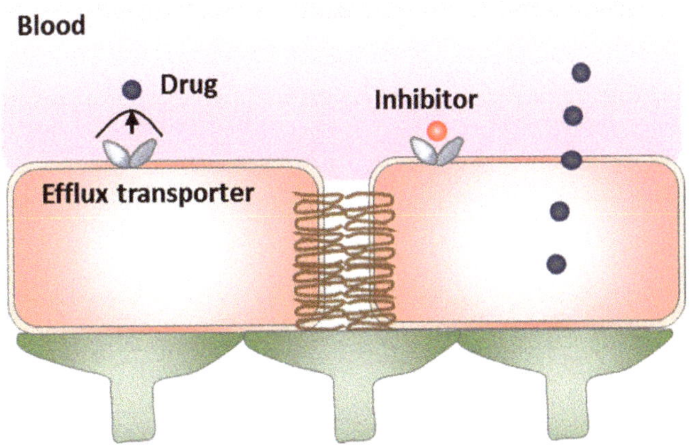

Figure 3. The strategy of directly inhibiting efflux transporters.

3.2. Targeting Regulatory Pathways of Efflux Transporters

Inhibiting the signal pathways intensifying Pgp expression and activity is supposed to overcome Pgp-mediated efflux and chemoresistance [90]. A number of "orphan" nuclear receptors are key transcriptional regulators and their expression at the BBB can upregulate Pgp, BCRP, and MRPs to respond to potentially harmful compounds. For example, pregnane X receptor (PXR) directly participates in Pgp upregulation by anticancer drugs [91–93]. Antagonists of these orphan nuclear receptors, such as ketoconazole, were shown to effectively inhibit rifampicin- and paclitaxel-induced Pgp upregulation, and sensitize brain cancers to anticancer drugs [94]. It is to be noted that these Pgp regulating mechanisms at the BBB likely exist in peripheral tissues. Strategies reversing Pgp upregulation might also reduce Pgp in other tissues and thereby cause unintended side effects.

The signaling pathway of glutamate/NMDA-R/COX-2/prostaglandin E2 EP1 receptor induces Pgp and BCRP overexpression at the BBB in epileptic brains (Figure 4). MK-801, an antagonist of N-methyl-D-aspartate receptor (NMDA-R), was proven to effectively prevent glutamate-induced Pgp upregulation [95]. However, the side effects severely restrict the development of this approach [96]. COX inhibition using indomethacin and celecoxib was proven to prevent seizure-induced Pgp overexpression and enhance delivery of antiepileptic drugs to the brain in epilepsy model with negligible effect on basal Pgp expression and transport activity [97–99]. Unfortunately, COX-2 inhibitors are also associated with an enhanced risk of cardiovascular and cerebrovascular events and the controversial impact on seizure thresholds and seizure severity [100]. Inhibiting the prostaglandin E2 EP1 receptor by SC-51089 was further demonstrated to abolish glutamate-induced Pgp increases at the BBB, and enhance antiepileptic drug efficacy [82,101]. Neurodegeneration aggravation after COX-2 inhibition can be attributed to the blocking of EP2, EP3, and EP4 downstream of prostaglandin E2 [102–104]. Therefore, antagonism of the prostaglandin E2 EP1 receptor may be the most promising approach to control Pgp expression and enhance entry of antiepileptic drugs to epileptic brains. Strategies of reversing Pgp upregulation in epilepsy can be extended to the application in treating brain ischemia, because the glutamate release and similar Pgp upregulation mechanisms also exists in brain ischemia [105]. In contrary, as a critical factor for intracranial clearance of amyloid β-protein (Aβ), Pgp expression at the BBB is often downregulated to promote intracranial Aβ accumulation in Alzheimer's disease [106–109]. Signaling pathways inducing Pgp upregulation may be carefully harnessed to treat Alzheimer's disease. For example, PXR ligands (e.g., hyperforin) and EP1 receptor agonists hold the potential for upregulating Pgp to interfere with Alzheimer's disease. In addition, strengthening the Wnt/β-catenin signaling may also be able to increase Pgp to reduce Aβ burden in Alzheimer's disease [110].

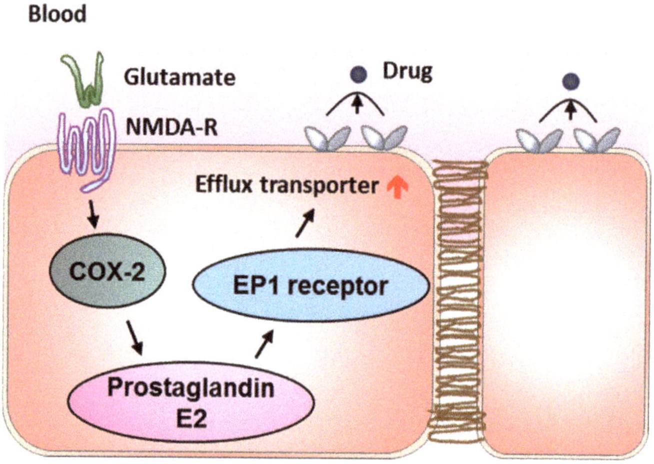

Figure 4. The signaling pathway of glutamate/NMDA-R/COX-2/prostaglandin E2 EP1 receptor induces the upregulation of efflux transports in epilepsy.

4. Modulation of Transcytosis

Receptor-mediated transcytosis is often used to mediate transcellular BBB crossing, owing to the extremely low paracellular BBB permeability controlled by the tight junctions and active efflux transporters. Receptor-specific ligands can be used to decorate drug delivery systems (e.g., multifunctional nanoparticles) to initiate transcellular transport across the BBB [8,49,111–117]. However, the density of these target receptors at the BBB is much lower than that of nutrient transporters (e.g., glucose transporter) [118]. More importantly, exclusively expressed Mfsd2a limits formation of caveolae-mediated transcytotic vesicles and the transcytosis rate at the BBB by regulating BBB endothelial lipid composition [1–6,119–121]. Therefore, the efficiency of transcellular transport at the BBB should be modulated to improve brain accumulation of ligand-modified drug delivery systems.

4.1. Upregulation of LRP1

Low-density lipoprotein receptor-related protein 1 (LRP1) is expressed at both luminal and abluminal sides of the BBB. While abluminal LRP1 is primarily responsible for clearing Aβ from the brain to blood [122], luminal LRP1 has been extensively studied to mediate drug delivery to the brain. Inspired by the fact that statins can suppress cholesterol synthesis and then induce compensatory expression of LRP1 [118,123–126], simvastatin-loaded nanoparticles were reported in our previous work to upregulate LRP1 at the BBB and boost LRP1-targeting chemotherapy efficiency against brain metastases from breast cancer [114]. In addition, LRP1 can respond to astrocytic apolipoprotein E to maintain the BBB integrity by suppressing the BBB-degrading pathway of activation of cyclophilin A-matrix metalloproteinase 9 [127,128]. More importantly, the diminishment of abluminal LRP1 is closely related to intracranial Aβ accumulation in Alzheimer's disease, and also to the aggregation of α-synuclein into Lewy bodies in Parkinson's disease [127,128]. Therefore, the strategy of upregulating LRP1, a potentially important therapeutic target of BBB breakdown-related diseases, holds the potential to be used to treat both Alzheimer's disease and Parkinson's disease. In fact, delivery of LRP1 gene to the BBB has been reported to facilitate Aβ clearance via upregulating LRP1 [127,129].

4.2. Inhibition of Mfsd2a

Reversible inhibition of Mfsd2a holds the potential to temporarily liberate the limited transcytosis at the BBB [2]. In our previous work, Mfsd2a inhibitor tunicamycin was delivered to the BBB and shown to be able to enhance brain accumulation of subsequent therapeutic nanoparticles and the efficiency in treating brain metastases from breast cancer in mice [117]. Owing to the crucial role of Mfsd2a in transporting essential fatty acids and promoting BBB formation and brain development, Mfsd2a knockout induces microcephaly, Allan-Herndon-Dudley syndrome, and other severe side effects (e.g., BBB breakdown, neuronal loss, cognitive impairment, intellectual disability, behavioral deficits, spasticity, and absent speech and so on) [4,121,127,128,130–132]. In clinical practice, the loss of BBB Mfsd2a is often found in Alzheimer's disease, traumatic brain injury, stroke, and brain tumor. Mfsd2a may be a potential therapeutic target for these diseases and remains to be explored further [130,131]. However, tunicamycin-mediated Mfsd2a inhibition is likely to be reversible, because the inhibition mechanism is supposed to be just physical binding and the inhibitor would dissociate from Mfsd2a after entering the brain [2]. Therefore, side effects associated with Mfsd2a deficiency could be avoided.

4.3. Upregulation of GLUT1

Glucose transporter 1 (GLUT1) at the BBB maintains the continuous high glucose and energy demands of the brain. Based on its essential role in transporting glucose and its participation in pathological processes of various brain diseases such as Alzheimer's disease, ischemia, and brain tumors, upregulation of GLUT1 has been proposed to treat hypoglycemic conditions, while its downregulation or inhibition could be used to cope with hyperglycemic conditions [133]. In addition to being direct therapeutic targets, wide expression of GLUT1 at the BBB has been extensively used to mediate drug delivery to the brain. GLUT1 upregulation at the luminal side of the BBB via hypoglycemia and its migration to the abluminal side were implemented via rapid glycemic increase after fasting [134]. Then, the brain accumulation of properly configured glucose nanoparticles was shown to reach 6% dose/g-brain in normal mice with glycemic control. Because Alzheimer's disease is characterized by reduced GLUT1 at the BBB and a reduction of glucose transport [129], this strategy of rapid glycemic increase after fasting holds the potential to treat Alzheimer's disease via upregulating GLUT1.

5. Multifunctional Strategies by Multiple BBB Modulation

All the above strategies increase BBB permeability via separately modulating tight junctions, active efflux, or transcytosis. In fact, there many other multifunctional strategies were also reported, which can simultaneously modulate multiple controlling factors and achieve theoretically higher BBB permeability for efficient drug delivery to the brain.

5.1. Focused Ultrasound

Low intensity focused ultrasound is a noninvasive technique that is combined with intravenously injected gaseous perfluorocarbon-filled microbubbles to transiently and focally modulate the BBB [135,136]. With the help of stable oscillation of microbubbles, the BBB is transiently and reversibly disrupted and characterized by (1) disintegration of tight junctions including claudin-5; (2) fenestration and channel formation; (3) Pgp suppression; and (4) upregulation of caveolin-1 and caveolae-mediated transcytotic vesicles, which jointly facilitate both paracellular transport and transcellular passage through the BBB [137–141]. Under the guidance by magnetic resonance imaging, microbubble-enhanced focused ultrasound can act on specific intracranial areas with negligible toxicity to adjacent normal brain cells [142–146]. Further, ultrasmall superparamagnetic iron oxide nanoparticles can be encapsulated into microbubbles and nanobubbles to increase the BBB disruption efficiency and monitor post-sonication BBB opening and drug delivery across the BBB [147,148]. Generally, microbubble-enhanced focused ultrasound is less invasive than BBB disruption induced by osmotic agents with minimal neurotoxicity, inflammation, and stroke occurrences in clinical settings [135,149–153]. However, increasing acoustic energy is associated with increasing risk of side effects including vascular damage, edema, parenchymal damage, microhemorrhage, and over-activation of the immune system (e.g., autoimmunity) [137,154,155]. Therefore, adjusting ultrasound parameters is necessary for reducing risks, especially for repeated treatments and the application of mediating drug delivery to Alzheimer's disease owing to Aβ-mediated resistance of BBB disruption [156,157].

5.2. Activating A2A Adenosine Receptor

A2A adenosine receptor interacts with G_s protein to activate adenylate cyclase and further increase intracellular cAMP [154]. It is located on platelets, leukocytes, blood vessels and intracranial regions such as striatum [158]. Its activation can inhibit platelet aggregation and regulate blood pressure through vasodilation [159]. Its expression can be altered by pathological conditions, e.g., upregulation on glial cells by hypoxia and inflammation and at the BBB by brain tumors [10,160], to protect against damage via reducing inflammation [161]. The activation of A2A adenosine receptor at the BBB can increase BBB permeability by rapid and reversible decrease of tight junction proteins (e.g., claudin-5), Pgp and BCRP [154,162]. Intravenous injection of clinically used regadenoson was shown to be able to increase intracranial concentrations of small molecules and macromolecules in preclinical studies [163–167]. However, regadenoson treatment at FDA-approved doses in humans (bolus injection of 0.4 mg) was found without increased intracranial concentrations of temozolomide in patients with recurrent glioblastoma [168,169], which may be attributed to the insufficient dose of this strategy for effective BBB modulation, and warrants the necessity of studies on whether higher dose or different agonists would be effective [154]. The alternative option of nanomedicine-mediated targeted agonist delivery holds the potential of not only enhancing selectivity, intensifying the BBB opening effect, and prolonging the BBB opening time window from up to 50 min to up to 2 h [170–174], but also avoiding affecting peripheral A2A adenosine receptors to minimize systemic side effects, e.g., excessive vasodilatation of the peripheral vascular bed, dizziness, and headaches [154].

5.3. Activating Potassium Channels

Blood vessel endothelium widely expresses potassium channels, especially ATP-dependent potassium channels (K_{ATP}) [175,176]. Activation of K_{ATP} can regulate vascular hyperpolarization, relaxation, dilatation and vessel permeability [175–178], making K_{ATP} a therapeutic target for hypertension. K_{ATP} is often upregulated in hypoxic environments including brain tumors and ischemia [178,179]. The regulatory effects on BTB permeability by activating the K_{ATP} are expected to be more significant than those of the BBB [176,180]. These effects include intensified paracellular diffusion and transcellular transport, which involve in downregulated tight junction proteins and upregulated caveolin-1 and caveolae-mediated transcytotic vesicles [176,181,182]. BTB modulation by strengthening the activation of K_{ATP} can be tightly controlled by inhibitors and has been used via minoxidil to increase Herceptin delivery to primary or metastatic brain tumors [183–186]. Although minoxidil was found to be nontoxic in both mice and rats [175], nonselective activation of K_{ATP} may induce pericardial effusion, cardiac tamponade, reflex tachycardia, myocardial necrosis, coronary arteriopathy, degeneration of renal tubules, hypotension, dermatologic reactions, and hypertrichosis [154,187]. Intracarotid injection rather intravenous infusion holds the potential of concentrating minoxidil to the brain and reducing effects on peripheral tissues. As an alternative approach, in our previous work, minoxidil was delivered by hyaluronic acid modified nanoparticles to specially intensify the activation of BTB K_{ATP} to enhance specific accumulation of subsequently injected therapeutic nanoparticles in brain metastases in mice [188].

5.4. Other Potential Multifunctional Strategies

As a key factor in hypertension, diabetes and aging, angiotensin-II can increase BBB permeability in both paracellular and transcellular manner by altering the distribution of tight junction proteins, decreasing Mfsd2a, and increasing caveolin-1 [189]. Thus, angiotensin-II can be used to open the BBB for increased drug delivery into the brain to treat various brain diseases. As a surgical technique, laser interstitial thermal therapy has been widely used to ablate brain tumors [190,191]. Interestingly, increasing data indicate that thermal therapy can disrupt the BBB via temporarily altering tight junctions and increasing transcytosis [190]. Although this technique is invasive and requires general anesthesia, combination of laser interstitial thermal therapy with other systemic therapies still holds the potential for synergistic therapeutic effect.

6. Conclusions and Future Perspectives

Modulation of the BBB, including tight junctions, active efflux transporters, and transcytotic vesicles, has been extensively studied to increase drug delivery to the brain. Although improved intracranial drug concentrations were often shown for almost all approaches, most of these studies were conducted preclinically and focused on brain tumors with very few exceptions on epilepsy. Side effects associated with these modulating strategies need to be carefully handled to extend these technologies to various brain diseases, including neurodegenerative diseases. First, although any delivery route can be used including intravenous, intracarotid or stereotactic administration, these BBB modulation approaches by themselves (e.g., radiation and various modulators) can be severely toxic. Second, besides the BBB's protective roles, BBB modulations are likely to impair the intracranial physiological functions of related targets, e.g., normal physiological actions of bradykinin B2 receptor, S1PR1, Pgp, Mfsd2a, LRP1, GLUT1, A2A adenosine receptor, and K_{ATP}. Third, increased drug concentrations in normal brain and peripheral tissues resulting from efflux inhibition or tight junction opening may worsen side effects of subsequent therapeutic drugs. Fourth, unwanted accumulation of endogenous neurotoxic blood components and xenobiotics in normal brain regions (even specific accumulation in diseased regions) may lead to severe neurological complications. Therefore, the modulation window of various modulation strategies should be carefully investigated for safe clinical translation, especially those multifunctional strategies that combine multiple BBB modulations.

Funding: This work was funded by the National Natural Science Foundation of China (81973254 and 32171381), the Natural Science Foundation of Jiangsu Province (BK20191421), the Suzhou Science and Technology Development Project (SYS2019033) and the Priority Academic Program Development of the Jiangsu Higher Education Institutes (PAPD).

Conflicts of Interest: The author declares that there are no conflict of interest.

References

1. Andreone, B.J.; Chow, B.W.; Tata, A.; Lacoste, B.; Ben-Zvi, A.; Bullock, K.; Deik, A.A.; Ginty, D.D.; Clish, C.B.; Gu, C. Blood-brain barrier permeability is regulated by lipid transport-dependent suppression of caveolae-mediated transcytosis. *Neuron* **2017**, *94*, 581–594.e585. [CrossRef]
2. Wang, J.Z.; Xiao, N.; Zhang, Y.Z.; Zhao, C.X.; Guo, X.H.; Lu, L.M. Mfsd2a-based pharmacological strategies for drug delivery across the blood-brain barrier. *Pharmacol. Res.* **2016**, *104*, 124–131. [CrossRef]
3. Knowland, D.; Arac, A.; Sekiguchi, K.J.; Hsu, M.; Lutz, S.E.; Perrino, J.; Steinberg, G.K.; Barres, B.A.; Nimmerjahn, A.; Agalliu, D. Stepwise recruitment of transcellular and paracellular pathways underlies blood-brain barrier breakdown in stroke. *Neuron* **2014**, *82*, 603–617. [CrossRef]
4. Ben-Zvi, A.; Lacoste, B.; Kur, E.; Andreone, B.J.; Mayshar, Y.; Yan, H.; Gu, C. Mfsd2a is critical for the formation and function of the blood-brain barrier. *Nature* **2014**, *509*, 507–511. [CrossRef] [PubMed]
5. Armulik, A.; Genove, G.; Mae, M.; Nisancioglu, M.H.; Wallgard, E.; Niaudet, C.; He, L.; Norlin, J.; Lindblom, P.; Strittmatter, K.; et al. Pericytes regulate the blood-brain barrier. *Nature* **2010**, *468*, 557–561. [CrossRef]
6. Daneman, R.; Zhou, L.; Kebede, A.A.; Barres, B.A. Pericytes are required for blood-brain barrier integrity during embryogenesis. *Nature* **2010**, *468*, 562–566. [CrossRef] [PubMed]
7. Arvanitis, C.D.; Ferraro, G.B.; Jain, R.K. The blood-brain barrier and blood-tumour barrier in brain tumours and metastases. *Nat. Rev. Cancer* **2020**, *20*, 26–41. [CrossRef]
8. Han, L.; Jiang, C. Evolution of blood-brain barrier in brain diseases and related systemic nanoscale brain-targeting drug delivery strategies. *Acta Pharm. Sin. B* **2021**, *11*, 2306–2325. [CrossRef] [PubMed]

9. Abbott, N.J.; Ronnback, L.; Hansson, E. Astrocyte-endothelial interactions at the blood-brain barrier. *Nat. Rev. Neurosci.* **2006**, *7*, 41–53. [CrossRef]
10. Gao, X.; Yue, Q.; Liu, Y.; Fan, D.; Fan, K.; Li, S.; Qian, J.; Han, L.; Fang, F.; Xu, F.; et al. Image-guided chemotherapy with specifically tuned blood brain barrier permeability in glioma margins. *Theranostics* **2018**, *8*, 3126–3137. [CrossRef] [PubMed]
11. Liu, J.; He, Y.; Zhang, J.; Li, J.; Yu, X.; Cao, Z.; Meng, F.; Zhao, Y.; Wu, X.; Shen, T.; et al. Functionalized nanocarrier combined seizure-specific vector with p-glycoprotein modulation property for antiepileptic drug delivery. *Biomaterials* **2016**, *74*, 64–76. [CrossRef] [PubMed]
12. Soffietti, R.; Ahluwalia, M.; Lin, N.; Ruda, R. Management of brain metastases according to molecular subtypes. *Nat. Rev. Neurol.* **2020**, *16*, 557–574. [CrossRef]
13. Luo, H.; Shusta, E.V. Blood-brain barrier modulation to improve glioma drug delivery. *Pharmaceutics* **2020**, *12*, 1085. [CrossRef]
14. Lochhead, J.J.; Yang, J.; Ronaldson, P.T.; Davis, T.P. Structure, function, and regulation of the blood-brain barrier tight junction in central nervous system disorders. *Front. Physiol.* **2020**, *11*, 914. [CrossRef] [PubMed]
15. Pandit, R.; Chen, L.; Gotz, J. The blood-brain barrier: Physiology and strategies for drug delivery. *Adv. Drug Deliv. Rev.* **2020**, *165–166*, 1–14. [CrossRef] [PubMed]
16. Bell, R.D.; Winkler, E.A.; Sagare, A.P.; Singh, I.; LaRue, B.; Deane, R.; Zlokovic, B.V. Pericytes control key neurovascular functions and neuronal phenotype in the adult brain and during brain aging. *Neuron* **2010**, *68*, 409–427. [CrossRef]
17. Yanagida, K.; Liu, C.H.; Faraco, G.; Galvani, S.; Smith, H.K.; Burg, N.; Anrather, J.; Sanchez, T.; Iadecola, C.; Hla, T. Size-selective opening of the blood-brain barrier by targeting endothelial sphingosine 1-phosphate receptor 1. *Proc. Natl. Acad. Sci. USA* **2017**, *114*, 4531–4536. [CrossRef] [PubMed]
18. Kodack, D.P.; Askoxylakis, V.; Ferraro, G.B.; Fukumura, D.; Jain, R.K. Emerging strategies for treating brain metastases from breast cancer. *Cancer Cell* **2015**, *27*, 163–175. [CrossRef]
19. Haluska, M.; Anthony, M.L. Osmotic blood-brain barrier modification for the treatment of malignant brain tumors. *Clin. J. Oncol. Nurs.* **2004**, *8*, 263–267. [CrossRef] [PubMed]
20. Kroll, R.A.; Neuwelt, E.A. Outwitting the blood-brain barrier for therapeutic purposes: Osmotic opening and other means. *Neurosurgery* **1998**, *42*, 1083–1099; discussion 1099–1100. [CrossRef]
21. Siegal, T.; Rubinstein, R.; Bokstein, F.; Schwartz, A.; Lossos, A.; Shalom, E.; Chisin, R.; Gomori, J.M. In vivo assessment of the window of barrier opening after osmotic blood-brain barrier disruption in humans. *J. Neurosurg.* **2000**, *92*, 599–605. [CrossRef] [PubMed]
22. van Vliet, E.A.; da Costa Araujo, S.; Redeker, S.; van Schaik, R.; Aronica, E.; Gorter, J.A. Blood-brain barrier leakage may lead to progression of temporal lobe epilepsy. *Brain J. Neurol.* **2007**, *130*, 521–534. [CrossRef] [PubMed]
23. Marchi, N.; Angelov, L.; Masaryk, T.; Fazio, V.; Granata, T.; Hernandez, N.; Hallene, K.; Diglaw, T.; Franic, L.; Najm, I.; et al. Seizure-promoting effect of blood-brain barrier disruption. *Epilepsia* **2007**, *48*, 732–742. [CrossRef]
24. Ikeda, M.; Bhattacharjee, A.K.; Kondoh, T.; Nagashima, T.; Tamaki, N. Synergistic effect of cold mannitol and na(+)/ca(2+) exchange blocker on blood-brain barrier opening. *Biochem. Biophys. Res. Commun.* **2002**, *291*, 669–674. [CrossRef]
25. Stapleton, S.; Jaffray, D.; Milosevic, M. Radiation effects on the tumor microenvironment: Implications for nanomedicine delivery. *Adv. Drug Deliv. Rev.* **2017**, *109*, 119–130. [CrossRef]
26. Brown, W.R.; Thore, C.R.; Moody, D.M.; Robbins, M.E.; Wheeler, K.T. Vascular damage after fractionated whole-brain irradiation in rats. *Radiat. Res.* **2005**, *164*, 662–668. [CrossRef] [PubMed]
27. van Vulpen, M.; Kal, H.B.; Taphoorn, M.J.; El-Sharouni, S.Y. Changes in blood-brain barrier permeability induced by radiotherapy: Implications for timing of chemotherapy? (review). *Oncol. Rep.* **2002**, *9*, 683–688. [CrossRef] [PubMed]
28. Crowe, W.; Wang, L.; Zhang, Z.; Varagic, J.; Bourland, J.D.; Chan, M.D.; Habib, A.A.; Zhao, D. Mri evaluation of the effects of whole brain radiotherapy on breast cancer brain metastasis. *Int. J. Radiat. Biol.* **2019**, *95*, 338–346. [CrossRef]
29. Teng, F.; Tsien, C.I.; Lawrence, T.S.; Cao, Y. Blood-tumor barrier opening changes in brain metastases from pre to one-month post radiation therapy. *Radiother. Oncol. J. Eur. Soc. Ther. Radiol. Oncol.* **2017**, *125*, 89–93. [CrossRef]
30. Bouchet, A.; Potez, M.; Coquery, N.; Rome, C.; Lemasson, B.; Brauer-Krisch, E.; Remy, C.; Laissue, J.; Barbier, E.L.; Djonov, V.; et al. Permeability of brain tumor vessels induced by uniform or spatially microfractionated synchrotron radiation therapies. *Int. J. Radiat. Oncol. Biol. Phys.* **2017**, *98*, 1174–1182. [CrossRef]
31. Lemasson, B.; Serduc, R.; Maisin, C.; Bouchet, A.; Coquery, N.; Robert, P.; Le Duc, G.; Tropres, I.; Remy, C.; Barbier, E.L. Monitoring blood-brain barrier status in a rat model of glioma receiving therapy: Dual injection of low-molecular-weight and macromolecular mr contrast media. *Radiology* **2010**, *257*, 342–352. [CrossRef]
32. Fang, L.; Sun, X.; Song, Y.; Zhang, Y.; Li, F.; Xu, Y.; Ma, S.; Lin, N. Whole-brain radiation fails to boost intracerebral gefitinib concentration in patients with brain metastatic non-small cell lung cancer: A self-controlled, pilot study. *Cancer Chemother. Pharmacol.* **2015**, *76*, 873–877. [CrossRef]
33. Zeng, Y.D.; Liao, H.; Qin, T.; Zhang, L.; Wei, W.D.; Liang, J.Z.; Xu, F.; Dinglin, X.X.; Ma, S.X.; Chen, L.K. Blood-brain barrier permeability of gefitinib in patients with brain metastases from non-small-cell lung cancer before and during whole brain radiation therapy. *Oncotarget* **2015**, *6*, 8366–8376. [CrossRef] [PubMed]
34. Miller, M.A.; Chandra, R.; Cuccarese, M.F.; Pfirschke, C.; Engblom, C.; Stapleton, S.; Adhikary, U.; Kohler, R.H.; Mohan, J.F.; Pittet, M.J.; et al. Radiation therapy primes tumors for nanotherapeutic delivery via macrophage-mediated vascular bursts. *Sci. Transl. Med.* **2017**, *9*. [CrossRef] [PubMed]

35. Le Pechoux, C.; Laplanche, A.; Faivre-Finn, C.; Ciuleanu, T.; Wanders, R.; Lerouge, D.; Keus, R.; Hatton, M.; Videtic, G.M.; Senan, S.; et al. Clinical neurological outcome and quality of life among patients with limited small-cell cancer treated with two different doses of prophylactic cranial irradiation in the intergroup phase iii trial (pci99-01, eortc 22003-08004, rtog 0212 and ifct 99-01). *Ann. Oncol. Off. J. Eur. Soc. Med Oncol.* **2011**, *22*, 1154–1163. [CrossRef]
36. Dietrich, J.; Monje, M.; Wefel, J.; Meyers, C. Clinical patterns and biological correlates of cognitive dysfunction associated with cancer therapy. *Oncologist* **2008**, *13*, 1285–1295. [CrossRef] [PubMed]
37. Emerich, D.F.; Dean, R.L.; Osborn, C.; Bartus, R.T. The development of the bradykinin agonist labradimil as a means to increase the permeability of the blood-brain barrier: From concept to clinical evaluation. *Clin. Pharmacokinet.* **2001**, *40*, 105–123. [CrossRef]
38. de Vries, N.A.; Beijnen, J.H.; Boogerd, W.; van Tellingen, O. Blood-brain barrier and chemotherapeutic treatment of brain tumors. *Expert Rev. Neurother.* **2006**, *6*, 1199–1209. [CrossRef] [PubMed]
39. Bartus, R.T.; Elliott, P.J.; Dean, R.L.; Hayward, N.J.; Nagle, T.L.; Huff, M.R.; Snodgrass, P.A.; Blunt, D.G. Controlled modulation of bbb permeability using the bradykinin agonist, rmp-7. *Exp. Neurol.* **1996**, *142*, 14–28. [CrossRef]
40. Sanovich, E.; Bartus, R.T.; Friden, P.M.; Dean, R.L.; Le, H.Q.; Brightman, M.W. Pathway across blood-brain barrier opened by the bradykinin agonist, rmp-7. *Brain Res.* **1995**, *705*, 125–135. [CrossRef]
41. Matsukado, K.; Inamura, T.; Nakano, S.; Fukui, M.; Bartus, R.T.; Black, K.L. Enhanced tumor uptake of carboplatin and survival in glioma-bearing rats by intracarotid infusion of bradykinin analog, rmp-7. *Neurosurgery* **1996**, *39*, 125–133; discussion 124–133. [CrossRef]
42. Borlongan, C.V.; Emerich, D.F. Facilitation of drug entry into the cns via transient permeation of blood brain barrier: Laboratory and preliminary clinical evidence from bradykinin receptor agonist, cereport. *Brain Res. Bull.* **2003**, *60*, 297–306. [CrossRef]
43. Ford, J.; Osborn, C.; Barton, T.; Bleehen, N.M. A phase i study of intravenous rmp-7 with carboplatin in patients with progression of malignant glioma. *Eur. J. Cancer* **1998**, *34*, 1807–1811. [CrossRef]
44. Warren, K.; Jakacki, R.; Widemann, B.; Aikin, A.; Libucha, M.; Packer, R.; Vezina, G.; Reaman, G.; Shaw, D.; Krailo, M.; et al. Phase ii trial of intravenous lobradimil and carboplatin in childhood brain tumors: A report from the children's oncology group. *Cancer Chemother. Pharmacol.* **2006**, *58*, 343–347. [CrossRef] [PubMed]
45. Prados, M.D.; Schold, S.C., Jr.; Fine, H.A.; Jaeckle, K.; Hochberg, F.; Mechtler, L.; Fetell, M.R.; Phuphanich, S.; Feun, L.; Janus, T.J.; et al. A randomized, double-blind, placebo-controlled, phase 2 study of rmp-7 in combination with carboplatin administered intravenously for the treatment of recurrent malignant glioma. *Neuro Oncol.* **2003**, *5*, 96–103. [CrossRef] [PubMed]
46. Deeken, J.F.; Loscher, W. The blood-brain barrier and cancer: Transporters, treatment, and trojan horses. *Clin. Cancer Res. Off. J. Am. Assoc. Cancer Res.* **2007**, *13*, 1663–1674. [CrossRef] [PubMed]
47. Riley, M.G.; Kim, N.N.; Watson, V.E.; Gobin, Y.P.; LeBel, C.P.; Black, K.L.; Bartus, R.T. Intra-arterial administration of carboplatin and the blood brain barrier permeabilizing agent, rmp-7: A toxicologic evaluation in swine. *J. Neurooncol.* **1998**, *36*, 167–178. [CrossRef]
48. Hashizume, K.; Black, K.L. Increased endothelial vesicular transport correlates with increased blood-tumor barrier permeability induced by bradykinin and leukotriene c4. *J. Neuropathol. Exp. Neurol.* **2002**, *61*, 725–735. [CrossRef] [PubMed]
49. Rozhkova, E.A. Nanoscale materials for tackling brain cancer: Recent progress and outlook. *Adv. Mater.* **2011**, *23*, H136–H150. [CrossRef] [PubMed]
50. Haseloff, R.F.; Dithmer, S.; Winkler, L.; Wolburg, H.; Blasig, I.E. Transmembrane proteins of the tight junctions at the blood-brain barrier: Structural and functional aspects. *Semin. Cell Dev. Biol.* **2015**, *38*, 16–25. [CrossRef] [PubMed]
51. Zihni, C.; Mills, C.; Matter, K.; Balda, M.S. Tight junctions: From simple barriers to multifunctional molecular gates. *Nat. Rev. Mol. Cell Biol.* **2016**, *17*, 564–580. [CrossRef] [PubMed]
52. Nitta, T.; Hata, M.; Gotoh, S.; Seo, Y.; Sasaki, H.; Hashimoto, N.; Furuse, M.; Tsukita, S. Size-selective loosening of the blood-brain barrier in claudin-5-deficient mice. *J. Cell Biol.* **2003**, *161*, 653–660. [CrossRef]
53. Campbell, M.; Kiang, A.S.; Kenna, P.F.; Kerskens, C.; Blau, C.; O'Dwyer, L.; Tivnan, A.; Kelly, J.A.; Brankin, B.; Farrar, G.J.; et al. Rnai-mediated reversible opening of the blood-brain barrier. *J. Gene Med.* **2008**, *10*, 930–947. [CrossRef] [PubMed]
54. Campbell, M.; Hanrahan, F.; Gobbo, O.L.; Kelly, M.E.; Kiang, A.S.; Humphries, M.M.; Nguyen, A.T.; Ozaki, E.; Keaney, J.; Blau, C.W.; et al. Targeted suppression of claudin-5 decreases cerebral oedema and improves cognitive outcome following traumatic brain injury. *Nat. Commun.* **2012**, *3*, 849. [CrossRef] [PubMed]
55. Tachibana, K.; Hashimoto, Y.; Shirakura, K.; Okada, Y.; Hirayama, R.; Iwashita, Y.; Nishino, I.; Ago, Y.; Takeda, H.; Kuniyasu, H.; et al. Safety and efficacy of an anti-claudin-5 monoclonal antibody to increase blood-brain barrier permeability for drug delivery to the brain in a non-human primate. *J. Control. Release Off. J. Control. Release Soc.* **2021**, *336*, 105–111. [CrossRef]
56. Hashimoto, Y.; Zhou, W.; Hamauchi, K.; Shirakura, K.; Doi, T.; Yagi, K.; Sawasaki, T.; Okada, Y.; Kondoh, M.; Takeda, H. Engineered membrane protein antigens successfully induce antibodies against extracellular regions of claudin-5. *Sci. Rep.* **2018**, *8*, 8383. [CrossRef]
57. Hashimoto, Y.; Shirakura, K.; Okada, Y.; Takeda, H.; Endo, K.; Tamura, M.; Watari, A.; Sadamura, Y.; Sawasaki, T.; Doi, T.; et al. Claudin-5-binders enhance permeation of solutes across the blood-brain barrier in a mammalian model. *J. Pharmacol. Exp. Ther.* **2017**, *363*, 275–283. [CrossRef] [PubMed]
58. Dithmer, S.; Staat, C.; Muller, C.; Ku, M.C.; Pohlmann, A.; Niendorf, T.; Gehne, N.; Fallier-Becker, P.; Kittel, A.; Walter, F.R.; et al. Claudin peptidomimetics modulate tissue barriers for enhanced drug delivery. *Ann. N. Y. Acad. Sci.* **2017**, *1397*, 169–184. [CrossRef]

59. Krug, S.M.; Amasheh, S.; Richter, J.F.; Milatz, S.; Gunzel, D.; Westphal, J.K.; Huber, O.; Schulzke, J.D.; Fromm, M. Tricellulin forms a barrier to macromolecules in tricellular tight junctions without affecting ion permeability. *Mol. Biol. Cell* **2009**, *20*, 3713–3724. [CrossRef] [PubMed]
60. Zeniya, S.; Kuwahara, H.; Daizo, K.; Watari, A.; Kondoh, M.; Yoshida-Tanaka, K.; Kaburagi, H.; Asada, K.; Nagata, T.; Nagahama, M.; et al. Angubindin-1 opens the blood-brain barrier in vivo for delivery of antisense oligonucleotide to the central nervous system. *J. Control. Release Off. J. Control. Release Soc.* **2018**, *283*, 126–134. [CrossRef] [PubMed]
61. Krug, S.M.; Hayaishi, T.; Iguchi, D.; Watari, A.; Takahashi, A.; Fromm, M.; Nagahama, M.; Takeda, H.; Okada, Y.; Sawasaki, T.; et al. Angubindin-1, a novel paracellular absorption enhancer acting at the tricellular tight junction. *J. Control. Release Off. J. Control. Release Soc.* **2017**, *260*, 1–11. [CrossRef]
62. Spampinato, S.F.; Obermeier, B.; Cotleur, A.; Love, A.; Takeshita, Y.; Sano, Y.; Kanda, T.; Ransohoff, R.M. Sphingosine 1 phosphate at the blood brain barrier: Can the modulation of s1p receptor 1 influence the response of endothelial cells and astrocytes to inflammatory stimuli? *PLoS ONE* **2015**, *10*, e0133392.
63. Fan, L.; Yan, H. Fty720 attenuates retinal inflammation and protects blood-retinal barrier in diabetic rats. *Investig. Ophthalmol. Vis. Sci.* **2016**, *57*, 1254–1263. [CrossRef]
64. Gril, B.; Paranjape, A.N.; Woditschka, S.; Hua, E.; Dolan, E.L.; Hanson, J.; Wu, X.; Kloc, W.; Izycka-Swieszewska, E.; Duchnowska, R.; et al. Reactive astrocytic s1p3 signaling modulates the blood-tumor barrier in brain metastases. *Nat. Commun.* **2018**, *9*, 2705. [CrossRef] [PubMed]
65. Dusaban, S.S.; Chun, J.; Rosen, H.; Purcell, N.H.; Brown, J.H. Sphingosine 1-phosphate receptor 3 and rhoa signaling mediate inflammatory gene expression in astrocytes. *J. Neuroinflammation* **2017**, *14*, 111. [CrossRef]
66. Sanna, M.G.; Vincent, K.P.; Repetto, E.; Nguyen, N.; Brown, S.J.; Abgaryan, L.; Riley, S.W.; Leaf, N.B.; Cahalan, S.M.; Kiosses, W.B.; et al. Bitopic sphingosine 1-phosphate receptor 3 (s1p3) antagonist rescue from complete heart block: Pharmacological and genetic evidence for direct s1p3 regulation of mouse cardiac conduction. *Mol. Pharmacol.* **2016**, *89*, 176–186. [CrossRef]
67. Iannitti, T.; Palmieri, B. An update on the therapeutic role of alkylglycerols. *Mar. Drugs* **2010**, *8*, 2267–2300. [CrossRef]
68. Erdlenbruch, B.; Alipour, M.; Fricker, G.; Miller, D.S.; Kugler, W.; Eibl, H.; Lakomek, M. Alkylglycerol opening of the blood-brain barrier to small and large fluorescence markers in normal and c6 glioma-bearing rats and isolated rat brain capillaries. *Br. J. Pharmacol.* **2003**, *140*, 1201–1210. [CrossRef] [PubMed]
69. Erdlenbruch, B.; Jendrossek, V.; Eibl, H.; Lakomek, M. Transient and controllable opening of the blood-brain barrier to cytostatic and antibiotic agents by alkylglycerols in rats. *Exp. Brain* **2000**, *135*, 417–422.
70. Erdlenbruch, B.; Jendrossek, V.; Kugler, W.; Eibl, H.; Lakomek, M. Increased delivery of erucylphosphocholine to c6 gliomas by chemical opening of the blood-brain barrier using intracarotid pentylglycerol in rats. *Cancer Chemother. Pharmacol.* **2002**, *50*, 299–304. [CrossRef] [PubMed]
71. Erdlenbruch, B.; Schinkhof, C.; Kugler, W.; Heinemann, D.E.; Herms, J.; Eibl, H.; Lakomek, M. Intracarotid administration of short-chain alkylglycerols for increased delivery of methotrexate to the rat brain. *Br. J. Pharmacol.* **2003**, *139*, 685–694. [CrossRef] [PubMed]
72. Kim, H.J.; Pyeun, Y.S.; Kim, Y.W.; Cho, B.M.; Lee, T.H.; Moon, T.Y.; Suh, K.T.; Park, B.R. A model for research on the blood-brain barrier disruption induced by unsaturated fatty acid emulsion. *Investig. Radiol.* **2005**, *40*, 270–276. [CrossRef]
73. Sztriha, L.; Betz, A.L. Oleic acid reversibly opens the blood-brain barrier. *Brain Res.* **1991**, *550*, 257–262. [CrossRef]
74. Zhou, W.; Chen, C.; Shi, Y.; Wu, Q.; Gimple, R.C.; Fang, X.; Huang, Z.; Zhai, K.; Ke, S.Q.; Ping, Y.F.; et al. Targeting glioma stem cell-derived pericytes disrupts the blood-tumor barrier and improves chemotherapeutic efficacy. *Cell Stem Cell* **2017**, *21*, 591–603 e594. [CrossRef] [PubMed]
75. Guerra, D.A.P.; Paiva, A.E.; Sena, I.F.G.; Azevedo, P.O.; Silva, W.N.; Mintz, A.; Birbrair, A. Targeting glioblastoma-derived pericytes improves chemotherapeutic outcome. *Angiogenesis* **2018**, *21*, 667–675. [CrossRef]
76. Rodriguez, P.L.; Jiang, S.; Fu, Y.; Avraham, S.; Avraham, H.K. The proinflammatory peptide substance p promotes blood-brain barrier breaching by breast cancer cells through changes in microvascular endothelial cell tight junctions. *Int. J. Cancer* **2014**, *134*, 1034–1044. [CrossRef] [PubMed]
77. Ferrero, E.; Zocchi, M.R.; Magni, E.; Panzeri, M.C.; Curnis, F.; Rugarli, C.; Ferrero, M.E.; Corti, A. Roles of tumor necrosis factor p55 and p75 receptors in tnf-alpha-induced vascular permeability. *Am. J. Physiol. Cell Physiol.* **2001**, *281*, C1173–C1179. [CrossRef] [PubMed]
78. Connell, J.J.; Chatain, G.; Cornelissen, B.; Vallis, K.A.; Hamilton, A.; Seymour, L.; Anthony, D.C.; Sibson, N.R. Selective permeabilization of the blood-brain barrier at sites of metastasis. *J. Natl. Cancer Inst.* **2013**, *105*, 1634–1643. [CrossRef]
79. Avraham, H.K.; Jiang, S.; Fu, Y.; Nakshatri, H.; Ovadia, H.; Avraham, S. Angiopoietin-2 mediates blood-brain barrier impairment and colonization of triple-negative breast cancer cells in brain. *J. Pathol.* **2014**, *232*, 369–381. [CrossRef]
80. Gurnik, S.; Devraj, K.; Macas, J.; Yamaji, M.; Starke, J.; Scholz, A.; Sommer, K.; Di Tacchio, M.; Vutukuri, R.; Beck, H.; et al. Angiopoietin-2-induced blood-brain barrier compromise and increased stroke size are rescued by ve-ptp-dependent restoration of tie2 signaling. *Acta Neuropathol.* **2016**, *131*, 753–773. [CrossRef]
81. Loscher, W.; Gericke, B. Novel intrinsic mechanisms of active drug extrusion at the blood-brain barrier: Potential targets for enhancing drug delivery to the brain? *Pharmaceutics* **2020**, *12*, 966. [CrossRef]
82. Potschka, H. Targeting regulation of abc efflux transporters in brain diseases: A novel therapeutic approach. *Pharmacol. Ther.* **2010**, *125*, 118–127. [CrossRef]

83. Bauer, B.; Hartz, A.M.; Fricker, G.; Miller, D.S. Modulation of p-glycoprotein transport function at the blood-brain barrier. *Exp. Biol. Med.* **2005**, *230*, 118–127. [CrossRef]
84. Fox, E.; Bates, S.E. Tariquidar (xr9576): A p-glycoprotein drug efflux pump inhibitor. *Expert Rev. Anticancer Ther.* **2007**, *7*, 447–459. [CrossRef]
85. Bors, L.A.; Erd, F. Overcoming the blood–brain barrier. Challenges and tricks for cns drug delivery. *Sci. Pharm.* **2019**, *87*, 6. [CrossRef]
86. Shan, Y.; Cen, Y.; Zhang, Y.; Tan, R.; Zhao, J.; Nie, Z.; Zhang, J.; Yu, S. Effect of p-glycoprotein inhibition on the penetration of ceftriaxone across the blood-brain barrier. *Neurochem. Res.* **2021**. [CrossRef] [PubMed]
87. Erdo, F.; Nagy, I.; Toth, B.; Bui, A.; Molnar, E.; Timar, Z.; Magnan, R.; Krajcsi, P. Abcb1a (p-glycoprotein) limits brain exposure of the anticancer drug candidate seliciclib in vivo in adult mice. *Brain Res. Bull.* **2017**, *132*, 232–236. [CrossRef]
88. Carcaboso, A.M.; Elmeliegy, M.A.; Shen, J.; Juel, S.J.; Zhang, Z.M.; Calabrese, C.; Tracey, L.; Waters, C.M.; Stewart, C.F. Tyrosine kinase inhibitor gefitinib enhances topotecan penetration of gliomas. *Cancer Res.* **2010**, *70*, 4499–4508. [CrossRef]
89. Choo, E.F.; Kurnik, D.; Muszkat, M.; Ohkubo, T.; Shay, S.D.; Higginbotham, J.N.; Glaeser, H.; Kim, R.B.; Wood, A.J.; Wilkinson, G.R. Differential in vivo sensitivity to inhibition of p-glycoprotein located in lymphocytes, testes, and the blood-brain barrier. *J. Pharmacol. Exp. Ther.* **2006**, *317*, 1012–1018. [CrossRef]
90. Ekins, S.; Ecker, G.F.; Chiba, P.; Swaan, P.W. Future directions for drug transporter modelling. *Xenobiotica; Fate Foreign Compd. Biol. Syst.* **2007**, *37*, 1152–1170. [CrossRef]
91. Harmsen, S.; Meijerman, I.; Beijnen, J.H.; Schellens, J.H. The role of nuclear receptors in pharmacokinetic drug-drug interactions in oncology. *Cancer Treat Rev.* **2007**, *33*, 369–380. [CrossRef]
92. Zastre, J.A.; Chan, G.N.; Ronaldson, P.T.; Ramaswamy, M.; Couraud, P.O.; Romero, I.A.; Weksler, B.; Bendayan, M.; Bendayan, R. Up-regulation of p-glycoprotein by hiv protease inhibitors in a human brain microvessel endothelial cell line. *J. Neurosci. Res.* **2009**, *87*, 1023–1036. [CrossRef]
93. Bauer, B.; Hartz, A.M.; Fricker, G.; Miller, D.S. Pregnane x receptor up-regulation of p-glycoprotein expression and transport function at the blood-brain barrier. *Mol. Pharmacol.* **2004**, *66*, 413–419.
94. Huang, H.; Wang, H.; Sinz, M.; Zoeckler, M.; Staudinger, J.; Redinbo, M.R.; Teotico, D.G.; Locker, J.; Kalpana, G.V.; Mani, S. Inhibition of drug metabolism by blocking the activation of nuclear receptors by ketoconazole. *Oncogene* **2007**, *26*, 258–268. [CrossRef]
95. Bankstahl, J.P.; Hoffmann, K.; Bethmann, K.; Loscher, W. Glutamate is critically involved in seizure-induced overexpression of p-glycoprotein in the brain. *Neuropharmacology* **2008**, *54*, 1006–1016. [CrossRef]
96. Loscher, W. Pharmacology of glutamate receptor antagonists in the kindling model of epilepsy. *Prog. Neurobiol.* **1998**, *54*, 721–741. [CrossRef]
97. Bauer, B.; Hartz, A.M.; Pekcec, A.; Toellner, K.; Miller, D.S.; Potschka, H. Seizure-induced up-regulation of p-glycoprotein at the blood-brain barrier through glutamate and cyclooxygenase-2 signaling. *Mol. Pharmacol.* **2008**, *73*, 1444–1453. [CrossRef]
98. Zibell, G.; Unkruer, B.; Pekcec, A.; Hartz, A.M.; Bauer, B.; Miller, D.S.; Potschka, H. Prevention of seizure-induced up-regulation of endothelial p-glycoprotein by cox-2 inhibition. *Neuropharmacology* **2009**, *56*, 849–855. [CrossRef]
99. van Vliet, E.A.; Zibell, G.; Pekcec, A.; Schlichtiger, J.; Edelbroek, P.M.; Holtman, L.; Aronica, E.; Gorter, J.A.; Potschka, H. Cox-2 inhibition controls p-glycoprotein expression and promotes brain delivery of phenytoin in chronic epileptic rats. *Neuropharmacology* **2010**, *58*, 404–412. [CrossRef]
100. Kulkarni, S.K.; Dhir, A. Cyclooxygenase in epilepsy: From perception to application. *Drugs Today* **2009**, *45*, 135–154. [CrossRef]
101. Pekcec, A.; Unkruer, B.; Schlichtiger, J.; Soerensen, J.; Hartz, A.M.; Bauer, B.; van Vliet, E.A.; Gorter, J.A.; Potschka, H. Targeting prostaglandin e2 ep1 receptors prevents seizure-associated p-glycoprotein up-regulation. *J. Pharmacol. Exp. Ther.* **2009**, *330*, 939–947. [CrossRef] [PubMed]
102. Ahmad, A.S.; Ahmad, M.; de Brum-Fernandes, A.J.; Dore, S. Prostaglandin ep4 receptor agonist protects against acute neurotoxicity. *Brain Res.* **2005**, *1066*, 71–77. [CrossRef]
103. Bilak, M.; Wu, L.; Wang, Q.; Haughey, N.; Conant, K.; St Hillaire, C.; Andreasson, K. Pge2 receptors rescue motor neurons in a model of amyotrophic lateral sclerosis. *Ann. Neurol.* **2004**, *56*, 240–248. [CrossRef] [PubMed]
104. McCullough, L.; Wu, L.; Haughey, N.; Liang, X.; Hand, T.; Wang, Q.; Breyer, R.M.; Andreasson, K. Neuroprotective function of the pge2 ep2 receptor in cerebral ischemia. *J. Neurosci. Off. J. Soc. Neurosci.* **2004**, *24*, 257–268. [CrossRef]
105. Spudich, A.; Kilic, E.; Xing, H.; Kilic, U.; Rentsch, K.M.; Wunderli-Allenspach, H.; Bassetti, C.L.; Hermann, D.M. Inhibition of multidrug resistance transporter-1 facilitates neuroprotective therapies after focal cerebral ischemia. *Nat. Neurosci.* **2006**, *9*, 487–488. [CrossRef]
106. Cirrito, J.R.; Deane, R.; Fagan, A.M.; Spinner, M.L.; Parsadanian, M.; Finn, M.B.; Jiang, H.; Prior, J.L.; Sagare, A.; Bales, K.R.; et al. P-glycoprotein deficiency at the blood-brain barrier increases amyloid-beta deposition in an alzheimer disease mouse model. *J. Clin. Investig.* **2005**, *115*, 3285–3290. [CrossRef]
107. Vogelgesang, S.; Cascorbi, I.; Schroeder, E.; Pahnke, J.; Kroemer, H.K.; Siegmund, W.; Kunert-Keil, C.; Walker, L.C.; Warzok, R.W. Deposition of alzheimer's beta-amyloid is inversely correlated with p-glycoprotein expression in the brains of elderly non-demented humans. *Pharmacogenetics* **2002**, *12*, 535–541. [CrossRef]
108. Deane, R.; Zlokovic, B.V. Role of the blood-brain barrier in the pathogenesis of alzheimer's disease. *Curr. Alzheimer Res.* **2007**, *4*, 191–197. [CrossRef]

109. Lee, G.; Bendayan, R. Functional expression and localization of p-glycoprotein in the central nervous system: Relevance to the pathogenesis and treatment of neurological disorders. *Pharm. Res.* **2004**, *21*, 1313–1330. [CrossRef]
110. Lim, J.C.; Kania, K.D.; Wijesuriya, H.; Chawla, S.; Sethi, J.K.; Pulaski, L.; Romero, I.A.; Couraud, P.O.; Weksler, B.B.; Hladky, S.B.; et al. Activation of beta-catenin signalling by gsk-3 inhibition increases p-glycoprotein expression in brain endothelial cells. *J. Neurochem.* **2008**, *106*, 1855–1865.
111. Ju, X.; Chen, H.; Miao, T.; Ni, J.; Han, L. Prodrug delivery using dual-targeting nanoparticles to treat breast cancer brain metastases. *Mol. Pharm.* **2021**, *18*, 2694–2702. [CrossRef]
112. Khan, N.U.; Ni, J.; Ju, X.; Miao, T.; Chen, H.; Han, L. Escape from abluminal lrp1-mediated clearance for boosted nanoparticle brain delivery and brain metastasis treatment. *Acta Pharm. Sin. B* **2021**, *11*, 1341–1354. [CrossRef]
113. Ni, J.; Miao, T.; Su, M.; Khan, N.U.; Ju, X.; Chen, H.; Liu, F.; Han, L. Psma-targeted nanoparticles for specific penetration of blood-brain tumor barrier and combined therapy of brain metastases. *J. Control. Release Off. J. Control. Release Soc.* **2021**, *329*, 934–947. [CrossRef]
114. Guo, Q.; Zhu, Q.; Miao, T.; Tao, J.; Ju, X.; Sun, Z.; Li, H.; Xu, G.; Chen, H.; Han, L. Lrp1-upregulated nanoparticles for efficiently conquering the blood-brain barrier and targetedly suppressing multifocal and infiltrative brain metastases. *J. Control. Release Off. J. Control. Release Soc.* **2019**, *303*, 117–129. [CrossRef]
115. Guo, Q.; Chang, Z.; Khan, N.U.; Miao, T.; Ju, X.; Feng, H.; Zhang, L.; Sun, Z.; Li, H.; Han, L. Nanosizing noncrystalline and porous silica material-naturally occurring opal shale for systemic tumor targeting drug delivery. *ACS Appl. Mater. Interfaces* **2018**, *10*, 25994–26004. [CrossRef] [PubMed]
116. Dong, A.; Han, L.; Shao, Z.; Fan, P.; Zhou, X.; Yuan, H. Glaucoma drainage device coated with mitomycin c loaded opal shale microparticles to inhibit bleb fibrosis. *ACS Appl. Mater. Interfaces* **2019**, *11*, 10244–10253. [CrossRef] [PubMed]
117. Ju, X.; Miao, T.; Chen, H.; Ni, J.; Han, L. Overcoming mfsd2a-mediated low transcytosis to boost nanoparticle delivery to brain for chemotherapy of brain metastases. *Adv. Healthc. Mater.* **2021**, *10*, e2001997. [CrossRef] [PubMed]
118. Uchida, Y.; Ohtsuki, S.; Katsukura, Y.; Ikeda, C.; Suzuki, T.; Kamiie, J.; Terasaki, T. Quantitative targeted absolute proteomics of human blood-brain barrier transporters and receptors. *J. Neurochem.* **2011**, *117*, 333–345. [CrossRef]
119. Nguyen, L.N.; Ma, D.; Shui, G.; Wong, P.; Cazenave-Gassiot, A.; Zhang, X.; Wenk, M.R.; Goh, E.L.; Silver, D.L. Mfsd2a is a transporter for the essential omega-3 fatty acid docosahexaenoic acid. *Nature* **2014**, *509*, 503–506. [CrossRef]
120. Bengmark, S. Gut microbiota, immune development and function. *Pharmacol. Res.* **2013**, *69*, 87–113. [CrossRef]
121. Alakbarzade, V.; Hameed, A.; Quek, D.Q.; Chioza, B.A.; Baple, E.L.; Cazenave-Gassiot, A.; Nguyen, L.N.; Wenk, M.R.; Ahmad, A.Q.; Sreekantan-Nair, A.; et al. A partially inactivating mutation in the sodium-dependent lysophosphatidylcholine transporter mfsd2a causes a non-lethal microcephaly syndrome. *Nat. Genet.* **2015**, *47*, 814–817. [CrossRef]
122. Zhao, Z.; Sagare, A.P.; Ma, Q.; Halliday, M.R.; Kong, P.; Kisler, K.; Winkler, E.A.; Ramanathan, A.; Kanekiyo, T.; Bu, G.; et al. Central role for picalm in amyloid-beta blood-brain barrier transcytosis and clearance. *Nat. Neurosci.* **2015**, *18*, 978–987. [CrossRef]
123. Andras, I.E.; Eum, S.Y.; Huang, W.; Zhong, Y.; Hennig, B.; Toborek, M. Hiv-1-induced amyloid beta accumulation in brain endothelial cells is attenuated by simvastatin. *Mol. Cell. Neurosci.* **2010**, *43*, 232–243. [CrossRef]
124. Zandl-Lang, M.; Fanaee-Danesh, E.; Sun, Y.; Albrecher, N.M.; Gali, C.C.; Cancar, I.; Kober, A.; Tam-Amersdorfer, C.; Stracke, A.; Storck, S.M.; et al. Regulatory effects of simvastatin and apoj on app processing and amyloid-beta clearance in blood-brain barrier endothelial cells. *Biochim. Biophys. Acta Mol. Cell Biol. Lipids* **2018**, *1863*, 40–60. [CrossRef]
125. Zlokovic, B.V.; Yamada, S.; Holtzman, D.; Ghiso, J.; Frangione, B. Clearance of amyloid beta-peptide from brain: Transport or metabolism? *Nat. Med.* **2000**, *6*, 718–719. [CrossRef]
126. Tobert, J.A. New developments in lipid-lowering therapy: The role of inhibitors of hydroxymethylglutaryl-coenzyme a reductase. *Circulation* **1987**, *76*, 534–538. [CrossRef] [PubMed]
127. Sweeney, M.D.; Zhao, Z.; Montagne, A.; Nelson, A.R.; Zlokovic, B.V. Blood-brain barrier: From physiology to disease and back. *Physiol. Rev.* **2019**, *99*, 21–78. [CrossRef] [PubMed]
128. Sweeney, M.D.; Sagare, A.P.; Zlokovic, B.V. Blood-brain barrier breakdown in alzheimer disease and other neurodegenerative disorders. *Nat. Rev. Neurol.* **2018**, *14*, 133–150. [CrossRef] [PubMed]
129. Winkler, E.A.; Nishida, Y.; Sagare, A.P.; Rege, S.V.; Bell, R.D.; Perlmutter, D.; Sengillo, J.D.; Hillman, S.; Kong, P.; Nelson, A.R.; et al. Glut1 reductions exacerbate alzheimer's disease vasculo-neuronal dysfunction and degeneration. *Nat. Neurosci.* **2015**, *18*, 521–530. [CrossRef]
130. Zhao, C.; Ma, J.; Wang, Z.; Li, H.; Shen, H.; Li, X.; Chen, G. Mfsd2a attenuates blood-brain barrier disruption after sub-arachnoid hemorrhage by inhibiting caveolae-mediated transcellular transport in rats. *Transl. Stroke Res.* **2020**, *11*, 1012–1027. [CrossRef]
131. Montagne, A.; Zhao, Z.; Zlokovic, B.V. Alzheimer's disease: A matter of blood-brain barrier dysfunction? *J. Exp. Med.* **2017**, *214*, 3151–3169. [CrossRef]
132. Guemez-Gamboa, A.; Nguyen, L.N.; Yang, H.; Zaki, M.S.; Kara, M.; Ben-Omran, T.; Akizu, N.; Rosti, R.O.; Rosti, B.; Scott, E.; et al. Inactivating mutations in mfsd2a, required for omega-3 fatty acid transport in brain, cause a lethal microcephaly syndrome. *Nat. Genet.* **2015**, *47*, 809–813. [CrossRef] [PubMed]
133. Patching, S.G. Glucose transporters at the blood-brain barrier: Function, regulation and gateways for drug delivery. *Mol. Neurobiol.* **2017**, *54*, 1046–1077. [CrossRef] [PubMed]
134. Anraku, Y.; Kuwahara, H.; Fukusato, Y.; Mizoguchi, A.; Ishii, T.; Nitta, K.; Matsumoto, Y.; Toh, K.; Miyata, K.; Uchida, S.; et al. Glycaemic control boosts glucosylated nanocarrier crossing the bbb into the brain. *Nat. Commun.* **2017**, *8*, 1001. [CrossRef]

135. Arsiwala, T.A.; Sprowls, S.A.; Blethen, K.E.; Adkins, C.E.; Saralkar, P.A.; Fladeland, R.A.; Pentz, W.; Gabriele, A.; Kielkowski, B.; Mehta, R.I.; et al. Ultrasound-mediated disruption of the blood tumor barrier for improved therapeutic delivery. *Neoplasia* **2021**, *23*, 676–691. [CrossRef]
136. Meng, Y.; Suppiah, S.; Surendrakumar, S.; Bigioni, L.; Lipsman, N. Low-intensity mr-guided focused ultrasound mediated disruption of the blood-brain barrier for intracranial metastatic diseases. *Front. Oncol.* **2018**, *8*, 338. [CrossRef]
137. Alonso, A. Ultrasound-induced blood-brain barrier opening for drug delivery. *Front. Neurol. Neurosci.* **2015**, *36*, 106–115. [PubMed]
138. Sheikov, N.; McDannold, N.; Sharma, S.; Hynynen, K. Effect of focused ultrasound applied with an ultrasound contrast agent on the tight junctional integrity of the brain microvascular endothelium. *Ultrasound Med. Biol.* **2008**, *34*, 1093–1104. [CrossRef] [PubMed]
139. Sheikov, N.; McDannold, N.; Vykhodtseva, N.; Jolesz, F.; Hynynen, K. Cellular mechanisms of the blood-brain barrier opening induced by ultrasound in presence of microbubbles. *Ultrasound Med. Biol.* **2004**, *30*, 979–989. [CrossRef] [PubMed]
140. Deng, J.; Huang, Q.; Wang, F.; Liu, Y.; Wang, Z.; Wang, Z.; Zhang, Q.; Lei, B.; Cheng, Y. The role of caveolin-1 in blood-brain barrier disruption induced by focused ultrasound combined with microbubbles. *J. Mol. Neurosci. MN* **2012**, *46*, 677–687. [CrossRef] [PubMed]
141. Aryal, M.; Fischer, K.; Gentile, C.; Gitto, S.; Zhang, Y.Z.; McDannold, N. Effects on p-glycoprotein expression after blood-brain barrier disruption using focused ultrasound and microbubbles. *PLoS ONE* **2017**, *12*, e0166061. [CrossRef] [PubMed]
142. Ahmed, N.; Gandhi, D.; Melhem, E.R.; Frenkel, V. Mri guided focused ultrasound-mediated delivery of therapeutic cells to the brain: A review of the state-of-the-art methodology and future applications. *Front. Neurol.* **2021**, *12*, 669449. [CrossRef]
143. Chen, K.T.; Lin, Y.J.; Chai, W.Y.; Lin, C.J.; Chen, P.Y.; Huang, C.Y.; Kuo, J.S.; Liu, H.L.; Wei, K.C. Neuronavigation-guided focused ultrasound (navifus) for transcranial blood-brain barrier opening in recurrent glioblastoma patients: Clinical trial protocol. *Ann. Transl. Med.* **2020**, *8*, 673. [CrossRef]
144. Appelboom, G.; Detappe, A.; LoPresti, M.; Kunjachan, S.; Mitrasinovic, S.; Goldman, S.; Chang, S.D.; Tillement, O. Stereotactic modulation of blood-brain barrier permeability to enhance drug delivery. *Neuro. Oncol.* **2016**, *18*, 1601–1609. [CrossRef] [PubMed]
145. McDannold, N.; Zhang, Y.; Supko, J.G.; Power, C.; Sun, T.; Vykhodtseva, N.; Golby, A.J.; Reardon, D.A. Blood-brain barrier disruption and delivery of irinotecan in a rat model using a clinical transcranial mri-guided focused ultrasound system. *Sci. Rep.* **2020**, *10*, 8766. [CrossRef] [PubMed]
146. Hersh, D.S.; Wadajkar, A.S.; Roberts, N.; Perez, J.G.; Connolly, N.P.; Frenkel, V.; Winkles, J.A.; Woodworth, G.F.; Kim, A.J. Evolving drug delivery strategies to overcome the blood brain barrier. *Curr. Pharm. Des.* **2016**, *22*, 1177–1193. [CrossRef]
147. Lammers, T.; Koczera, P.; Fokong, S.; Gremse, F.; Ehling, J.; Vogt, M.; Pich, A.; Storm, G.; van Zandvoort, M.; Kiessling, F. Theranostic uspio-loaded microbubbles for mediating and monitoring blood-brain barrier permeation. *Adv. Funct. Mater.* **2015**, *25*, 36–43. [CrossRef]
148. Huang, H.Y.; Liu, H.L.; Hsu, P.H.; Chiang, C.S.; Tsai, C.H.; Chi, H.S.; Chen, S.Y.; Chen, Y.Y. A multitheragnostic nanobubble system to induce blood-brain barrier disruption with magnetically guided focused ultrasound. *Adv. Mater.* **2015**, *27*, 655–661. [CrossRef] [PubMed]
149. Song, Z.; Wang, Z.; Shen, J.; Xu, S.; Hu, Z. Nerve growth factor delivery by ultrasound-mediated nanobubble destruction as a treatment for acute spinal cord injury in rats. *Int. J. Nanomed.* **2017**, *12*, 1717–1729. [CrossRef] [PubMed]
150. Kinoshita, M.; McDannold, N.; Jolesz, F.A.; Hynynen, K. Noninvasive localized delivery of herceptin to the mouse brain by mri-guided focused ultrasound-induced blood-brain barrier disruption. *Proc. Natl. Acad. Sci. USA* **2006**, *103*, 11719–11723. [CrossRef] [PubMed]
151. Choi, J.J.; Selert, K.; Gao, Z.; Samiotaki, G.; Baseri, B.; Konofagou, E.E. Noninvasive and localized blood-brain barrier disruption using focused ultrasound can be achieved at short pulse lengths and low pulse repetition frequencies. *J. Cereb. Blood Flow Metab.* **2011**, *31*, 725–737. [CrossRef]
152. Baseri, B.; Choi, J.J.; Tung, Y.S.; Konofagou, E.E. Multi-modality safety assessment of blood-brain barrier opening using focused ultrasound and definity microbubbles: A short-term study. *Ultrasound Med. Biol.* **2010**, *36*, 1445–1459. [CrossRef]
153. Hynynen, K.; McDannold, N.; Vykhodtseva, N.; Jolesz, F.A. Noninvasive mr imaging-guided focal opening of the blood-brain barrier in rabbits. *Radiology* **2001**, *220*, 640–646. [CrossRef]
154. Wala, K.; Szlasa, W.; Saczko, J.; Rudno-Rudzinska, J.; Kulbacka, J. Modulation of blood-brain barrier permeability by activating adenosine a2 receptors in oncological treatment. *Biomolecules* **2021**, *11*, 633. [CrossRef]
155. Sassaroli, E.; O'Neill, B.E. Modulation of the interstitial fluid pressure by high intensity focused ultrasound as a way to alter local fluid and solute movement: Insights from a mathematical model. *Phys. Med. Biol.* **2014**, *59*, 6775–6795. [CrossRef] [PubMed]
156. Burgess, A.; Nhan, T.; Moffatt, C.; Klibanov, A.L.; Hynynen, K. Analysis of focused ultrasound-induced blood-brain barrier permeability in a mouse model of alzheimer's disease using two-photon microscopy. *J. Control. Release Off. J. Control. Release Soc.* **2014**, *192*, 243–248. [CrossRef] [PubMed]
157. McMahon, D.; Poon, C.; Hynynen, K. Evaluating the safety profile of focused ultrasound and microbubble-mediated treatments to increase blood-brain barrier permeability. *Expert Opin. Drug Deliv.* **2019**, *16*, 129–142. [CrossRef] [PubMed]
158. Effendi, W.I.; Nagano, T.; Kobayashi, K.; Nishimura, Y. Focusing on adenosine receptors as a potential targeted therapy in human diseases. *Cells* **2020**, *9*, 785. [CrossRef]

159. Ledent, C.; Vaugeois, J.M.; Schiffmann, S.N.; Pedrazzini, T.; El Yacoubi, M.; Vanderhaeghen, J.J.; Costentin, J.; Heath, J.K.; Vassart, G.; Parmentier, M. Aggressiveness, hypoalgesia and high blood pressure in mice lacking the adenosine a2a receptor. *Nature* **1997**, *388*, 674–678. [CrossRef]
160. Bynoe, M.S.; Viret, C.; Yan, A.; Kim, D.G. Adenosine receptor signaling: A key to opening the blood-brain door. *Fluids Barriers CNS* **2015**, *12*, 20. [CrossRef] [PubMed]
161. Bobermin, L.D.; Roppa, R.H.A.; Quincozes-Santos, A. Adenosine receptors as a new target for resveratrol-mediated glioprotection. *Biochim. Biophys. Acta Mol. Basis Dis.* **2019**, *1865*, 634–647. [CrossRef]
162. Kim, D.G.; Bynoe, M.S. A2a adenosine receptor modulates drug efflux transporter p-glycoprotein at the blood-brain barrier. *J. Clin. Investig.* **2016**, *126*, 1717–1733. [CrossRef]
163. Jackson, S.; Anders, N.M.; Mangraviti, A.; Wanjiku, T.M.; Sankey, E.W.; Liu, A.; Brem, H.; Tyler, B.; Rudek, M.A.; Grossman, S.A. The effect of regadenoson-induced transient disruption of the blood-brain barrier on temozolomide delivery to normal rat brain. *J. Neurooncol.* **2016**, *126*, 433–439. [CrossRef]
164. Vezina, A.; Manglani, M.; Morris, D.; Foster, B.; McCord, M.; Song, H.; Zhang, M.; Davis, D.; Zhang, W.; Bills, J.; et al. Adenosine a2a receptor activation enhances blood-tumor barrier permeability in a rodent glioma model. *Mol. cancer Res. MCR* **2021**. [CrossRef] [PubMed]
165. Kim, D.G.; Bynoe, M.S. A2a adenosine receptor regulates the human blood-brain barrier permeability. *Mol. Neurobiol.* **2015**, *52*, 664–678. [CrossRef] [PubMed]
166. Carman, A.J.; Mills, J.H.; Krenz, A.; Kim, D.G.; Bynoe, M.S. Adenosine receptor signaling modulates permeability of the blood-brain barrier. *J. Neurosci. Off. J. Soc. Neurosci.* **2011**, *31*, 13272–13280. [CrossRef] [PubMed]
167. Pak, R.W.; Kang, J.; Valentine, H.; Loew, L.M.; Thorek, D.L.J.; Boctor, E.M.; Wong, D.F.; Kang, J.U. Voltage-sensitive dye delivery through the blood brain barrier using adenosine receptor agonist regadenoson. *Biomed. Opt. Express* **2018**, *9*, 3915–3922. [CrossRef] [PubMed]
168. Jackson, S.; Weingart, J.; Nduom, E.K.; Harfi, T.T.; George, R.T.; McAreavey, D.; Ye, X.; Anders, N.M.; Peer, C.; Figg, W.D.; et al. The effect of an adenosine a2a agonist on intra-tumoral concentrations of temozolomide in patients with recurrent glioblastoma. *Fluids Barriers CNS* **2018**, *15*, 2. [CrossRef]
169. Jackson, S.; George, R.T.; Lodge, M.A.; Piotrowski, A.; Wahl, R.L.; Gujar, S.K.; Grossman, S.A. The effect of regadenoson on the integrity of the human blood-brain barrier, a pilot study. *J. Neurooncol.* **2017**, *132*, 513–519. [CrossRef]
170. Meng, L.; Wang, C.; Lu, Y.; Sheng, G.; Yang, L.; Wu, Z.; Xu, H.; Han, C.; Lu, Y.; Han, F. Targeted regulation of blood-brain barrier for enhanced therapeutic efficiency of hypoxia-modifier nanoparticles and immune checkpoint blockade antibodies for glioblastoma. *ACS Appl. Mater. Interfaces* **2021**, *13*, 11657–11671. [CrossRef]
171. Han, L.; Cai, Q.; Tian, D.; Kong, D.K.; Gou, X.; Chen, Z.; Strittmatter, S.M.; Wang, Z.; Sheth, K.N.; Zhou, J. Targeted drug delivery to ischemic stroke via chlorotoxin-anchored, lexiscan-loaded nanoparticles. *Nanomedicine* **2016**, *12*, 1833–1842. [CrossRef] [PubMed]
172. Han, L.; Kong, D.K.; Zheng, M.Q.; Murikinati, S.; Ma, C.; Yuan, P.; Li, L.; Tian, D.; Cai, Q.; Ye, C.; et al. Increased nanoparticle delivery to brain tumors by autocatalytic priming for improved treatment and imaging. *ACS Nano* **2016**, *10*, 4209–4218. [CrossRef]
173. Zou, Y.; Liu, Y.; Yang, Z.; Zhang, D.; Lu, Y.; Zheng, M.; Xue, X.; Geng, J.; Chung, R.; Shi, B. Effective and targeted human orthotopic glioblastoma xenograft therapy via a multifunctional biomimetic nanomedicine. *Adv. Mater.* **2018**, *30*, e1803717. [CrossRef]
174. Gao, X.; Qian, J.; Zheng, S.; Changyi, Y.; Zhang, J.; Ju, S.; Zhu, J.; Li, C. Overcoming the blood-brain barrier for delivering drugs into the brain by using adenosine receptor nanoagonist. *ACS Nano* **2014**, *8*, 3678–3689. [CrossRef] [PubMed]
175. Khaitan, D.; Reddy, P.L.; Ningaraj, N. Targeting brain tumors with nanomedicines: Overcoming blood brain barrier challenges. *Curr. Clin. Pharmacol.* **2018**, *13*, 110–119. [CrossRef]
176. Ningaraj, N.S.; Rao, M.K.; Black, K.L. Adenosine 5′-triphosphate-sensitive potassium channel-mediated blood-brain tumor barrier permeability increase in a rat brain tumor model. *Cancer Res.* **2003**, *63*, 8899–8911.
177. Brayden, J.E. Functional roles of katp channels in vascular smooth muscle. *Clin. Exp. Pharmacol. Physiol.* **2002**, *29*, 312–316. [CrossRef]
178. Kitazono, T.; Faraci, F.M.; Taguchi, H.; Heistad, D.D. Role of potassium channels in cerebral blood vessels. *Stroke* **1995**, *26*, 1713–1723. [CrossRef]
179. Ruoslahti, E. Specialization of tumour vasculature. *Nat. Rev. Cancer* **2002**, *2*, 83–90. [CrossRef]
180. Ningaraj, N.S.; Sankpal, U.T.; Khaitan, D.; Meister, E.A.; Vats, T.S. Modulation of kca channels increases anticancer drug delivery to brain tumors and prolongs survival in xenograft model. *Cancer Biol. Ther.* **2009**, *8*, 1924–1933. [CrossRef]
181. Gu, Y.T.; Xue, Y.X.; Wang, Y.F.; Wang, J.H.; Chen, X.; ShangGuan, Q.R.; Lian, Y.; Zhong, L.; Meng, Y.N. Minoxidil sulfate induced the increase in blood-brain tumor barrier permeability through ros/rhoa/pi3k/pkb signaling pathway. *Neuropharmacology* **2013**, *75*, 407–415. [CrossRef] [PubMed]
182. Gu, Y.T.; Xue, Y.X.; Zhang, H.; Li, Y.; Liang, X.Y. Adenosine 5′-triphosphate-sensitive potassium channel activator induces the up-regulation of caveolin-1 expression in a rat brain tumor model. *Cell. Mol. Neurobiol.* **2011**, *31*, 629–634. [CrossRef]
183. Tinker, A.; Aziz, Q.; Thomas, A. The role of atp-sensitive potassium channels in cellular function and protection in the cardiovascular system. *Br. J. Pharmacol.* **2014**, *171*, 12–23. [CrossRef]
184. Rich, J.N.; Bigner, D.D. Development of novel targeted therapies in the treatment of malignant glioma. *Nat. Rev. Drug Discov.* **2004**, *3*, 430–446. [CrossRef]

185. Lockman, P.R.; Mittapalli, R.K.; Taskar, K.S.; Rudraraju, V.; Gril, B.; Bohn, K.A.; Adkins, C.E.; Roberts, A.; Thorsheim, H.R.; Gaasch, J.A.; et al. Heterogeneous blood-tumor barrier permeability determines drug efficacy in experimental brain metastases of breast cancer. *Clin. Cancer Res. Off. J. Am. Assoc. Cancer Res.* **2010**, *16*, 5664–5678. [CrossRef]
186. Gallo, J.M.; Li, S.; Guo, P.; Reed, K.; Ma, J. The effect of p-glycoprotein on paclitaxel brain and brain tumor distribution in mice. *Cancer Res* **2003**, *63*, 5114–5117.
187. Hanton, G.; Sobry, C.; Dagues, N.; Rochefort, G.Y.; Bonnet, P.; Eder, V. Cardiovascular toxicity of minoxidil in the marmoset. *Toxicol. Lett.* **2008**, *180*, 157–165. [CrossRef]
188. Miao, T.T.; Ju, X.F.; Zhu, Q.N.; Wang, Y.M.; Guo, Q.; Sun, T.; Lu, C.Z.; Han, L. Nanoparticles surmounting blood-brain tumor barrier through both transcellular and paracellular pathways to target brain metastases. *Adv. Funct. Mater.* **2019**, *29*, 201900259. [CrossRef]
189. Guo, S.; Som, A.T.; Arai, K.; Lo, E.H. Effects of angiotensin-ii on brain endothelial cell permeability via pparalpha regulation of para- and trans-cellular pathways. *Brain Res.* **2019**, *1722*, 146353. [CrossRef]
190. Patel, B.; Yang, P.H.; Kim, A.H. The effect of thermal therapy on the blood-brain barrier and blood-tumor barrier. *Int. J. Hyperth.* **2020**, *37*, 35–43. [CrossRef]
191. Ashraf, O.; Patel, N.V.; Hanft, S.; Danish, S.F. Laser-induced thermal therapy in neuro-oncology: A review. *World Neurosurg.* **2018**, *112*, 166–177. [CrossRef] [PubMed]

pharmaceutics

MDPI

Review

Status Quo and Trends of Intra-Arterial Therapy for Brain Tumors: A Bibliometric and Clinical Trials Analysis

Julian S. Rechberger [1,2,*], Frederic Thiele [3] and David J. Daniels [1,4]

[1] Department of Neurologic Surgery, Mayo Clinic, Rochester, MN 55905, USA; Daniels.David@mayo.edu
[2] Mayo Clinic Graduate School of Biomedical Sciences, Mayo Clinic, Rochester, MN 55905, USA
[3] Department of Neurology, Mayo Clinic, Rochester, MN 55905, USA; Thiele.Frederic@mayo.edu
[4] Department of Molecular Pharmacology and Experimental Therapeutics, Mayo Clinic, Rochester, MN 55905, USA
* Correspondence: rechberger.julian@mayo.edu

Abstract: Intra-arterial drug delivery circumvents the first-pass effect and is believed to increase both efficacy and tolerability of primary and metastatic brain tumor therapy. The aim of this update is to report on pertinent articles and clinical trials to better understand the research landscape to date and future directions. Elsevier's Scopus and ClinicalTrials.gov databases were reviewed in August 2021 for all possible articles and clinical trials of intra-arterial drug injection as a treatment strategy for brain tumors. Entries were screened against predefined selection criteria and various parameters were summarized. Twenty clinical trials and 271 articles satisfied all inclusion criteria. In terms of articles, 201 (74%) were primarily clinical and 70 (26%) were basic science, published in a total of 120 different journals. Median values were: publication year, 1986 (range, 1962–2021); citation count, 15 (range, 0–607); number of authors, 5 (range, 1–18). Pertaining to clinical trials, 9 (45%) were phase 1 trials, with median expected start and completion years in 2011 (range, 1998–2019) and 2022 (range, 2008–2025), respectively. Only one (5%) trial has reported results to date. Glioma was the most common tumor indication reported in both articles (68%) and trials (75%). There were 215 (79%) articles investigating chemotherapy, while 13 (65%) trials evaluated targeted therapy. Transient blood–brain barrier disruption was the commonest strategy for articles (27%) and trials (60%) to optimize intra-arterial therapy. Articles and trials predominately originated in the United States (50% and 90%, respectively). In this bibliometric and clinical trials analysis, we discuss the current state and trends of intra-arterial therapy for brain tumors. Most articles were clinical, and traditional anti-cancer agents and drug delivery strategies were commonly studied. This was reflected in clinical trials, of which only a single study had reported outcomes. We anticipate future efforts to involve novel therapeutic and procedural strategies based on recent advances in the field.

Keywords: brain tumor; glioma; drug delivery; injection; intra-arterial; chemotherapy; targeted therapy; immunotherapy; nanoparticles; treatment

Citation: Rechberger, J.S.; Thiele, F.; Daniels, D.J. Status Quo and Trends of Intra-Arterial Therapy for Brain Tumors: A Bibliometric and Clinical Trials Analysis. *Pharmaceutics* **2021**, *13*, 1885. https://doi.org/10.3390/pharmaceutics13111885

Academic Editors: Jingyuan Wen and Yuan Huang

Received: 20 September 2021
Accepted: 4 November 2021
Published: 6 November 2021

1. Introduction

Conventional treatment options for brain tumors rely on surgery, radiotherapy, and systemic pharmacotherapy. Oral and intravenous drug administration is often associated with poor brain distribution and bioavailability, limiting therapeutic effect, and contributing to unsatisfactory clinical outcomes [1–6]. High-grade gliomas, including glioblastoma and H3K27-altered diffuse midline glioma, with a median survival of approximately 12–15 months after diagnosis, stand a grim example of this failure to develop effective treatments [7–11]. In this multiomics era of biomedical research, insights into biological aspects of cancer have allowed us to identify potential targets that could improve the clinical course of these devastating diseases [12–15]. The first-pass effect and the blood–brain barrier (BBB), however, remain significant obstacles for therapeutic access to the brain and hinder novel therapies from unfolding pharmacologic potential [16–20].

One proposed solution to overcome these hurdles comprises strategies to minimize systemic drug exposure and modulate the BBB, which could expand the spectrum of usable drugs and potentially improve therapeutic efficacy and tolerability. Intra-arterial injection into intracranial vessels is one such strategy, with the potential to increase drug responses to primary and metastatic brain tumors [21–30]. Intra-arterial infusion of anti-cancer therapies can be combined with concurrent administration of a variety of agents, including chemical reagents, penetration drug carriers, or microbubbles for focused ultrasound, to selectively open the BBB in areas of interest [17,25,31,32]. By accessing intracranial vessels through peripheral arteries and directly administering BBB-disrupting and therapeutic agents into the arterial supply to the brain, intra-arterial injection facilitates greatly improved local drug delivery, increased intra-tumoral concentration, and lowered systemic exposure [33–37].

Since it was first described more than half a century ago, there have been considerable efforts not only to explore the biological mechanisms behind intra-arterial therapy but also to evaluate its applicability to a wide range of diseases. To date, multiple research studies are quoted to have investigated intra-arterial drug administration, yet there has been little, if any, translational impact observed for brain tumors [31,34,38–43]. Therefore, it is important to characterize how impactful the literature and previous clinical trials have been to predict where this drug delivery approach is heading. The aim of this study was to analyze the bibliometric parameters of available articles and evaluate registered clinical trials that have incorporated intra-arterial drug injection as a treatment strategy for brain tumors. This will provide a profile of the most impactful articles and trials to better inform clinicians of the current research landscape of intra-arterial drug delivery. Furthermore, this will enable future clinical trials to optimize and justify their design based on previous experiences to maximize trial discoveries and outcomes.

2. Methodology

The search strategy was designed to capture all possible Scopus-indexed articles and ClinicalTrials.gov-registered clinical trials referring to intra-arterial therapies for the treatment of brain tumors. Elsevier's Scopus facilitates access to peer-reviewed articles from approximately 22,000 journals. It offers one of the largest scientific literature capture reaches of biomedical electronic research databases [44]. ClinicalTrials.gov is a database provided by the US National Library of Medicine that contains referenced clinical trials on a wide range of conditions and diseases conducted around the world. It has been shown to have entries on 388,133 research studies from all 50 states of the USA and 219 countries worldwide [45,46]. Both databases were searched and screened independently by two investigators (J.S.R. and F.T.). We searched Scopus for referenced articles from its date of inception to August 2021 using the following string of search terms: (intra-arterial) AND (therapy OR treatment) AND (brain tumor OR glioma). The ClinicalTrials.gov portal was searched in August 2021 using "brain tumor", "glioma", and "intra-arterial injection" search terms for Condition or disease and Intervention/treatment, respectively. Any discrepancies were resolved by discussion until consensus was reached. Publications were limited to the English language.

To be included in our subsequent analyses, articles and clinical trials were required to investigate (1) intra-arterial administration of (2) therapeutics as (3) a treatment strategy for (4) tumors related to (5) the brain. In the case of articles and research studies that explored intra-arterial injection as a purely diagnostic tool, focused on diseases other than primary or secondary brain tumors, or investigated tumors of other organ systems, these were not included due to lack of specificity. Assessment of articles and trials to satisfy these criteria was performed independently by two investigators (J.S.R and F.T.), with any discrepancies resolved by discussion. There was no location restriction for eligible database entries.

The following validated article variables were then extracted from the Scopus database: article title, year, authors, number of authors, country of correspondence of the senior author, journal, Scopus citations, document type, study type, tumor type, therapy type, and type of treatment strategy for optimizing intra-arterial administration. Regarding the latter variable, 5 categories were defined: (1) nanoparticles, (2) transient BBB disruption, (3) transient cerebral hypoperfusion or flow arrest, (4) superselective intra-arterial cerebral infusion, and (5) the combination of imaging techniques with intra-arterial infusion of contrast agents or labeled therapeutic agents. With respect to study type, articles were dichotomized to be either basic science (BSc) or clinical (CL). BSc articles were ones primarily describing nonpatient investigations, such as in vitro and in vivo models, whereas CL articles were ones focusing on patient outcomes, including feasibility, safety, and survival. Clinical trial outcomes extracted from ClinicalTrials.gov included National Clinical Trial (NCT) number, title, sponsor, institution of correspondence, country of origin of the corresponding institution, number of institutions involved, involvement of outside countries, status, availability of results, type of condition, type of primary intervention, primary and secondary outcome measurements, gender enrollment, age of enrollment, number of patients enrolled, study phases, study type, start year, completion year, year of the first release of results, and last updated year [47]. Missing data were denoted as "not reported". All data analyses, including the generation of figures and tables, were performed using Pandas 1.3.2 (i.e., Python Data Analysis Library), an open-source data analysis and manipulation tool that is built on top of the Python programming language [48]. No statistical comparisons were conducted.

3. Results

3.1. Article Characteristics

A total of 546 articles were retrieved from Scopus after the initial database search. We screened titles and abstracts to obtain 357 articles not meeting any exclusion criteria. Full-text evaluation yielded 271 articles that were finally included in our study (Figure 1). A summary of the whole article cohort is provided in Table 1, and detailed results can be found in Tables S1–S13, Supplementary Materials. We identified 227 (84%) as original articles and 44 (16%) as review articles. There were 70 BSc articles (26%) and 201 CL articles (74%). Fifty-four (20%) were published open access, and therefore freely accessible online (Table S1). The most common articles for intra-arterial drug delivery in brain tumors were for gliomas (*n*= 184, 68%), including glioblastoma, gliosarcoma, diffuse intrinsic pontine glioma and glioma without further specification, brain metastasis (*n* = 12, 4%), and lymphoma (*n* = 5, 2%). Sixty-six articles reported inclusion of multiple tumor types (24%) (Table S2).

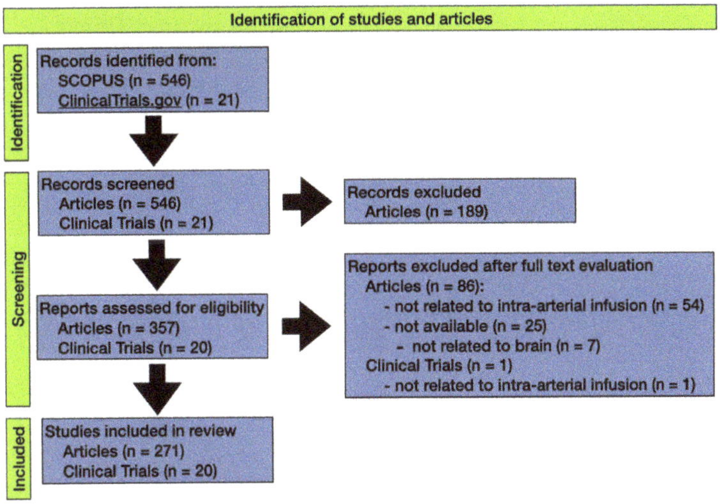

Figure 1. Methodological approach to identify articles and clinical trials on intra-arterial brain tumor therapy via databases and registers.

Table 1. Summary of article characteristics.

Parameter	Outcome (n = 271 Publications) *
Publication Type	
Original articles	227 (84%)
Review articles	44 (16%)
Clinical articles	201 (74%)
Basic science articles	70 (26%)
Open access	54 (20%)
Year of publication	
Range in years	1962–2021
Peak year	1986
Number of publications in peak year	17
Median publications per year	5
Citations	
Median	15
Most cited publication (n)	Primary central nervous system lymphoma (607)
Most cited original article (n)	Safety and efficacy of a multicenter study using intraarterial chemotherapy in conjunction with osmotic opening of the blood–brain barrier for the treatment of patients with malignant brain tumors (300)
Most cited review article (n)	Primary central nervous system lymphoma (607)
Authors	
Median number of authors per publication	5
Most authored publications (n)	Neuwelt E.A. (14)
Most first authored publications (n)	Nakagawa H. (7)
Most senior authored publications (n)	Neuwelt E.A. (8), Boockvar J.A. (8)
Country of correspondence	
Total countries involved	20
Countries with most publications	
US	135 (50%)
Japan	46 (17%)
Canada	19 (7%)
Contributing journals	
Total number of journals involved	120
Journals with most publications	
Journal of Neuro-Oncology	48 (18%)
Japanese Journal of Cancer and Chemotherapy	14 (5%)
Neurosurgery	13 (5%)
Tumor type #	
Most common	
Glioma (combined)	184 (68%)
Multiple (>1 tumor type)	66 (24%)
Therapies #	
Chemotherapy	215 (79%)
Targeted Therapy	40 (15%)
Immunotherapy	13 (5%)
Radiosensitizing/neutron capture therapy	17 (6%)
Stem cell therapy	5 (2%)
Treatment strategies #	
Number of publications using:	
Nanoparticles	17 (6%)
Transient blood–brain barrier disruption	74 (27%)
Transient cerebral hypoperfusion or flow arrest	6 (2%)
Superselective intra-arterial cerebral infusion	27 (10%)
Imaging techniques with contrast or labelled therapeutic agents	13 (5%)

* Categorical data reported as n (% total). # Does not sum to 271 as studies could report more than one tumor type and therapeutic approach.

The median citation count was 15 (range, 0–607), with the most-cited article to date a review by Hochberg et al. [49], published in 1988 with 607 citations ("Primary central nervous system lymphoma" in the *Journal of Neurosurgery*). The most cited original article was the CL study by Doolittle et al. [34], published in 2000 with 300 citations ("Safety and efficacy of a multicenter study using intraarterial chemotherapy in conjunction with osmotic opening of the blood–brain barrier for the treatment of patients with malignant brain tumors" in Cancer). Matsukado et al. [50] published in 1996 the most-cited BSc article with 151 citations ("Enhanced tumor uptake of carboplatin and survival in glioma-bearing rats by intracarotid infusion of bradykinin analog, RMP-7" in Neurosurgery) (Table S3).

With regard to contributing authors, the median number of authors for original and review articles was five (range, 1–18). The most authored article was the original, CL study by Angelov et al. [51], published in 2009 with 18 authors ("Blood–brain barrier disruption and intra-arterial methotrexate-based therapy for newly diagnosed primary CNS lymphoma: A multi-institutional experience" in the *Journal of Clinical Oncology*). The highest number of authors for BSc articles was 12: Liu et al. [52] published their manuscript in 1991 ("Effects of intracarotid and intravenous infusion of human TNF and LT on established intracerebral rat gliomas" in Lymphokine and Cytokine Research) whereas the article by Mao et al. [53] was published in 2020 ("Peritumoral administration of IFNβ upregulated mesenchymal stem cells inhibits tumor growth in an orthotopic, immunocompetent rat glioma model" in Journal for ImmunoTherapy of Cancer). The most authored review article was by Aoki et al. [54], published in 1993 with 13 authors ("Supraophthalmic chemotherapy with long tapered catheter: Distribution evaluated with intraarterial and intravenous Tc-99m HMPAO" in Radiology). The authors with the most senior-authored articles overall were E.A. Neuwelt and J.A. Boockvar, who both contributed eight articles [34,36,37,51,55–66] (Table S4).

All articles were published between 1962 and 2021 (Figure 2), with a median of 5 publications per year. The peak year (median) with most-published articles was 17 (6%) articles published in 1986. Original articles and reviews peaked with respect to their annual publication number in 1986 and 2020, respectively. Most BSc articles were published in 1999, while CL articles had their peak year in 1986 (Table S5).

A total of 20 countries were denoted as the location for correspondence of all articles (Figure 3). The USA was the country with the highest contribution, with 135 articles (50%), followed by Japan and Canada, with 46 (17%) and 19 (7%), respectively. The USA was the most common country of correspondence for all document and study types (Table S6).

One hundred and twenty journals contributed to articles of intra-arterial therapy for the treatment of brain tumors. The most common ones were the *Journal of Neuro-Oncology*, with 48 (18%) articles, the *Japanese Journal of Cancer and Chemotherapy* ($n = 14$, 5%), and *Neurosurgery* ($n = 13$, 5%). The journal publishing most original studies, review articles, BSc articles, and CL articles was the *Journal of Neuro-Oncology* (Table S7).

In terms of therapy types used with intra-arterial delivery, general chemotherapy was the most common, with 215 (79%) articles, followed by targeted therapy ($n = 40$, 15%), and radiosensitizing or neutron capture therapy ($n = 17$, 6%). The number of articles per therapy type per year of publication is illustrated in Figure 4. Chemotherapy was the top therapeutic strategy in all but three years (1973, 2014, and 2017). The most commonly studied chemotherapeutic agents included i.a. carmustine ($n = 29$, 13%), i.a. nimustine ($n = 20$, 9%), and i.a. cisplatin ($n = 23$, 11%). Twenty-three articles (11%) mentioned the general concept of intra-arterial chemotherapy without further specification (Tables S8–S12).

At least 1 additional treatment strategy for optimizing intra-arterial drug delivery was evaluated in 104 articles (Figure 5). The most common strategy was transient BBB disruption, mentioned in 74 articles (27%). Transient BBB disruption was followed by superselective intra-arterial cerebral infusion ($n = 27$, 10%), and nanoparticles ($n = 17$, 6%). Among BBB-opening modalities, mannitol was the most common one, referenced in 48 articles (65%), followed by bradykinin/RMP-7 ($n = 16$, 22%) (Table S13).

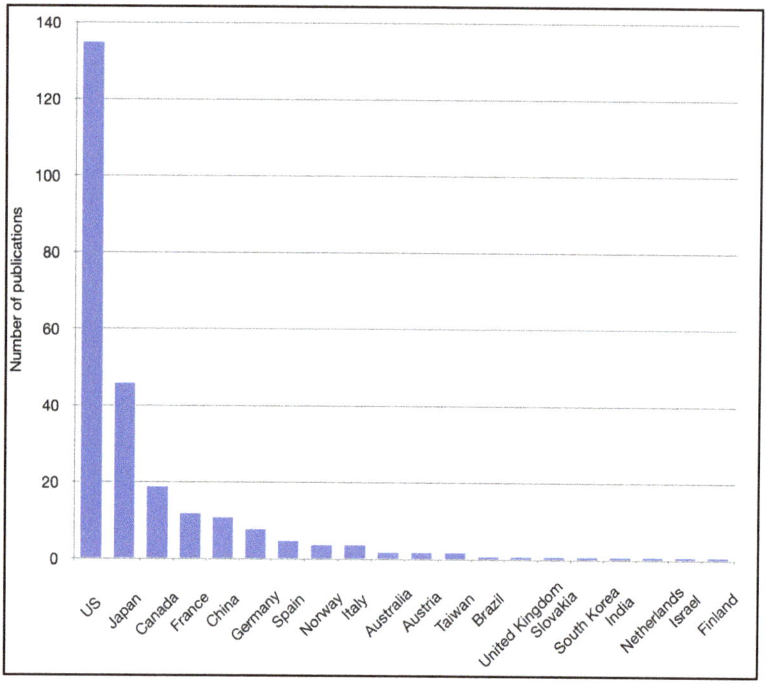

Figure 2. Distribution of articles about intra-arterial drug delivery for the treatment of brain tumors based on the country of correspondence.

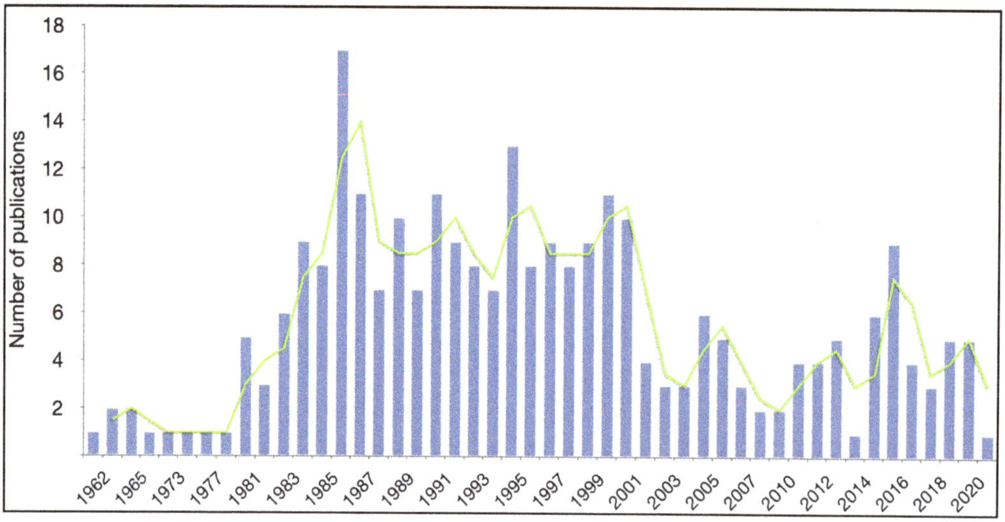

Figure 3. Distribution of articles about intra-arterial drug delivery for the treatment of brain tumors based on the year of publication.

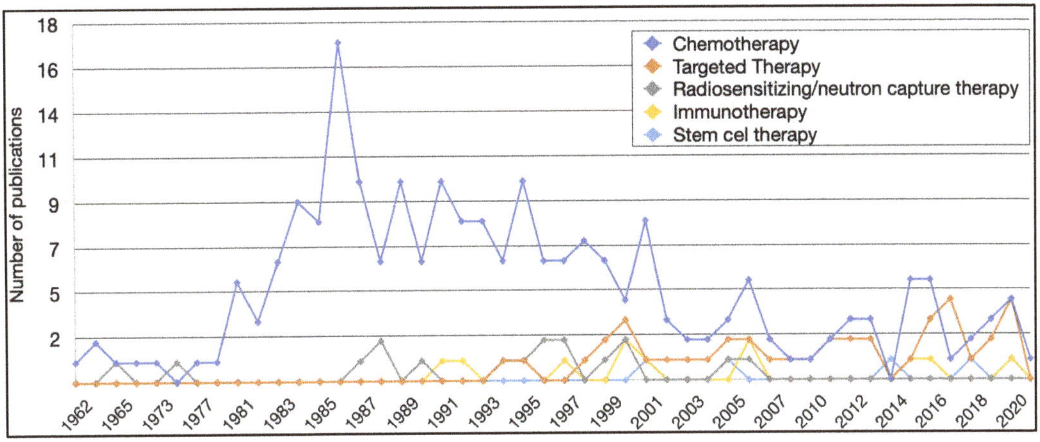

Figure 4. Different therapy types investigated in articles of intra-arterial drug delivery for the treatment of brain tumors based on the year of publication.

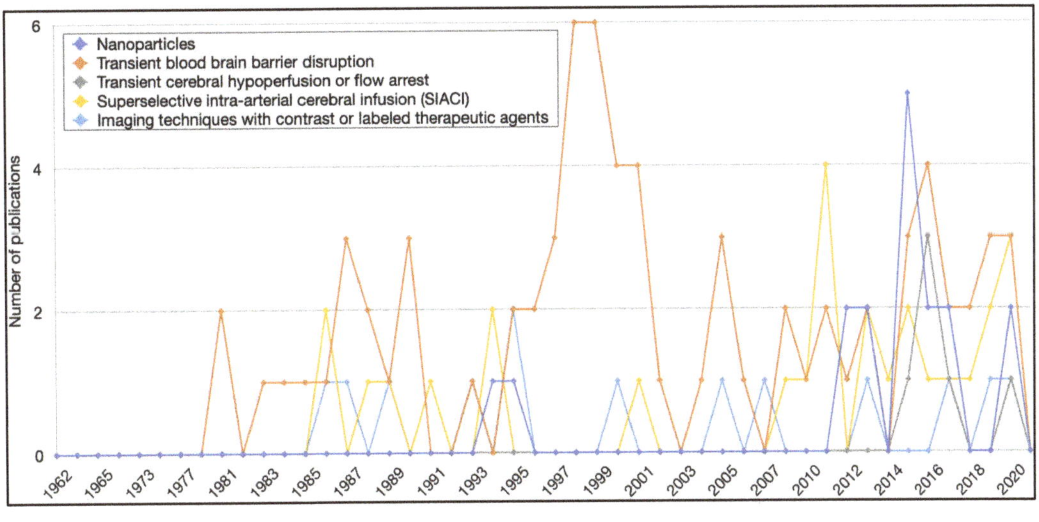

Figure 5. Treatment strategies to optimize intra-arterial drug delivery for the treatment of brain tumors in pertinent articles based on the year of publication.

3.2. Clinical Trial Characteristics

The initial search of the ClinicalTrials.gov portal yielded 21 clinical trials for screening. One trial was excluded because it did not investigate intra-arterial drug injection, but rather looked at cerebral blood perfusion changes during emergence from general anesthesia for craniotomy using an intra-arterial pressure line [67]. Consequently, 20 trials were included in our study, all of which were interventional in nature. Included trials have been summarized in Table 2, with individual details listed in Tables S14–S24.

Glioblastoma was the most common brain tumor indications for trials involving intra-arterial drug delivery (*n*= 13, 65%), followed by anaplastic astrocytoma (*n* = 8, 40%) (Table S14). The median commencement year was 2011, with trials reporting start dates between 1998 and 2019. As for expected completion year, the median was 2022 (range, 2008–2025) (Table S15). As of August 2021, 6 (30%) trials are reported to have completed recruiting patients, 8 (40%) are still recruiting, and 2 (10%) are active but not recruiting. Two (10%) trials are declared as suspended (Table S16).

All trials reported target enrollment sizes between 3 and 60 patients, with the Portland-based trial "NCT00075387: Combination Chemotherapy With or Without Sodium Thiosulfate in Preventing Low Platelet Count While Treating Patients With Malignant Brain Tumors" [68] targeting the most ($n = 60$). This trial has an estimated study completion date in spring 2023 (Table S17). With regard to age of enrollment, the median minimum patient age was 18 years (range, 1 month–18 years), with 18 (90%) of trials using this threshold. The median maximum patient age was 99 years (range 17–120 years), with 2 (10%) trials focusing solely on the pediatric demographic while 18 (90%) also included adult patients (Table S18).

Table 2. Summary of clinical trial characteristics.

Parameter	Outcome (n = 20 Trials) *
Time (expected)	
Start year	2011 (1998–2019)
Completion year	2022 (2008–2025)
Results first posted	2015 ^
Last updated	2020 (2013–2021)
Status	
Current status as of August 2021	
Recruiting	8 (40%)
Completed	6 (30%)
Suspended	2 (10%)
Active, not recruiting	2 (10%)
Terminated	1 (5%)
Unknown status	1 (5%)
Study results available	1 (5%)
Cohort	
Minimum age of enrollment (years)	18 (0–18)
Maximum age of enrollment (years)	99 (17–120)
Design	
Interventional studies	20 (100%)
Phase	
Phase 1	9 (45%)
Phase 1 + Phase 2	8 (40%)
Phase 2	3 (15%)
Outcomes #	
Primary	
Safety and toxicity	11 (55%)
PFS	6 (35%)
OS	5 (25%)
Secondary	
PFS	11 (55%)
Safety and toxicity	9 (45%)
OS	8 (40%)
QOL	5 (25%)
Location and funding	
Two most common corresponding institutes	
Northwell Health	10 (50%)
OHSU Knight Cancer Institute	3 (15%)
Trials per Country	
US	18 (90%)
China, Canada	1 (5%) each
Number of sites involved	1 (1–2)

Table 2. *Cont.*

Parameter	Outcome (n = 20 Trials) *
Therapies #	
Number of research studies using:	
Targeted Therapy	13 (65%)
Chemotherapy	8 (40%)
Treatment mechanism #	
Number of research studies using:	
Superselective intra-arterial cerebral Infusion [1]	13 (65%)
Transient blood–brain barrier disruption using mannitol [2]	12 (60%)
Three most common conditions #	
Glioblastoma	13 (65%)
Anaplastic Astrocytoma	8 (40%)
Brain Metastasis	3 (15%)

PFS, progression-free survival; OS, overall survival; QOL, quality of life. * Continuous data reported as the median (range) and categorical data reported as n (% total). ^ Only 1 trial. # Does not sum to 20 as trials could report more than one condition, outcome, and therapeutic approach. [1] Superselective intra-arterial cerebral infusion into a major tumor feeding artery was performed using neurovascular microcatheter systems under fluoroscopic guidance to increase the concentration of drug delivered to the tumor while sparing the patient of systemic side effects. [2] Temporary opening of the blood–brain barrier was achieved by treating patients with an intra-arterial infusion of the osmotic agent mannitol followed by intra-arterial administration of therapeutic agents (mannitol 20–25%; 3–12.5 mL over 2 min).

Phase category was reported for all clinical trials included in this study. With 9 (45%) trials, phase 1 was the most common phase design. Eight (40%) trials were registered as both phase 1 and 2. A total of 3 (15%) trials were exclusively phase 2. Two phase 2 studies were randomized. Allocation was non-randomized in 4 phase 1 trials, while allocation type was not available for all other trials (Table S19).

In terms of the different types of primary intervention, therapeutic drug alone was the most common, with 14 (70%) trials. Combinations of radiation and drug therapy as well as therapeutic drug and psychological assessments were applied in 2 (10%) trials each. Investigations of biological agents alone (n = 1, 5%) and in combination with drug therapy (n = 1, 5%) were also reported (Table S20). Overall, there were 20 different types of primary intervention combinations evaluated in clinical trials of intra-arterial therapy for brain tumors (Table S21). Based on our original classification, targeted therapy was the therapeutic strategy most commonly investigated (n = 13, 65%), followed by chemotherapy (n = 8, 40%). Of these, i.a. bevacizumab (n = 5, 25%), i.a. cetuximab (n = 3, 15%), and i.a. melphalan (n = 2, 10%) were most common (Table S22). Transient BBB disruption was used in 12 (60%) trials. Thirteen (65%) trials explored superselective intra-arterial cerebral infusion as a strategy to optimize intra-arterial administration (Table S23).

Feasibility, safety, and toxicity of a treatment or intervention was the most common primary outcome reported (n = 11, 55%). With respect to other primary outcomes, 6 (35%) trials reported progression-free survival and 5 (25%) reported overall survival. One study (5%) reported tumor response and intracellular carboplatin accumulation as primary outcome measurement. The most common secondary outcome reported was progression-free survival 11 (55%), followed by feasibility, safety, and toxicity (n = 9, 45%) and overall survival (n = 8, 40%) (Table S24).

As of August 2021, only 1 (5%) trial has posted results (NCT00362817: Carboplatin and Temozolomide (Temodar) for Recurrent and Symptomatic Residual Brain Metastases) [69]. This study started recruiting patients in 2004 and reported results in 2015. Seventeen patients older than 18 years, who had all received prior systemic chemotherapy for primary cancers in parts of the body other than the brain, were enrolled to investigate the use of intra-arterial carboplatin and oral temozolomide for the treatment of recurrent and symptomatic residual brain metastases. In terms of primary outcome, the reported response rate, evaluated by MRI criteria (MacDonald criteria), was approximately 43%. Secondary outcome measures included 25 weeks overall survival, 23 weeks progression-free survival, and no incidence of CNS toxicities or CNS tumor-related deaths. In 7 (41%) cases, systemic disease progression was determined as cause of death (Table 3).

Table 3. Summary of clinical trial with reported results.

Parameter	Outcome
NCT number	NCT00362817
Title	Carboplatin and Temozolomide (Temodar) for Recurrent and Symptomatic Residual Brain Metastases
Location	Ohio State University, Columbus, Ohio, United States
Start date	October 2004
Finish date	January 2008
Results first posted	May 2015
Enrolment size	17
Age range (years)	18 and older
Primary outcome	
Response rate	42.8%
Secondary outcome	
Overall survival in weeks	25.2
Time to progression in weeks (mean)	22.6
Incidence of CNS toxicities	0
Cause of death	CNS tumor = 0, systemic disease progression = 7

A total of 10 different institutions coordinated all 20 clinical trials on intra-arterial therapeutic delivery to brain tumors. Three different countries were listed as the location for correspondence of all trials, with the USA contributing 18 (90%) trials. The Lenox Hill Brain Tumor Center, located in New York City, coordinated the most trials (n = 10, 50%) [70–79]. The only other institution coordinating more than one trial was the OHSU Knight Cancer Institute in Portland, OR (n = 3, 15%) [68,80,81]. Only two trials had corresponding institutions outside the USA, with the Beijing YouAn Hospital (China) and the Centre hospitalier universitaire de Sherbrooke (Canada) both coordinating one (5%) trial [82,83] (Table S25). The median number of institutions involved was one (range, 1–3), with 18 (95%) studies involving a single institution. All trials were conducted in a single country.

4. Discussion

The intention of this study was to identify and characterize the published literature and registered clinical trials on intra-arterial drug administration for brain tumor treatment. We identified 271 articles and 20 trials to meet our inclusion criteria. These numbers are reflected in the quoted numbers reported by recently published reviews [31,84], even though this is the first study to offer a precise number of clinical trials involving intra-arterial brain tumor therapy, highlighting a previously unreported area in the field as to how many distinct trials have officially been registered and conducted since the technique was first described in 1950 [85]. The complexity of successfully translating intra-arterial drug delivery into the clinic is demonstrated by the fact that in the last 20 years, only 6 trials eligible for this review have completed recruitment [69,74,76,77,82,86], and results of just a single study are publicly available at the ClinicalTrials.gov portal as of August 2021 [69]. Despite these findings, given the discovery of novel biological and molecular features of brain tumors potentially amenable to therapy [12,13,87,88], we posit that more tumor-specific intra-arterial interventions will emerge in future trials to add to the current body of research studies.

The development of intra-arterial technologies was historically driven by the need to minimize the systemic toxicity of traditional anti-cancer agents and propelled by advances in endovascular techniques; however, very few studies took into consideration the pharmacokinetic characteristics underlying intra-arterial drug delivery [89]. Although the neuro-oncological application of intra-arterial technology has been established by impactful CL articles [34,38,85], accurate and reliable pharmacological models to optimize the method, rate, and duration of drug injection for high local extraction and systemic clearance may be lacking to date [90]. Furthermore, biological hurdles to intra-arterial therapy of brain tumors, including the vascular heterogeneity within the tumor microenvironment, have to be considered in ongoing research efforts and future refinements [91]. The lack of effective therapies to be delivered by the intra-arterial route and reported in BSc articles could in part explain why CL articles and clinical trials remain without definitive success. Consequently, we expect to observe an increase in BSc articles in the future as our understanding of this technology and our ability to modify relevant drug properties continue to grow.

For those within the field of intra-arterial therapy for brain tumor treatment, it is not surprising that E.A. Neuwelt and J.A. Boockvar were identified as particularly impactful authors who pioneered the field and spearheaded recent advances of this drug delivery technique in terms of preclinical and clinical research. The portfolio of both these authors was predominantly focused on CL articles and clinical trials based in the USA. When considering all articles included in this study, E.A. Neuwelt was the author of most with 14 articles overall, of which he senior-authored 8 CL articles [34,51,55–60,92–94]. Through the Neuro-Oncology Blood-Brain Barrier Program at OHSU, he was also involved in initiating 3 clinical trials that are currently being conducted at the OHSU Knight Cancer Institute [68,80,81]. J.A. Boockvar authored 10 articles overall, serving as the corresponding author of 5 original and 3 review CL articles [35–37,61–66,95]. In his role as vice chair of neurosurgery at Lenox Hill Hospital, he has also been in charge of 10 clinical trials that were registered to evaluate intra-arterial brain tumor therapies, including bevacizumab, cetuximab, trastuzumab, and temozolomide alone or in combination with carboplatin, radiotherapy, and/or mannitol, for conditions such as glioblastoma, anaplastic astrocytoma, vestibular schwannoma, and brain metastasis [70–79]. Collectively, the clinical trials overseen by J.A. Boockvar and E.A. Neuwelt account for more than half of all trials included in this study. The general focus of both authors on translational research is largely reflected in the current research landscape of intra-arterial drug delivery for brain tumors, highlighting their significant impact on the field.

When Perese et al. [96] first proposed the intra-arterial route as a drug delivery strategy for treating patients with malignant brain tumors, they posited that this technology could be used to deliver large concentrations of a variety of anti-cancer agents to the brain without causing much systemic reaction. More than a half-century later, based on this study of pertinent articles and clinical trials, it appears their vision has, in part, been realized, but new hurdles have emerged. The largest indication for intra-arterial administration was chemotherapy, with 215 of 271 articles describing its BSc or CL use. Indeed, intra-arterial chemotherapy allowed relatively high dosing while minimizing systemic toxicity [41,59,63,64]. However, articles on chemotherapeutic drugs peaked over three decades ago, possibly indicating that these therapies were lacking efficacy with intra-arterial use. Furthermore, several articles alluded to chemotherapy-related safety concerns, some of which were unique to the intra-arterial delivery route [38,58,60,93]. This could explain why only a few traditional chemotherapeutics, all of which had previously demonstrated safety and efficacy in preclinical models and via other drug delivery strategies, have found their way to clinical trials. The fact that targeted therapy was the most commonly used therapy type in clinical trials could suggest a paradigm shift towards novel therapeutic strategies. Based on exciting developments in modern neuro-oncology, involving precision medicine [97], immunotherapy [98], and stem cell technology [99], we anticipate an increased number of articles and clinical trials investigating these therapies with intra-arterial injection in the future [100].

As effective treatment modalities for different types of brain tumors are desperately needed, it is not surprising that a number of technologies to improve the therapeutic effect of intra-arterial drug delivery have been proposed [24,30]. BBB penetrance, targeting, and accuracy of intra-arterial administration are of major interest, which is underscored by the high number of articles and clinical trials exploring strategies to account for these parameters. We found chemical reagents, and mannitol in particular, to be the oldest and most common approach to open the BBB. However, the capability of mannitol and newer agents, such as the bradykinin agonist RMP-7, to permeabilize the BBB is limited [50,63,101]. Focused ultrasound is a non-invasive strategy for disrupting BBB tight junctions in a reversible and controlled fashion and has the potential to be used with intra-arterial technologies [32,102,103]. The scientific complexity of this concept is underlined by the fact that of all 271 articles included in this study, only 2 review articles described focused ultrasound in combination with intra-arterial drug delivery [20,104]. Although mentioned by only a small proportion of articles, superselective intra-arterial cerebral infusion into the tumor-feeding arteries was reported in 13 of 20 clinical trials. This possibly indicates a trend towards using this advanced endovascular procedure to reduce neurotoxic side effects and ensure targeted intra-arterial therapy [35–37,61,63–65,95]. It is interesting to observe that several articles published in recent years investigated nanoparticles. The attraction of nanotechnology for intra-arterial drug delivery is multifold. Various authors noted these small particles could not only be loaded with different therapies, including small-molecule inhibitors, gene therapies or siRNAs, but could also be modified to cross the BBB through a variety of transport mechanisms and remain at the target site for longer periods of time to allow for a gradual release of loaded therapeutics [23,105–113].

We speculate that future refinements of intra-arterial brain tumor therapy will come from multiple angles. From a therapeutic perspective, studies to date are using mostly approved agents, as they are easier to translate; however, certain novel compounds may have superior pharmacokinetics and be ultimately more useful for intra-arterial drug delivery. Disease-specific drugs will enhance efficacy and minimize systemic and CNS-related side effects [87]. Drug modification or loading into nanoparticles can allow for improved BBB penetration, tumor targeting, and drug-tumor contact time of active compounds [114–116]. Labeled therapeutic agents as well as theragnostic nanoparticles have the potential to be used with advanced imaging techniques [50,106,109]. From a procedural point of view, optimizing currently available endovascular technologies and combining them with innovative strategies, such as superselective intra-arterial cerebral infusion or transient cerebral hypoperfusion/flow arrest, is crucial to ensure procedural safety and effect [31,61,89]. With regard to clinical trials, it will be important to move from phase 1 and 2 to phase 3 trials and to evaluate novel drugs and procedures in the context of randomized patient allocations. This will help to ensure the validity of conclusions not only from a feasibility and safety perspective but also in terms of efficacy. The inability of the vast majority of clinical trials to report results suggests that a collaborative approach may be necessary to improve the fate of future trials. Therefore, we stress the importance of intra- and inter-institutional collaboration in preclinical and clinical research for progress within the field of intra-arterial brain tumor therapy.

The intra-arterial therapeutic concept constitutes only one of many technologies to facilitate drug delivery to the brain and brain tumors. An enhanced understanding of the BBB physiology has led to the development of a multitude of noninvasive and invasive strategies to target tumor cells present beyond this barrier. Locoregional invasive technologies, in particular, are a remarkably fast-evolving segment within the neurooncology field. These technologies are based on local delivery of therapeutics directly to the brain, thereby bypassing the BBB entirely and facilitating smaller initial drug dosage and minimal systemic absorption. They include drug delivery to the cerebrospinal fluid via intrathecal or intraventricular injections and interstitial delivery via biodegradable polymers or catheters [17]. Diffusion-based approaches such as intracavitary wafers placed at the time of tumor resection, intrathecal injection using the Ommaya reservoir, and intraventricular injection via lumbar puncture are limited by the restricted tissue penetrance of most therapeutic agents into structures not immediately adjacent to the brain surface, hindering them from reaching deep and infiltrative tumor cells [21,27,117]. However, molecularly engineered cells, especially chimeric antigen receptor (CAR) T-cells and natural killer cells, feature enhanced tumor-homing abilities and have shown promise in preclinical and clinical investigations of these strategies in various brain tumors [118–126]. In contrast to locoregional therapies, intra-arterial administration takes advantage of the branched blood vessel system that is feeding into brain tumors, thereby reaching even distant, infiltrative tumor cells, and enabling site-directed infiltration of cell-based therapies or diffusion of macromolecules [127].

Direct interstitial drug infusion to brain tumors is achieved by placing one or multiple catheters under stereotactic guidance into the bulk tumor. These cannulas can be connected to osmotic or mechanical pumps and allow for direct, targeted delivery [28,29]. The former can provide continuous drug delivery at a set infusion rate, whereby the infusion is driven by an osmotic pressure gradient [128]. Convection-enhanced delivery (CED), which describes direct interstitial infusion under a mechanical pressure gradient, has further advantages, including a larger, more homogeneous volume of drug distribution [129]. This technology is currently being used in multiple clinical trials for brain tumors like glioblastoma and diffuse intrinsic pontine glioma (DIPG) [130–138]. In addition to technical and procedural challenges, such as catheter design and placement, tracking of infusate distribution, prevention of reflux along the canula tract, and reduction in edema and mechanical tissue damage, the success of CED is hampered by the potential requirement of repetitive infusions [139,140]. Almost 100 clinical trials for DIPG have failed, and it has recently been shown that the brain half-life of panobinostat, a small molecule inhibitor, after CED is only 2.9 h [141,142]. Intra-arterial technologies address some of these pitfalls, allowing for repeated and prolonged therapeutic administration to ensure pharmacologic effect, but are accompanied by their own constraints, as discussed above. Consequently, a "one size fits all" approach may not be effective, and a rational combination of therapeutics and their delivery strategies should be considered. In this way, a comprehensive treatment regime to attain optimal concentrations in brain tumors over a prolonged period of time while minimizing off-target effects could be established.

There are certain limitations that are inherent to bibliometric and clinical trials analyses. First, Elsevier's Scopus and ClinicalTrials.gov are only two of many databases for articles and clinical trials, respectively. With both of them being US-based, this may have influenced the predominance of US-based literature and trials in this study. There is validity to the argument that our representation of the research landscape of intra-arterial brain tumor therapy would have been more comprehensive if additional registries would have been included. Even though both Scopus and ClinicalTrials.gov constitute major databases in their respective field, holding registrations from journals and institutions around the world, there is a distinct possibility that this study is an underestimate of all articles and trials evaluating intra-arterial brain tumor treatments. Second, since our therapy type and treatment strategy classifications were solely based on the literature and our own experience, it is unclear whether the presented categories and proportions optimally reflect the current status and trends of the field. It is possible that more refined categorizations would have led to a better representation. Finally, article and clinical trial parameters, e.g., citation count and number of institutions involved, are regularly updated to rigorously reflect the current state of affairs. As it is difficult to continue updating these parameters once they have been extracted, our study represents the status quo and trends of articles and clinical trials on intra-arterial drug delivery for brain tumor treatment as of August 2021. We anticipate that analyses in the future will confirm whether these were accurate.

5. Conclusions

In this bibliometric and clinical trials analysis, we identified, characterized, and analyzed available parameters of preclinical and clinical research on intra-arterial therapy for brain tumors. Overall, 271 articles and 20 clinical trials were sufficiently specific for inclusion. Among articles, most were CL and chemotherapy was the most common therapeutic modality. With respect to treatment strategies for optimizing intra-arterial drug delivery, transient blood–brain barrier disruption using mannitol was the most frequently studied. These trends were reflected in clinical trials, but unfortunately only a single phase 1/phase 2 study has reported outcomes to date. Given the longstanding history of intra-arterial brain tumor therapy research, our results mandate the consideration of novel therapeutic and procedural strategies, including precision medicine, nanoparticles, and superselective intra-arterial cerebral infusion, to foster the preclinical research basis and set the stage for more robust, systematic clinical trials in the future.

Supplementary Materials: The following are available online at https://www.mdpi.com/article/10.3390/pharmaceutics13111885/s1, Table S1. Articles on intra-arterial therapy for brain tumors based on publication type; Table S2. Classification of tumors investigated in articles on intra-arterial therapy for brain tumors; Table S3. Citations for articles on intra-arterial therapy for brain tumors; Table S4. Authors of articles on intra-arterial therapy for brain tumors; Table S5. Years of publications of intra-arterial therapy for brain tumors differentiated by article type; Table S6. Involvement of countries in articles on intra-arterial therapy for brain tumors; Table S7. Involvement of journals in articles on intra-arterial therapy for brain tumors; Table S8. Investigated chemotherapies and application ways in articles on intra-arterial therapy for brain tumors; Table S9. Investigated targeted therapies in articles on intra-arterial therapy for brain tumors; Table S10. Investigated immunotherapies in articles on intra-arterial therapy for brain tumors; Table S11. Investigated radiosensitizing/neutron capture therapies in articles on intra-arterial therapy for brain tumors; Table S12. Investigated stem cell therapies in articles on intra-arterial therapy for brain tumors; Table S13. Investigated treatment strategies in articles on intra-arterial therapy for brain tumors; Table S14. Tumor types investigated in clinical trials on intra-arterial therapy for brain tumors; Table S15. Timeline of clinical trials on intra-arterial therapy for brain tumors, including start year, completion year, year of the first release of results, and last updated year; Table S16. Recruitment status of clinical trials on intra-arterial therapy for brain tumors; Table S17. Number of patients enrolled in clinical trials intra-arterial therapy for brain tumors; Table S18. Minimum and maximum age of enrollment in clinical trials on intra-arterial therapy for brain tumors; Table S19. Distribution of the different study phases of clinical trials on intra-arterial therapy for brain tumors; Table S20. Type of primary intervention investigated by the clinical trials on intra-arterial therapy for brain tumors; Table S21. Detailed primary interventions applied by the clinical trials on intra-arterial therapy for brain tumors; Table S22. Therapies investigated in clinical trials on intra-arterial therapy for brain tumors; Table S23. Treatment strategies investigated in clinical trials on intra-arterial therapy for brain tumors; Table S24. Different outcome measurements of clinical trials on intra-arterial therapy for brain tumors with respect to primary and secondary outcome, overall survival, progression-free survival, safety aspects, and quality of life; Table S25. Sponsors, institutions and countries involved in clinical trials on intra-arterial therapy for brain tumors.

Author Contributions: Conceptualization, J.S.R. and D.J.D.; methodology, J.S.R.; software, F.T.; validation, J.S.R. and D.J.D.; formal analysis, J.S.R. and F.T.; investigation, J.S.R.; resources, J.S.R.; data curation, J.S.R. and F.T.; writing—original draft preparation, J.S.R.; writing—review and editing, F.T. and D.J.D.; visualization, F.T.; supervision, D.J.D.; project administration, J.S.R. All authors have read and agreed to the published version of the manuscript.

Funding: This research received no external funding.

Institutional Review Board Statement: Not applicable.

Informed Consent Statement: Not applicable.

Data Availability Statement: All data supporting reported results can be found in the manuscript and supplementary materials to the manuscript.

Acknowledgments: No individuals other than the listed co-authors contributed to this publication.

Conflicts of Interest: The authors declare no conflict of interest.

References

1. Parrish, K.E.; Sarkaria, J.N.; Elmquist, W.F. Improving drug delivery to primary and metastatic brain tumors: Strategies to overcome the blood-brain barrier. *Clin. Pharmacol. Ther.* **2015**, *97*, 336–346. [CrossRef] [PubMed]
2. Omuro, A.; DeAngelis, L.M. Glioblastoma and other malignant gliomas: A clinical review. *JAMA* **2013**, *310*, 1842–1850. [CrossRef] [PubMed]
3. Tzika, A.A.; Astrakas, L.G.; Zarifi, M.K.; Zurakowski, D.; Poussaint, T.Y.; Goumnerova, L.; Tarbell, N.J.; Black, P.M. Spectroscopic and perfusion magnetic resonance imaging predictors of progression in pediatric brain tumors. *Cancer* **2004**, *100*, 1246–1256. [CrossRef] [PubMed]
4. Arvold, N.D.; Lee, E.Q.; Mehta, M.P.; Margolin, K.; Alexander, B.M.; Lin, N.U.; Anders, C.K.; Soffietti, R.; Camidge, D.R.; Vogelbaum, M.A.; et al. Updates in the management of brain metastases. *Neuro Oncol.* **2016**, *18*, 1043–1065. [CrossRef] [PubMed]
5. Nayak, L.; Lee, E.Q.; Wen, P.Y. Epidemiology of brain metastases. *Curr. Oncol. Rep.* **2012**, *14*, 48–54. [CrossRef] [PubMed]
6. Pitz, M.W.; Desai, A.; Grossman, S.A.; Blakeley, J.O. Tissue concentration of systemically administered antineoplastic agents in human brain tumors. *J. Neuro-Oncol.* **2011**, *104*, 629–638. [CrossRef] [PubMed]
7. Stupp, R.; Mason, W.P.; van den Bent, M.J.; Weller, M.; Fisher, B.; Taphoorn, M.J.; Belanger, K.; Brandes, A.A.; Marosi, C.; Bogdahn, U.; et al. Radiotherapy plus concomitant and adjuvant temozolomide for glioblastoma. *N. Engl. J. Med.* **2005**, *352*, 987–996. [CrossRef]
8. Sun, T.; Wan, W.; Wu, Z.; Zhang, J.; Zhang, L. Clinical outcomes and natural history of pediatric brainstem tumors: With 33 cases follow-ups. *Neurosurg. Rev.* **2013**, *36*, 311–319; discussion 319–320. [CrossRef]
9. Cohen, K.J.; Jabado, N.; Grill, J. Diffuse intrinsic pontine gliomas-current management and new biologic insights. Is there a glimmer of hope? *Neuro Oncol.* **2017**, *19*, 1025–1034. [CrossRef]
10. Frazier, J.L.; Lee, J.; Thomale, U.W.; Noggle, J.C.; Cohen, K.J.; Jallo, G.I. Treatment of diffuse intrinsic brainstem gliomas: Failed approaches and future strategies. *J. Neurosurg. Pediatr.* **2009**, *3*, 259–269. [CrossRef]
11. Vanan, M.I.; Eisenstat, D.D. DIPG in Children—What Can We Learn from the Past? *Front. Oncol.* **2015**, *5*, 237. [CrossRef]
12. Schwartzentruber, J.; Korshunov, A.; Liu, X.Y.; Jones, D.T.; Pfaff, E.; Jacob, K.; Sturm, D.; Fontebasso, A.M.; Quang, D.A.; Tönjes, M.; et al. Driver mutations in histone H3.3 and chromatin remodelling genes in paediatric glioblastoma. *Nature* **2012**, *482*, 226–231. [CrossRef]
13. Wu, G.; Broniscer, A.; McEachron, T.A.; Lu, C.; Paugh, B.S.; Becksfort, J.; Qu, C.; Ding, L.; Huether, R.; Parker, M.; et al. Somatic histone H3 alterations in pediatric diffuse intrinsic pontine gliomas and non-brainstem glioblastomas. *Nat. Genet.* **2012**, *44*, 251–253. [CrossRef]
14. Zorzan, M.; Giordan, E.; Redaelli, M.; Caretta, A.; Mucignat-Caretta, C. Molecular targets in glioblastoma. *Future Oncol.* **2015**, *11*, 1407–1420. [CrossRef]
15. Wei, W.; Shin, Y.S.; Xue, M.; Matsutani, T.; Masui, K.; Yang, H.; Ikegami, S.; Gu, Y.; Herrmann, K.; Johnson, D.; et al. Single-Cell Phosphoproteomics Resolves Adaptive Signaling Dynamics and Informs Targeted Combination Therapy in Glioblastoma. *Cancer Cell* **2016**, *29*, 563–573. [CrossRef]
16. Cardoso, F.L.; Brites, D.; Brito, M.A. Looking at the blood-brain barrier: Molecular anatomy and possible investigation approaches. *Brain Res. Rev.* **2010**, *64*, 328–363. [CrossRef]
17. Griffith, J.I.; Rathi, S.; Zhang, W.; Zhang, W.; Drewes, L.R.; Sarkaria, J.N.; Elmquist, W.F. Addressing BBB Heterogeneity: A New Paradigm for Drug Delivery to Brain Tumors. *Pharmaceutics* **2020**, *12*, 1205. [CrossRef] [PubMed]
18. Kumar Yadav, S.; Kumar Srivastava, A.; Dev, A.; Kaundal, B.; Roy Choudhury, S.; Karmakar, S. Nanomelatonin triggers superior anticancer functionality in a human malignant glioblastoma cell line. *Nanotechnology* **2017**, *28*, 365102. [CrossRef] [PubMed]
19. Abbott, N.J.; Patabendige, A.A.; Dolman, D.E.; Yusof, S.R.; Begley, D.J. Structure and function of the blood-brain barrier. *Neurobiol. Dis.* **2010**, *37*, 13–25. [CrossRef]
20. van Tellingen, O.; Yetkin-Arik, B.; de Gooijer, M.C.; Wesseling, P.; Wurdinger, T.; de Vries, H.E. Overcoming the blood-brain tumor barrier for effective glioblastoma treatment. *Drug Resist. Updates* **2015**, *19*, 1–12. [CrossRef] [PubMed]
21. Fowler, M.J.; Cotter, J.D.; Knight, B.E.; Sevick-Muraca, E.M.; Sandberg, D.I.; Sirianni, R.W. Intrathecal drug delivery in the era of nanomedicine. *Adv. Drug Deliv Rev.* **2020**, *165–166*, 77–95. [CrossRef]
22. Gutenberg, A.; Bock, H.C.; Brück, W.; Doerner, L.; Mehdorn, H.M.; Roggendorf, W.; Westphal, M.; Felsberg, J.; Reifenberger, G.; Giese, A. MGMT promoter methylation status and prognosis of patients with primary or recurrent glioblastoma treated with carmustine wafers. *Br. J. Neurosurg.* **2013**, *27*, 772–778. [CrossRef] [PubMed]
23. Householder, K.T.; Dharmaraj, S.; Sandberg, D.I.; Wechsler-Reya, R.J.; Sirianni, R.W. Fate of nanoparticles in the central nervous system after intrathecal injection in healthy mice. *Sci. Rep.* **2019**, *9*, 12587. [CrossRef] [PubMed]
24. Kroll, R.A.; Neuwelt, E.A. Outwitting the blood-brain barrier for therapeutic purposes: Osmotic opening and other means. *Neurosurgery* **1998**, *42*, 1083–1099; discussion 1099–1100. [CrossRef] [PubMed]
25. Marcucci, F.; Corti, A.; Ferreri, A.J.M. Breaching the Blood-Brain Tumor Barrier for Tumor Therapy. *Cancers* **2021**, *13*, 2391. [CrossRef] [PubMed]
26. Niwińska, A.; Rudnicka, H.; Murawska, M. Breast cancer leptomeningeal metastasis: The results of combined treatment and the comparison of methotrexate and liposomal cytarabine as intra-cerebrospinal fluid chemotherapy. *Clin. Breast Cancer* **2015**, *15*, 66–72. [CrossRef]

27. Wait, S.D.; Prabhu, R.S.; Burri, S.H.; Atkins, T.G.; Asher, A.L. Polymeric drug delivery for the treatment of glioblastoma. *Neuro Oncol.* **2015**, *17* (Suppl. 2), ii9–ii23. [CrossRef]
28. Bobo, R.H.; Laske, D.W.; Akbasak, A.; Morrison, P.F.; Dedrick, R.L.; Oldfield, E.H. Convection-enhanced delivery of macromolecules in the brain. *Proc. Natl. Acad. Sci. USA* **1994**, *91*, 2076–2080. [CrossRef]
29. Lonser, R.R.; Sarntinoranont, M.; Morrison, P.F.; Oldfield, E.H. Convection-enhanced delivery to the central nervous system. *J. Neurosurg.* **2015**, *122*, 697–706. [CrossRef]
30. Kunigelis, K.E.; Vogelbaum, M.A. Therapeutic Delivery to Central Nervous System. *Neurosurg. Clin. N. Am.* **2021**, *32*, 291–303. [CrossRef]
31. Huang, R.; Boltze, J.; Li, S. Strategies for Improved Intra-arterial Treatments Targeting Brain Tumors: A Systematic Review. *Front. Oncol.* **2020**, *10*, 1443. [CrossRef]
32. Sheikov, N.; McDannold, N.; Sharma, S.; Hynynen, K. Effect of focused ultrasound applied with an ultrasound contrast agent on the tight junctional integrity of the brain microvascular endothelium. *Ultrasound Med. Biol* **2008**, *34*, 1093–1104. [CrossRef] [PubMed]
33. Bellavance, M.A.; Blanchette, M.; Fortin, D. Recent advances in blood-brain barrier disruption as a CNS delivery strategy. *AAPS J.* **2008**, *10*, 166–177. [CrossRef]
34. Doolittle, N.D.; Miner, M.E.; Hall, W.A.; Siegal, T.; Jerome, E.; Osztie, E.; McAllister, L.D.; Bubalo, J.S.; Kraemer, D.F.; Fortin, D.; et al. Safety and efficacy of a multicenter study using intraarterial chemotherapy in conjunction with osmotic opening of the blood-brain barrier for the treatment of patients with malignant brain tumors. *Cancer* **2000**, *88*, 637–647. [CrossRef]
35. Boockvar, J.A.; Tsiouris, A.J.; Hofstetter, C.P.; Kovanlikaya, I.; Fralin, S.; Kesavabhotla, K.; Seedial, S.M.; Pannullo, S.C.; Schwartz, T.H.; Stieg, P.; et al. Safety and maximum tolerated dose of superselective intraarterial cerebral infusion of bevacizumab after osmotic blood-brain barrier disruption for recurrent malignant glioma. Clinical article. *J. Neurosurg.* **2011**, *114*, 624–632. [CrossRef] [PubMed]
36. Riina, H.A.; Knopman, J.; Greenfield, J.P.; Fralin, S.; Gobin, Y.P.; Tsiouris, A.J.; Souweidane, M.M.; Boockvar, J.A. Balloon-assisted superselective intra-arterial cerebral infusion of bevacizumab for malignant brainstem glioma. A technical note. *Interv. Neuroradiol.* **2010**, *16*, 71–76. [CrossRef] [PubMed]
37. Chakraborty, S.; Filippi, C.G.; Wong, T.; Ray, A.; Fralin, S.; Tsiouris, A.J.; Praminick, B.; Demopoulos, A.; McCrea, H.J.; Bodhinayake, I.; et al. Superselective intraarterial cerebral infusion of cetuximab after osmotic blood/brain barrier disruption for recurrent malignant glioma: Phase I study. *J. Neurooncol.* **2016**, *128*, 405–415. [CrossRef]
38. Hochberg, F.H.; Pruitt, A.A.; Beck, D.O.; DeBrun, G.; Davis, K. The rationale and methodology for intra-arterial chemotherapy with BCNU as treatment for glioblastoma. *J. Neurosurg.* **1985**, *63*, 876–880. [CrossRef]
39. Ashby, L.S.; Shapiro, W.R. Intra-arterial cisplatin plus oral etoposide for the treatment of recurrent malignant glioma: A phase II study. *J. Neurooncol.* **2001**, *51*, 67–86. [CrossRef]
40. Mortimer, J.E.; Crowley, J.; Eyre, H.; Weiden, P.; Eltringham, J.; Stuckey, W.J. A phase II randomized study comparing sequential and combined intraarterial cisplatin and radiation therapy in primary brain tumors. A Southwest Oncology Group study. *Cancer* **1992**, *69*, 1220–1223. [CrossRef]
41. Imbesi, F.; Marchioni, E.; Benericetti, E.; Zappoli, F.; Galli, A.; Corato, M.; Ceroni, M. A randomized phase III study: Comparison between intravenous and intraarterial ACNU administration in newly diagnosed primary glioblastomas. *Anticancer Res.* **2006**, *26*, 553–558. [PubMed]
42. Stewart, D.J.; Belanger, J.M.; Grahovac, Z.; Curuvija, S.; Gionet, L.R.; Aitken, S.E.; Hugenholtz, H.; Benoit, B.G.; DaSilva, V.F. Phase I study of intracarotid administration of carboplatin. *Neurosurgery* **1992**, *30*, 512–516; discussion 516–517. [CrossRef]
43. Theodotou, C.; Shah, A.H.; Hayes, S.; Bregy, A.; Johnson, J.N.; Aziz-Sultan, M.A.; Komotar, R.J. The role of intra-arterial chemotherapy as an adjuvant treatment for glioblastoma. *Br. J. Neurosurg.* **2014**, *28*, 438–446. [CrossRef]
44. Falagas, M.E.; Pitsouni, E.I.; Malietzis, G.A.; Pappas, G. Comparison of PubMed, Scopus, Web of Science, and Google Scholar: Strengths and weaknesses. *FASEB J.* **2008**, *22*, 338–342. [CrossRef]
45. Pfiffner, P.B.; Oh, J.; Miller, T.A.; Mandl, K.D. ClinicalTrials.gov as a data source for semi-automated point-of-care trial eligibility screening. *PLoS ONE* **2014**, *9*, e111055. [CrossRef] [PubMed]
46. Huser, V.; Cimino, J.J. Linking ClinicalTrials.gov and PubMed to track results of interventional human clinical trials. *PLoS ONE* **2013**, *8*, e68409. [CrossRef] [PubMed]
47. Lim, K.J.; Yoon, D.Y.; Yun, E.J.; Seo, Y.L.; Baek, S.; Gu, D.H.; Yoon, S.J.; Han, A.; Ku, Y.J.; Kim, S.S. Characteristics and trends of radiology research: A survey of original articles published in AJR and Radiology between 2001 and 2010. *Radiology* **2012**, *264*, 796–802. [CrossRef]
48. McKinney, W. Data Structures for Statistical Computing in Python. In Proceedings of the 9th Python in Science Conference, Austin, TX, USA, 28 June–3 July 2010; Volume 445, pp. 56–61. [CrossRef]
49. Hochberg, F.H.; Miller, D.C. Primary central nervous system lymphoma. *J. Neurosurg.* **1988**, *68*, 835–853. [CrossRef]
50. Matsukado, K.; Inamura, T.; Nakano, S.; Fukui, M.; Bartus, R.T.; Black, K.L. Enhanced tumor uptake of carboplatin and survival in glioma-bearing rats by intracarotid infusion of bradykinin analog, RMP-7. *Neurosurgery* **1996**, *39*, 125–133; discussion 133–124. [CrossRef]

51. Angelov, L.; Doolittle, N.D.; Kraemer, D.F.; Siegal, T.; Barnett, G.H.; Peereboom, D.M.; Stevens, G.; McGregor, J.; Jahnke, K.; Lacy, C.A.; et al. Blood-brain barrier disruption and intra-arterial methotrexate-based therapy for newly diagnosed primary CNS lymphoma: A multi-institutional experience. *J. Clin. Oncol.* **2009**, *27*, 3503–3509. [CrossRef]
52. Liu, S.K.; Jakowatz, J.G.; Pollack, R.B.; Ceraldi, C.; Yamamoto, R.; Dett, C.; Lopez, F.; Camacho, C.; Carson, W.E.; Sentovich, S.M.; et al. Effects of intracarotid and intravenous infusion of human TNF and LT on established intracerebral rat gliomas. *Lymphokine Cytokine Res.* **1991**, *10*, 189–194.
53. Mao, J.; Cao, M.; Zhang, F.; Zhang, J.; Duan, X.; Lu, L.; Yang, Z.; Zhang, X.; Zhu, W.; Zhang, Q.; et al. Peritumoral administration of IFNβ upregulated mesenchymal stem cells inhibits tumor growth in an orthotopic, immunocompetent rat glioma model. *J. Immunother Cancer* **2020**, *8*, e000164. [CrossRef]
54. Aoki, S.; Terada, H.; Kosuda, S.; Shitara, N.; Fujii, H.; Suzuki, K.; Kutsukake, Y.; Tanaka, J.; Sasaki, Y.; Okubo, T.; et al. Supraophthalmic chemotherapy with long tapered catheter: Distribution evaluated with intraarterial and intravenous Tc-99m HMPAO. *Radiology* **1993**, *188*, 347–350. [CrossRef] [PubMed]
55. Dahlborg, S.A.; Petrillo, A.; Crossen, J.R.; Roman-Goldstein, S.; Doolittle, N.D.; Fuller, K.H.; Neuwelt, E.A. The potential for complete and durable response in nonglial primary brain tumors in children and young adults with enhanced chemotherapy delivery. *Cancer J. Sci. Am.* **1998**, *4*, 110–124. [PubMed]
56. Roman-Goldstein, S.; Mitchell, P.; Crossen, J.R.; Williams, P.C.; Tindall, A.; Neuwelt, E.A. MR and cognitive testing of patients undergoing osmotic blood-brain barrier disruption with intraarterial chemotherapy. *Am. J. Neuroradiol.* **1995**, *16*, 543–553.
57. Uluc, K.; Siler, D.A.; Lopez, R.; Varallyay, C.; Netto, J.P.; Firkins, J.; Lacy, C.; Huddleston, A.; Ambady, P.; Neuwelt, E.A. Long-Term Outcomes of Intra-Arterial Chemotherapy for Progressive or Unresectable Pilocytic Astrocytomas: Case Studies. *Neurosurgery* **2021**, *88*, E336–E342. [CrossRef]
58. Muldoon, L.L.; Pagel, M.A.; Netto, J.P.; Neuwelt, E.A. Intra-arterial administration improves temozolomide delivery and efficacy in a model of intracerebral metastasis, but has unexpected brain toxicity. *J. Neurooncol.* **2016**, *126*, 447–454. [CrossRef]
59. Osztie, E.; Várallyay, P.; Doolittle, N.D.; Lacy, C.; Jones, G.; Nickolson, H.S.; Neuwelt, E.A. Combined intraarterial carboplatin, intraarterial etoposide phosphate, and IV Cytoxan chemotherapy for progressive optic-hypothalamic gliomas in young children. *Am. J. Neuroradiol.* **2001**, *22*, 818–823. [PubMed]
60. Doolittle, N.D.; Muldoon, L.L.; Brummett, R.E.; Tyson, R.M.; Lacy, C.; Bubalo, J.S.; Kraemer, D.F.; Heinrich, M.C.; Henry, J.A.; Neuwelt, E.A. Delayed sodium thiosulfate as an otoprotectant against carboplatin-induced hearing loss in patients with malignant brain tumors. *Clin. Cancer Res.* **2001**, *7*, 493–500.
61. Kulason, K.O.; Schneider, J.R.; Chakraborty, S.; Filippi, C.G.; Pramanik, B.; Wong, T.; Fralin, S.; Tan, K.; Ray, A.; Alter, R.A.; et al. Superselective intraarterial cerebral infusion of cetuximab with blood brain barrier disruption combined with Stupp Protocol for newly diagnosed glioblastoma. *J. Exp. Ther. Oncol.* **2018**, *12*, 223–229.
62. Shin, B.J.; Burkhardt, J.K.; Riina, H.A.; Boockvar, J.A. Superselective intra-arterial cerebral infusion of novel agents after blood-brain disruption for the treatment of recurrent glioblastoma multiforme: A technical case series. *Neurosurg. Clin. N. Am.* **2012**, *23*, 323–329. [CrossRef]
63. D'Amico, R.S.; Khatri, D.; Reichman, N.; Patel, N.V.; Wong, T.; Fralin, S.R.; Li, M.; Ellis, J.A.; Ortiz, R.; Langer, D.J.; et al. Super selective intra-arterial cerebral infusion of modern chemotherapeutics after blood-brain barrier disruption: Where are we now, and where we are going. *J. Neurooncol.* **2020**, *147*, 261–278. [CrossRef]
64. Riina, H.A.; Fraser, J.F.; Fralin, S.; Knopman, J.; Scheff, R.J.; Boockvar, J.A. Superselective intraarterial cerebral infusion of bevacizumab: A revival of interventional neuro-oncology for malignant glioma. *J. Exp. Ther. Oncol.* **2009**, *8*, 145–150.
65. Faltings, L.; Kulason, K.O.; Patel, N.V.; Wong, T.; Fralin, S.; Li, M.; Schneider, J.R.; Filippi, C.G.; Langer, D.J.; Ortiz, R.; et al. Rechallenging Recurrent Glioblastoma with Intra-Arterial Bevacizumab with Blood Brain-Barrier Disruption Results in Radiographic Response. *World Neurosurg.* **2019**, *131*, 234–241. [CrossRef] [PubMed]
66. Burkhardt, J.K.; Riina, H.A.; Shin, B.J.; Moliterno, J.A.; Hofstetter, C.P.; Boockvar, J.A. Intra-arterial chemotherapy for malignant gliomas: A critical analysis. *Interv. Neuroradiol.* **2011**, *17*, 286–295. [CrossRef]
67. Huashan Hospital. Cerebral Blood Perfusion Changes after General Anesthesia for Craniotomy. Available online: https://ClinicalTrials.gov/show/NCT01642147 (accessed on 3 August 2021).
68. OHSU Knight Cancer Institute; Oregon Health and Science University. Combination Chemotherapy With or Without Sodium Thiosulfate in Preventing Low Platelet Count While Treating Patients With Malignant Brain Tumors. Available online: https://ClinicalTrials.gov/show/NCT00075387 (accessed on 3 August 2021).
69. Ohio State University Comprehensive Cancer Center. Carboplatin and Temozolomide (Temodar) for Recurrent and Symptomatic Residual Brain Metastases. Available online: https://ClinicalTrials.gov/show/NCT00362817 (accessed on 3 August 2021).
70. Northwell Health; Feinstein Institute for Medical Research; Hofstra North Shore. Super-Selective Intraarterial Cerebral Infusion of Bevacizumab (Avastin) for Treatment of Vestibular Schwannoma. Available online: https://ClinicalTrials.gov/show/NCT01083966 (accessed on 3 August 2021).
71. Northwell Health; Feinstein Institute for Medical Research. Repeated Super-Selective Intraarterial Cerebral Infusion of Bevacizumab (Avastin) for Treatment of Newly Diagnosed GBM. Available online: https://ClinicalTrials.gov/show/NCT01811498 (accessed on 3 August 2021).
72. Northwell Health. Super-Selective Intra-arterial Repeated Infusion of Cetuximab for the Treatment of Newly Diagnosed Glioblastoma. Available online: https://ClinicalTrials.gov/show/NCT02861898 (accessed on 3 August 2021).

73. Northwell Health. Super Selective Intra-Arterial Repeated Infusion of Cetuximab (Erbitux) with Reirradiation for Treatment of Relapsed/Refractory GBM, AA, and AOA. Available online: https://ClinicalTrials.gov/show/NCT02800486 (accessed on 3 August 2021).
74. Northwell Health. Super-Selective Intraarterial Cerebral Infusion of Cetuximab (Erbitux) for Treatment of Relapsed/Refractory GBM and AA. Available online: https://ClinicalTrials.gov/show/NCT01238237 (accessed on 3 August 2021).
75. Northwell Health. Super-Selective Intra-Arterial Cerebral Infusion of Trastuzumab for the Treatment of Cerebral Metastases of HER2/Neu Positive Breast Cancer. Available online: https://ClinicalTrials.gov/show/NCT02571530 (accessed on 3 August 2021).
76. Northwell Health. Super-Selective Intraarterial Intracranial Infusion of Avastin (Bevacizumab). Available online: https://ClinicalTrials.gov/show/NCT00968240 (accessed on 3 August 2021).
77. Northwell Health; Feinstein Institute for Medical Research; Hofstra North Shore. Super-Selective Intraarterial Cerebral Infusion Of Temozolomide (Temodar) For Treatment Of Newly Diagnosed GBM And AA. Available online: https://ClinicalTrials.gov/show/NCT01180816 (accessed on 3 August 2021).
78. Northwell Health; Feinstein Institute for Medical Research. Repeated Super-Selective Intraarterial Cerebral Infusion of Bevacizumab (Avastin) for Treatment of Relapsed GBM and AA. Available online: https://ClinicalTrials.gov/show/NCT01269853 (accessed on 3 August 2021).
79. Northwell Health. Repeated Super-Selective Intraarterial Cerebral Infusion of Bevacizumab Plus Carboplatin For Treatment Of Relapsed/Refractory GBM And Anaplastic Astrocytoma. Available online: https://ClinicalTrials.gov/show/NCT01386710 (accessed on 3 August 2021).
80. OHSU Knight Cancer Institute; National Cancer Institute (NCI). Melphalan with BBBD in Treating Patients with Brain Malignancies. Available online: https://ClinicalTrials.gov/show/NCT00253721 (accessed on 3 August 2021).
81. OHSU Knight Cancer Institute; National Institute of Neurological Disorders and Stroke (NINDS); Oregon Health and Science University. Melphalan, Carboplatin, Mannitol, and Sodium Thiosulfate in Treating Patients With Recurrent or Progressive CNS Embryonal or Germ Cell Tumors. Available online: https://ClinicalTrials.gov/show/NCT00983398 (accessed on 3 August 2021).
82. Huazhong University of Science and Technology; Beijing Tiantan Hospital; Beijing Chao Yang Hospital; Beijing Friendship Hospital. ADV-TK Improves Outcome of Recurrent High-Grade Glioma. Available online: https://ClinicalTrials.gov/show/NCT00870181 (accessed on 3 August 2021).
83. Université de Sherbrooke. IA Carboplatin + Radiotherapy in Relapsing GBM. Available online: https://ClinicalTrials.gov/show/NCT03672721 (accessed on 3 August 2021).
84. Srinivasan, V.M.; Lang, F.F.; Chen, S.R.; Chen, M.M.; Gumin, J.; Johnson, J.; Burkhardt, J.K.; Kan, P. Advances in endovascular neuro-oncology: Endovascular selective intra-arterial (ESIA) infusion of targeted biologic therapy for brain tumors. *J. Neurointerv. Surg.* **2020**, *12*, 197–203. [CrossRef]
85. Klopp, C.T.; Alford, T.C.; Bateman, J.; Berry, G.N.; Winship, T. Fractionated intra-arterial cancer; chemotherapy with methyl bis amine hydrochloride; a preliminary report. *Ann. Surg* **1950**, *132*, 811–832. [CrossRef] [PubMed]
86. Sidney Kimmel Comprehensive Cancer Center at Johns Hopkins; Solving Kids' Cancer. Intra-Arterial Chemotherapy for the Treatment of Progressive Diffuse Intrinsic Pontine Gliomas (DIPG). Available online: https://ClinicalTrials.gov/show/NCT01688401 (accessed on 3 August 2021).
87. Louis, D.N.; Perry, A.; Wesseling, P.; Brat, D.J.; Cree, I.A.; Figarella-Branger, D.; Hawkins, C.; Ng, H.K.; Pfister, S.M.; Reifenberger, G.; et al. The 2021 WHO Classification of Tumors of the Central Nervous System: A summary. *Neuro Oncol.* **2021**, *23*, 1231–1251. [CrossRef]
88. Sharma, P.; Debinski, W. Receptor-Targeted Glial Brain Tumor Therapies. *Int J. Mol. Sci.* **2018**, *19*, 3326. [CrossRef] [PubMed]
89. Joshi, S.; Ellis, J.A.; Ornstein, E.; Bruce, J.N. Intraarterial drug delivery for glioblastoma mutiforme: Will the phoenix rise again? *J. Neurooncol.* **2015**, *124*, 333–343. [CrossRef] [PubMed]
90. Hsieh, C.H.; Chen, Y.F.; Chen, F.D.; Hwang, J.J.; Chen, J.C.; Liu, R.S.; Kai, J.J.; Chang, C.W.; Wang, H.E. Evaluation of pharmacokinetics of 4-borono-2-(18)F-fluoro-L-phenylalanine for boron neutron capture therapy in a glioma-bearing rat model with hyperosmolar blood-brain barrier disruption. *J. Nucl. Med.* **2005**, *46*, 1858–1865. [PubMed]
91. Yuan, F.; Salehi, H.A.; Boucher, Y.; Vasthare, U.S.; Tuma, R.F.; Jain, R.K. Vascular permeability and microcirculation of gliomas and mammary carcinomas transplanted in rat and mouse cranial windows. *Cancer Res.* **1994**, *54*, 4564–4568.
92. Neuwelt, E.A.; Barnett, P.A.; McCormick, C.I.; Remsen, L.G.; Kroll, R.A.; Sexton, G. Differential permeability of a human brain tumor xenograft in the nude rat: Impact of tumor size and method of administration on optimizing delivery of biologically diverse agents. *Clin. Cancer Res.* **1998**, *4*, 1549–1555.
93. Neuwelt, E.A.; Pagel, M.A.; Hasler, B.P.; Deloughery, T.G.; Muldoon, L.L. Therapeutic efficacy of aortic administration of N-acetylcysteine as a chemoprotectant against bone marrow toxicity after intracarotid administration of alkylators, with or without glutathione depletion in a rat model. *Cancer Res.* **2001**, *61*, 7868–7874.
94. Neuwelt, E.A.; Hill, S.A.; Frenkel, E.P.; Diehl, J.T.; Maravilla, K.R.; Vu, L.H.; Clark, W.K.; Rapoport, S.I.; Barnett, P.A.; Lewis, S.E.; et al. Osmotic blood-brain barrier disruption: Pharmacodynamic studies in dogs and a clinical phase I trial in patients with malignant brain tumors. *Cancer Treat. Rep.* **1981**, *65* (Suppl. 2), 39–43.
95. Rajappa, P.; Krass, J.; Riina, H.A.; Boockvar, J.A.; Greenfield, J.P. Super-selective basilar artery infusion of bevacizumab and cetuximab for multiply recurrent pediatric ependymoma. *Interv. Neuroradiol.* **2011**, *17*, 459–465. [CrossRef]

96. Perese, D.M.; Day, C.E.; Chardach, W.M. Chemotherapy of brain tumors by intra-arterial infusion. *J. Neurosurg.* **1962**, *19*, 215–219. [CrossRef]
97. Campanella, R.; Guarnaccia, L.; Caroli, M.; Zarino, B.; Carrabba, G.; La Verde, N.; Gaudino, C.; Rampini, A.; Luzzi, S.; Riboni, L.; et al. Personalized and translational approach for malignant brain tumors in the era of precision medicine: The strategic contribution of an experienced neurosurgery laboratory in a modern neurosurgery and neuro-oncology department. *J. Neurol. Sci.* **2020**, *417*, 117083. [CrossRef] [PubMed]
98. Rahman, M.; Parney, I. Journal of Neuro Oncology: Immunotherapy for brain tumors. *J. Neurooncol.* **2021**, *151*, 1. [CrossRef] [PubMed]
99. Luzzi, S.; Giotta Lucifero, A.; Brambilla, I.; Trabatti, C.; Mosconi, M.; Savasta, S.; Foiadelli, T. The impact of stem cells in neuro-oncology: Applications, evidence, limitations and challenges. *Acta Biomed.* **2020**, *91*, 51–60. [CrossRef]
100. Wen, P.Y.; Weller, M.; Lee, E.Q.; Alexander, B.M.; Barnholtz-Sloan, J.S.; Barthel, F.P.; Batchelor, T.T.; Bindra, R.S.; Chang, S.M.; Chiocca, E.A.; et al. Glioblastoma in adults: A Society for Neuro-Oncology (SNO) and European Society of Neuro-Oncology (EANO) consensus review on current management and future directions. *Neuro Oncol.* **2020**, *22*, 1073–1113. [CrossRef]
101. Bartus, R.T.; Elliott, P.; Hayward, N.; Dean, R.; McEwen, E.L.; Fisher, S.K. Permeability of the blood brain barrier by the bradykinin agonist, RMP-7: Evidence for a sensitive, auto-regulated, receptor-mediated system. *Immunopharmacology* **1996**, *33*, 270–278. [CrossRef]
102. Englander, Z.K.; Wei, H.J.; Pouliopoulos, A.N.; Bendau, E.; Upadhyayula, P.; Jan, C.I.; Spinazzi, E.F.; Yoh, N.; Tazhibi, M.; McQuillan, N.M.; et al. Focused ultrasound mediated blood-brain barrier opening is safe and feasible in a murine pontine glioma model. *Sci. Rep.* **2021**, *11*, 6521. [CrossRef]
103. Columbia University; Focused Ultrasound Foundation. Non-Invasive Focused Ultrasound (FUS) with Oral Panobinostat in Children with Progressive Diffuse Midline Glioma (DMG). Available online: https://clinicaltrials.gov/ct2/show/NCT04804709 (accessed on 30 October 2021).
104. Drapeau, A.; Fortin, D. Chemotherapy Delivery Strategies to the Central Nervous System: Neither Optional nor Superfluous. *Curr. Cancer Drug Targets* **2015**, *15*, 752–768. [CrossRef]
105. Charest, G.; Sanche, L.; Fortin, D.; Mathieu, D.; Paquette, B. Glioblastoma treatment: Bypassing the toxicity of platinum compounds by using liposomal formulation and increasing treatment efficiency with concomitant radiotherapy. *Int. J. Radiat. Oncol. Biol. Phys.* **2012**, *84*, 244–249. [CrossRef] [PubMed]
106. He, H.; David, A.; Chertok, B.; Cole, A.; Lee, K.; Zhang, J.; Wang, J.; Huang, Y.; Yang, V.C. Magnetic nanoparticles for tumor imaging and therapy: A so-called theranostic system. *Pharm. Res.* **2013**, *30*, 2445–2458. [CrossRef] [PubMed]
107. Joshi, S.; Singh-Moon, R.P.; Ellis, J.A.; Chaudhuri, D.B.; Wang, M.; Reif, R.; Bruce, J.N.; Bigio, I.J.; Straubinger, R.M. Cerebral hypoperfusion-assisted intra-arterial deposition of liposomes in normal and glioma-bearing rats. *Neurosurgery* **2015**, *76*, 92–100. [CrossRef]
108. Joshi, S.; Cooke, J.R.; Chan, D.K.; Ellis, J.A.; Hossain, S.S.; Singh-Moon, R.P.; Wang, M.; Bigio, I.J.; Bruce, J.N.; Straubinger, R.M. Liposome size and charge optimization for intraarterial delivery to gliomas. *Drug Deliv. Transl. Res.* **2016**, *6*, 225–233. [CrossRef] [PubMed]
109. Nguyen, J.; Cooke, J.R.N.; Ellis, J.A.; Deci, M.; Emala, C.W.; Bruce, J.N.; Bigio, I.J.; Straubinger, R.M.; Joshi, S. Cationizable lipid micelles as vehicles for intraarterial glioma treatment. *J. Neurooncol.* **2016**, *128*, 21–28. [CrossRef]
110. Nguyen, J.; Hossain, S.S.; Cooke, J.R.N.; Ellis, J.A.; Deci, M.B.; Emala, C.W.; Bruce, J.N.; Bigio, I.J.; Straubinger, R.M.; Joshi, S. Flow arrest intra-arterial delivery of small TAT-decorated and neutral micelles to gliomas. *J. Neurooncol.* **2017**, *133*, 77–85. [CrossRef]
111. Rainov, N.G.; Zimmer, C.; Chase, M.; Kramm, C.M.; Chiocca, E.A.; Weissleder, R.; Breakefield, X.O. Selective uptake of viral and monocrystalline particles delivered intra-arterially to experimental brain neoplasms. *Hum. Gene Ther.* **1995**, *6*, 1543–1552. [CrossRef]
112. McCrorie, P.; Vasey, C.E.; Smith, S.J.; Marlow, M.; Alexander, C.; Rahman, R. Biomedical engineering approaches to enhance therapeutic delivery for malignant glioma. *J. Control. Release* **2020**, *328*, 917–931. [CrossRef] [PubMed]
113. A Power, E.; Rechberger, J.S.; Lu, V.M.; Daniels, D.J. The emerging role of nanotechnology in pursuit of successful drug delivery to H3K27M diffuse midline gliomas. *Nanomedicine* **2021**, *16*. [CrossRef]
114. Zhao, M.; van Straten, D.; Broekman, M.L.D.; Préat, V.; Schiffelers, R.M. Nanocarrier-based drug combination therapy for glioblastoma. *Theranostics* **2020**, *10*, 1355–1372. [CrossRef] [PubMed]
115. Anselmo, A.C.; Mitragotri, S. Nanoparticles in the clinic: An update. *Bioeng. Transl. Med.* **2019**, *4*, e10143. [CrossRef] [PubMed]
116. Bredlau, A.L.; Dixit, S.; Chen, C.; Broome, A.M. Nanotechnology Applications for Diffuse Intrinsic Pontine Glioma. *Curr Neuropharmacol* **2017**, *15*, 104–115. [CrossRef]
117. El-Khouly, F.E.; van Vuurden, D.G.; Stroink, T.; Hulleman, E.; Kaspers, G.J.L.; Hendrikse, N.H.; Veldhuijzen van Zanten, S.E.M. Effective Drug Delivery in Diffuse Intrinsic Pontine Glioma: A Theoretical Model to Identify Potential Candidates. *Front. Oncol.* **2017**, *7*, 254. [CrossRef]
118. Brown, C.E.; Alizadeh, D.; Starr, R.; Weng, L.; Wagner, J.R.; Naranjo, A.; Ostberg, J.R.; Blanchard, M.S.; Kilpatrick, J.; Simpson, J.; et al. Regression of Glioblastoma after Chimeric Antigen Receptor T-Cell Therapy. *N. Engl. J. Med.* **2016**, *375*, 2561–2569. [CrossRef]

119. Donovan, L.K.; Delaidelli, A.; Joseph, S.K.; Bielamowicz, K.; Fousek, K.; Holgado, B.L.; Manno, A.; Srikanthan, D.; Gad, A.Z.; Van Ommeren, R.; et al. Locoregional delivery of CAR T cells to the cerebrospinal fluid for treatment of metastatic medulloblastoma and ependymoma. *Nat. Med.* **2020**, *26*, 720–731. [CrossRef]
120. Mount, C.W.; Majzner, R.G.; Sundaresh, S.; Arnold, E.P.; Kadapakkam, M.; Haile, S.; Labanieh, L.; Hulleman, E.; Woo, P.J.; Rietberg, S.P.; et al. Potent antitumor efficacy of anti-GD2 CAR T cells in H3-K27M(+) diffuse midline gliomas. *Nat. Med.* **2018**, *24*, 572–579. [CrossRef] [PubMed]
121. Theruvath, J.; Sotillo, E.; Mount, C.W.; Graef, C.M.; Delaidelli, A.; Heitzeneder, S.; Labanieh, L.; Dhingra, S.; Leruste, A.; Majzner, R.G.; et al. Locoregionally administered B7-H3-targeted CAR T cells for treatment of atypical teratoid/rhabdoid tumors. *Nat. Med.* **2020**, *26*, 712–719. [CrossRef]
122. Vora, P.; Venugopal, C.; Salim, S.K.; Tatari, N.; Bakhshinyan, D.; Singh, M.; Seyfrid, M.; Upreti, D.; Rentas, S.; Wong, N.; et al. The Rational Development of CD133-Targeting Immunotherapies for Glioblastoma. *Cell Stem Cell* **2020**, *26*, 832–844.e836. [CrossRef] [PubMed]
123. Ingegnere, T.; Mariotti, F.R.; Pelosi, A.; Quintarelli, C.; De Angelis, B.; Tumino, N.; Besi, F.; Cantoni, C.; Locatelli, F.; Vacca, P.; et al. Human CAR NK Cells: A New Non-viral Method Allowing High Efficient Transfection and Strong Tumor Cell Killing. *Front. Immunol.* **2019**, *10*, 957. [CrossRef]
124. Kennis, B.A.; Michel, K.A.; Brugmann, W.B.; Laureano, A.; Tao, R.H.; Somanchi, S.S.; Einstein, S.A.; Bravo-Alegria, J.B.; Maegawa, S.; Wahba, A.; et al. Monitoring of intracerebellarly-administered natural killer cells with fluorine-19 MRI. *J. Neurooncol.* **2019**, *142*, 395–407. [CrossRef] [PubMed]
125. Oh, S.; Lee, J.H.; Kwack, K.; Choi, S.W. Natural Killer Cell Therapy: A New Treatment Paradigm for Solid Tumors. *Cancers* **2019**, *11*, 1534. [CrossRef] [PubMed]
126. City of Hope Medical Center; National Cancer Institute (NCI); Food and Drug Administration (FDA). Genetically Modified T-cells in Treating Patients with Recurrent or Refractory Malignant Glioma. Available online: https://ClinicalTrials.gov/show/NCT02208362 (accessed on 30 October 2021).
127. Hanahan, D.; Weinberg, R.A. Hallmarks of cancer: The next generation. *Cell* **2011**, *144*, 646–674. [CrossRef]
128. Occhiogrosso, G.; Edgar, M.A.; Sandberg, D.I.; Souweidane, M.M. Prolonged convection-enhanced delivery into the rat brainstem. *Neurosurgery* **2003**, *52*, 388–393; discussion 393–384. [CrossRef]
129. Rechberger, J.S.; Power, E.A.; Lu, V.M.; Zhang, L.; Sarkaria, J.N.; Daniels, D.J. Evaluating infusate parameters for direct drug delivery to the brainstem: A comparative study of convection-enhanced delivery versus osmotic pump delivery. *Neurosurg. Focus* **2020**, *48*, E2. [CrossRef] [PubMed]
130. Therapeutics, Y.-M.; Labcorp Drug Development; Invicro. 131I-Omburtamab Delivered by Convection-Enhanced Delivery in Patients with Diffuse Intrinsic Pontine Glioma. Available online: https://ClinicalTrials.gov/show/NCT05063357 (accessed on 30 October 2021).
131. OncoSynergy, Inc.; Infuseon Therapeutics, Inc. Convection-Enhanced Delivery of OS2966 for Patients with High-grade Glioma Undergoing a Surgical Resection. Available online: https://ClinicalTrials.gov/show/NCT04608812 (accessed on 30 October 2021).
132. Istari Oncology, Inc. EAP for the Treatment of Glioblastoma with PVSRIPO. Available online: https://ClinicalTrials.gov/show/NCT04599647 (accessed on 30 October 2021).
133. Bigner, D.; Rockefeller University. Phase 1 Trial of D2C7-IT in Combination with 2141-V11 for Recurrent Malignant Glioma. Available online: https://ClinicalTrials.gov/show/NCT04547777 (accessed on 30 October 2021).
134. Istari Oncology, I. LUMINOS-101: PVSRIPO and Pembrolizumab in Patients with Recurrent Glioblastoma. Available online: https://ClinicalTrials.gov/show/NCT04479241 (accessed on 30 October 2021).
135. Zacharoulis, S.; Columbia University. CED of MTX110 Newly Diagnosed Diffuse Midline Gliomas. Available online: https://ClinicalTrials.gov/show/NCT04264143 (accessed on 30 October 2021).
136. Bigner, D.; Istari Oncology, Inc.; National Cancer Institute (NCI); Genentech, Inc. D2C7-IT with Atezolizumab for Recurrent Gliomas. Available online: https://ClinicalTrials.gov/show/NCT04160494 (accessed on 30 October 2021).
137. Therapeutics, P.; National Cancer Institute (NCI). Maximum Tolerated Dose, Safety, and Efficacy of Rhenium Nanoliposomes in Recurrent Glioma (ReSPECT). Available online: https://ClinicalTrials.gov/show/NCT01906385 (accessed on 30 October 2021).
138. Therapeutics, Y.-M.; Memorial Sloan Kettering Cancer Center. Convection-Enhanced Delivery of 124I-Omburtamab for Patients with Non-Progressive Diffuse Pontine Gliomas Previously Treated with External Beam Radiation Therapy. Available online: https://ClinicalTrials.gov/show/NCT01502917 (accessed on 30 October 2021).
139. Kunwar, S.; Chang, S.; Westphal, M.; Vogelbaum, M.; Sampson, J.; Barnett, G.; Shaffrey, M.; Ram, Z.; Piepmeier, J.; Prados, M.; et al. Phase III randomized trial of CED of IL13-PE38QQR vs Gliadel wafers for recurrent glioblastoma. *Neuro Oncol.* **2010**, *12*, 871–881. [CrossRef]
140. D'Amico, R.S.; Aghi, M.K.; Vogelbaum, M.A.; Bruce, J.N. Convection-enhanced drug delivery for glioblastoma: A review. *J. Neurooncol.* **2021**, *151*, 415–427. [CrossRef] [PubMed]
141. Rechberger, J.S.; Lu, V.M.; Zhang, L.; Power, E.A.; Daniels, D.J. Clinical trials for diffuse intrinsic pontine glioma: The current state of affairs. *Childs Nerv. Syst.* **2020**, *36*, 39–46. [CrossRef] [PubMed]
142. Singleton, W.G.B.; Bienemann, A.S.; Woolley, M.; Johnson, D.; Lewis, O.; Wyatt, M.J.; Damment, S.J.P.; Boulter, L.J.; Killick-Cole, C.L.; Asby, D.J.; et al. The distribution, clearance, and brainstem toxicity of panobinostat administered by convection-enhanced delivery. *J. Neurosurg. Pediatr.* **2018**, *22*, 288–296. [CrossRef] [PubMed]

pharmaceutics

Systematic Review

Ultrasound-Mediated Blood–Brain Barrier Disruption for Drug Delivery: A Systematic Review of Protocols, Efficacy, and Safety Outcomes from Preclinical and Clinical Studies

Kushan Gandhi [1,2], Anita Barzegar-Fallah [1,2], Ashik Banstola [1,2], Shakila B. Rizwan [2,3] and John N. J. Reynolds [1,2,*]

[1] Department of Anatomy, School of Biomedical Sciences, University of Otago, Dunedin 9016, New Zealand; ganku455@student.otago.ac.nz (K.G.); anita.fallah@postgrad.otago.ac.nz (A.B.-F.); ashik.banstola@otago.ac.nz (A.B.)
[2] Brain Health Research Centre, University of Otago, Dunedin 9016, New Zealand; shakila.rizwan@otago.ac.nz
[3] School of Pharmacy, University of Otago, Dunedin 9016, New Zealand
* Correspondence: john.reynolds@otago.ac.nz; Tel.: +64-3479-5781; Fax: +64-3479-7254

Abstract: Ultrasound-mediated blood–brain barrier (BBB) disruption has garnered focus as a method of delivering normally impenetrable drugs into the brain. Numerous studies have investigated this approach, and a diverse set of ultrasound parameters appear to influence the efficacy and safety of this approach. An understanding of these findings is essential for safe and reproducible BBB disruption, as well as in identifying the limitations and gaps for further advancement of this drug delivery approach. We aimed to collate and summarise protocols and parameters for achieving ultrasound-mediated BBB disruption in animal and clinical studies, as well as the efficacy and safety methods and outcomes associated with each. A systematic search of electronic databases helped in identifying relevant, included studies. Reference lists of included studies were further screened to identify supplemental studies for inclusion. In total, 107 articles were included in this review, and the following parameters were identified as influencing efficacy and safety outcomes: microbubbles, transducer frequency, peak-negative pressure, pulse characteristics, and the dosing of ultrasound applications. Current protocols and parameters achieving ultrasound-mediated BBB disruption, as well as their associated efficacy and safety outcomes, are identified and summarised. Greater standardisation of protocols and parameters in future preclinical and clinical studies is required to inform robust clinical translation.

Keywords: focused ultrasound; blood–brain barrier opening; therapeutic agent delivery; ultrasound parameters; ultrasound safety; review

Citation: Gandhi, K.; Barzegar-Fallah, A.; Banstola, A.; Rizwan, S.B.; Reynolds, J.N.J. Ultrasound-Mediated Blood–Brain Barrier Disruption for Drug Delivery: A Systematic Review of Protocols, Efficacy, and Safety Outcomes from Preclinical and Clinical Studies. *Pharmaceutics* **2022**, *14*, 833. https://doi.org/10.3390/pharmaceutics14040833

Academic Editors: Jingyuan Wen and Yuan Huang

Received: 13 March 2022
Accepted: 6 April 2022
Published: 11 April 2022
Corrected: 20 December 2022

1. Introduction

1.1. The Blood–Brain Barrier and Drug Delivery

The blood–brain barrier (BBB) is a selectively permeable structure that restricts the passage of solutes from the brain's microvasculature into its extracellular space. Anatomically, the BBB is composed of the apical and basal membranes of the cerebrovascular endothelial cells (CECs), an associated basement membrane containing embedded pericytes, and perivascular foot-like processes of astrocytes ensheathing the abluminal capillary surface collectively referred to as the neurovascular unit [1] (see Figure 1). The CECs express a limited range of membrane carrier proteins and numerous membrane efflux pumps and have a dense number of tight junctions linking them to other CECs. This combined structural arrangement restricts the movement of most hydrophilic and high molecular weight molecules (exceeding 400 to 500 Da) [2], inflammatory cells, and pathogens, thereby providing a vital function in maintaining homeostasis and preventing the entry of harmful substances into the brain. The BBB, therefore, grants a significant survival advantage, but it also poses a disadvantage in its inability to allow most therapeutic agents to penetrate it, rendering 98% of small-molecule agents and 100% of large-molecule agents unable to enter the brain parenchyma [3]. As a result, there is a significant limitation to the pharmacological agents available in the treatment of central nervous system (CNS) conditions, including brain malignancies, dementias, and other neurodegenerative conditions.

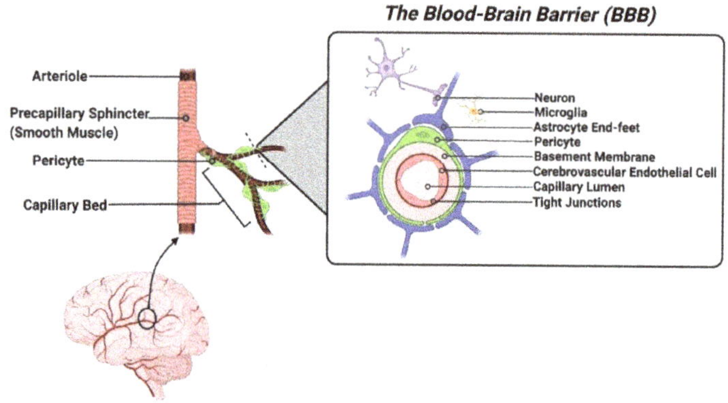

Figure 1. Schematic representation of the anatomical structure of the blood–brain barrier (BBB) and the accompanying neurovascular unit. Note the abluminal CEC surface is ensheathed by a basement membrane embedded with pericytes. (*Created with Biorender.com* (accessed on 12 March 2022)).

1.2. Ultrasound-Mediated Drug Delivery and the BBB

An approach to overcoming the challenge posed by the BBB is to temporarily induce BBB disruption, in a controlled and targeted manner, to enhance the uptake of therapeutic agents into desired target locations in the brain. A minimally invasive strategy that has been employed to achieve this is via the application of ultrasound. The use of transcranial ultrasound for enhancing drug delivery in the CNS also extends beyond BBB disruption, including in functioning as an external trigger to initiate drug release from nanoparticles [4] at targeted areas of the BBB in diseases such as epilepsy [5]. While the use of ultrasound in disrupting the BBB was first described in the 1950s [6], it is within the last 20 years [7] that this technique has garnered significant research interest in improving drug delivery to the brain. Subsequently, numerous preclinical animal studies, as well as several phase I/II clinical trials [8–11] (ClinicalTrials.gov identifier numbers: NCT03321487, NCT03322813, NCT02253212, NCT03608553, NCT03626896, NCT02343991, NCT02986932, NCT03712293), assessing the feasibility of this drug delivery approach have emerged. While the exact mechanisms underlying ultrasound-mediated BBB disruption are not yet well defined, the mechanical bioeffects of ultrasound exposure are thought to predominate. When exposed to ultrasound, dissolved gas bubbles within the vasculature experience a phenomenon known as cavitation, where they experience oscillatory changes in their volume, expanding in volume with rarefactions (low sonic pressure), and contracting with compressions (high sonic pressure) of the ultrasound waves [7]. Gas bubbles may also experience an acoustic radiation force, where they gain additional translational movement towards the direction of the ultrasound beam. These effects together are thought to contribute to the observed reduction in tight junction proteins between CECs of the BBB [12], the reduced expression of P-glycoprotein drug efflux pumps along the CEC membrane [13–15], and the increased formation of transcytotic vesicles across the CECs [16]. To enhance these mechanical effects ultrasound contrast agents or microbubbles (preformed gas-filled bubbles, typically of 1 to 6 μm in diameter) are co-administered, thereby increasing the number of available echogenic centres that can induce a mechanical effect within the cerebral vasculature, and thus reducing the threshold of ultrasound intensity required for BBB permeabilisation. Furthermore, magnetic resonance imaging (MRI) has been coupled with ultrasound and microbubbles, as a way of ensuring precise targeting [17] of the ultrasound beam to specific regions within the brain, confining drug penetration to these foci only, e.g., tumour sites for glioma patients.

1.3. Challenges with Ultrasound-Mediated BBB Disruption

Though numerous studies have achieved variable levels of successful ultrasound-mediated BBB disruption, it has become clear that the extent of BBB disruption is greatly influenced by the choice of ultrasound parameters, as well as the type and dose of microbubbles used alongside each sonication [18]. Unfortunately, ultrasound-mediated BBB disruption has potential adverse effects, including haemorrhagic change (ranging from sparse erythrocyte extravasation to gross intracerebral haemorrhaging) [19], oedema [9,20–26], inflammation [26,27], neuronal ischaemia [28,29], and tissue apoptosis [23,27,28,30–34]. The occurrence of these adverse effects is theorised to be due to excessive mechanical activity, where sonicated bubbles within the vasculature experience inertial, non-stable cavitation, rapidly imploding to exert excessive endothelial force, causing the extravasation of fluid, erythrocytes, and leucocytes into the surrounding tissue. Additionally, these effects may contribute to direct neuronal and glial injury. This has precipitated a large body of both preclinical and clinical studies demonstrating ultrasound-mediated BBB disruption with a range of sonication parameters, accompanied by a diverse set of reported safety outcomes. Ultimately, this has made selecting an appropriate sonication protocol that provides both successful and safe BBB disruption a difficult task. Previous narrative reviews of this body of evidence have been conducted but only broadly summarise key ultrasound-related parameters and their associated effects on the efficacy and safety of ultrasound-mediated BBB disruption. A systematic review of such literature and a published database of individual sonication paradigms and their consequential safety outcomes has yet to be conducted. The results of this systematic review will aim to inform future researchers of methods, sonication protocols, and the parameters that influence BBB disruption, as well as the safety outcomes associated with each, across a variety of experimental models (rodents, rabbits, sheep, pigs, non-human primates (NHPs)) and humans.

2. Materials and Methods

The systematic review was conducted according to the Preferred Reporting Items for Systematic Reviews and Meta-analyses (PRISMA) guidelines [35,36], PRISMA's checklist or PRISMA Flow Diagram for systematic reviews has been completed and is available as Table S1 in Supplementary Materials. This systematic review was not registered.

2.1. Eligibility Criteria

All studies with (i) clearly outlined sonication protocols (containing the relevant terms below), where (ii) ultrasound was applied to the brain of in vivo animal or human participants and where (iii) successful BBB disruption was achieved and confirmed using a reliable method, were included within this systematic review. Additionally, included studies had to have conducted appropriate safety assessments and reported any adverse effects associated with each protocol achieving successful BBB disruption. Only sonication protocols achieving confirmed BBB disruption, with corresponding safety assessments, were included within the data collection process. Protocols where the primary aim was applying ultrasound for cellular, viral, or gene delivery; neuromodulation; stimulation; or tissue ablation were excluded. Studies not published in English and review papers were also excluded.

2.2. Information Sources

This systematic review was based on searches from the following online search databases: PubMed, Medline, and EMBASE. A complete search of databases was conducted on 22 September 2021 to include any subsequent articles published within this timeframe. Additional articles were identified from reviewing the reference lists of relevant articles identified via the initial database search, as well as via Google Scholar alerts from the date of the initial search. A complete search of databases was conducted by K.G.

2.3. *Search Strategy*

The following MeSH terms were used to identify relevant articles:

1. 'Ultrasound' OR 'focused ultrasound' OR 'MRI-guided ultrasound' OR 'MR-guided focused ultrasound';
2. 'Blood brain barrier' OR 'BBB';
3. 'Disruption' OR 'permeabilisation' OR 'permeabilization' OR 'opening';
4. 'Drug delivery'.

2.4. *Study Selection*

Citations identified from the searches of the three databases were collated into a combined EndNote (X9) library and were de-duplicated as per a published protocol [37]. All unique citations were then screened for inclusion according to the eligibility criteria. Citation screening was conducted by K.G. in the following sequence: initially by their titles, then by their abstracts, and finally by reviewing the entire text. K.G., A.B.-F., and A.B. independently identified additional studies from Google Scholar alerts and from reviewing the reference list of relevant articles identified via the database search.

2.5. *Data Items and Collection Process*

From each included study, the following data items were extracted: (1) species of in vivo subject; (2) type of ultrasound transducer used; (3) methods for assessing BBB disruption; (4) methods for assessing safety; (5) microbubbles used (type, dose, administration protocol); (6) sonication parameters (frequency, peak negative pressure in situ, continuous or pulsated delivery, sonication duration, number of sonications, interstimulus interval, number of independent sessions, intersession interval). The extracted data items were then tabulated (Table S2—Supplementary Materials). Additional summary tables regarding methods used to assess BBB disruption efficacy Table 1) and safety, as well as microbubble and ultrasound parameters influencing ultrasound-mediated BBB disruption are also included in this systematic review. K.G. conducted all data extraction and collection.

3. Results

3.1. *Included Studies*

A total of 1480 citations were identified after the initial literature search from the three databases (Figure 2). After de-duplication, 882 unique citations were identified and were subsequently screened, in order, by their title and abstract, and then by a full-text review of the remaining articles ($n = 100$). After completing the screening process, a total of 76 studies were identified and included for data extraction and synthesis. An additional 31 studies were identified and included from Google Scholar alerts and after screening reference lists of included studies. Ultimately, a total of 107 studies were eligible for inclusion in our qualitative comparison and analysis.

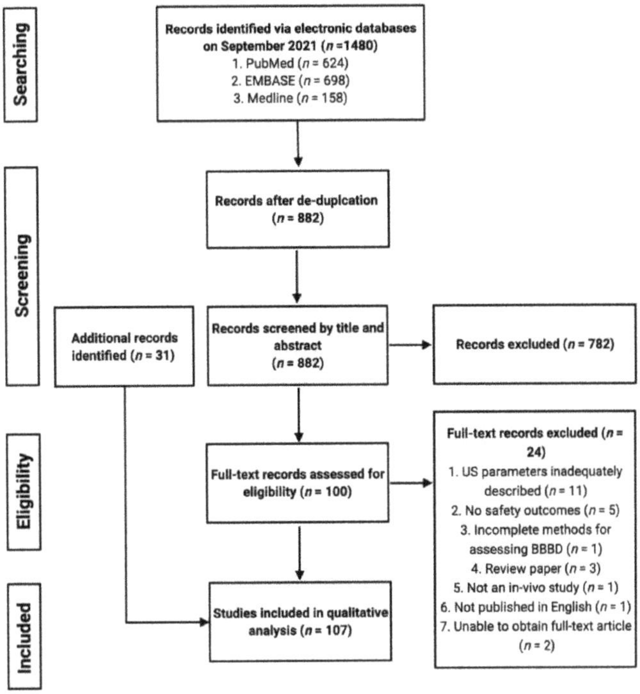

Figure 2. Flowchart highlighting the screening and selection process for studies included within this systematic review. (*Created with Biorender.com* (accessed on 12 March 2022)).

3.2. Ultrasound Devices

A range of commercial (e.g., FUS Instruments, Imasonic, Riverside Research Institute, Sonic Concepts) and in-house manufactured ultrasound devices were utilised in the included study protocols, with the majority of these being single-element or single piezoelectric devices. In recent times, multi-element devices have been developed to overcome associated concerns around ultrasound attenuation and beam defocussing, providing better transcranial transmission. These devices have been tested in preclinical animal models as well as in many ongoing and published clinical trials. In addition, we identified a protocol utilising two single-element transducers in tandem [38], and two that even used diagnostic [39,40], imaging transducers to disrupt the BBB. A comparative figure highlighting therapeutic ultrasound devices identified amongst included literature is shown in Figure 3.

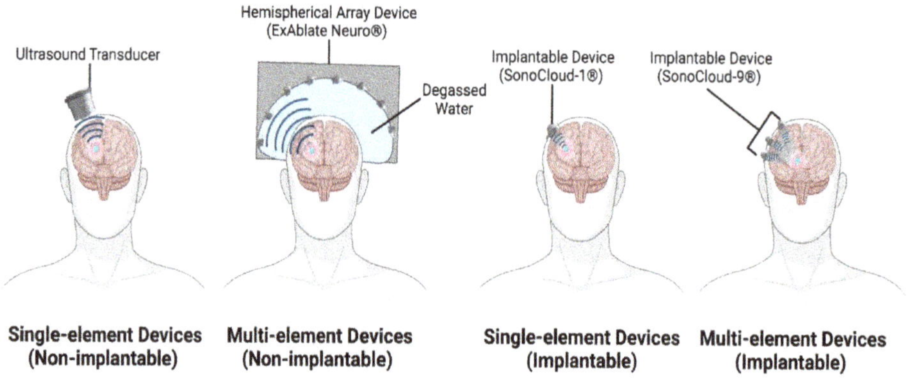

Figure 3. Comparison of therapeutic ultrasound devices used for BBB disruption. (*Created with Biorender.com* (accessed on 12 March 2022)).

3.2.1. Single-Element Ultrasound Devices

While single-element devices are smaller, and more accessible for testing in preclinical studies, their application in clinical studies has been more limited due to the attenuation and defocussing resulting from the application of a single ultrasound beam [41]. A strategy employed [9] to circumvent this issue has been to create a bony window in the calvaria and apply ultrasound directly through it, thereby reducing attenuation of the ultrasound beam at the bone interface [42]. Two animal studies directly compared this strategy with application through intact bone, with one highlighting no difference with the use of a 260 kHz transducer in rabbits [30] and the other highlighting significant improvements with the use of a 28 kHz transducer in pigs [23]. The SonoCloud-1®, a single-element device manufactured by CarThera, is one such example that requires implantation via a burr hole in the skull. Currently, this is the only implantable device we identified amongst all included protocols, and it has demonstrated efficacy in disrupting the BBB in both animal [20,43,44] and clinical studies [9]. Dual single-element transducers were employed in a couple of studies [38,45] to initiate BBB disruption using a lower frequency transducer, while a higher frequency transducer was employed in an attempt to stimulate the transport of a therapeutic agent into the brain parenchyma.

3.2.2. Multi-Element Ultrasound Devices

Multi-element array devices confer the benefit of being able to treat multiple, separate tissue foci simultaneously, as well as providing greater spatial coverage than single-element devices [46]. Additionally, multi-element phased array devices confer the ability to alter the phase and amplitude of individual transducers, correcting for aberrations to the ultrasound beam as it surpasses more complex skull surfaces, such as the human calvaria [46,47]. An emerging leader in this category of devices is the ExAblate® system (manufactured by InSightec), a 1024-element phased array device, initially designed for the thermal ablation of tissue, prior to being applied in rat [48,49], NHP [50], and clinical studies [8,10,11,51–53] to disrupt and open the BBB. The ExAblate® system functions with a large, stereotactically positioned helmet that is coupled to an MRI system to help plan sonication targets and monitor the procedure. A second multi-element phased array system—NaviFUS® (produced by NaviFUS corporation)—is a 256-element phased array device that has also demonstrated its ability to disrupt the BBB in a recent clinical trial [54]. While this device and the ExAblate® share similarities in their appearance, NaviFUS® does not require stereotactic positioning and relies on traditional, neurosurgical, navigation to help plan and guide ultrasound beams to sonication targets. The SonoCloud-9® (manufactured by CarThera) is an iteration of the SonoCloud-1® and functions as an implantable grid of nine interconnected transducer elements. As yet, no published study has employed the

SonoCloud-9® for in vivo BBB disruption, but ongoing clinical trials exist (NCT03744026, NCT04614493, NCT04528680).

3.2.3. Diagnostic Ultrasound Devices

Disruption of the BBB was also achieved using diagnostic ultrasound imaging devices in mice [39,40], albeit with much broader and less well-defined tissue coverage as compared to the prior mentioned therapeutic ultrasound devices. This is partly due to the higher central frequencies (2–10 MHz) that diagnostic devices tend to operate with, often resulting in greater aberration and defocussing of the penetrating ultrasound beam [39].

3.2.4. Implantable Ultrasound Devices

Nearly all identified ultrasound devices were non-implantable and usually required precise (e.g., stereotactic, neuronavigation, MRI-guided) positioning over the cranium of each subject prior to sonication. Implantable devices (SonoCloud® devices) are highly portable and eliminate the need for repeat repositioning, at the cost of requiring more invasive, surgical placement. Non-implantable devices have the advantage of being surgically non-invasive and can be repositioned for targeting multiple sites, at the cost of longer ultrasound sessions, during which subjects are not ambulatory [55]. A recent review [55] suggested that non-implantable, extracranial devices were not appropriate for targeting superficial lesions, a claim not supported by findings from identified protocols that achieved successful and safe BBB disruption in superficial cortical regions (e.g., primary motor cortex [8,56], primary visual cortex [24], prefrontal cortex [10,57]) using both single-element and multi-element phased array devices.

3.3. Methods for Assessing Successful BBB Disruption and Opening

3.3.1. MRI

The majority of identified protocols confirmed BBB disruption and its subsequent opening via contrast-enhanced T1-weighted MRI (CE-T1 MRI). The fundamentals of CE-T1 MRI involve taking T1 images prior to sonication, administering a gadolinium contrast agent, and then acquiring T1 images post-sonication. The molecular weight (~0.5 to 1.1 kDA) and hydrophilicity of gadolinium contrast agents make them incapable of passing the BBB in normal circumstances. Therefore, an opening in the BBB will result in visible extravasation of these agents into the cerebral interstitium, marked by hyperintensity on a post-sonication T1 image (see Figure 4). MRI quantification methods used in identified studies can be broadly summarised as follows: (1) T1 mapping to estimate the concentration and spatial distribution of the contrast agent [58,59]; (2) calculating vascular transfer coefficients of contrast agents after dynamic contrast-enhanced T1 imaging [60]; (3) or calculating changes in contrast signal enhancement [31]. The ability to observe BBB disruption in vivo is conferred by CE-T1 MRI, without requiring postmortem histological analysis. Multiple investigations have shown correlative relationships between the extravasation of the MRI contrast agent and that of histological tracers [61,62] and some therapeutic agents, including Herceptin [31], doxorubicin [63], and nanoparticles [23,38]. A few studies have employed the use of T2/T2* weighted MRI to track the uptake of superparamagnetic iron oxide (SPIO)-labelled drug molecules into sonicated brain parenchyma. This MRI technique provides a more sensitive method for assessing drug uptake by allowing the real-time, direct visualisation [23,64,65] of drug extravasation into the brain, as opposed to the use of a proxy marker (gadolinium contrast agent). Additionally, studies have used CE-T1 MRI to track the reversibility of BBB opening after sonication, unsurprisingly concluding that the duration of BBB opening, and thus the reversal time, increases with the initial degree of BBB disruption [66].

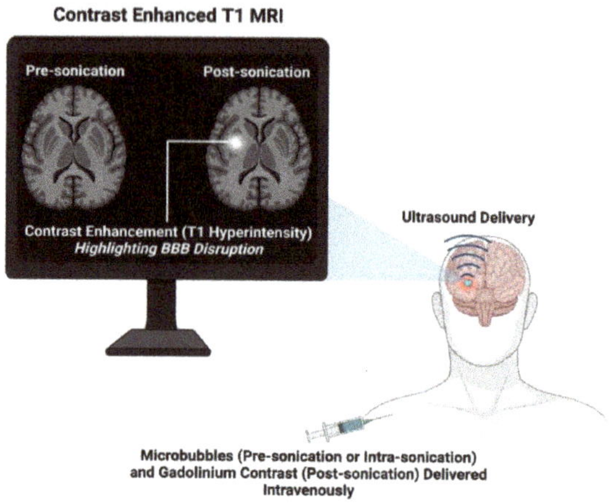

Figure 4. Representative cartoon highlighting the assessment and confirmation of ultrasound-mediated BBB disruption using CE-T1 MRI. (*Created with Biorender.com* (accessed on 12 March 2022)).

3.3.2. Tracer Molecules

Tracer molecules, including Evans/trypan blue (67 kDa when albumin-bound), fluorescein (333 Da), fluorescently labelled dextrans (3 to 2000 kDa), horseradish peroxidase (44 kDa), and antibodies (either endogenous or exogenously administered), are molecules incapable of surpassing the BBB and are widely administered to assess its opening. These molecules are readily available and cheap and can be observed macroscopically (Evans and trypan blue) or microscopically (fluorescein, dextrans, horseradish peroxidase), and their cerebral uptake can be quantified to confirm the degree of successful BBB opening. Additionally, tracer molecules come in various molecular weights, meaning their extravasation can better delineate the size of molecular weight therapeutics that could pass the disrupted BBB. Rodent studies [67,68] have highlighted differences in the extravasation of variable-sized dextrans after BBB opening with equivalent parameter sonications, where lower molecular weight dextrans (3 to 70 kDa) have significant extravasation, while higher (500 to 2000 kDa) weight dextrans have minimal extravasation. Therefore, the use of variable molecular weight tracer molecules gives an advantage over CE-T1 MRI, the latter of which only indicates BBB opening to a potential maximum threshold equal to the molecular weight of the injected gadolinium contrast agent. Due to the tissue analysis required for assessing tracer uptake, these methods are almost exclusively used in preclinical, animal studies and are harder to conduct in human trials due to the necessity of a brain biopsy. Interestingly, one clinical trial [51] did microscopically assess fluorescein uptake into resected, sonicated tumour/peritumoral tissue, reporting a 2.2-fold increase in comparison to non-sonicated tumour tissue.

3.3.3. Therapeutic Agent Quantification

Another approach in assessing BBB opening is to directly assess the cerebral uptake of normally impenetrable therapeutic agents, e.g., antibodies and chemotherapeutic agents. This has been done by quantifying the concentration of therapeutics from tissue homogenates via high powered liquid chromatography, liquid chromatography–mass spectrometry, or fluorometry or by labelling therapeutic molecules with fluorescent [38,69], radioactive, or magnetic markers [23] in order to more sensitively visualise the extent of tissue penetration and the location of therapeutic accumulation. Ultimately, this latter approach is the most direct method of ascertaining the clinical efficacy of ultrasound as a novel technique for enhancing therapeutic delivery to the brain. Only one [11] identified clinical trial reported any data on quantified therapeutic uptake after BBB disruption. More of these investigations are required to supplement concurrent CE-T1 MRI assessments in human trials to further validate the efficacy of this novel approach to drug delivery. Furthermore, the timing of drug administration relative to the application of ultrasound appears to influence drug uptake into the targeted brain region [70,71].

3.3.4. Comparing BBB Disruption between Studies

While a diverse range of reliably proven methods for assessing BBB opening exist, a standard protocol for conducting each does not, complicating the comparative analysis of successful BBB opening between studies. Of note amongst included studies was the variation in dose, administration time, and route of delivery of contrast agents, tracer dyes, exogenous antibodies, and/or therapeutic agents between studies. Investigations have noted significant variation in the extravasation of these agents as a response to altered administration times [37,66] relative to each sonication and to the route of chosen delivery [72] (e.g., intravenous vs. intraperitoneal). In addition, there exists a range of MRI parameters and quantification methods for the uptake of contrast and tracer agents utilised between studies, further complicating the ability to perform external comparisons between study protocols. As a result of the observed heterogeneity in specific BBB disruption assessment protocols, the 'Comparative Degree of Observed BBB Disruption' column (Table S2—Supplementary Materials) qualitatively highlights relative differences in BBB disruption achieved between different parameters investigated within the same study, as opposed to parameters between different studies. A comparison of methods used to assess BBB disruption across included protocols is presented in Table 1.

Table 1. Summary of the methods used by included protocols in assessing the extent of BBB disruption.

In Vivo Subject	Study and Year Published	Assessments of BBB Disruption and Opening							
		MRI	Tracer Molecules						Quantified Therapeutic Uptake
			EB	TB	Fl	FD	HRP	Antibodies	
Mouse	Baghirov et al., 2018 [38]	X							X (Polymeric nanoparticles)
	Baseri et al., 2010 [73]	X				X			
	Bing et al., 2009 [39]	X							
	Chen et al., 2013 [74]					X			
	Chen et al., 2014 [67]					X			
	Choi et al., 2010 [75]					X			
	Choi et al., 2011 [76]					X			
	Choi et al., 2011 [60]	X				X			
	Choi et al., 2008 [77]	X							
	Choi et al., 2010 [68]					X			
	Englander et al., 2021 [78]	X	X						X (Etoposide)
	Jordao et al., 2013 [61]	X						X (Anti-endogenous IgG and IgM)	
	Kinoshita et al., 2006 [31]	X		X					X (Herceptin)
	Kinoshita et al., 2006 [62]	X		X				X (Anti-D4 IgG)	
	Lapin et al., 2020 [79]	X							
	Liu et al., 2014 [80]	X	X						X (Temozolomide)
	McDannold et al., 2017 [81]	X							
	McMahon et al., 2020 [59]	X				X		X (Anti-albumin IgG)	
	Morse et al., 2022 [82]								X (Fluorescently labelled, unloaded liposomes)
	Morse et al., 2019 [83]					X		X (Anti-albumin IgG)	
	Olumolade et al., 2016 [84]	X							
	Omata et al., 2019 [85]		X			X			
	Raymond et al., 2007 [86]		X			X			
	Raymond et al., 2008 [87]	X	X	X				X (Anti-amyloid + anti-endogenous IgG)	
	Samiotaki et al., 2012 [66]	X							
	Shen et al., 2016 [69]		X						X (Fluorescently labelled, unloaded liposomes)
	Sierra et al., 2017 [88]	X			X				
	Vlachos et al., 2011 [72]	X							
	Wu et al., 2014 [89]								X (Liposomal doxorubicin)
	Zhang, D. et al., 2020 [43]			X					X (Paclitaxel—free and protein-bound)
	Zhao, B. et al., 2018 [40]		X						

Table 1. *Cont.*

In Vivo Subject	Study and Year Published	Assessments of BBB Disruption and Opening							
		MRI	Tracer Molecules						Quantified Therapeutic Uptake
			EB	TB	Fl	FD	HRP	Antibodies	
Rat	Ali et al., 2018 [90]	X	X						X (Doxorubicin)
	Aryal et al., 2017 [15]	X		X					
	Aryal et al., 2015 [91]	X		X					X (Doxorubicin)
	Aryal et al., 2015 [70]	X		X					X (Doxorubicin)
	Aslund et al., 2017 [92]	X							X (Pegylated macromolecule)
	Cho et al., 2016 [14]	X	X						
	Chopra et al., 2010 [93]	X							
	Fan et al., 2016 [64]	X							X (SPIO-labelled, doxorubicin-loaded microbubbles)
	Fan et al., 2014 [45]		X						X (Carmustine loaded microbubbles)
	Fan et al., 2015 [94]		X						X (Carmustine loaded microbubbles)
	Goutal et al., 2018 [95]	X	X						
	Han et al., 2021 [96]	X							
	Huh et al., 2020 [97]	X							
	Jung et al., 2019 [98]	X	X						X (Doxorubicin)
	Kobus et al., 2016 [99]	X							
	Kovacs et al., 2017 [27]	X						X (Anti-albumin IgG)	
	Kovacs et al., 2018 [100]	X							
	Liu et al., 2009 [65]	X	X						
	Liu et al., 2010 [101]	X	X						X (Carmustine)
	Liu et al., 2010 [102]		X						
	Liu et al., 2008 [32]	X	X						
	Liu et al., 2010 [103]	X							
	Marty et al., 2012 [58]	X							
	McDannold et al., 2019 [48]	X							X (Carboplatin)
	McDannold et al., 2020 [49]	X							X (Irinotecan and SN-38)
	McDannold et al., 2011 [104]	X		X					
	Mcmahon et al., 2017 [26]	X							
	Mcmahon et al., 2020 [105]	X	X						
	Mcmahon et al., 2020 [106]	X							
	O'Reilly et al., 2017 [107]	X							
	O'Reilly et al., 2011 [108]	X							
	Park et al., 2017 [109]	X		X					X (Doxorubicin)
	Park et al., 2012 [71]	X		X					X (Doxorubicin)
	Shin et al., 2018 [19]		X						
	Song et al., 2017 [110]		X						
	Treat et al., 2007 [63]	X	X						X (Doxorubicin)
	Tsai et al., 2018 [33]		X						
	Wei et al., 2013 [111]	X	X						X (Temozolomide)
	Wu et al., 2017 [112]	X	X						
	Yang et al., 2013 [113]	X	X						
	Yang et al., 2014 [114]	X	X						
	Yang et al., 2012 [34]	X	X						
	Yang et al., 2011 [115]	X	X						
	Yang et al., 2012 [116]	X	X						
	Zhang, Y. et al., 2016 [117]	X							
Rabbit	Beccaria et al., 2013 [20]	X	X						
	Chopra et al., 2010 [93]	X							
	Hynyen et al., 2005 [28]	X					X		
	Hynyen et al., 2006 [30]	X					X		
	McDannold et al., 2006 [118]	X							
	McDannold et al., 2007 [25]	X							
	McDannold et al., 2008 [119]	X							
	McDannold et al., 2008 [120]	X							
	Mei et al., 2009 [121]	X	X						X (Methotrexate)
	Wang et al., 2009 [122]	X	X						
Dog	O'Reilly et al., 2017 [123]	X							
Pig	Liu et al., 2011 [23]	X	X						X (SPIO nanoparticles)
Sheep	Pelekanos et al., 2018 [29]		X					X (Anti-endogenous IgG)	
Non-Human Primate (NHP)	Yoon et al., 2019 [124]	X							
	Arvantis et al., 2012 [50]	X							
	Downs et al., 2015 [21,22]	X							
	Goldwirt et al., 2016 [44]	X							X (Carboplatin)
	Horodyckid et al., 2017 [56]	X							
	Marquet et al., 2014 [125]	X							
	Marquet et al., 2011 [24]	X							
	McDannold et al., 2012 [126]	X		X					
	Pouliopoulos et al., 2019 [57]	X							
	Wu et al., 2016 [127]	X							

Table 1. *Cont.*

In Vivo Subject	Study and Year Published	Assessments of BBB Disruption and Opening							
		MRI	Tracer Molecules						Quantified Therapeutic Uptake
			EB	TB	Fl	FD	HRP	Antibodies	
Human	Abrahao et al., 2019 [8]	X							
	Anastasiadis et al., 2021 [51]	X			X				
	Chen et al., 2021 [54]	X							
	Gasca-Salas et al., 2021 [52]	X							
	Idbaidh et al., 2019 [9]	X							
	Lipsman et al., 2018 [10]	X							
	Mainprize et al., 2019 [11]	X							X (Liposomal doxorubicin and temozolomide)
	Park et al., 2020 [53]	X							

EB: Evans blue; TB: trypan blue; FL: fluorescein; FD: fluorescently labelled dextrans; HRP: horseradish peroxidase.

3.4. Methods of Assessing Safety Outcomes

The safety of ultrasound-mediated BBB disruption is crucial for this technology to receive mainstream clinical adoption in the treatment of CNS disease; thus, in this review, it was essential to only include ultrasound protocols with a corresponding safety assessment. The techniques employed by studies to analyse safety outcomes can be broadly characterised into five categories: macroscopic, histological, biochemical, electrophysiological, and behavioural safety assessments. Histological and macroscopic assessments have undoubtedly been the most extensively conducted techniques amongst included literature, as they highlight detailed changes in tissue architecture and can be readily conducted in preclinical animal studies. When comparing safety outcomes between studies employing different ultrasound protocols and parameters, the time of safety data acquisition is vital [17]. Studies have highlighted how MRI and histological adverse safety events may progress or regress with the time interval from sonication to MRI acquisition [32,71] or tissue extraction [59,88]. For this reason, we have included, when available, the timing of MRI or histological safety data acquisition from the last sonication, for each included protocol within this study (Table S2—Supplementary Materials). A detailed summary of specific safety investigations employed across included studies is presented in Table 2.

3.4.1. Macroscopic Assessments

MRI techniques, most commonly T2, T2*, and susceptibility-weighted imaging (SWI), have been employed to detect evidence of oedematous (hyperintensities on T2) [21,22] and haemorrhagic (hypointensities on T2* and SWI) [50] change within the sonicated brain. Currently, the clinical application of ultrasound-mediated BBB disruption has relied on MRI, serving as an assessment technique for confirming in vivo BBB opening (as previously discussed). It also provides the ability to observe changes in tissue health and to track the progression of any of these changes serially, for hours and days following sonication [10,21,22,80]. In clinical trials, ultrasound-mediated BBB disruption has been generally well tolerated, but MRI findings have also shown transient oedematous [8,9] and microhaemorrhagic change [10], observed in a small subset of patients only. A few rodent studies [27,103] also utilised T2* MRI to image the extravasation of superparamagnetic-labelled macrophages into the sonicated tissue when assessing for an inflammatory reaction to ultrasound-mediated BBB disruption. Thermometry is another macroscopic safety assessment identified amongst protocols, playing a role in the monitoring of unwanted thermogenic bioeffects from ultrasound application. Methods of thermometry included ex vivo calvaria thermometry [29], the use of in situ thermal probes [89,98], and real-time MR thermometry [8,10,52]. Generally, temperature elevations did not exceed 1.5 °C in most studies employing in vivo thermometry [8,10,52,98]. One study investigated the application of continuous ultrasound to induce a hyperthermic effect in mice, noting a temperature elevation of 13 °C over a 10 min period of sonication [89]. Positron emission tomography (PET) scanning has also been conducted in a handful of NHP and clinical studies, revealing no changes in glucose uptake and metabolism [52,56] in sonicated tissue following multiple ultrasound sessions. Direct visualisation (without imaging) of gross haemorrhage in brain tissue has been reported with significant BBB disruption in animal studies [19] after applying more intense (higher pressure) ultrasound or over prolonged sonication periods.

3.4.2. Histological Assessments

Basic histological stains, most notably haematoxylin and eosin, Cresyl violet/Luxol fast blue, and Perl's Prussian Blue, have been readily utilised to confirm microscopic changes to tissue architecture, haemorrhagic change, and iron deposition. Immunolabelling of specific proteins has allowed for the investigation of more specific histological changes associated with ultrasound-mediated BBB disruption, including potential reactive astrogliosis (glial fibrillary acid protein or GFAP), microglial activation (Iba-1), and neurogenesis (BrdU) macrophage (CD68+) and T lymphocyte (ICAM-1, CD-4, CD-8) infiltration. Additionally, immunolabelling of endothelial markers (RECA-1 and CD-31) has allowed for the screening of direct endothelial damage [14] and assessing tissue vascular density when comparing BBB opening between sonicated tumour and normal tissue [54]. Major reported histopathological findings include a continuum of haemorrhagic change within the brain parenchyma [19], oedema [9,20–26], neuronal ischaemia [28,29], tissue apoptosis [23,27,28,30–34], immune cell infiltration, and gliosis. Reported histopathological outcomes have been identified at a variety of endpoints, from immediately following [115] to months after initial sonication [123], highlighting both the potential acuteness and chronicity at which ultrasound-mediated BBB disruption may exert unwanted biological effects. Histopathological assessments generally reinforce pathological findings on MRI, but in some studies [62,92,93], they appear to highlight pathological change in the absence of any on MRI, despite equivalent timing of data acquisition, suggesting higher sensitivity for adverse pathological change.

3.4.3. Biochemical Assessments

Biochemical assessments, namely polymerase chain reaction, Western blotting and enzyme-linked immunosorbent assays, have been employed in a handful of rat investigations [26,27,100,105] to track changes in the expression of proinflammatory genes and proteins following ultrasound-mediated BBB disruption. Of note, these studies have shown an upregulation in the transcriptomic expression of proinflammatory genes related to the NF-kB [26,27] (e.g., Ccl2, Ilα, Ilβ, Selp, Tnf, Icam1) and AkT/GSKβ pathways [27] with larger doses of administered microbubbles. Furthermore, temporal changes in the proteomic expression of Iba1 (activated microglia) and GFAP (reactive astrocyte marker) have been described over a time course of 15 days [61]. Serum biochemical analysis was employed as a safety assessment in one study, which reported an increase in fibrinogen levels 8 days after sonication in animals exposed to the highest intensity ultrasound, likely attributable to the corresponding histological findings [33]. These findings have generated a link between ultrasound-mediated BBB disruption and subsequent proinflammatory changes, and further work is required in assessing the significance and potentially deleterious effect this may have on the health of the sonicated brain.

3.4.4. Electrophysiological Assessments

Electrophysiological investigations following ultrasound-mediated BBB disruption, including electroencephalography, electromyography, and somatosensory evoked potentials, have been occasionally used within the identified literature, appearing in two NHP [21,56] studies and a clinical trial [8]. One NHP study reported no abnormal electroencephalographic waveform changes, nor any to the somatosensory evoked potentials from the median or popliteal nerves, following repeated BBB disruption of the primary motor cortex over a 15-day period [56]. No differences in electromyographic signals from the temporalis muscle of NHPs following repeat BBB disruption of basal ganglia structures were noted in another investigation [21] either. In a clinical trial involving BBB disruption of the primary motor cortex in ALS patients, electroencephalographic readings also remained unchanged after repeat sonications [8]. Although reassuring, these data are generated from a very small sample size. Given the emerging role of ultrasound in the field of neuromodulation [128], it is surprising to see the relative lack of neuro-electrophysiological analyses conducted across current literature.

3.4.5. Physical and Behavioural Assessments

Physical and behavioural assessments have been employed to monitor safety outcomes following ultrasound-mediated BBB disruption in a range of experimental models, including in rodent, dog, NHP, and human studies. Adverse motor outcomes in rodents have been assessed via rotarod and pinch grip tests, as well as via gross motor observations, and outcomes have included periods of hypoactivity, tremor, and ataxia in rodents [33,84] that underwent higher intensity sonications. Conversely, glioma-implanted rodents sonicated with similar intensity ultrasound and lower microbubble doses have exhibited no changes in motor coordination or grip strength following ultrasound with lower intensity ultrasound [78,90]. Other reported motor outcomes include mildly altered reaction times in one NHP study [21] and reversible, mild upper-limb hemiplegia in another NHP study [24]. Physiological outcomes have been reported, including transient, microbubble-associated tachycardia [78] and tachypnoea [56] in some rat and NHP studies, but these do not appear to be corroborated by other preclinical [22] and clinical studies. Detailed neurological testing following sonication in aged canines has also been conducted, yielding no changes in neurological or mental status [123]. Additionally, long-term cognitive testing in NHPs [22] via reward-based reaction and visual dot motion tasks has been conducted, revealing no significant changes to cognitive decision-making abilities, but potentially eliciting a reduction in motivation. Overall, motor and behavioural changes following BBB disruption in preclinical models appear to be mild.

In clinical trials, physical findings most frequently included pain associated with setting up and stabilising the patient's head into the phased array transducer [8,10,11] or minimal irritation from connecting the implanted transducer to its electrical supply [9]. In one trial [9], a single patient experienced a transient facial palsy that occurred immediately following three separate sonications, resolving within two hours after steroid administration. Clinical trials have also incorporated neuropsychological assessments (e.g., Mini Mental State Exam, Montreal Cognitive Assessment) to assess potential alterations in cognition after BBB disruption in patients with Parkinson's disease dementia [52], Alzheimer's dementia [10], and ALS [8]. In summary, the occurrence of adverse physical and behavioural outcomes following ultrasound-mediated BBB disruption in humans has been infrequent and predominantly transient when present. Once again, these data are limited due to small patient sample sizes and the lack of sham or control groups. Additionally, significant patient neurological comorbidity in these trials makes it difficult to directly attribute adverse events to ultrasound-mediated BBB disruption.

Table 2. Summary of safety assessments conducted by included protocols.

In Vivo Subject	Study Reference	Safety Assessments															
		Macroscopic				Histological									Biochemical	Electrophysiological	Physical/ Behvaioural
		MRI	PET	ΔT	Gross	H/E	TUNEL	VF	LB	CV	PB	GFAP	Iba1	Other			
	[38]	X				X											
	[73]	X			X	X											
	[39]					X											
	[74]					X											
	[67]					X											
	[75]					X											
Mouse	[76]					X											
	[60]					X	X										
	[77]	X				X											
	[68]					X											
	[78]	X				X											X
	[61]											X	X	X	X (PCR + WB)		
	[31]				X	X	X	X									
	[62]				X	X											

Table 2. *Cont.*

In Vivo Subject	Study Reference	Safety Assessments															
		Macroscopic				Histological									Biochemical	Electrophysiological	Physical/ Behvaioural
		MRI	PET	ΔT	Gross	H/E	TUNEL	VF	LB	CV	PB	GFAP	Iba1	Other			
	[79]	X															
	[80]					X											
	[81]					X											
	[59]	X				X											
	[82]					X											
	[83]					X											
	[84]					X			X	X							X
	[85]					X								X			
	[86]				X	X								X			
	[87]					X											
	[66]					X											
	[69]					X											
	[88]	X				X							X				
	[72]	X				X											
Mouse	[89]			X	X		X										
	[43]					X											
	[40]					X								X			
	[90]					X								X			X
	[15]	X				X											
	[91]	X				X											
	[70]	X				X											
	[92]	X				X											
	[14]	X				X								X			
	[93]	X				X											
	[64]					X											
	[45]	X				X	X										
	[94]					X											
	[95]	X	X														
	[96]	X				X						X		X	X (AQP-4)		
	[97]					X											
	[98]	X		X		X											
	[99]	X				X						X					
	[27]					X	X					X	X	X	X (ELISA, PCR, WB)		
	[100]	X				X						X	X	X	X (WB)		
	[65]	X			X	X					X						
	[101]	X				X											
	[102]					X											
	[32]	X				X	X										
	[103]	X									X			X			
Rat	[58]	X															
	[48]	X				X			X								
	[49]	X				X											
	[104]				X	X											
	[26]	X				X									X (PCR)		
	[105]	X				X									X (PCR)		
	[106]	X										X		X	X (ELISA)		
	[107]	X				X											
	[108]	X				X											
	[109]	X				X											
	[71]	X				X											
	[19]				X	X											
	[110]				X									X			
	[63]				X	X											
	[33]					X	X					X			X (Plasma fibrinogen)		X
	[111]	X				X											
	[112]	X				X											
	[113]					X											
	[114]					X											
	[34]					X	X										
	[115]					X											
	[116]					X	X										
	[117]	X									X		X				
	[20]	X				X											
	[93]	X				X											
	[28]					X	X	X									
	[30]					X	X	X									
	[118]					X											
Rabbit	[25]	X				X											
	[119]					X											
	[120]					X											
	[121]					X											
	[122]				X												
Dog	[123]	X					X				X		X				X
Pig	[23]	X				X					X						
Sheep	[29]			X	X	X		X				X					
	[124]	X				X		X	X								
	[50]	X				X				X							
	[21,22]	X														X (EMG)	X
	[44]	X															
	[56]	X	X			X					X			X		X (EEG, SSEP)	X
NHP	[125]	X															
	[24]	X															X
	[126]	X				X	X		X	X							X
	[57]	X															
	[127]	X															
	[8]	X		X												X (EEG)	X
	[51]	X				X								X			X
	[54]	X												X			X
Human	[52]	X	X	X													X
	[9]	X															X
	[10]	X	X	X													X
	[11]	X															X
	[53]	X															X

***PET:** positron emission tomography; **ΔT:** thermometry; **H/E:** haematoxylin and eosin; **TUNEL:** terminal deoxynucleotidyl transferase dUTP nick end labelling; **VF:** vanadium acid fuchsin; **LB:** Luxol fast blue; **CV:** Cresyl violet; **PB:** Perl's Prussian blue; **Iba1:** ionized calcium-binding adaptor molecule 1; **GFAP:** glial fibrillary acidic protein; **PCR:** polymerase chain reaction; **WB:** Western blotting; **ELISA:** enzyme-linked immunosorbent assay; **EMG:** electromyogram; **EEG:** electroencephalography; **SSEP:** somatosensory evoked potentials*

3.5. Parameters Influencing Ultrasound-Mediated BBB Disruption

After an extensive review of all protocols identified amongst included studies, the following parameter domains have been frequently investigated to assess their influence on the efficacy and safety of ultrasound-mediated BBB disruption: microbubbles, transducer frequency, peak negative pressure (PNP), pulsed delivery parameters (see Figure 5), the duration of each sonication, and the dosing of ultrasound application. The transducer frequency defines the frequency of the generated ultrasound wave, and the PNP reflects the amplitude or intensity of the wave. Detailed parameters from each included study are listed in Table S2 (Supplementary Materials), and a summary of the influence of each parameter domain is listed in Tables 3 and 4.

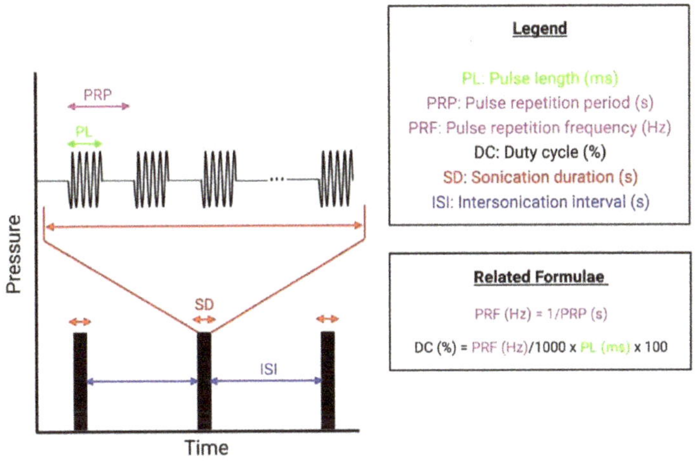

Figure 5. Overview of the pulsed delivery paradigm used for US delivery. (*Created with Biorender.com* (accessed on 12 March 2022)).

3.5.1. Microbubbles

Five major commercially available microbubble formulations—Definity®/Luminity®, Optison®, SonoVue®/Lumason®, Sonazoid®, and Usphere®—have been utilised in studies investigating ultrasound-mediated BBB disruption. For reference, a comparison of these microbubble formulations, as well as their frequency of use and typical dosing in included studies, is included in Table 3. In addition, a handful of studies used in-house microbubbles, some of which were drug-loaded [38,45,64,94], in an attempt to further potentiate localised mechanical effects to move therapeutics across the BBB. Studies have also demonstrated the potential of BBB disruption without microbubble administration [65,89]; however, this was accomplished with a significant thermogenic effect [89] or by using higher intensity ultrasound waves [65]. Direct comparisons of microbubble administration against no administration have shown significant improvements in BBB disruption when microbubbles are administered, at unifying parameters [90]. Without microbubbles, markedly higher PNP sonications are required to achieve equitable BBB disruption, at the cost of poorer safety outcomes [32,65]. A previous review [17] commented on the complexities of assessing the effect of microbubbles on BBB disruption, referencing the lack of an accepted protocol for handling and administering microbubbles, as well as the intersubjective differences in cardiovascular function that result in variable microbubble concentrations at target locations. While most investigations employing commercially available microbubbles have cited adherence to manufacturer instructions on handling and preparation of microbubbles, pre-activation vial temperature [129] and time between decanting/administration [130] have been shown to alter the size distribution when using Definity® microbubbles. As for the intersubject variability in cardiovascular function, this holds true for any administered agent that relies on the cardiovascular system for transport and accumulation in specific tissue vasculature and is a variable accounted for across the large number of studies included in this review. According to the review of the included literature, current in vivo evidence suggests the following microbubble-related factors influence the degree of BBB disruption and its safety: (1) microbubble characteristics, (2) dosing, and (3) timing/method of administration.

Microbubble Characteristics

A comparison of three commercially available microbubble formulations (SonoVue® vs. Definity® vs. Usphere™) in rats found comparable BBB opening and safety results between Definity® and Upshere™, while sonications with SonoVue® yielded significantly greater BBB opening than the other two microbubble formulations, at the lowest investigated ultrasound intensity [112]. More specific rodent investigations [85] sought to compare the effect of differing microbubble gas core composition (C_3F- vs. C_4F_{10}- vs. SF_6-filled), by administering equal doses of in-house microbubbles with identical shell composition and sizes. C_3F_8- and C_4F_{10}-filled microbubbles yielded significantly greater BBB disruption than SF_6-filled ones, suggesting that microbubble gas composition specifically influences the ability to induce BBB disruption. These findings correlated with additional comparative findings where Sonazoid® (C_4F_{10}-filled) microbubbles yielded significantly greater BBB disruption than comparably sized SonoVue® (SF_6) microbubbles, at unifying doses, administration timing, and ultrasound exposure parameters. The influence of microbubble size or diameter has also been investigated across three studies that directly compared compositionally identical, in-house microbubbles of different average diameters (1 to 2 μm vs. 4 to 5 μm [75]; 1 to 2 μm vs. 4 to 5 μm vs. 6 to 8 μm [66,72]; 2 μm vs. 6 μm [110]). Findings concluded that larger diameter microbubbles caused a linear increase in BBB disruption [72], resulting in more prolonged [66] BBB opening, while only mildly elevating the potential for tissue damage [72]. This trend was supported by another study [45] that compared SonoVue® (2.5 μm) with in-house (1.1 μm) microbubbles of similar composition. Additionally, increased proinflammatory gene expression has been observed in one study with the use of larger (4.2 μm vs. 1 to 1.5 μm) microbubbles, albeit with differing gas compositions [105]. Based on these data, the administration of larger diameter microbubbles appears to reduce the threshold for achieving BBB opening, requiring lower PNP sonications. Ultimately, a range of microbubble formulations have been used for safe ultrasound-mediated BBB disruption with an appropriate selection of sonication parameters, but differences in the efficacy of each microbubble formulation do appear and are likely attributable to variations in microbubble characteristics between formulations. Thus far, only Definity® [8,131] and SonoVue® [9,54] microbubbles have been used in clinical trials, likely due to their FDA approval and frequent use in preclinical studies.

Microbubble Dosing

The association between microbubble dosing, BBB disruption, and subsequent safety outcomes has been studied in numerous investigations with rodent and rabbit subjects [19,26,33,34,40,62,63,76,79,110,113,120]. The consensus from these findings is that using escalating microbubble dose only mildly increases the disruption and opening of the BBB, an effect that is often statistically insignificant when quantified [19,60,120]. Additionally, there seems to be an upper threshold microbubble dose for which subsequent administration of larger doses seems to cause BBB disruption to plateau [132] or paradoxically decrease [33,34,79] in rodents. Aberrations in this trend were noted when a range of microbubble doses were investigated in combination with (1) non-pulsed, unfocused ultrasound from a diagnostic, imaging transducer [39]; and (2) pulsed ultrasound, using a focused transducer [63]. In these studies, a significant positive correlation between microbubble dose and degree of BBB disruption was established, albeit with extensive tissue damage at higher doses. From available data, we can conclude that escalating microbubble dose may yield mildly elevated BBB disruption, usually up to a certain upper threshold dose, and with some heterogeneity in this trend observed among a few of the identified investigations. On the other hand, there seems to be a more consistent relationship between escalating microbubble doses and the increased risk of adverse safety outcomes reported by these same studies. This includes numerous reports of significant tissue damage [33,34,79], increased expression of proinflammatory genes associated with the NF-kB pathway [26], and greater cellular apoptosis [33,34].

Timing and Method of Microbubble Administration

In all identified protocols, microbubbles were administered via an intravenous route and were usually administered immediately prior to or at the onset of ultrasound application. As per the method of administration, evidence [79,108] has suggested that a prolonged intravenous infusion across the entire sonication period yields more reproducible and consistent, but not necessarily greater, BBB disruption when multiple cerebral foci are targeted [126]. It is theorised these differences can be attributed to the rapidly changing intravascular concentration of microbubbles attributed to bolus dosing, versus more stable microbubble availability attributable to infusion dosing [17]. Conversely, one rodent study assessed the extent of microbubble administration over 30 and 180 s infusion periods, reporting no significant difference in the extent of BBB disruption [76]. There is also some evidence to support that an infusion administration may yield less oedematous foci on T2 MRI, as compared to bolus administration [108]. More recent clinical trials have adopted microbubble infusion protocols continuously throughout the applied sonications [131,133].

Table 3. Comparison of five major commercially available microbubble formulations used in studies for ultrasound-mediated BBB disruption (information sourced from manufacturer) and typical doses.

Agent	Manufacturer	Shell Composition	Gas Core Composition	Mean Bubble Diameter (μm)	Bubble Concentration (Bubbles/mL)	Use in Identified Studies
Definity®/Luminity®	Lantheus Medical Imaging	Lipid	C_3F_8	1.1–3.3	1.2×10^{10}	Used in n = 42 preclinical studies (typical doses: 10–20 μL/kg) and n = 6 clinical studies (typical dose: 4 μL/kg)
Optison®	GE Healthcare	Protein	C_3F_8	3.0–4.5	$5–8 \times 10^8$	Used in n = 14 preclinical studies (typical doses: 50–100 μL/kg but significantly varied in mice studies)
SonoVue®/Lumason®	Bracco Diagnostics	Lipid	SF_6	1.5–2.5	$1.5–5.6 \times 10^8$	Used in n = 29 preclinical studies (typical doses 25–150 μL/kg) and n = 2 clinical studies (typical dose: 100 μL/kg)
Usphere Prime®	Trust Bio-sonics	Lipid	C_3F_8	1.0	2.8×10^{10}	Used in n = 1 preclinical study
Sonazoid®	GE Healthcare	Lipid	C_4F_{10}	2.0–3.0	9×10^8	Used in n = 1 preclinical study

3.5.2. Transducer Frequency

While a range of transducer frequencies, from 28 kHz [23,102] to 10 MHz [45], have been applied to disrupt and open the BBB, the majority of these protocols have employed frequencies that fall within a narrower range of 0.2 to 1.5 MHz amongst in vivo subjects. Among clinical trials, data currently exist for the application of only three ultrasound frequencies—ExAblate® Neuro (0.22 MHz), SonoCloud-1® (1.05 MHz), and NaviFUS® (0.5 MHz). In general, lower frequency ultrasound application (e.g., 28 kHz) has been shown to have greater tissue penetration, but a wider tissue focus, resulting in less targeted, ill-defined BBB disruption [102]. Conversely, higher frequency ultrasound beams tend to be more collimated, less tissue penetrative [94], and more likely to undergo tissue attenuation, resulting in greater beam aberration [134] and thermal energy liberation in the surrounding tissue, especially at the bony interface of the skull. We identified four preclinical, parametric studies that directly investigated the effect of altering the central frequency of a single-element transducer on BBB disruption efficacy and safety outcomes [19,45,94,119].

McDannold et al. [119] evaluated sonications of a variety of frequencies (0.26 MHz [30,118] vs. 0.69 MHz [25,28,120] vs. 1.63 MHz [7] vs. 2.04 MHz [119]) from multiple rabbit investigations. In their comparison, escalating frequencies had a higher threshold for BBB opening, requiring more intense, higher PNP ultrasound to achieve BBB disruption. This led to the conclusion that the threshold for successful BBB disruption was more appropriately dependent on the mechanical index (MI)—a ratio of the PNP over the square root of the transducer frequency. An estimated MI of 0.46 was identified as a threshold at which successful BBB disruption was achieved across all tested frequencies. Following up on this work, subsequent investigations comparing sonications with 1 MHz vs. 10 MHz [45,94] and 0.5 MHz vs. 1.6 MHz [19] ultrasound transducers have been conducted in rats. Findings from these studies support the notion that significantly higher PNP sonications are required to achieve BBB disruption with escalating frequencies, further consolidating the idea of an MI-dependent threshold. However, an MI threshold for BBB disruption was not observed when comparing 1 MHz to 10 MHz sonications [45,94], as was observed between frequencies used in other studies [19,119], and this may be due to the larger difference in frequencies tested between these studies. Lower frequency sonications, both at an equivalent MI [45,94] and at equivalent PNPs [19], produced a much larger area of BBB disruption, accompanied by off-target involvement, upon gross evaluation of Evans blue extravasation. This is believed to be due to the production of standing waves [135], enhanced reflection of ultrasound waves at the skull, and re-penetration into the brain's parenchyma [94].

Despite requiring greater PNPs to achieve BBB disruption, higher frequency sonications show mild to significantly favourable safety outcomes over lower frequency sonications, when observed 2–6 h after sonication. After applying higher frequency sonications, *McDannold* et al. [119] reported a subtle reduction in microhaemorrhagic damage in tissue sonicated with 2.04 MHz as compared to 0.26 MHz ultrasound but an increased density of these red blood cell extravasations relative to the area of tissue region exposed to the ultrasound. *Fan* et al. [45,94] highlighted significantly greater haemorrhagic and oedematous change on MRI, gross, and microscopic examinations in brains sonicated with frequencies of 1 MHz than 10 MHz, both when controlling for MI [94] and PNP [45]. It is important to note that *McDannold* et al. [119] *and Fan* et al. [45] both applied ultrasound to rabbits and rodents via a craniotomy site, thereby reducing the potential of beam defocussing and attenuation from transcranial application.

3.5.3. Peak Negative Pressure

The effect of PNP has been directly examined in a plethora of studies, including in rodents [15,19,31–33,45,62,63,65,69,80,81,87,88,93,94,101,112], rabbits [20,25,28,30,118], sheep [29,124], and even clinical trials [9]. Unfortunately, the accurate determination of PNP remains challenging [18] as in vivo PNP is difficult to measure; instead, in vitro pressures are measured and combined with skull attenuation coefficients to provide an estimate of the in vivo PNP [31]. While this may impede comparisons of PNPs between studies, data and trends from within studies can be useful in determining optimal parameters for safe and effective BBB disruption. We found that sonication PNPs at which safe and effective BBB disruption has been accomplished ranged from 0.2 to 0.5 MPa in most preclinical animal studies (see Table 4), with some utilising higher PNPs safely with higher frequency transducers (>1 MHz) [32,45,94,103]. It has been difficult to establish a narrow range of PNPs routinely used amongst clinical trials, as in their design they each test a range of PNPs across repeated sonications, ranging from 0.48 to 1.15 MPa [9,54], and 2.5 [10] to 60 W [52] of applied power.

General findings suggest that a threshold PNP is required for a given frequency of applied ultrasound (threshold MI), after which BBB disruption is achieved [67,88]. There is then a narrow therapeutic window at which a positive dose–response relationship exists, where raising the applied PNP improves the degree of BBB disruption, without materially impacting safety [19,25,32]. After this, continued elevations in PNP confer improvements in BBB disruption and opening, but also worsen safety outcomes, achieving a state of dose-limiting toxicity [65,68,73]. Eventually, a plateau is obtained [32,63], at which further escalations in PNP cause insignificant improvements to BBB disruption, while continuing to worsen safety outcomes [25,32]. After surpassing the threshold PNP required for BBB opening, and prior to this relationship plateauing, preclinical studies have identified linear relationships with escalating PNP and the volume of BBB opening on MRI [66,72,75], the extravasation of dextrans [67], and the uptake of therapeutic agents such as Herceptin [31]. Clinical trials in glioblastoma patients have also shown an increasing degree of BBB disruption with escalating PNP sonications [9,54], albeit with increased incidence of oedema [9]. Interestingly, one study noted that the uptake of a chemotherapeutic agent, BCNU, increased as the sonication PNP was raised from 0.45 to 0.62 MPa, peaked at 0.62 MPa, but decreased with subsequent elevations in PNP (0.98 and 1.38 MPa), despite an increase in contrast enhancement on MRI at these higher pressures [101]. The PNP has also been shown to influence the size [69] and molecular weight [67] of agents capable of passing through the BBB, with current evidence suggesting that higher, and therefore less safe, PNPs are required for transporting larger substances. Additionally, sonications of increasing PNP have been shown to prolong the reversibility or closure time following the disruption and opening of the BBB [65,66]. Furthermore, one study reported the effect of BBB disruption produced with PNPs of 0.55 and 0.81 MPa on downregulating the immunohistochemical expression of a key cerebrovascular drug-efflux pump—P-glycoprotein—for 48 and 72 h after sonication, respectively [15]. This finding suggests that increasing the PNP of ultrasound may go beyond exerting mechanical effects on the BBB and may additionally cause biochemical changes that favour drug accumulation in the brain.

The increasing presence of adverse safety events associated with escalating PNPs has been proposed to be due to the increased frequency of inertial cavitation in microbubbles. These events are demonstrated by the presence of broad or wide-band acoustic emissions from sonicated microbubbles, detected via a receiving ultrasound transducer element [30,45,67,112]. Collectively, this monitoring process is known as passive cavitation detection or acoustic emissions monitoring and has resulted in a paradigm shift in sonication delivery, where a dynamic power ramp technique is utilised to determine optimal PNP as opposed to applying static PNP sonications. Here, power is incrementally escalated to produce sonications of graduating PNP, and this power is stabilised when ultraharmonic and subharmonic signals (indicating stable cavitation) are detected, or the power is reduced if any wide-band emissions (indicating inertial cavitation) are detected. This variable power ramp delivery protocol has been applied successfully to produce safe BBB disruption in rodent [26,93], NHP [50,126], and clinical studies [10].

3.5.4. Pulse Characteristics

Amongst identified investigations, ultrasound is typically delivered in a non-continuous, pulsed manner, with a small minority applying a continuous ultrasound scheme [40,89,121,122]. A pulsed delivery approach has been adopted as a mainstay to limit the exposure time to ultrasound in delicate brain tissue and has been shown to significantly reduce the thermogenic effect [89] associated with the continuous application of ultrasound. Of the four studies that applied a continuous ultrasound paradigm, one study was able to disrupt the BBB reproducibly, without adverse histopathological events, using a diagnostic, imaging ultrasound transducer [40]. We identified two primary variables that have intimately influenced the efficacy and safety of ultrasound-mediated BBB disruption: the length or duration of each pulse, consisting of one or more excitatory cycles of acoustic pressure waves, and the pulse repetition frequency, how frequently these series of pulses repeat (see Figure 5). Additionally, more novel iterations in discontinuous ultrasound delivery have emerged, including the delivery of ultrasound bursts (consisting of shorter, phasic pulses) over more commonly used tonic pulses (consisting of a longer pulse) [59,60,83,108].

Pulse Length

While pulse lengths as low as 0.35 μs [39] and as high as 100 ms [19,23,102] have been used to disrupt the BBB via pulsed ultrasound, a majority of preclinical studies appear to use pulses of 10 ms in length. In clinical studies, pulse lengths of 2 to 3 ms [8,10,11,53] have been used with the ExAblate® Neuro device, and pulse lengths of 10 ms [54] and 23.8 ms [9] have been used with the NaviFUS® and SonoCloud-1® devices, respectively. We identified six parametric, preclinical studies that directly investigated the efficacy and safety outcomes of a range of pulse lengths. Escalating pulse length from 0.1 to 10 ms appeared to consistently increase BBB disruption in all six studies; in two studies, subsequently higher pulse length appeared to yield no significant improvements in BBB disruption efficacy, whilst simultaneously worsening safety outcomes [7,76]. Three studies did not corroborate this plateauing effect with sonications of pulse length >10 ms, highlighting a larger area of BBB disruption following sonications of 50 [102] and 100 ms [19,102] pulses, respectively. This effect may be attributable to the use of a diagnostic, imaging transducer, operating at a lower central frequency (28 kHz), delivering higher MI (MI = 4.78) sonications in two of the three studies by *Liu* et al. [23,102]. However, the transducer type and parameters utilised by *Shin* et al. [19] were comparable to the two studies that did highlight a plateauing effect with lengthening pulses >10 ms, making this previously described trend [7,18,120] less definitive. The threshold PNP required to successfully open the BBB has been shown to decrease with escalating pulse lengths from 0.1 to 10 ms in one study [120], likely due to the greater cumulative effect from more prolonged ultrasound pulses. Additionally, with sonications of pulse lengths ≥10 ms, the spatial distribution of tracers appears more heterogeneous, with significantly greater accumulation around blood vessels and less even parenchymal distribution than is observed with pulse lengths <10 ms [76,83]. Nonetheless, from the currently available literature, it appears that sonications of pulse lengths ≤10 ms appear to provide the greatest efficacy and safety benefits for ultrasound-mediated BBB disruption, when controlling for all other parameters.

Phasic vs. Tonic Pulses

More recently, the use of rapid, short pulse sonications or phasic pulses consisting of bursts (as opposed to more continuous tonic pulses) has been investigated for its potential to disrupt and open the BBB more homogeneously. Benefits of phasic pulses are theorised to occur via increased intraburst microbubble transit time, and the reduction in standing waves afforded with shorter, phasic pulse sequences [60,108]. Reports of ultrasound-mediated BBB disruption with phasic pulses have explored the use of pulse lengths ranging from 2.3 to 5 μs in length. Direct comparisons between phasic and tonic pulse sequences in mice have had mixed results, with some studies [82,83] reporting safer BBB disruption, with improved homogeneity and improved BBB reversibility, and another [59] reporting worse safety outcomes, with no improvements in the homogeneity or reversibility of BBB disruption with phasic pulsed schemes. These conflicting findings may be attributable to the differences in ultrasound frequency (1 [83] vs. 1.78 MHz [59]), microbubble type, and administration method (30 s infusion [83] vs. bolus [59]) between these studies. All studies thus far have exhibited a lower degree of BBB disruption with phasic pulses at unifying parameters, suggesting this protocol may provide a more conservative opening of the BBB. The use of phasic pulse regimens could provide safer, better-distributed delivery of therapeutics into the CNS, but it currently requires further investigation across a broader set of parameters for more conclusive data.

Pulse Repetition Frequency

Most sonication protocols that we identified utilised pulse repetition frequencies that fell within a range of 1–10 Hz in preclinical and clinical studies that employed single-element ultrasound transducers [9,54]. Clinical trials utilising the ExAblate® multi-element, phased array device appear to utilise pulse repetition frequency of 30 to 31 Hz instead. The effect of pulse repetition frequency on BBB disruption efficacy and safety has been studied in a limited fashion, by five parametric studies that investigated this relationship [19,60,76,108,120]. Evidence from these studies appears to suggest a threshold pulse repetition frequency, and therefore a minimum number of pulses over a given duration of sonication, required to achieve successful BBB disruption [76]. After surpassing a relatively low pulse repetition frequency threshold, the effect of escalating pulse repetition frequencies has been inconsistent. Two studies reported no statistically significant improvement in BBB disruption minutes following tonic pulsed sonications of pulse repetition frequency 1–25 Hz [76] and 0.5 to 5 Hz [120], respectively. Contrary to these findings, three studies have reported significantly improved BBB disruption with escalating pulse repetition frequencies, both with longer, tonic pulsed sonications (pulse repetition frequency 1 to 5 Hz) [19] and with shorter, phasic pulsed sonications as part of a burst sequence (pulse repetition frequencies 6250 to 100,000 Hz [60] and 1 to 166,666 Hz [108]). Safety outcomes from escalating pulse repetition frequencies were either mildly improved [108] or showed no significant differences [19,60,76,120] within hours following the last sonication. These inconsistencies warrant further parametric study into the effect of using higher pulse repetition frequency sonications and may help in further optimisation of safer parameters.

3.5.5. Sonication Duration

The sonication duration is another parameter that tends to affect the efficacy and safety of ultrasound-mediated BBB disruption, as it describes the time of exposure to ultrasound in one given application. Amongst all the study protocols we reviewed, the majority of sonication durations fell between 0.5 and 2 min, and this remained consistent in the protocols of clinical studies as well. Sonication durations as low as 6 s [121,122], with non-pulsed ultrasound, and as high as 20 min [93], with pulsed ultrasound, have also been shown to induce sufficient BBB disruption. From parametric studies, there appears to be a positive correlation between increasing sonication duration and the degree of BBB disruption, with the eventual trade-off being worsening safety outcomes following exposure to excessively long sonications both with pulsed [19,20,102] and continuous delivery ultrasound-mediated BBB disruption [40,121]. Additional data suggest that eventually a threshold is reached, where the effect of increasing the sonication duration saturates [93,115], and excessive tissue damage is observed [93]. Interestingly, one investigation digressed from this trend, where significant changes in the sonication duration resulted in mild but statistically insignificant increases in BBB disruption, without any observed histopathological change [76]. The authors of this study hypothesised that this was due to the fact BBB disruption saturating potential had already been achieved using the lowest tested sonication duration of 30 s, and this may be attributed to the higher frequency of pulsed ultrasound used, as compared to the other parametric studies identified.

3.5.6. Dosing (Number and Frequency) of Ultrasound Applications

In this review, we divided the application of ultrasound into two categories—a sonication and a session. A session was defined as an application period, consisting of one ultrasound sonication or numerous ultrasound sonications separated by an interval of usually minutes to an hour (intersonication interval). Sessions are usually separated by a larger interval of time, on the timescale of days to weeks apart (intersession interval). The partition of ultrasound applications into these categories helps in understanding the effect of cumulative ultrasound acutely (after multiple sonications) and chronically (after multiple sessions). Ultimately, multiple sonications, and multiple sessions of ultrasound-mediated BBB disruption over months to years, would need to be safely tolerated if this approach is to achieve widescale clinical use for improving drug delivery in patients with CNS malignancies, dementias, and other neurodegenerative diseases.

Ultrasound Sonications

Repeating an ultrasound sonication once (double sonication) has been shown to significantly improve the magnitude of BBB duration and duration of BBB opening when compared to a single sonication [71,115] at the same target site. Additionally, the choice of the intersonication interval may influence the penetration and uptake of drugs into the brain, and specific drug half-lives may need to be considered when determining the most appropriate intersonication interval [71]. Unfortunately, efficacy data from more than repeat sonications are non-existent, as no further studies have directly compared the effect of an equivalent single sonication against more than two repeat sonications. Other studies, both preclinical and clinical [9,52], have tested a greater range of repeat sonications but have not adequately reported group-specific data on BBB disruption efficacy. When directly compared, the safety of double sonications appears to be similar to [71] or slightly worse than [115] a single sonication. Indirect comparisons from two different studies that utilised equivalent ultrasound parameters highlighted worsening MRI and histological safety outcomes after increasing the number of sonications per session from two [48] to four [49], over three weekly ultrasound sessions. Safety outcomes from other protocols employing repeat sonications have been generally favourable, but also variable, with some studies reporting worsening outcomes [33,93] but most reporting no differences in healthy [84,109], aging [29], and glioma animal models [43,78] and clinical [8,11,54] studies. Additional evidence also suggests that multiple, lower PNP/MI sonications can produce a greater area of BBB disruption than a single, higher PNP/MI sonication, with improved safety outcomes [103].

Ultrasound Sessions

The effect of multiple, repeat ultrasound sessions on the degree of BBB disruption is unclear, as the few identified studies that directly compared single against multiple ultrasound session applications did not investigate differences in the efficacy of BBB disruption between these groups [43,93]. In addition, studies that conducted multiple, repeat sessions of ultrasound-mediated BBB disruption (Table 4) have not sought to investigate the potential of a cumulative effect of these sessions on the long-term integrity and permeability of the BBB. Subsequent ultrasound sessions have been shown to require sonications with gradually escalating PNPs in order to achieve BBB disruption in animal models [93,99,100]. This is likely attributable to the general growth and the increase in skull thickness observed in animal models [70,71,99] and has not been a finding corroborated in adult clinical trials [9,53]. Adverse radiographic safety outcomes following long-term, repeat ultrasound sessions have been generally favourable in NHP [70,84] and clinical studies [9,53]. However, transient MRI lesions (suggestive of microhaemorrhagic and oedematous change) have developed following repeat sessions in some NHP [21,22] and human [9,10] subjects. Long-term behavioural and clinical evaluations appear to be favourable in rodents [84], NHPs [21,22], and humans [52]. Histopathological investigation of these NHP and human studies has been limited, and only half of NHP [50,56,126] and no human studies investigated any histological outcomes following repeat sessions of ultrasound-mediated BBB disruption. Adverse histological outcomes in NHPs have ranged from minimal to moderate microhaemorrhagic change and, in one study [126], occurred despite the absence of any MRI abnormalities. Rodent investigations [99,100] have observed worsening adverse safety events after numerous, weekly ultrasound sessions. These include permanent structural changes on MRI (microhaemorrhagic/oedematous lesion, enlarged ventricles), histopathological evidence of macrophage infiltration, increasing accumulation of phosphorylated tau [100], and evidence of neurogenesis [100]. Furthermore, one study reported worsening tissue damage after multi-session ultrasound applications coupled with liposomal doxorubicin delivery in a glioma rodent model [70]. Interestingly, no tissue damage was observed after multiple ultrasound sessions without liposomal doxorubicin co-administration [70], suggesting that the repeat co-administration of certain chemotherapeutic drugs may either directly damage surrounding tissue or lower the threshold for inertial cavitation-induced ultrasound damage. These study findings, as well as the occurrence of a sparse number of transient MRI abnormalities in NHP and clinical studies with already limited sample sizes, highlight uncertainty around the chronic safety of ultrasound-mediated BBB disruption on tissue health, challenging the narrative that repeat sessions of ultrasound-mediated BBB disruption are generally safe, as presented in prior reviews [17,18].

4. Discussion

After an extensive systematic review of currently available literature, we feel we have comprehensively summarised the parameters used in published protocols of ultrasound-mediated BBB disruption for enhanced drug delivery, as well as the subsequent effects on efficacy and safety (Table S2—Supplementary Materials). We have also listed parameter ranges at which effective BBB disruption has been conducted with the most favourable safety outcomes (Table 4). The heterogeneity in protocols used to ultrasonically disrupt the BBB in included studies is apparent; thus, more rigorous standardisation is required, especially in the setting of clinical trials. In addition, we have identified several areas related to the procedure itself, as well as the techniques used to analyse its efficacy and safety, where the body of current knowledge is less established.

Firstly, in relation to the procedure of ultrasound-mediated BBB disruption, an emerging subset of investigations in this field have proposed the benefit of shorter, phased pulses of ultrasound over longer, tonic pulsed schemes that have predominated thus far. The use of phasic pulses may improve the homogeneity and safety of ultrasound-mediated BBB disruption, at the cost of opening the BBB to a smaller degree. As a result, this ultrasound pulse protocol may be applicable in frequent sessions of BBB disruption for the delivery of therapeutics for less aggressive, chronic CNS conditions, but further work is required to translate these findings beyond the subset of rodent studies currently available. Advances in microbubbles, namely in designing and testing microbubbles with more optimal characteristics (larger diameters and C_3H_8 or C_4H_{10} gas filling) may also play a role in enhancing the efficacy and safety of ultrasound-mediated BBB disruption.

Secondly, the methods used to confirm ultrasound-mediated BBB disruption have relied upon the visualisation of proxy markers, mainly histological tracers or gadolinium-based MRI contrast agents. While these tracers have been essential in demonstrating proof of concept of ultrasound-mediated BBB disruption, they are ultimately not the intended therapeutic molecules needing to be delivered into the CNS. Studies have identified that the molecular weight, half-life, and timing of administration [70,71] influence the ability of a drug to traverse a disrupted BBB following ultrasound, and thus more research is required to track the uptake and transport of drug molecules not only across the BBB but to desired target cells.

Thirdly, the type of safety assessments conducted throughout the investigations we identified have overwhelmingly focused on structural alterations in sonicated neural tissue, both at gross and microscopic anatomical levels (e.g., haemorrhagic, cellular, and oedematous change). This has created a gap in our understanding of the physiological changes that follow ultrasound-mediated BBB disruption and, of note, the possibility of long-term inflammatory changes persisting after the passing of cerebrovascular contents through the BBB. Current proteomic and transcriptomic analyses seem to suggest an upregulation of proinflammatory genes following ultrasound-mediated BBB disruption, but the effect of this, if any, on neural tissue functioning remains to be seen. Electrophysiological changes following parameters used for ultrasound-mediated BBB disruption is another understudied area, particularly as neuromodulation and stimulation is an emerging area of therapeutic ultrasound research [128]. Surprisingly, none of the studies we identified sought to assess the impact of ultrasound delivery on the cranial bone and surrounding soft-tissue structures (skin, connective tissue, galea), even though most protocols involve ultrasound application transcranially, and the cranium remains the first point of tissue contact with the ultrasound beam.

After reviewing studies that repeatedly disrupted the BBB over chronic testing periods, we feel there is insufficient evidence to suggest that ultrasound can be frequently and chronically applied without exhibiting some degree of damage. NHP and human studies trialling chronic sessions of ultrasound-mediated BBB disruption have reported the presence of some adverse events, mainly transient MRI, and behavioural/clinical abnormalities. Conversely, rodent studies have highlighted permanent MRI and histological adverse changes from chronic exposure. While these differences in safety outcomes may be attributable to interstudy protocol variability, or anatomical differences between humans, NHPs, and rodents, a definitive suggestion of repeatably safe ultrasound-mediated BBB disruption is difficult to make given the limited and conflicting dataset. While some adverse events, whether transient or permanent, may be an acceptable risk when treating advanced CNS conditions, the prevalence and long-term impact of any adverse event on pre-existing neurological morbidity are currently not known in humans. Additionally, current NHP and clinical evidence is limited, both by small sample sizes (n<10 in most studies) and the sparsity of histological and biochemical safety analyses. Pharmacological strategies such as dexamethasone administration in an attempt to attenuate inflammatory response following ultrasound-mediated BBB disruption may also play an important role in the clinical adoption of this technique in treating chronic CNS conditions [106] and therefore represent another area of further research. Emerging evidence on the benefit of real-time imaging techniques such as Doppler [136] and photoacoustic imaging [136,137] may provide further technological advances in the clinical confirmation of ultrasound-mediated BBB opening without the need for MRI.

5. Conclusions

Greater standardisation of protocols and parameters used in preclinical and clinical studies investigating ultrasound-mediated BBB disruption is required for advancing clinical translation. Future studies should strive to further characterise the efficacy of ultrasound-mediated BBB disruption. This should focus on not only the opening of the BBB to MRI contrast agents, but also the delivery of intended drug molecules and their subsequent benefit in outcomes related to CNS conditions (e.g., reduced tumour progression and improved survival rates with high-grade cancers, reduced cognitive decline in dementia). Currently, numerous, larger clinical trials involving CNS cancer [138] (NCT04440358, NCT04528680, NCT04614493, NCT03744026, NCT04804709) and dementia (NCT04118764) patients are ongoing. The data from these trials will hopefully provide greater clarity to our overall understanding of the long-term safety, tolerability, and efficacy of cumulative ultrasound-mediated BBB disruption and enhanced drug delivery in patients with advanced CNS conditions.

Table 4. Summary of safe and effective parameters used in identified studies and reported relationships between parameter escalation and BBB disruption efficacy and safety outcomes.

Parameter	Safe and Effective Parameters Commonly Used	Parameters Compared	Reported Effects on BBBD (Efficacy Outcomes)	Reported Safety Outcomes
Transducer Frequency	Preclinical: 0.20–1.50 MHz Clinical: 0.22, 0.50, and 1.05 MHz	0.26, 0.69, 1.63, 2.04 MHz [119]	Increasing frequency: greater PNP required to achieve BBBD [19,45,94,119]; smaller foci/area of BBBD [19,45,94]	Increasing frequency: increased density of microhaemorrhagic activity [119]; decreased haemorrhagic [19,45,94] and oedematous activity [45]
		1 and 10 MHz [45,94]		
		0.5 and 1.6 MHz [19]		
PNP	Preclinical: 0.2–0.5 MPa with <1 MHz transducers Clinical: 0.48–1.15 MPa and 2.5–60 W power	0.30, 0.46, 0.61, 0.75, 0.98 MPa [73]	Increasing PNP: increasing BBBD after surpassing threshold PNP [9,15,45,65,73]; eventual saturation point in BBBD [32]; prolonged BBB opening [65,66]; prolonged P-glycoprotein downregulation [15]	Increasing PNP: increased haemorrhagic [15,19,65,66,73,93] and microhaemorrhagic change [73,93]; neuropil loss; neuronal loss [73,93] and necrosis [93]; evidence of apoptosis [45]; cerebral oedema [9,45]; hypoactivity/ataxia/tremor [33]
		0.55, 0.81 MPa [15]		
		0.27, 0.39, 0.59, 0.78 MPa [93]		
		0.3, 0.5, 1.0, 1.5, 2.0, 2.5, 4.5 MPa [45,94]		
		1.1, 1.9, 2.45, and 3.5 MPa [65]		

Table 4. *Cont.*

Parameter	Safe and Effective Parameters Commonly Used	Parameters Compared	Reported Effects on BBBD (Efficacy Outcomes)	Reported Safety Outcomes
PNP	Preclinical: 0.2–0.5 MPa with <1 MHz transducers Clinical: 0.48–1.15 MPa and 2.5–60 W power	0.45, 0.62, 0.98, 1.32 MPa [101]		
		0.55, 0.78, 1.1, 1.9, 2.45, 3.47, 4.9 MPa [32]		
		0.2, 0.3, 0.6, 1.5 MPa [19]		
		0.30, 0.51, 0.89 MPa [33]		
		0.4, 0.5 0.8, 1.1, 1.4, 2.3, 3.1 MPa [28]		
		0.2, 0.4, 0.5, 0.8, 1.1, 1.8 MPa [25]		
		0.78, 0.90, 1.03, 1.15 MPa [9]		
PL	Preclinical: 10 ms Clinical: 2–3, 10, and 23.6 ms	0.1, 0.2, 1.0, 2.0, 10, 20, 30 ms [76]	Increasing PL: increasing BBBD with PL 0.1–10 ms; statistically non-significant increase in BBBD after PL > 10 ms [7,76]; decreased PNP threshold (PL = 0.1–10 ms) [120]; heterogeneous distribution of BBBD/greater perivascular accumulation of tracer [76]	Increasing PL: no microhaemorrhagic change with PL ≤ 10 ms [19,120]; significant haemorrhagic change with PL = 100 ms [19,23]; evidence of apoptosis with PL = 100 ms [23]
		1, 10, 100 ms [19]		
		10, 100 ms [7]		
		0.1, 1, 10 ms [120]		
		30, 100 ms [23]		
		10, 50 and 100 ms [102]		
PRF	Preclinical: 1–10 Hz Clinical: 1–10 Hz and 30–31 Hz	0.1, 1, 1, 10, 25 Hz[76]	Increasing PRF: no BBBD with PRF = 0.1 Hz [76]; inconsistent improvements in BBBD with tonic pulsed sequences, some being statistically significant [19] and others not [76,120]; improvements in BBBD with rapid, phasic pulses [60,108]	Increasing PRF: no increase in adverse safety outcomes, via MRI [108] and histology [19,60,76,108,120]
		0.5, 1, 2, 5 Hz [120]		
		1, 2, 5 Hz [19]		
		1, 1667, 3333, 16,667, 166,667 Hz [108]		
		6250, 25,000, 100,000 Hz [60]		
SD	Preclinical: 30–120 sClinical: 30–120 s; 150–270 s in one study	30, 660 s [76]	Increasing SD: improved BBBD with pulsed [19,93,102] and continuously [40,121] applied US; plateauing effect thereafter [93,115]; one study reported no improvement in BBBD [76]	Increasing SD: minimal change in adverse safety outcomes with small increases, and significantly worsening safety outcomes with excessive increases [19,40,93,102,121]; no increase in histopathological outcomes in one study [76]
		240, 360, 480, 600 s [102]		
		30, 60, 120, 300 s [19]		
		30, 180, 300, 600, 1200 s [93]		
		60, 120, 180, 240 s[40]		
		6, 8 and 10 s [121]		
Dosing (Number and Frequency) of Sonications	Preclinical: 1–13 sonications/session (ISI = 5 min) Clinical: 1–8 sonications/session (ISI not stated) *ISIs are listed within brackets*	1, 2 (10 min), 2 (120 min) sonications [71]	Increasing sonication #: increase in BBBD [71,115]; improved doxorubicin uptake with shorter ISI [71]	Increasing sonication #: no [71] or mild [115] histopathological change (increased neuropil vacuolation)
		1, 2 (20 min), 2 (40 min) sonications [115]		

Table 4. *Cont.*

Parameter	Safe and Effective Parameters Commonly Used	Parameters Compared	Reported Effects on BBBD (Efficacy Outcomes)	Reported Safety Outcomes
Dosing (Number and Frequency) of Sessions	Preclinical: 1–27 Clinical: 1–10 sessions *Intersession intervals are listed within brackets*	2–10, 2–6 sessions (biweekly and monthly) [84]	Increasing session #: higher PNP sonications required to achieve similar BBBD, but likely due to animal model growth [84] as not observed in developed adult clinical trials [9,11]	Increasing session #: no adverse safety outcomes [53,123]; transient MRI changes [9,21,22]; cortical atrophy, ventricular dilation, and lesion formation on MRI [100]; increased phosphorylated tau deposition [100]; increased neurogenesis [100] no change in motor and behavioural outcomes in rodents [84]; increased tissue damage and macrophage infiltration with doxorubicin co-delivery [70,91]; increasing number of apoptotic cells (significantly larger microbubble dose) [33]; mild increase in white matter vacuolation and mild neuronal injury (significantly larger microbubble dose) [43]
		1, 8 (3 days) sessions [43]		
		1, 4 (weekly) sessions [123]		
		1, 6 (weekly) sessions [100]		
		1, 3 (weekly) sessions [93]		
		1, 3 (weekly) sessions [70,91]		
		1, 2 (2 days), 3 (2 days) sessions [33]		
		3 (monthly), 6 (monthly) sessions [53]		
		4–27 (varying intersession intervals) sessions [21,22]		
		1–10 (monthly) sessions [9]		

***US:** ultrasound; **BBBD:** blood–brain barrier disruption; **PL:** pulse length; **PRF:** pulse repetition frequency; **SD:** sonication duration; **ISI:** intersonication interval.*

Supplementary Materials: The following supporting information can be downloaded at: https://www.mdpi.com/article/10.3390/pharmaceutics14040833/s1, PRISMA 2020 Guidelines for Reporting Systematic Reviews, Table S1: PRISMA 2020 checklist for this systematic review; Extracted Data from Included Studies, Table S2: Ultrasound protocol and parameter data from included studies, tabulated with efficacy and safety outcomes.

Author Contributions: Conceptualisation, K.G.; methodology, K.G.; data curation, K.G., A.B.-F. and A.B.; investigation, K.G. and A.B.-F.; formal analysis, K.G.; visualisation, K.G. and A.B.; resources, K.G. and J.N.J.R.; supervision, S.B.R. and J.N.J.R.; writing—original draft preparation, K.G.; writing—reviewing and editing, A.B.-F., A.B., S.B.R. and J.N.J.R. All authors have read and agreed to the published version of the manuscript.

Funding: This research was funded by the Ministry of Business, Innovation and Employment (contract UOOX1602). K.G. was partly funded by an Otago Medical School doctoral stipend. A.B.F. was sponsored by a doctoral scholarship from the Anatomy Department of the University of Otago.

Institutional Review Board Statement: Not applicable.

Informed Consent Statement: Not applicable.

Data Availability Statement: All data supporting reported results can be found in the manuscript and supplementary materials of the manuscript.

Conflicts of Interest: The authors declare no conflict of interest.

References

1. Ballabh, P.; Braun, A.; Nedergaard, M. The blood-brain barrier: An overview: Structure, regulation, and clinical implications. *Neurobiol. Dis.* **2004**, *16*, 1–13. [CrossRef] [PubMed]
2. Vykhodtseva, N.; McDannold, N.; Hynynen, K. Progress and problems in the application of focused ultrasound for blood-brain barrier disruption. *Ultrasonics* **2008**, *48*, 279–296. [CrossRef] [PubMed]
3. Pardridge, W.M. Drug and gene targeting to the brain with molecular Trojan horses. *Nat. Rev. Drug Discov.* **2002**, *1*, 131–139. [CrossRef] [PubMed]

4. Mackay, S.M.; Myint, M.A.; Easingwood, R.A.; Hegh, D.Y.; Wickens, J.R.; Hyland, B.I.; Jameson, G.N.L.; Reynolds, J.N.J.; Tan, E.W. Dynamic control of neurochemical release with ultrasonically-sensitive nanoshell-tethered liposomes. *Commun. Chem.* **2019**, *2*, 122. [CrossRef]
5. Nakano, T.; Rizwan, S.B.; Myint, D.M.; Gray, J.; Mackay, S.M.; Harris, P.; Perk, C.G.; Hyland, B.I.; Empson, R.; Tan, E.W.; et al. An On-Demand Drug Delivery System for Control of Epileptiform Seizures. *Pharmaceutics* **2022**, *14*, 468. [CrossRef]
6. Bakay, L.; Ballantine, T., Jr.; Hueter, T.F.; Sosa, D. Ultrasonically produced changes in the blood-brain barrier. *AMA Arch. Neurol. Psychiatry* **1956**, *76*, 457–467. [CrossRef]
7. Hynynen, K.; McDannold, N.; Vykhodtseva, N.; Jolesz, F.A. Jolesz. Noninvasive MR imaging-guided focal opening of the blood-brain barrier in rabbits. *Radiology* **2001**, *220*, 640–646. [CrossRef]
8. Abrahao, A.; Meng, Y.; Llinas, M.; Huang, Y.; Hamani, C.; Mainprize, T.; Aubert, I.; Heyn, C.; Black, S.E.; Hynynen, K.; et al. First-in-human trial of blood-brain barrier opening in amyotrophic lateral sclerosis using MR-guided focused ultrasound. *Nat. Commun.* **2019**, *10*, 4373. [CrossRef]
9. Idbaih, A.; Canney, M.; Belin, L.; Desseaux, C.; Vignot, A.; Bouchoux, G.; Asquier, N.; Law-Ye, B.; Leclercq, D.; Bissery, A.; et al. Safety and Feasibility of Repeated and Transient Blood-Brain Barrier Disruption by Pulsed Ultrasound in Patients with Recurrent Glioblastoma. *Clin. Cancer Res.* **2019**, *25*, 3793–3801. [CrossRef]
10. Lipsman, N.; Meng, Y.; Bethune, A.J.; Huang, Y.; Lam, B.; Masellis, M.; Herrmann, N.; Heyn, C.; Aubert, I.; Boutet, A.; et al. Blood-brain barrier opening in Alzheimer's disease using MR-guided focused ultrasound. *Nat. Commun.* **2018**, *9*, 2336. [CrossRef]
11. Mainprize, T.; Lipsman, N.; Huang, Y.; Meng, Y.; Bethune, A.; Ironside, S.; Heyn, C.; Alkins, R.; Trudeau, M.; Sahgal, A.; et al. Blood-Brain Barrier Opening in Primary Brain Tumors with Non-invasive MR-Guided Focused Ultrasound: A Clinical Safety and Feasibility Study. *Sci. Rep.* **2019**, *9*, 321. [CrossRef] [PubMed]
12. Sheikov, N.; McDannold, N.; Sharma, S.; Hynynen, K. Effect of focused ultrasound applied with an ultrasound contrast agent on the tight junctional integrity of the brain microvascular endothelium. *Ultrasound Med. Biol.* **2008**, *34*, 1093–1104. [CrossRef] [PubMed]
13. Choi, H.; Lee, E.H.; Han, M.; An, S.H.; Park, J. Diminished Expression of P-glycoprotein Using Focused Ultrasound Is Associated With JNK-Dependent Signaling Pathway in Cerebral Blood Vessels. *Front. Neurosci.* **2019**, *13*, 1350. [CrossRef] [PubMed]
14. Cho, H.S.; Lee, H.; Han, M.; Choi, J.R.; Lee, T.; Ahn, S.; Chang, Y.; Park, J. Localised down-regulation of p-glycoprotein by Focused Ultrasound and Microbubbles induced Blood-Brain Barrier Disruption in Rat Brain. *J. Ther. Ultrasound* **2016**, *5* (Suppl. S1), 16–17.
15. Aryal, M.; Fischer, K.; Gentile, C.; Gitto, S.; Zhang, Y.Z.; McDannold, N. Effects on P-Glycoprotein Expression after Blood-Brain Barrier Disruption Using Focused Ultrasound and Microbubbles. *PLoS ONE* **2017**, *12*, e0166061. [CrossRef]
16. Sheikov, N.; McDannold, N.; Jolesz, F.; Zhang, Y.Z.; Tam, K.; Hynynen, K. Brain arterioles show more active vesicular transport of blood-borne tracer molecules than capillaries and venules after focused ultrasound-evoked opening of the blood-brain barrier. *Ultrasound Med. Biol.* **2006**, *32*, 1399–1409. [CrossRef]
17. McMahon, D.; Poon, C.; Hynynen, K. Evaluating the safety profile of focused ultrasound and microbubble-mediated treatments to increase blood-brain barrier permeability. *Expert Opin. Drug Deliv.* **2019**, *16*, 129–142. [CrossRef]
18. Aryal, M.; Arvanitis, C.D.; Alexander, P.M.; McDannold, N. Ultrasound-mediated blood-brain barrier disruption for targeted drug delivery in the central nervous system. *Adv. Drug Deliv. Rev.* **2014**, *72*, 94–109. [CrossRef]
19. Shin, J.; Kong, C.; Cho, J.S.; Lee, J.; Koh, C.S.; Yoon, M.S.; Na, Y.C.; Chang, W.S.; Chang, J.W. Focused ultrasound-mediated noninvasive blood-brain barrier modulation: Preclinical examination of efficacy and safety in various sonication parameters. *Neurosurg. Focus* **2018**, *44*, E15. [CrossRef]
20. Beccaria, K.; Canney, M.; Goldwirt, L.; Fernandez, C.; Adam, C.; Piquet, J.; Autret, G.; Clement, O.; Lafon, C.; Chapelon, J.-Y.; et al. Opening of the blood-brain barrier with an unfocused ultrasound device in rabbits. *J. Neurosurg.* **2013**, *119*, 887–898. [CrossRef]
21. Downs, M.E.; Buch, A.; Karakatsani, M.E.; Konofagou, E.E.; Ferrera, V.P. Blood-Brain Barrier Opening in Behaving Non-Human Primates via Focused Ultrasound with Systemically Administered Microbubbles. *Sci. Rep.* **2015**, *5*, 15076. [CrossRef] [PubMed]
22. Downs, M.E.; Buch, A.; Sierra, C.; Karakatsani, M.E.; Teichert, T.; Chen, S.; Konofagou, E.E.; Ferrera, V.P. Long-Term Safety of Repeated Blood-Brain Barrier Opening via Focused Ultrasound with Microbubbles in Non-Human Primates Performing a Cognitive Task. *PLoS ONE* **2015**, *10*, e0125911.
23. Liu, H.-L.; Chen, P.-Y.; Yang, H.-W.; Wu, J.-S.; Tseng, I.-C.; Ma, Y.-J.; Huang, C.-Y.; Tsai, H.-C.; Chen, S.-M.; Lu, Y.-J.; et al. In Vivo MR quantification of superparamagnetic iron oxide nanoparticle leakage during low-frequency-ultrasound-induced blood-brain barrier opening in swine. *J. Magn. Reson. Imaging* **2011**, *34*, 1313–1324. [CrossRef] [PubMed]
24. Marquet, F.; Tung, Y.S.; Teichert, T.; Ferrera, V.P.; Konofagou, E.E. Noninvasive, transient and selective blood-brain barrier opening in non-human primates in vivo. *PLoS ONE* **2011**, *6*, e22598. [CrossRef] [PubMed]
25. McDannold, N.; Vykhodtseva, N.; Hynynen, K. Use of Ultrasound Pulses Combined with Definity for Targeted Blood-Brain Barrier Disruption: A Feasibility Study. *Ultrasound Med. Biol.* **2007**, *33*, 584–590. [CrossRef] [PubMed]
26. McMahon, D.; Hynynen, K. Acute Inflammatory Response Following Increased Blood-Brain Barrier Permeability Induced by Focused Ultrasound is Dependent on Microbubble Dose. *Theranostics* **2017**, *7*, 3989–4000. [CrossRef]
27. Kovacs, Z.I.; Kim, S.; Jikaria, N.; Qureshi, F.; Milo, B.; Lewis, B.K.; Bresler, M.; Burks, S.R.; Frank, J.A. Disrupting the blood-brain barrier by focused ultrasound induces sterile inflammation. *Proc. Natl. Acad. Sci. USA* **2017**, *114*, E75–E84. [CrossRef]
28. Hynynen, K.; McDannold, N.; Sheikov, N.A.; Jolesz, F.A.; Vykhodtseva, N. Local and reversible blood-brain barrier disruption by noninvasive focused ultrasound at frequencies suitable for trans-skull sonications. *Neuroimage* **2005**, *24*, 12–20. [CrossRef]

29. Pelekanos, M.; Leinenga, G.; Odabaee, M.; Odabaee, M.; Saifzadeh, S.; Steck, R.; Gotz, J. Establishing sheep as an experimental species to validate ultrasound-mediated blood-brain barrier opening for potential therapeutic interventions. *Theranostics* **2018**, *8*, 2583–2602. [CrossRef]
30. Hynynen, K.; McDannold, N.; Vykhodtseva, N.; Raymond, S.; Weissleder, R.; Jolesz, F.A.; Sheikov, N. Focal disruption of the blood-brain barrier due to 260-kHz ultrasound bursts: A method for molecular imaging and targeted drug delivery. *J. Neurosurg.* **2006**, *105*, 445–454. [CrossRef]
31. Kinoshita, M.; McDannold, N.; Jolesz, F.A.; Hynynen, K. Noninvasive localized delivery of Herceptin to the mouse brain by MRI-guided focused ultrasound-induced blood-brain barrier disruption. *Proc. Natl. Acad. Sci. USA* **2006**, *103*, 11719–11723. [CrossRef] [PubMed]
32. Liu, H.L.; Wai, Y.Y.; Chen, W.S.; Chen, J.C.; Hsu, P.H.; Wu, X.Y.; Huang, W.C.; Yen, T.C.; Wang, J.J. Hemorrhage detection during focused-ultrasound induced blood-brain-barrier opening by using susceptibility-weighted magnetic resonance imaging. *Ultrasound Med. Biol.* **2008**, *34*, 598–606. [CrossRef] [PubMed]
33. Tsai, H.C.; Tsai, C.H.; Chen, W.S.; Inserra, C.; Wei, K.C.; Liu, H.L. Safety evaluation of frequent application of microbubble-enhanced focused ultrasound blood-brain-barrier opening. *Sci. Rep.* **2018**, *8*, 17720. [CrossRef] [PubMed]
34. Yang, F.Y.; Lee, P.Y. Efficiency of drug delivery enhanced by acoustic pressure during blood-brain barrier disruption induced by focused ultrasound. *Int. J. Nanomed.* **2012**, *7*, 2573–2582. [CrossRef]
35. Liberati, A.; Altman, D.G.; Tetzlaff, J.; Mulrow, C.; Gotzsche, P.C.; Ioannidis, J.P.; Clarke, M.; Devereaux, P.J.; Kleijnen, J.; Moher, D. The PRISMA statement for reporting systematic reviews and meta-analyses of studies that evaluate healthcare interventions: Explanation and elaboration. *BMJ* **2009**, *339*, b2700. [CrossRef]
36. Moher, D.; Liberati, A.; Tetzlaff, J.; Altman, D.G.; Group, P. Preferred reporting items for systematic reviews and meta-analyses: The PRISMA statement. *BMJ* **2009**, *339*, b2535. [CrossRef]
37. Bramer, W.M.; Giustini, D.; de Jonge, G.B.; Holland, L.; Bekhuis, T. De-duplication of database search results for systematic reviews in EndNote. *J. Med. Libr. Assoc.* **2016**, *104*, 240–243. [CrossRef]
38. Baghirov, H.; Snipstad, S.; Sulheim, E.; Berg, S.; Hansen, R.; Thorsen, F.; Morch, Y.; Davies, C.L.; Aslund, A.K.O. Ultrasound-mediated delivery and distribution of polymeric nanoparticles in the normal brain parenchyma of a metastatic brain tumour model. *PLoS ONE* **2018**, *13*, e0191102. [CrossRef]
39. Bing, K.F.; Howles, G.P.; Qi, Y.; Palmeri, M.L.; Nightingale, K.R. Blood-Brain Barrier (BBB) Disruption Using a Diagnostic Ultrasound Scanner and Definity in Mice. *Ultrasound Med. Biol.* **2009**, *35*, 1298–1308. [CrossRef]
40. Zhao, B.; Chen, Y.; Liu, J.; Zhang, L.; Wang, J.; Yang, Y.; Lv, Q.; Xie, M. Blood-brain barrier disruption induced by diagnostic ultrasound combined with microbubbles in mice. *Oncotarget* **2018**, *9*, 4897–4914. [CrossRef]
41. Kyriakou, A.; Neufeld, E.; Werner, B.; Paulides, M.M.; Szekely, G.; Kuster, N. A review of numerical and experimental compensation techniques for skull-induced phase aberrations in transcranial focused ultrasound. *Int. J. Hyperth.* **2014**, *30*, 36–46. [CrossRef] [PubMed]
42. Beccaria, K.; Canney, M.; Bouchoux, G.; Puget, S.; Grill, J.; Carpentier, A. Blood-brain barrier disruption with low-intensity pulsed ultrasound for the treatment of pediatric brain tumors: A review and perspectives. *Neurosurg. Focus* **2020**, *48*, E10. [CrossRef] [PubMed]
43. Zhang, D.Y.; Dmello, C.; Chen, L.; Arrieta, V.A.; Gonzalez-Buendia, E.; Kane, J.R.; Magnusson, L.P.; Baran, A.; James, C.D.; Horbinski, C.; et al. Ultrasound-mediated Delivery of Paclitaxel for Glioma: A Comparative Study of Distribution, Toxicity, and Efficacy of Albumin-bound Versus Cremophor Formulations. *Clin. Cancer Res.* **2020**, *26*, 477–486. [CrossRef] [PubMed]
44. Goldwirt, L.; Canney, M.; Horodyckid, C.; Poupon, J.; Mourah, S.; Vignot, A.; Chapelon, J.Y.; Carpentier, A. Enhanced brain distribution of carboplatin in a primate model after blood-brain barrier disruption using an implantable ultrasound device. *Cancer Chemother. Pharmacol.* **2016**, *77*, 211–216. [CrossRef]
45. Fan, C.H.; Liu, H.L.; Ting, C.Y.; Lee, Y.H.; Huang, C.Y.; Ma, Y.J.; Wei, K.C.; Yen, T.C.; Yeh, C.K. Submicron-bubble-enhanced focused ultrasound for blood-brain barrier disruption and improved CNS drug delivery. *PLoS ONE* **2014**, *9*, e96327. [CrossRef]
46. Hynynen, K.; Jones, R.M. Image-guided ultrasound phased arrays are a disruptive technology for non-invasive therapy. *Phys. Med. Biol.* **2016**, *61*, R206–R248. [CrossRef]
47. Timbie, K.F.; Mead, B.P.; Price, R.J. Drug and gene delivery across the blood-brain barrier with focused ultrasound. *J. Control. Release* **2015**, *219*, 61–75. [CrossRef]
48. McDannold, N.; Zhang, Y.; Supko, J.G.; Power, C.; Sun, T.; Peng, C.; Vykhodtseva, N.; Golby, A.J.; Reardon, D.A. Acoustic feedback enables safe and reliable carboplatin delivery across the blood-brain barrier with a clinical focused ultrasound system and improves survival in a rat glioma model. *Theranostics* **2019**, *9*, 6284–6299. [CrossRef]
49. McDannold, N.; Zhang, Y.; Supko, J.G.; Power, C.; Sun, T.; Vykhodtseva, N.; Golby, A.J.; Reardon, D.A. Blood-brain barrier disruption and delivery of irinotecan in a rat model using a clinical transcranial MRI-guided focused ultrasound system. *Sci. Rep.* **2020**, *10*, 8766. [CrossRef]
50. Arvanitis, C.D.; Livingstone, M.S.; Vykhodtseva, N.; McDannold, N. Controlled ultrasound-induced blood-brain barrier disruption using passive acoustic emissions monitoring. *PLoS ONE* **2012**, *7*, e45783. [CrossRef]
51. Anastasiadis, P.; Gandhi, D.; Guo, Y.; Ahmed, A.K.; Bentzen, S.M.; Arvanitis, C.; Woodworth, G.F. Localized blood-brain barrier opening in infiltrating gliomas with MRI-guided acoustic emissions-controlled focused ultrasound. *Proc. Natl. Acad. Sci. USA* **2021**, *118*, e2103280118. [CrossRef] [PubMed]

52. Gasca-Salas, C.; Fernández-Rodríguez, B.; Pineda-Pardo, J.A.; Rodríguez-Rojas, R.; Obeso, I.; Hernández-Fernández, F.; del Álamo, M.; Mata, D.; Guida, P.; Ordás-Bandera, C.; et al. Blood-brain barrier opening with focused ultrasound in Parkinson's disease dementia. *Nat. Commun.* **2021**, *12*, 779. [CrossRef] [PubMed]
53. Park, S.H.; Kim, M.J.; Jung, H.H.; Chang, W.S.; Choi, H.S.; Rachmilevitch, I.; Zadicario, E.; Chang, J.W. Safety and feasibility of multiple blood-brain barrier disruptions for the treatment of glioblastoma in patients undergoing standard adjuvant chemotherapy. *J. Neurosurg.* **2020**, *134*, 475–483. [CrossRef]
54. Chen, K.T.; Chai, W.Y.; Lin, Y.J.; Lin, C.J.; Chen, P.Y.; Tsai, H.C.; Huang, C.Y.; Kuo, J.S.; Liu, H.L.; Wei, K.C. Neuronavigation-guided focused ultrasound for transcranial blood-brain barrier opening and immunostimulation in brain tumors. *Sci. Adv.* **2021**, *7*, eabd0772. [CrossRef] [PubMed]
55. Beccaria, K.; Canney, M.; Bouchoux, G.; Desseaux, C.; Grill, J.; Heimberger, A.B.; Carpentier, A. Ultrasound-induced blood-brain barrier disruption for the treatment of gliomas and other primary CNS tumors. *Cancer Lett.* **2020**, *479*, 13–22. [CrossRef]
56. Horodyckid, C.; Canney, M.; Vignot, A.; Boisgard, R.; Drier, A.; Huberfeld, G.; François, C.; Prigent, A.; Santin, M.D.; Adam, C.; et al. Safe long-term repeated disruption of the blood-brain barrier using an implantable ultrasound device: A multiparametric study in a primate model. *J. Neurosurg.* **2017**, *126*, 1351–1361. [CrossRef]
57. Pouliopoulos, A.N.; Wu, S.Y.; Burgess, M.T.; Karakatsani, M.E.; Kamimura, H.A.S.; Konofagou, E.E. A Clinical System for Non-invasive Blood-Brain Barrier Opening Using a Neuronavigation-Guided Single-Element Focused Ultrasound Transducer. *Ultrasound Med. Biol.* **2020**, *46*, 73–89. [CrossRef] [PubMed]
58. Marty, B.; Larrat, B.; Van Landeghem, M.; Robic, C.; Robert, P.; Port, M.; Le Bihan, D.; Pernot, M.; Tanter, M.; Lethimonnier, F.; et al. Dynamic study of blood-brain barrier closure after its disruption using ultrasound: A quantitative analysis. *J. Cereb. Blood Flow Metab.* **2012**, *32*, 1948–1958. [CrossRef]
59. McMahon, D.; Deng, L.; Hynynen, K. Comparing rapid short-pulse to tone burst sonication sequences for focused ultrasound and microbubble-mediated blood-brain barrier permeability enhancement. *J. Control. Release* **2020**, *329*, 696–705. [CrossRef]
60. Choi, J.J.; Selert, K.; Vlachos, F.; Wong, A.; Konofagou, E.E. Noninvasive and localized neuronal delivery using short ultrasonic pulses and microbubbles. *Proc. Natl. Acad. Sci. USA* **2011**, *108*, 16539–16544. [CrossRef]
61. Jordao, J.F.; Thévenot, E.; Markham-Coultes, K.; Scarcelli, T.; Weng, Y.-Q.; Xhima, K.; O'Reilly, M.; Huang, Y.; McLaurin, J.; Hynynen, K.; et al. Amyloid-beta plaque reduction, endogenous antibody delivery and glial activation by brain-targeted, transcranial focused ultrasound. *Exp. Neurol.* **2013**, *248*, 16–29. [CrossRef] [PubMed]
62. Kinoshita, M.; McDannold, N.; Jolesz, F.A.; Hynynen, K. Targeted delivery of antibodies through the blood-brain barrier by MRI-guided focused ultrasound. *Biochem. Biophys. Res. Commun.* **2006**, *340*, 1085–1090. [CrossRef]
63. Treat, L.H.; McDannold, N.; Vykhodtseva, N.; Zhang, Y.; Tam, K.; Hynynen, K. Targeted delivery of doxorubicin to the rat brain at therapeutic levels using MRI-guided focused ultrasound. *Int. J. Cancer* **2007**, *121*, 901–907. [CrossRef] [PubMed]
64. Fan, C.H.; Cheng, Y.H.; Ting, C.Y.; Ho, Y.J.; Hsu, P.H.; Liu, H.L.; Yeh, C.K. Ultrasound/Magnetic Targeting with SPIO-DOX-Microbubble Complex for Image-Guided Drug Delivery in Brain Tumors. *Theranostics* **2016**, *6*, 1542–1556. [CrossRef]
65. Liu, H.L.; Hsu, P.H.; Chu, P.C.; Wai, Y.Y.; Chen, J.C.; Shen, C.R.; Yen, T.C.; Wang, J.J. Magnetic resonance imaging enhanced by superparamagnetic iron oxide particles: Usefulness for distinguishing between focused ultrasound-induced blood-brain barrier disruption and brain hemorrhage. *J. Magn. Reson. Imaging* **2009**, *29*, 31–38. [CrossRef] [PubMed]
66. Samiotaki, G.; Vlachos, F.; Tung, Y.S.; Konofagou, E.E. A quantitative pressure and microbubble-size dependence study of focused ultrasound-induced blood-brain barrier opening reversibility in vivo using MRI. *Magn. Reson. Med.* **2012**, *67*, 769–777. [CrossRef] [PubMed]
67. Chen, H.; Konofagou, E.E. The size of blood-brain barrier opening induced by focused ultrasound is dictated by the acoustic pressure. *J. Cereb. Blood Flow Metab.* **2014**, *34*, 1197–1204. [CrossRef] [PubMed]
68. Choi, J.J.; Wang, S.; Tung, Y.S.; Morrison, B., III; Konofagou, E.E. Molecules of various pharmacologically-relevant sizes can cross the ultrasound-induced blood-brain barrier opening in vivo. *Ultrasound Med. Biol.* **2010**, *36*, 58–67. [CrossRef]
69. Shen, Y.; Guo, J.; Chen, G.; Chin, C.T.; Chen, X.; Chen, J.; Wang, F.; Chen, S.; Dan, G. Delivery of liposomes with different sizes to mice brain after sonication by focused ultrasound in the presence of microbubbles. *Ultrasound Med. Biol.* **2016**, *42*, 1499–1511. [CrossRef]
70. Aryal, M.; Vykhodtseva, N.; Zhang, Y.Z.; McDannold, N. Multiple sessions of liposomal doxorubicin delivery via focused ultrasound mediated blood-brain barrier disruption: A safety study. *J. Control. Release* **2015**, *204*, 60–69. [CrossRef]
71. Park, J.; Zhang, Y.; Vykhodtseva, N.; Jolesz, F.A.; McDannold, N.J. The kinetics of blood brain barrier permeability and targeted doxorubicin delivery into brain induced by focused ultrasound. *J. Control. Release* **2012**, *162*, 134–142. [CrossRef] [PubMed]
72. Vlachos, F.; Tung, Y.S.; Konofagou, E. Permeability dependence study of the focused ultrasound-induced blood-brain barrier opening at distinct pressures and microbubble diameters using DCE-MRI. *Magn. Reson. Med.* **2011**, *66*, 821–830. [CrossRef] [PubMed]
73. Baseri, B.; Choi, J.J.; Tung, Y.S.; Konofagou, E.E. Multi-modality safety assessment of blood-brain barrier opening using focused ultrasound and definity microbubbles: A short-term study. *Ultrasound Med. Biol.* **2010**, *36*, 1445–1459. [CrossRef] [PubMed]
74. Chen, C.C.; Sheeran, P.S.; Wu, S.Y.; Olumolade, O.O.; Dayton, P.A.; Konofagou, E.E. Targeted drug delivery with focused ultrasound-induced blood-brain barrier opening using acoustically-activated nanodroplets. *J. Control. Release* **2013**, *172*, 795–804. [CrossRef] [PubMed]

75. Choi, J.J.; Feshitan, J.A.; Baseri, B.; Wang, S.; Tung, Y.S.; Borden, M.A.; Konofagou, E.E. Microbubble-size dependence of focused ultrasound-induced blood-brain barrier opening in mice in vivo. *IEEE Trans. Biomed. Eng.* **2010**, *57*, 145–154. [CrossRef] [PubMed]
76. Choi, J.J.; Selert, K.; Gao, Z.; Samiotaki, G.; Baseri, B.; Konofagou, E.E. Noninvasive and localized blood-brain barrier disruption using focused ultrasound can be achieved at short pulse lengths and low pulse repetition frequencies. *J. Cereb. Blood Flow Metab.* **2011**, *31*, 725–737. [CrossRef] [PubMed]
77. Choi, J.J.; Wang, S.; Brown, T.R.; Small, S.A.; Duff, K.E.; Konofagou, E.E. Noninvasive and transient blood-brain barrier opening in the hippocampus of Alzheimer's double transgenic mice using focused ultrasound. *Ultrason. Imaging* **2008**, *30*, 189–200. [CrossRef]
78. Englander, Z.K.; Wei, H.-J.; Pouliopoulos, A.N.; Bendau, E.; Upadhyayula, P.; Jan, C.-I.; Spinazzi, E.F.; Yoh, N.; Tazhibi, M.; McQuillan, N.M.; et al. Focused ultrasound mediated blood-brain barrier opening is safe and feasible in a murine pontine glioma model. *Sci. Rep.* **2021**, *11*, 6521. [CrossRef]
79. Lapin, N.A.; Gill, K.; Shah, B.R.; Chopra, R. Consistent opening of the blood brain barrier using focused ultrasound with constant intravenous infusion of microbubble agent. *Sci. Rep.* **2020**, *10*, 16546. [CrossRef]
80. Liu, H.L.; Huang, C.Y.; Chen, J.Y.; Wang, H.Y.; Chen, P.Y.; Wei, K.C. Pharmacodynamic and therapeutic investigation of focused ultrasound-induced blood-brain barrier opening for enhanced temozolomide delivery in glioma treatment. *PLoS ONE* **2014**, *9*, e114311.
81. McDannold, N.; Zhang, Y.; Vykhodtseva, N. The Effects of Oxygen on Ultrasound-Induced Blood-Brain Barrier Disruption in Mice. *Ultrasound Med. Biol.* **2017**, *43*, 469–475. [CrossRef] [PubMed]
82. Morse, S.V.; Mishra, A.; Chan, T.G.; R, T.M.d.R.; Choi, J.J. Liposome delivery to the brain with rapid short-pulses of focused ultrasound and microbubbles. *J. Control. Release* **2022**, *341*, 605–615. [CrossRef] [PubMed]
83. Morse, S.V.; Pouliopoulos, A.N.; Chan, T.G.; Copping, M.J.; Lin, J.; Long, N.J.; Choi, J.J. Rapid Short-pulse Ultrasound Delivers Drugs Uniformly across the Murine Blood-Brain Barrier with Negligible Disruption. *Radiology* **2019**, *291*, 459–466. [CrossRef]
84. Olumolade, O.O.; Wang, S.; Samiotaki, G.; Konofagou, E.E. Longitudinal Motor and Behavioral Assessment of Blood-Brain Barrier Opening with Transcranial Focused Ultrasound. *Ultrasound Med. Biol.* **2016**, *42*, 2270–2282. [CrossRef]
85. Omata, D.; Maruyama, T.; Unga, J.; Hagiwara, F.; Munakata, L.; Kageyama, S.; Shima, T.; Suzuki, Y.; Maruyama, K.; Suzuki, R. Effects of encapsulated gas on stability of lipid-based microbubbles and ultrasound-triggered drug delivery. *J. Control. Release* **2019**, *311*, 65–73. [CrossRef] [PubMed]
86. Raymond, S.B.; Skoch, J.; Hynynen, K.; Bacskai, B.J. Multiphoton imaging of ultrasound/Optison mediated cerebrovascular effects in vivo. *J. Cereb. Blood Flow Metab.* **2007**, *27*, 393–403. [CrossRef]
87. Raymond, S.B.; Treat, L.H.; Dewey, J.D.; McDannold, N.J.; Hynynen, K.; Bacskai, B.J. Ultrasound enhanced delivery of molecular imaging and therapeutic agents in Alzheimer's disease mouse models. *PLoS ONE* **2008**, *3*, e2175. [CrossRef]
88. Sierra, C.; Acosta, C.; Chen, C.; Wu, S.Y.; Karakatsani, M.E.; Bernal, M.; Konofagou, E.E. Lipid microbubbles as a vehicle for targeted drug delivery using focused ultrasound-induced blood-brain barrier opening. *J. Cereb. Blood Flow Metab.* **2017**, *37*, 1236–1250. [CrossRef]
89. Wu, S.K.; Chiang, C.F.; Hsu, Y.H.; Lin, T.H.; Liou, H.C.; Fu, W.M.; Lin, W.L. Short-time focused ultrasound hyperthermia enhances liposomal doxorubicin delivery and antitumor efficacy for brain metastasis of breast cancer. *Int. J. Nanomed.* **2014**, *9*, 4485–4494.
90. Alli, S.; Figueiredo, C.A.; Golbourn, B.; Sabha, N.; Wu, M.Y.; Bondoc, A.; Luck, A.; Coluccia, D.; Maslink, C.; Smith, C.; et al. Brainstem blood brain barrier disruption using focused ultrasound: A demonstration of feasibility and enhanced doxorubicin delivery. *J. Control. Release* **2018**, *281*, 29–41. [CrossRef]
91. Aryal, M.; Park, J.; Vykhodtseva, N.; Zhang, Y.Z.; McDannold, N. Enhancement in blood-tumor barrier permeability and delivery of liposomal doxorubicin using focused ultrasound and microbubbles: Evaluation during tumor progression in a rat glioma model. *Phys. Med. Biol.* **2015**, *60*, 2511–2527. [CrossRef] [PubMed]
92. Aslund, A.K.; Snipstad, S.; Healey, A.; Kvale, S.; Torp, S.H.; Sontum, P.C.; Davies, C.L.; van Wamel, A. Efficient Enhancement of Blood-Brain Barrier Permeability Using Acoustic Cluster Therapy (ACT). *Theranostics* **2017**, *7*, 23–30. [CrossRef] [PubMed]
93. Chopra, R.; Vykhodtseva, N.; Hynynen, K. Influence of exposure time and pressure amplitude on blood-brain-barrier opening using transcranial ultrasound exposures. *ACS Chem. Neurosci.* **2010**, *1*, 391–398. [CrossRef] [PubMed]
94. Fan, C.H.; Ting, C.Y.; Chang, Y.C.; Wei, K.C.; Liu, H.L.; Yeh, C.K. Drug-loaded bubbles with matched focused ultrasound excitation for concurrent blood-brain barrier opening and brain-tumor drug delivery. *Acta Biomater.* **2015**, *15*, 89–101. [CrossRef]
95. Goutal, S.; Gerstenmayer, M.; Auvity, S.; Caille, F.; Meriaux, S.; Buvat, I.; Larrat, B.; Tournier, N. Physical blood-brain barrier disruption induced by focused ultrasound does not overcome the transporter-mediated efflux of erlotinib. *J. Control. Release* **2018**, *292*, 210–220. [CrossRef]
96. Han, M.; Seo, H.; Choi, H.; Lee, E.H.; Park, J. Localized Modification of Water Molecule Transport after Focused Ultrasound-Induced Blood-Brain Barrier Disruption in Rat Brain. *Front. Neurosci.* **2021**, *15*, 685977. [CrossRef]
97. Huh, H.; Park, T.Y.; Seo, H.; Han, M.; Jung, B.; Choi, H.J.; Lee, E.H.; Pahk, K.J.; Kim, H.; Park, J. A local difference in blood-brain barrier permeability in the caudate putamen and thalamus of a rat brain induced by focused ultrasound. *Sci. Rep.* **2020**, *10*, 19286. [CrossRef]
98. Jung, B.; Huh, H.; Lee, E.H.; Han, M.; Park, J. An advanced focused ultrasound protocol improves the blood-brain barrier permeability and doxorubicin delivery into the rat brain. *J. Control. Release* **2019**, *315*, 55–64. [CrossRef]

99. Kobus, T.; Vykhodtseva, N.; Pilatou, M.; Zhang, Y.; McDannold, N. Safety Validation of Repeated Blood-Brain Barrier Disruption Using Focused Ultrasound. *Ultrasound Med. Biol.* **2016**, *42*, 481–492. [CrossRef]
100. Kovacs, Z.I.; Tu, T.W.; Sundby, M.; Qureshi, F.; Lewis, B.K.; Jikaria, N.; Burks, S.R.; Frank, J.A. MRI and histological evaluation of pulsed focused ultrasound and microbubbles treatment effects in the brain. *Theranostics* **2018**, *8*, 4837–4855. [CrossRef]
101. Liu, H.L.; Hua, M.Y.; Chen, P.Y.; Chu, P.C.; Pan, C.H.; Yang, H.W.; Huang, C.Y.; Wang, J.J.; Yen, T.C.; Wei, K.C. Blood-brain barrier disruption with focused ultrasound enhances delivery of chemotherapeutic drugs for glioblastoma treatment. *Radiology* **2010**, *255*, 415–425. [CrossRef] [PubMed]
102. Liu, H.L.; Pan, C.H.; Ting, C.Y.; Hsiao, M.J. Opening of the blood-brain barrier by low-frequency (28-kHz) ultrasound: A novel pinhole-assisted mechanical scanning device. *Ultrasound Med. Biol.* **2010**, *36*, 325–335. [CrossRef] [PubMed]
103. Liu, H.L.; Wai, Y.Y.; Hsu, P.H.; Lyu, L.A.; Wu, J.S.; Shen, C.R.; Chen, J.C.; Yen, T.C.; Wang, J.J. In Vivo assessment of macrophage CNS infiltration during disruption of the blood-brain barrier with focused ultrasound: A magnetic resonance imaging study. *J. Cereb. Blood Flow Metab.* **2010**, *30*, 177–186. [CrossRef] [PubMed]
104. McDannold, N.; Zhang, Y.; Vykhodtseva, N. Blood-brain barrier disruption and vascular damage induced by ultrasound bursts combined with microbubbles can be influenced by choice of anesthesia protocol. *Ultrasound Med. Biol.* **2011**, *37*, 1259–1270. [CrossRef]
105. McMahon, D.; Lassus, A.; Gaud, E.; Jeannot, V.; Hynynen, K. Microbubble formulation influences inflammatory response to focused ultrasound exposure in the brain. *Sci. Rep.* **2020**, *10*, 21534. [CrossRef]
106. McMahon, D.; Oakden, W.; Hynynen, K. Investigating the effects of dexamethasone on blood-brain barrier permeability and inflammatory response following focused ultrasound and microbubble exposure. *Theranostics* **2020**, *10*, 1604–1618. [CrossRef]
107. O'Reilly, M.A.; Hough, O.; Hynynen, K. Blood-Brain Barrier Closure Time After Controlled Ultrasound-Induced Opening Is Independent of Opening Volume. *J. Ultrasound Med.* **2017**, *36*, 475–483. [CrossRef]
108. O'Reilly, M.A.; Waspe, A.C.; Ganguly, M.; Hynynen, K. Focused-ultrasound disruption of the blood-brain barrier using closely-timed short pulses: Influence of sonication parameters and injection rate. *Ultrasound Med. Biol.* **2011**, *37*, 587–594. [CrossRef]
109. Park, J.; Aryal, M.; Vykhodtseva, N.; Zhang, Y.Z.; McDannold, N. Evaluation of permeability, doxorubicin delivery, and drug retention in a rat brain tumor model after ultrasound-induced blood-tumor barrier disruption. *J. Control. Release* **2017**, *250*, 77–85. [CrossRef]
110. Song, K.H.; Fan, A.C.; Hinkle, J.J.; Newman, J.; Borden, M.A.; Harvey, B.K. Microbubble gas volume: A unifying dose parameter in blood-brain barrier opening by focused ultrasound. *Theranostics* **2017**, *7*, 144–152. [CrossRef]
111. Wei, K.C.; Chu, P.-C.; Wang, H.-Y.J.; Huang, C.-Y.; Chen, P.-Y.; Tsai, H.-C.; Lu, Y.-J.; Lee, P.-Y.; Tseng, I.-C.; Feng, L.-Y.; et al. Focused ultrasound-induced blood-brain barrier opening to enhance temozolomide delivery for glioblastoma treatment: A preclinical study. *PLoS ONE* **2013**, *8*, e58995. [CrossRef] [PubMed]
112. Wu, S.K.; Chu, P.C.; Chai, W.Y.; Kang, S.T.; Tsai, C.H.; Fan, C.H.; Yeh, C.K.; Liu, H.L. Characterization of Different Microbubbles in Assisting Focused Ultrasound-Induced Blood-Brain Barrier Opening. *Sci. Rep.* **2017**, *7*, 46689. [CrossRef] [PubMed]
113. Yang, F.Y.; Chen, C.C.; Kao, Y.H.; Chen, C.L.; Ko, C.E.; Horng, S.C.; Chen, R.C. Evaluation of Dose Distribution of Molecular Delivery after Blood-Brain Barrier Disruption by Focused Ultrasound with Treatment Planning. *Ultrasound Med. Biol.* **2013**, *39*, 620–627. [CrossRef] [PubMed]
114. Yang, F.Y.; Ko, C.E.; Huang, S.Y.; Chung, I.F.; Chen, G.S. Pharmacokinetic changes induced by focused ultrasound in glioma-bearing rats as measured by dynamic contrast-enhanced MRI. *PLoS ONE* **2014**, *9*, e92910. [CrossRef]
115. Yang, F.Y.; Lin, Y.S.; Kang, K.H.; Chao, T.K. Reversible blood-brain barrier disruption by repeated transcranial focused ultrasound allows enhanced extravasation. *J. Control. Release* **2011**, *150*, 111–116. [CrossRef]
116. Yang, F.Y.; Wang, H.E.; Lin, G.L.; Lin, H.H.; Wong, T.T. Evaluation of the increase in permeability of the blood-brain barrier during tumor progression after pulsed focused ultrasound. *Int. J. Nanomed.* **2012**, *7*, 723–730. [CrossRef]
117. Zhang, Y.; Tan, H.; Bertram, E.H.; Aubry, J.-F.; Lopes, M.-B.; Roy, J.; Dumont, E.; Xie, M.; Zuo, Z.; Klibanov, A.L.; et al. Non-Invasive, Focal Disconnection of Brain Circuitry Using Magnetic Resonance-Guided Low-Intensity Focused Ultrasound to Deliver a Neurotoxin. *Ultrasound Med. Biol.* **2016**, *42*, 2261–2269. [CrossRef]
118. McDannold, N.; Vykhodtseva, N.; Hynynen, K. Targeted disruption of the blood-brain barrier with focused ultrasound: Association with cavitation activity. *Phys. Med. Biol.* **2006**, *51*, 793–807. [CrossRef]
119. McDannold, N.; Vykhodtseva, N.; Hynynen, K. Blood-brain barrier disruption induced by focused ultrasound and circulating preformed microbubbles appears to be characterized by the mechanical index. *Ultrasound Med. Biol.* **2008**, *34*, 834–840. [CrossRef]
120. McDannold, N.; Vykhodtseva, N.; Hynynen, K. Effects of acoustic parameters and ultrasound contrast agent dose on focused-ultrasound induced blood-brain barrier disruption. *Ultrasound Med. Biol.* **2008**, *34*, 930–937. [CrossRef]
121. Mei, J.; Cheng, Y.; Song, Y.; Yang, Y.; Wang, F.; Liu, Y.; Wang, Z. Experimental study on targeted methotrexate delivery to the rabbit brain via magnetic resonance imaging-guided focused ultrasound. *J. Ultrasound Med.* **2009**, *28*, 871–880. [CrossRef] [PubMed]
122. Wang, F.; Cheng, Y.; Mei, J.; Song, Y.; Yang, Y.Q.; Liu, Y.; Wang, Z. Focused ultrasound microbubble destruction-mediated changes in blood-brain barrier permeability assessed by contrast-enhanced magnetic resonance imaging. *J. Ultrasound Med.* **2009**, *28*, 1501–1509. [CrossRef]
123. O'Reilly, M.A.; Jones, R.M.; Barrett, E.; Schwab, A.; Head, E.; Hynynen, K. Investigation of the Safety of Focused Ultrasound-Induced Blood-Brain Barrier Opening in a Natural Canine Model of Aging. *Theranostics* **2017**, *7*, 3573–3584. [CrossRef] [PubMed]

124. Yoon, K.; Lee, W.; Chen, E.; Lee, J.E.; Croce, P.; Cammalleri, A.; Foley, L.; Tsao, A.L.; Yoo, S.S. Localized Blood-Brain Barrier Opening in Ovine Model Using Image-Guided Transcranial Focused Ultrasound. *Ultrasound Med. Biol.* **2019**, *45*, 2391–2404. [CrossRef] [PubMed]
125. Marquet, F.; Teichert, T.; Wu, S.Y.; Tung, Y.S.; Downs, M.; Wang, S.; Chen, C.; Ferrera, V.; Konofagou, E.E. Real-time, transcranial monitoring of safe blood-brain barrier opening in non-human primates. *PLoS ONE* **2014**, *9*, e84310. [CrossRef] [PubMed]
126. McDannold, N.; Arvanitis, C.D.; Vykhodtseva, N.; Livingstone, M.S. Temporary disruption of the blood-brain barrier by use of ultrasound and microbubbles: Safety and efficacy evaluation in rhesus macaques. *Cancer Res.* **2012**, *72*, 3652–3663. [CrossRef]
127. Wu, S.Y.; Sanchez, C.S.; Samiotaki, G.; Buch, A.; Ferrera, V.P.; Konofagou, E.E. Characterizing Focused-Ultrasound Mediated Drug Delivery to the Heterogeneous Primate Brain In Vivo with Acoustic Monitoring. *Sci. Rep.* **2016**, *6*, 37094. [CrossRef]
128. Pasquinelli, C.; Hanson, L.G.; Siebner, H.R.; Lee, H.J.; Thielscher, A. Safety of transcranial focused ultrasound stimulation: A systematic review of the state of knowledge from both human and animal studies. *Brain Stimul.* **2019**, *12*, 1367–1380. [CrossRef]
129. Helfield, B.L.; Huo, X.; Williams, R.; Goertz, D.E. The effect of preactivation vial temperature on the acoustic properties of Definity. *Ultrasound Med. Biol.* **2012**, *38*, 1298–1305. [CrossRef]
130. Goertz, D.E.; de Jong, N.; van der Steen, A.F. Attenuation and size distribution measurements of Definity and manipulated Definity populations. *Ultrasound Med. Biol.* **2007**, *33*, 1376–1388. [CrossRef]
131. Meng, Y.; Reilly, R.M.; Pezo, R.C.; Trudeau, M.; Sahgal, A.; Singnurkar, A.; Perry, J.; Myrehaug, S.; Pople, C.B.; Davidson, B.; et al. MR-guided focused ultrasound enhances delivery of trastuzumab to Her2-positive brain metastases. *Sci. Transl. Med.* **2021**, *13*, eabj4011. [CrossRef] [PubMed]
132. Bing, C.; Hong, Y.; Hernandez, C.; Rich, M.; Cheng, B.; Munaweera, I.; Szczepanski, D.; Xi, Y.; Bolding, M.; Exner, A.; et al. Characterization of different bubble formulations for blood-brain barrier opening using a focused ultrasound system with acoustic feedback control. *Sci. Rep.* **2018**, *8*, 7986. [CrossRef] [PubMed]
133. Park, S.H.; Baik, K.; Jeon, S.; Chang, W.S.; Ye, B.S.; Chang, J.W. Extensive frontal focused ultrasound mediated blood-brain barrier opening for the treatment of Alzheimer's disease: A proof-of-concept study. *Transl. Neurodegener.* **2021**, *10*, 44. [CrossRef]
134. Yin, X.; Hynynen, K. A numerical study of transcranial focused ultrasound beam propagation at low frequency. *Phys. Med. Biol.* **2005**, *50*, 1821–1836. [CrossRef] [PubMed]
135. O'Reilly, M.A.; Huang, Y.; Hynynen, K. The impact of standing wave effects on transcranial focused ultrasound disruption of the blood-brain barrier in a rat model. *Phys. Med. Biol.* **2010**, *55*, 5251–5267. [CrossRef]
136. Le Floc'h, J.; Lu, H.D.; Lim, T.L.; Demore, C.; Prud'homme, R.K.; Hynynen, K.; Foster, F.S. Transcranial Photoacoustic Detection of Blood-Brain Barrier Disruption Following Focused Ultrasound-Mediated Nanoparticle Delivery. *Mol. Imaging Biol.* **2020**, *22*, 324–334. [CrossRef]
137. Wang, P.H.; Liu, H.L.; Hsu, P.H.; Lin, C.Y.; Wang, C.R.; Chen, P.Y.; Wei, K.C.; Yen, T.C.; Li, M.L. Gold-nanorod contrast-enhanced photoacoustic micro-imaging of focused-ultrasound induced blood-brain-barrier opening in a rat model. *J. Biomed. Opt.* **2012**, *17*, 061222. [CrossRef]
138. Meng, Y.; Pople, C.B.; Budiansky, D.; Li, D.; Suppiah, S.; Lim-Fat, M.J.; Perry, J.; Sahgal, A.; Lipsman, N. Current state of therapeutic focused ultrasound applications in neuro-oncology. *J. Neurooncol.* **2022**, *156*, 49–59. [CrossRef]

MDPI
St. Alban-Anlage 66
4052 Basel
Switzerland
Tel. +41 61 683 77 34
Fax +41 61 302 89 18
www.mdpi.com

Pharmaceutics Editorial Office
E-mail: pharmaceutics@mdpi.com
www.mdpi.com/journal/pharmaceutics

MDPI
St. Alban-Anlage 66
4052 Basel
Switzerland
Tel. +41 61 683 77 34
Fax +41 61 302 89 18
www.mdpi.com

Pharmaceutics Editorial Office
E-mail: pharmaceutics@mdpi.com
www.mdpi.com/journal/pharmaceutics

MDPI